£144.00 ✓

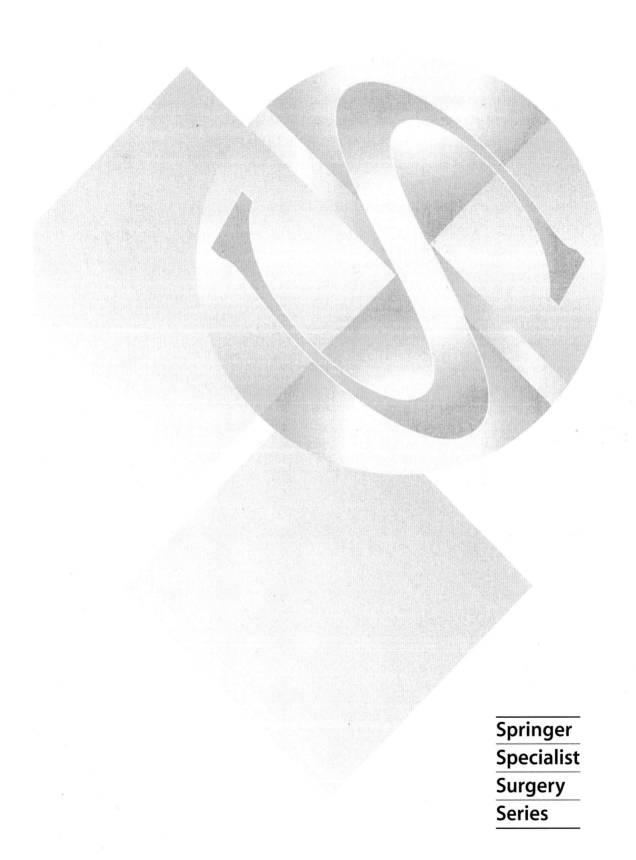

Springer
Specialist
Surgery
Series

Other titles in this series:

Transplantation Surgery, edited by Hakim & Danovitch, 2001

Neurosurgery: Principles and Practice, edited by Moore & Newell, 2004

Upper Gastrointestinal Surgery, edited by Fielding & Hallissey, 2005

Tumor Neurosurgery, edited by Moore & Newell, 2006

Vascular Surgery, edited by Davies & Brophy, 2006

Endocrine Surgery: Principles & Practice, edited by Hubbard, Inabnet & Lo, 2009

Coloproctology, edited by Zbar & Wexner, 2010

Christopher R. Chapple and William D. Steers (Eds.)

Practical Urology: Essential Principles and Practice

With 269 Illustrations

Series Editor: John Lumley

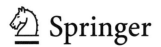 Springer

Editors

Christopher R. Chapple, BSc, MD, FRCS(Urol)
Department of Urology
Sheffield Teaching Hospitals
UK

William D. Steers, MD, FACS
Department of Urology
University of Virginia School of Medicine
Charlottesville, VA
USA

ISBN 978-1-84882-033-3   e-ISBN 978-1-84882-034-0
DOI 10.1007/978-1-84882-034-0
Springer London Dordrecht Heidelberg New York

British Library Cataloguing in Publication Data
A catalogue record for this book is available from the British Library

Library of Congress Control Number: 2011922046

Cover design: eStudioCalamar, Figueres/Berlin

Printed on acid-free paper

Springer is part of Springer Science+Business Media (www.springer.com)

Preface and Acknowledgments

One of the many characteristics that distinguishes training in surgery from merely an apprenticeship is a clear and integrated understanding not only of the basis of disease, but its clinical management. The practice of urology is therefore grounded in scientific principles, but also incorporates the important "crafts" of both medicine and surgery.

With this in mind, clearly, urology benefits from both courses and programs that incorporate scientific principles and basic pathophysiology into their curricula. Although basic science courses for trainees are held annually in both North America and Europe, a text acting as a repository of this information is lacking. In years past, textbooks such as Chisholm's *Scientific Foundations of Urology* have appeared only to go out of print. This book contains a concise summary of this basic information presented by the best of educators in North America and Europe, many of whom contribute to those basic science courses sponsored by the European Association of Urology or the American Urological Association. While not covering all aspects of urology, the topics included represent those often most confusing to trainees. We would like to thank our publisher and authors for their commitment to this project and dedicate this book to the next generation of urologists and urologic researchers who hopefully will use this information as their first primer for understanding urological disease.

Christopher R. Chapple
Sheffield, UK

William D. Steers
VA, USA

Contents

Preface and Acknowledgements v

Contributors... xi

Part I Basic Sciences In Urology

1. Embryology for Urologists 3
   Bernhard T. Mittemeyer and Allan L. Haynes Jr.

2. Gross and Laparoscopic Anatomy of the Upper Urinary
   Tract and Retroperitoneum 29
   John N. Kabalin

3. Gross and Laparoscopic Anatomy of the Lower Urinary
   Tract and Pelvis... 43
   Bastian Amend and Arnulf Stenzl

4. Anatomy of the Male Reproductive System 57
   Klaus Steger and Wolfgang Weidner

5. Imaging of the Upper Tracts.................................... 69
   Ferekh Salim

6. Principles of Bacterial Urinary Tract Infections and Antimicrobials.... 91
   *Florian M.E. Wagenlehner, Wolfgang Weidner,
   and Kurt G. Naber*

7. An Overview of Renal Physiology 105
   Mitchell H. Rosner

8. Ureteral Physiology and Pharmacology........................ 115
   Daniel M. Kaplon and Stephen Y. Nakada

9. Physiology and Pharmacology of the Bladder..................... 123
   Karl-Erik Andersson

10. Pharmacology of Sexual Function............................ 139
   Andreas Meissner and Martin C. Michel

11. Metabolic Evaluation and Medical Management of Stone Disease..... 147
   Dorit E. Zilberman, Michael N. Ferrandino,
   and Glenn M. Preminger

12. Molecular Biology for Urologists............................. 161
   Peter E. Clark

13. Chemotherapeutic Agents for Urologic Oncology 175
   Hendrik Van Poppel and Filip Ameye

14. Tumor and Transplant Immunology........................... 187
   Sean C. Kumer and Kenneth L. Brayman

15. Pathophysiology of Renal Obstruction........................ 197
   Glenn M. Cannon and Richard S. Lee

16. Pathophysiology of Lower Urinary Tract Obstruction.............. 207
   Marcus J. Drake and Ahmed M. Shaban

17. Urologic Endocrinology 219
   Paolo Verze and Vincenzo Mirone

18. Physiology and Pharmacology of the Prostate 239
   William D. Steers

19. Wound Healing and Principles of Plastic Surgery................. 249
   Timothy O. Davies and Gerald H. Jordan

20. Overview of the Evaluation of Lower Urinary Tract
    Dysfunction... 261
    Christopher R. Chapple and Altaf Mangera

21. Urologic Instrumentation: Endoscopes and Lasers 283
    Erica H. Lambert, Nicole L. Miller, and S. Duke Herrell

Part II Clinical Urologic Practice

22. Prostatitis and Male Chronic Pelvic Pain Syndrome.................. 295
    J. Curtis Nickel

23. Disorders of Scrotal Contents: Orchitis, Epididymitis, Testicular
    Torsion, Torsion of the Appendages, and Fournier's Gangrene........ 309
    Parviz K. Kavoussi and Raymond A. Costabile

24. Nonbacterial Infections of the Genitourinary Tract.................. 323
    Ryan N. Fogg and Jack H. Mydlo

25. Sexually Transmitted Infections................................... 339
    Tara Lee Frenkl and Jeannette M. Potts

26. Hematuria: Evaluation and Management........................... 351
    Richard J. Bryant and James W.F. Catto

27. Benign Prostatic Hyperplasia (BPH)............................. 361
    Andrea Tubaro and Cosimo de Nunzio

28. Practical Guidelines for the Treatment of Erectile Dysfunction
    and Peyronie's Disease.. 373
    Christian Gratzke, Karl-Erik Andersson, Thorsten Diemer,
    Wolfgang Weidner, and Christian G. Stief

29. Premature Ejaculation... 385
    Chris G. McMahon

30. The Role of Interventional Management for Urinary Tract Calculi 403
    Kenneth J. Hastie

31. Current Concepts of Anterior Urethral Pathology: Management
    and Future Directions... 415
    Altaf Mangera and Christopher R. Chapple

32. Urinary Incontinence 437
    Priya Padmanabhan and Roger Dmochowski

33. Neurogenic Bladder.. 453
    William D. Steers

34. Pelvic Prolapse 465
    Rashel M. Haverkorn and Philippe E. Zimmern

35. Urinary Tract Fistula 481
    Brett D. Lebed and Eric S. Rovner

36. Urologic Trauma.. 497
    Bradley D. Figler and Viraj A. Master

37. Bladder Cancer... 511
    Evelyn C.C. Cauberg, Jean J.M.C.H. de la Rosette,
    and Theo M. de Reijke

38. Prostate Cancer.. 527
    Charles D. Scales Jr. and Judd W. Moul

39. The Management of Testis Cancer.............................. 539
    Noel W. Clarke

Index 551

Contributors

Bastian Amend, MD
Department of Urology, University Hospital,
University of Tuebingen, Tuebingen, Germany

Filip Ameye, MD, PhD
Consultant Urologist, University of Hospital
Gasthuisberg, Katholieke Universiteit Leuven,
Herestraat 49, B 3000 Leuven, Belgium

Karl-Erik Andersson, MD, PhD
Institute for Regenerative Medicine, Wake
Forest University Medical School, Winston
Salem, NC, USA

Kenneth L. Brayman, MD, PhD
Division of Transplant Surgery, Department
of Surgery, University of Virginia,
Charlottesville, VA, USA

Richard J. Bryant, BMedSci(Hons),
MBChB(Hons), MRCSEd, PhD
Nuffield Department of Surgical Sciences,
University of Oxford, John Radcliffe Hospital,
Oxford, UK

Glenn M. Cannon, Jr., MD
Department of Urology, Children's Hospital
Boston, Harvard Medical School,
Boston, MA, USA

James W. F. Catto, Mb, ChB, PhD, FRCS(Urol)
Academic Urology Unit, University of
Sheffield, Royal Hallamshire Hospital,
Sheffield, UK

Evelyne C.C. Cauberg, MD
Department of Urology, Academic Medical
Center, University of Amsterdam, Amsterdam,
The Netherlands

Christopher R. Chapple, BSc MD, FRCS(Urol)
Department of Urology, Sheffield Teaching
Hospitals, Sheffield, UK

Peter E. Clark, MD
Department of Urologic Surgery, Vanderbilt
University Medical Center, Nashville, TN, USA

Noel W. Clarke, MBBS, ChM, FRCS(Urol)
Departments of Surgery and Urology,
Manchester University, Christie and Salford
Royal Hospitals, Manchester, UK

Raymond A. Costabile, MD
Prof. Jay Y. Gillenwater
Department of Urology, University of Virginia
School of Medicine, Charlottesville, VA, USA

Timothy O. Davies, MD
Division of Urology, McMaster University/
Henderson Hospital, Hamilton, ON, Canada

Jean J. M. C. H. de la Rosette, MD, PhD
Department of Urology, Academic Medical
Center, Amsterdam, The Netherlands

Theo M. de Reijke, MD, PhD, FEBU
Department of Urology, Academic Medical
Center, Amsterdam, The Netherlands

Thorsten Diemer, Priv.-Doz., Dr. Med.
Department of Urology, University-Hospital
Giessen and Marburg GmbH, Justus-Liebig-
University Giessen, Giessen, Germany

Roger Dmochowski, MD, FACS
Department of Urology, Vanderbilt University
Medical Center, Nashville, TN, USA

Marcus J. Drake, MA, DM, FRCS(Urol)
University of Bristol, Bristol Urological
Institute, Southmead Hospital, Bristol, UK

Michael N. Ferrandino
Division of Urologic Surgery, Duke
Comprehensive Kidney Stone Center, Duke
University Medical Center, Durham, NC, USA

Bradley D. Figler, MD
Department of Urology, Emory University,
Atlanta, GA, USA

Ryan N. Fogg, MD
Department of Urology, Temple University
School of Medicine, Philadelphia, PA, USA

Tara Lee Frenkl, MD, MPH
Department of Surgery, Division of Urology,
University of Pennsylvania, Philadelphia, PA,
USA

Christian Gratzke, MD
Department of Urology, University-Hospital
Grosshadern, Ludwig-Maximilians-University
Munich, Munich, Germany

Kenneth J. Hastie
Department of Urology, Royal Hallamshire
Hospital, Sheffield, UK

Rashel M. Haverkorn, MD
Department of Urology, Female Pelvic
Medicine, Reconstructive Surgery, and
Neurourology, UT Southwestern Medical
Center, Dallas, TX, USA

Allan L. Haynes, Jr., MD, FACS
Department of Urology, Texas Tech University
Health Sciences Center, School of Medicine,
Lubbock, TX, USA

S. Duke Herrell
Department of Urologic Surgery, Vanderbilt
University Medical Center, Nashville, TN, USA

Gerald H. Jordan, MD
Department of Urology, Sentara Medical
Group/Eastern Virginia Medical School,
Norfolk, VA, USA

John N. Kabalin, MD, FACS
Section of Urologic Surgery, University of
Nebraska College of Medicine, Scottsbluff, NE,
USA

Daniel M. Kaplon, MD
Department of Urology, University of
Wisconsin Hospital and Clinics, Madison, WI,
USA

Parviz K. Kavoussi, MD
Department of Urology, University of Virginia
School of Medicine, Charlottesville, VA, USA

Sean C. Kumer, MD, PhD
Division of Transplant Surgery, Department of
Surgery, University of Virginia, Charlottesville,
VA, USA

Erica H. Lambert
Department of Urologic Surgery, Vanderbilt
University Medical Center, Nashville, TN, USA

Brett D. Lebed, MD
Department of Urology, Medical University of
South Carolina, Charleston, SC, USA

Richard S. Lee, MD
Department of Urology, Children's Hospital
Boston, Boston, MA, USA

Altaf Mangera
Department of Urology, Sheffield Teaching
Hospitals, Sheffield, UK

Viraj A. Master, MD, PhD, FACS
Department of Urology, Emory University,
Atlanta, GA, USA

Chris G. McMahon, MBBS, FAChSHM
University of Sydney, Australian Centre for
Sexual Health, Suite 2-4, Berry Road Medical
Centre, 1a Berry Road, St Leonards,
NSW 2065, Australia

Andreas Meissner, MD
Department of Urology, Academic Medical
Center, University of Amsterdam, Amsterdam,
The Netherlands

Martin C. Michel, MD
Department of Pharmacology &
Pharmacotherapy, Academic Medical Center,
University of Amsterdam, Amsterdam, The
Netherlands

Nicole L. Miller
Department of Urologic Surgery, Vanderbilt
University Medical Center, Nashville, TN, USA

Vincenzo Mirone, MD
Department of Urology, University of Naples,
AOU "Federico II", Naples, Italy

Bernhard T. Mittemeyer, MD, FACS
Department of Urology, Texas Tech University
Health Sciences Center, School of Medicine,
Lubbock, TX, USA

Judd W. Moul, MD
Department of Surgery, Duke University
Medical Center, Durham, NC, USA

Jack H. Mydlo, MD
Department of Urology, Temple
University School of Medicine,
Philadelphia, PA, USA

Kurt G. Naber, MD, PhD
Technical University of Munich, Munich,
Germany

Stephen Y. Nakada, MD
Department of Urology, University of
Wisconsin Hospital and Clinics, Madison,
WI, USA

J. Curtis Nickel, MD
Department of Urology, CIHR Canada
Research Chair in Urologic Pain and
Inflammation, Queen's University,
Kingston General Hospital, Kingston,
ON, Canada

Cosimo de Nunzio
Department of Urology, La Sapienza
University – Sant'Andrea Hospital, Rome, Italy

Priya Padmanabhan, MD, MPH
Female Urology and Reconstructive Surgery,
University of Kansas Medical Center, Kansas
City, KS, USA

Jeannette M. Potts, MD
Department of Urology, University Hospitals,
Case Western Reserve University, School of
Medicine, Cleveland, OH, USA

Glenn M. Preminger, MD
Division of Urologic Surgery, Duke University
Medical Center, Durham, NC, USA

Mitchell H. Rosner, MD
Division of Nephrology, Department of
Medicine/Nephrology, University of Virginia
Health System, Charlottesville, VA, USA

Eric S. Rovner, MD
Department of Urology, Medical University of
South Carolina, Charleston, SC, USA

Ferekh Salim, MBChB, MRCP(UK), FRCR
Department of Medical Imaging, Sheffield
Teaching Hospitals, Sheffield, UK

Charles D. Scales, Jr., MD
Division of Urology, Department of Surgery,
Duke University Medical Center, Durham, NC,
USA

Ahmed M. Shaban
Bristol Urological Institute, Southmead
Hospital, Bristol, UK

William D. Steers, MD, FACS
Department of Urology, University of Virginia
School of Medicine, Charlottesville, VA, USA

Klaus Steger, PhD
Department of Urology and Pediatric Urology,
Justus Liebig University, Giessen, Germany

Arnulf Stenzl, MD
Department of Urology, University Hospital,
University of Tuebingen, Tuebingen, Germany

Christian G. Stief
Department of Urology, University-Hospital
Grosshadern, Ludwig-Maximilians-University
Munich, Munich, Germany

Andrea Tubaro
Department of Urology, La Sapienza
University – Sant'Andrea Hospital, Rome, Italy

Hendrik Van Poppel, MD, PhD
Department of Urology, University Hospitals
Leuven, Campus Gasthuisberg, Leuven,
Belgium

Paolo Verze, MD, PhD
Department of Urology, University of Naples,
AOU "Federico II", Naples, Italy

Florian M.E. Wagenlehner, MD, PhD
Department of Urology, Pediatric Urology
and Andrology , Justus-Liebig-University,
Giessen, Germany

Wolfgang Weidner, MD
Department of Urology, Pediatric Urology
and Andrology, University Hospital Giessen
and Marburg GmbH, Giessen, Germany

Dorit E. Zilberman, MD
Department of Surgery/Urology, Duke
University Medical Center, Durham, NC, USA

Philippe E. Zimmern, MD
Department of Urology, University of Texas
Southwestern Medical Center at Dallas,
Dallas, TX, USA

Part I

Basic Sciences In Urology

1

Embryology for Urologists

Bernhard T. Mittemeyer and Allan L. Haynes Jr.

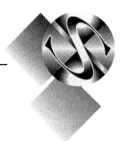

Introduction

The embryology of the genito-urinary tract is fascinating and is an integral part of our daily practice. As practitioners of our "art" we generally do not think of the underlying embryological development until we see a problem. In fact, as clinicians and surgeons in both our adult and pediatric practice, we often, if not daily, hear about, see in consultation, care for, or operate on patients with problems that have an embryological anomalous basis. Unfortunately, most of us were glad when "embryology" was behind us and while we generally know how to correct the problem we do not really recall how or why it occurred.

The purpose of this chapter is to present a short, practical, in-the-trenches guide to the embryology we deal with as urologists. It is in no way intended to replace the very interesting and more detailed explanations of these embryological events as described in the several excellent embryology textbooks available to us. (See references.) It is however a succinct presentation of the basic embryological knowledge that you might need to better understand the patients' problem, further evaluate, direct therapy, and explain to your patient why the problem occurred and why and how it may or may not need treatment. It is also intended to be a fun and easy way to review the underlying cause of the many problems we see on a daily or regular basis.

This chapter is based and modeled after the annual lecture presentation given at the annual Basic Science and Review courses sponsored by the AUA and EUA. Many of the pictures used in that lecture presentation come from Netter's medical illustrations in Ciba's book two and six. In addition to the pictures presented in this text, the reader is encouraged to review those illustrations to provide a visual description of the embryology presented. Finally, I should note that while we address each individual area of embryological development separately (kidneys, ureters, bladder, etc.) as well as their more common associated anomalies, the reader must visualize and recognize that the ongoing development is bilateral and overlapping.

Incidence of Congenital Anomalies

Congenital anomalies of the genito-urinary tract are common and an estimated 10% occur in the population in general. If other systems are congenitally abnormal, the incidence of the genito-urinary tract being involved increases to 30%, and if one genito-urinary anomaly exists, there is a 75% chance that a coexisting

C.R. Chapple and W.D. Steers (eds.), *Practical Urology: Essential Principles and Practice*,
DOI: 10.1007/978-1-84882-034-0_1, © Springer-Verlag London Limited 2011

anomaly is present elsewhere in the GU tract. These anomalies can be present in several ways:

1. They can be clinically obvious, as in hypospadias, epispadias, and bladder extrophy.
2. They may not be clinically obvious, but suspected, in newborns with Potter's facies, oligohydramnios, prune belly, single umbilical artery, and imperforate anus.
3. They may not be clinically obvious or suspected, but coincidentally found, as in patients with horseshoe kidneys, congenital solitary kidney, or duplex collecting systems.
4. Finally, they may not be clinically obvious, or suspected, or coincidentally found, but found because of symptoms of obstruction, stasis, infection, or stone formation, which prompt urological evaluation.

Congenital anomalies are thus extremely important and must not only be recognized, but understood in the urological practice.

Renal Development

Basic to normal renal development is the presence of a urogenital ridge – also known as the Wolffian body (see Fig. 1.1). It contains the nephric, gonadal, and genital ductal primordia. Within this urogenital ridge, three distinct and

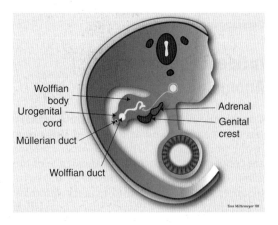

Figure 1.1. Relationship of Wolffian body with gonadal and adrenal primordia.

progressive stages of renal development occur. They are the pronephros, mesonephros, and metanephros.

Pronephros

The pronephros is the earliest nephric stage in man and corresponds to the mature structure of the most primitive vertebrates. It is the principal excretory organ during the first 4 weeks of embryonic life. It consists of six to ten pairs of tubules, which join to form the pronephric duct, which grows caudad. This pronephric duct eventually reaches and opens into the cloaca, which is the terminal portion of the hindgut. Being a vestigial structure, the pronephros disappears at about the fourth week of embryonic life (see Fig. 1.2).

Mesonephros

The second stage of nephric development is the mesonephros. It is the principal excretory organ during the fourth to eighth week of embryonic life. When the mesonephric tubules from the mesonephros become connected to this pronephric duct, its name is changed to mesonephric or Wolffian duct. This single structure gives rise to the entire male genital tract and "gives birth" to the ureter, which, in turn, is essential in the development of a normal kidney. Thus, in this early embryonic stage, faulty development of the mesonephric duct is probably related to the development of many of the genitourinary anomalies.

Metanephros

The metanephros is the third and final phase of the nephric systems and the primordium of the normal kidney. Its normal differentiation into the metanephrogenic blastema is entirely dependent upon the normal development and cranial growth of the ureteral bud into this mass of tissue. The metanephros thus caps this invaginating and branching ureteral bud and gives rise to the true renal cortex – that is, the glomeruli, proximal convoluted tubules, Henle's loop, and the distal convoluted tubules.

Figure 1.2. Renal and mesonephric duct development.

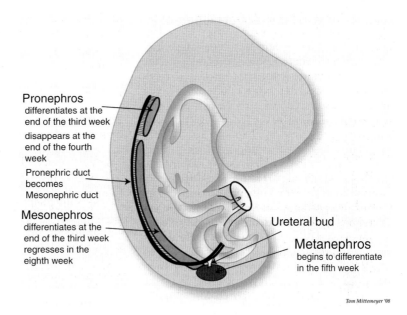

Pronephros
differentiates at the end of the third week

disappears at the end of the fourth week

Pronephric duct becomes Mesonephric duct

Mesonephros
differentiates at the end of the third week regresses in the eighth week

Ureteral bud

Metanephros
begins to differentiate in the fifth week

Tom Mittemeyer '08

Development of the Collecting System

The ureteral bud arises from the dorsal surface of the mesonephric duct a short distance from the cloacal wall. It initially bifurcates into two branches, which are the forerunners of the major calyces, with the point of bifurcation eventually forming the renal pelvis (see Fig. 1.3).

Between these two primary divisions of the ureter one or two additional divisions usually occur to form additional major calyces. From the ampullary enlargement of each of these primary divisions, two to four secondary tubules develop. These in turn give rise to tertiary tubules and the process is repeated until the fifth month of fetal life, when an estimated 12 generations of tubules have developed.

The pelvis and the primary as well as secondary tubules enlarge greatly during this development. The primary divisions become the major calyces, and the secondary divisions give rise to the minor calyces. The tubules of the third and fourth order are absorbed into the walls of the enlarging secondary tubules so that the tubules of the fifth order (a total of 20–30 in number) open into the minor calyces as papillary ducts. The remaining order of tubules constitutes the collecting tubules which form the greater part of the medulla of

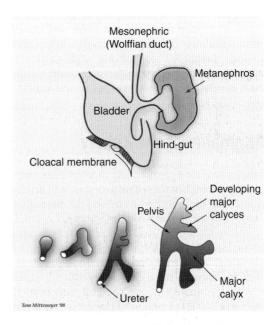

Mesonephric (Wolffian duct)

Metanephros

Bladder

Hind-gut

Cloacal membrane

Developing major calyces

Pelvis

Ureter

Major calyx

Tom Mittemeyer '08

Figure 1.3. Ureteral bud and renal collecting system development.

the adult kidney. Remember, at the point the collecting tubules meet and fuse with distal convoluted tubules (ureteral bud meets metanephrogenic blastema) is where congenital renal cystic disease has its origin.

Critical Steps in Further Development

While differentiating into this "final stage kidney," during the 9th to 12th weeks of fetal life, the metanephros undergoes three critical steps in further development. These include ascendance, rotation, and revascularization. First, the kidneys ascend from the level of the fourth lumbar vertebral level to the first lumbar or 12th thoracic level. This ascent of the kidney is due to both cephalad migration as well as the differential growth of the caudal part of the fetus. Second, in addition to ascent, the kidneys also undergo an approximate 90° rotation from a plane with the pelvis anterior to one with the pelvis lying medial and somewhat posterior. Third, as each kidney ascends and rotates, it is successively supplied by arteries which are located higher and higher on the urogenital ridge. They can arise from the iliac, middle sacral, lower aorta, and inferior mesenteric artery, and eventually from the final position on the aorta just below the superior mesenteric artery.

Failure of any of these progressive steps to occur in proper sequence and order will result in anomalous development. Such anomalies include anomalies of volume and structure, anomalies of number, anomalies of location, anomalies of rotation, anomalies of form, and anomalies of the vessels.

Anomalies of the Kidney

While there are a great variety of anomalies associated with each of these categories, we will briefly discuss the more common and serious anomalies associated with renal maldevelopment.

Before discussing renal agenesis, aplasia, and hypoplasia, it is important to reiterate that the presence of a normal ureteral bud is a prerequisite to normal renal development. In other words, the quality of the ureteral bud reflects not only the development of the ureter itself but also the appearance and development of the bladder trigone and kidney as well.

Renal Agenesis

It therefore stands to reason that in the vast majority of cases of renal agenesis, a ureteral bud abnormality existed and could be due to any of the following:

1. Absence of the entire genito-urinary ridge.
2. Failure of mesonephric duct development.
3. Failure of ureteral bud development from the mesonephric duct.
4. Failure of the ureteral bud to reach the metanephros.
5. Failure of the vascular supply to invade the metanephrogenic blastema.

Clinically, if agenesis is due to ureteral bud absence, a hemitrigone would be seen cystoscopically. On the other hand, if the ureteral bud develops normally but the metanephros fails, a normal trigone would be visualized and a blind ending ureter should be identifiable on retrograde urography. In patients with renal agenesis secondary to absence of the mesonephric duct proper, the genital duct apparatus would also be absent on the ipsilateral side. Furthermore, if the entire genito-urinary ridge failed to develop, not only the kidney, ureter, and genital duct structures, but the testis as well would be absent on the ipsilateral side.

Renal agenesis can be unilateral or bilateral. The unilateral absence of a kidney is not uncommon and occurs in approximately one of every 500 births. Bilateral agenesis is fortunately quite rare and, when present, is classically seen in association with the typical Potter's facies. In such cases, other anomalies are almost always present and generally incompatible with life. It is noteworthy that in unilateral renal agenesis the existing kidney is normally larger than a kidney which has hypertrophied because of destruction of its mate by injury or disease.

Renal Aplasia

In the patient with renal aplasia, nephrogenic tissue is present but it has failed to develop. These very small kidneys generally do not function and the ureter is generally equally poorly developed. Embryologically, they are best explained by inadequate stimulation of the metanephros by a bud of poor quality or inadequate vascularization of the metanephrogenic blastema. Again, the opposite kidney is usually significantly hypertrophied.

Renal Hypoplasia

In renal hypoplasia, the kidney is grossly normal but small. Microscopically, the kidneys are also normal but there is a reduced quantity of tissue. Once again, they are usually associated with a corresponding poorly developed ureter and trigone. Inadequate ureteral bud development or vascularization is again thought to play a major role in their etiology. Renal hypoplasia is usually unilateral but can be bilateral and may be confused with chronic pyelonephritis. An important point to remember in renal hypoplasia is that these kidneys usually are unable to hypertrophy with contralateral nephrectomy.

Renal Ectopia

Renal ectopia can be simple or crossed. The ectopic kidney can be normal or hypoplastic and is usually malrotated with the pelvis lying anterior or posterior from the norm. The usual cause is arrest of normal upward migration by abnormal persistence of vascular attachments which then prevent normal ascendance of the developing kidney from its pelvic fetal location to its normal position high in the retroperitoneum. Thus, aberrant renal vascularity is almost always present and can originate from any nearby major artery such as the aorta, the iliacs, the middle sacral, or inferior mesenteric arteries. Simple ectopia is not uncommon, occurs in approximately one of every 800 patients, and is three times more common on the left side.

In crossed ectopia, there is an 85% incidence of fusion with the contralateral kidney, which is generally in a normal position. A variety of configurations or shapes may occur, but the fusion is generally pole to pole. As in simple ectopia, the blood supply is aberrant. The ureters, however, generally enter the bladder in a normal position.

Renal Fusion

Renal fusion can take many shapes or forms. The lump or cake kidney is a solid, irregular, or lobulated organ which is usually quite low in position with an aberrant blood supply. Again, as in ectopia, the ureters generally enter the bladder in a normal manner because, as you recall, the ureteral bud arises from the mesonephric duct to enter the metanephros and ascends into a normal or abnormal position.

Such ascendance does not change the location of the ureteral opening in the urogental sinus, i.e. the trigone.

Horseshoe kidneys are examples of abnormal fusion where the lower and occasionally upper poles of the two renal blastemas are fused by an isthmus composed of either solid parenchymal tissue or a fibrous band which crosses in front of the aorta and vena cava. In a rare instance, the isthmus may be situated behind or between the great vessels.

This abnormal fusion of the right and left metanephros generally occurs between the fourth and eighth week of fetal development while the mesonephros is the functional renal unit and prevents normal ascent and rotation of the kidneys. The fusion and lack of rotation explain the anterior position of the ureters in such patients. The horseshoe kidney is typically located with the isthmus overlying the L-3 or L-4 level. In about 5% of patients, the upper poles are fused. When both poles are fused, the finding is described as a doughnut kidney. As might be expected, the blood supply is very anomalous in these cases. Twenty-five percent of these patients remain asymptomatic throughout life, and when symptoms do occur they are generally related to obstruction and its aftermath of the ureters as they cross the isthmus.

Ureteral Development

The next major area of discussion deals with the ureters and particularly their assumption of a normal position in the developing urogenital sinus (see Fig. 1.4). You will recall that the ureteral bud originally sprouted from the dorsal surface of the mesonephric duct just proximal to its junction with the cloaca. Because of the manner of growth and absorption of the mesonephric duct into the developing urogenital sinus, the ureter gradually assumes a more lateral and eventual anterior position on the mesonephric duct.

With continued expansion of the urogenital sinus, the mesonephric duct with its ureteral bud is literally absorbed. They eventually separate from each other through a somewhat complicated form of growth with the ureteral orifice moving in a lateral and cephalad direction while the mesonephric duct, which has now separated from the ureteral bud, continues to move in a

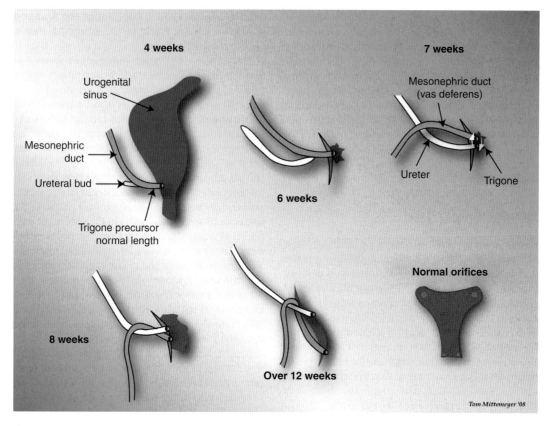

Figure 1.4. Normal ureteral development.

medial and caudal direction. In other words, the ureters migrate laterally and cranially while that portion of the urogenital sinus which receives the mesonephric ducts remains in close proximity to the midline and migrates distally. On completion of urogenital sinus development and differentiation, the orifices of the mesonephric ducts are thus eventually located on the floor of the prostatic urethra where they will serve as the opening of the ejaculatory ducts in the male (or their embryological remnants in the female).

Thus, a portion of the area bounded by the ureteral orifices and the openings of the mesonephric ducts, that is, the openings of the ejaculatory ducts – from an embryological standpoint – is thought to be of mesodermal origin while the remainder of the bladder is of endodermal origin. In the male, this area of mesonephric or mesodermal tissue includes the trigone of the bladder and the floor of the proximal portion of the prostatic urethra. In the female, it includes

the trigone, the floor of the entire urethra and a portion of the vestibule.

With this basic understanding of both normal ureteral development as well as the anatomic positioning of the kidneys as discussed previously, we can now discuss variations in development of the ureters which give rise to anomalies of the ureter and which are so often seen in association with genito-urinary pathology. While there are large a number of possible anomalies which can be associated with ureteral maldevelopment, we will concentrate on the more common and more interesting groups of such anomalies which can occur.

Anomalies of Origin

Anomalies of origin include ureteral agenesis, aplasia, and hypoplasia. In agenesis, no ureteral bud developed from the mesonephric duct and the ureter is thus absent. In aplasia, the ureteral bud is of very poor quality and the ureter is generally nothing more than a fibrous cord. In hypoplasia it may be a thin-walled tube. These ureteral anomalies thus represent varying degrees of ureteral bud development which will in turn determine the appearance of the vesical trigone, ureteral orifice, and kidneys. In other words, the clinical appearance of the ureteral orifice, trigone, and kidney normally parallel the extent of ureteral development. These corresponding structures may thus be absent, aplastic, or hypoplastic, as discussed earlier under renal development.

Anomalies of Number

Ureteral anomalies of number are among the most interesting from both a pathological and embryological standpoint (see Fig. 1.5). Whereas ureteral triplication is extremely rare, duplication of one or both ureters is quite common, and in a large autopsy series the incidence was as high as one in 160 cases. Logically, duplication is more often incomplete than complete as described below and unilateral involvement is

six times more common than bilateral involvement. It is definitely more common in females, and because of associated symptoms of obstruction or reflux it is generally diagnosed in childhood rather than in later life.

Incomplete Ureteral Duplication

The embryological explanation of incomplete ureteral duplication is simple and differs totally from the explanation for complete duplication. In incomplete duplication, premature bifurcation or splitting of the ureteral bud occurs after it arises from the mesonephric duct. If such branching occurs just below the normal point of bifurcation as it enters into the metanephros, the condition is called "bifid pelvis." Such premature splitting can occur anywhere along the course of ureteral bud development. If it occurs very early in its growth from the mesonephric duct, the point of bifurcation may actually be within the intravesical ureter that is within the developing bladder wall. Although such patients may be diagnosed to have completely duplicated ureters on radiography, cystoscopy would reveal a single ureteral orifice within the bladder.

Complete Ureteral Duplication

As noted previously, the embryological explanation of complete ureteral duplication differs totally from that of incomplete duplication. Specifically, two separate ureteral buds sprout from the respective mesonephric duct (see Fig. 1.6). Logically, the ureteral buds which sprout from the higher level of the mesonephric duct invaginate into the upper portion of the adjacent metanephros while the lower ureteral bud invaginates into the lower portion of the metanephros. One would thus expect the upper ureteral orifice to be associated with the ureter that drains the upper renal pelvis while the lower ureteral orifice in the bladder drains the ureter of the lower renal pelvis. However, this is not so and, in fact, the opposite is true. In reality, the ureteral orifice serving the lower renal pelvis is always situated cranially and laterally to the ureteral orifice serving the upper renal pelvis.

This is known as the Weigert-Meyer Law. Only rare instances have been reported in which this rule does not hold true. This is so because, as

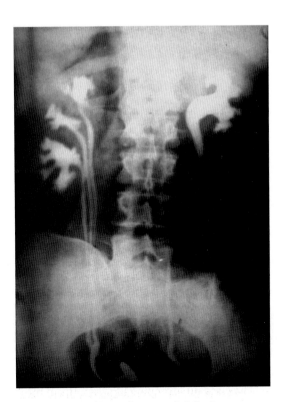

Figure 1.5. X-ray of incomplete ureteral triplication.

Figure 1.6. Ureteral duplication.

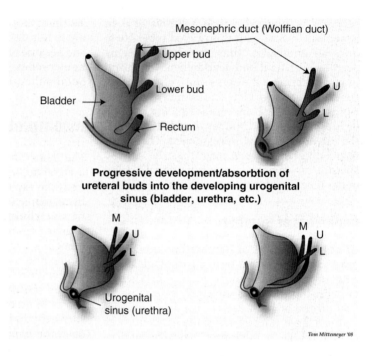

mentioned previously, the portion of the urinary bladder which received the mesonephric duct with its attached ureteral bud or buds grows in an uneven manner so that the ureter, once absorbed into the bladder wall, migrates laterally and cranially, while the rest of the mesonephric duct with the attached upper bud grows medially and distally. It thus stands to reason that the lower ureteral bud, which is absorbed into the bladder first, assumes a more lateral and cephalad position than the upper ureteral bud which is carried distally and medially by the migrating mesonephric duct. Only as still more of the duct is absorbed into the bladder or urethra does this ureter attain its independent opening. It can, of course, be so high in position that it never leaves the mesonephric duct in which case it will empty into the ejaculatory duct or the higher structures to which of the embryological mesonephric duct gives rise or its embryological remnants in the female (Gartner's Duct).

Clinically, because of their anatomic position, one or both of these duplicated ureteral orifices are often associated with either vesicoureteral reflux (ureter draining the lower renal segment), or ureteroceles and ureteral ectopia with stenosis and severe dilatation (ureter draining the upper renal segment). The paired ureters normally

course downward side by side to the level of the bony pelvis and, just prior to reaching the bladder, the ureter from the upper renal pelvis passes beneath its mate to enter the bladder at a lower and more medial position. Since this ureter draining the upper renal pelvis normally opens in the more dense trigonal tissue, it is often associated with stenosis and secondary ureteral dilatation or a ureterocele. It can, of course have an extra vesical entry; in which case it is generally much more obstructed and dilated.

Similarly, it is these ureters which are often associated with a ureterocele. On the other hand, the ureter draining the lower renal segment empties high and laterally into the bladder wall and is thus often off the trigone. It therefore has a relatively short segment, and by virtue of its lateral position is more subject to vesicoureteral reflux.

Clinical symptoms and signs associated with ureteral duplication are then generally related to obstruction or reflux, and these findings are best demonstrated by three classical radiographic findings which include (see Fig 1.7):

1. Non-visualization of a relatively large renal area (severely obstructed upper renal segment).
2. The classical "drooping lily" sign (from pressure above).

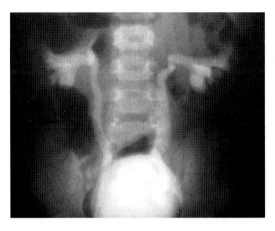

Figure 1.7. X-ray of ureteral duplication with "drooping lily" sign.

3. The finding of a dilated, often refluxing laterally displaced ureter by it severely dilated obstructed mate which drains the upper renal segment.

Ureteral Ectopia

Ureteral orifices which drain other than in their normal position on the trigone are considered to be ectopic. The vast majority or 80% of these are associated with a duplicated renal collecting system as discussed above, and if this is the case, both could be ectopic. If only one is ectopic, it is generally the ureter draining the upper renal segment.

Embryology of Ectopia

The ectopic ureter can best be explained embryologically as follows. If the point of origin of the ureteral bud from the mesonephric duct is closer to the urogenital sinus (developing bladder) than normal, it will enter the bladder earlier and thus be positioned at a point more cephalad and lateral to the normal position on the trigone. On the other hand, if the point of origin of the ureteral bud is higher on the mesonephric duct than normal, it will be carried more medially and distally with the mesonephric duct and may, in fact, never enter the bladder proper.

Inasmuch as the mesonephric duct contributes to the formation of the trigone and posterior urethra and then gives rise to the entire ejaculatory duct, seminal vesicles, vas deferens and epididymis in the male, ureteral ectopia may occur at any of these sites – depending upon how high the uretral bud was positioned on the mesonephric duct.

Similarly, location of ectopic ureteral orifices in the vesical neck, urethra or vestibule of the female are explained on the basis of their mesonephric duct origin and its contribution to the urogenital sinus. Since vestigal remnants of the mesonephric duct in the female may be found along a line running from the hymen (homologue of the verumontanum) through the anterolateral walls of the vagina, the cervix, the wall of the uterus, and between the layers of the broad ligament to the ovaries, it is feasible that ectopic orifices could in fact drain into any of these embryological remnants which include the epoöphoron, paroöphoron, and Gartner's duct. Such a location would be extremely uncommon and of so, the obstruction is usually so great that the renal segment is non-functioning.

Clinical Correlation

If the ectopic orifice is outside the bladder, the location depends on the sex of the patient.

Location of Ectopic Ureteral Orifices – Male (in Descending Order According to Incidence)

Vesical neck and prostatic urethra
Seminal vesicles
Vas Deferens
Ejaculatory duct
Rarely in the rectum

Location of Ectopic Ureteral Orifices – Female

In the female, the location of the ectopic ureteral orifices, are generally divided equally between the vesical neck and urethra, the vestibule, and the vagina.

Vesical neck and urethra
Vestibule
Vagina
Cervix, uterus and rectum

Logically, in the male, the vesical neck and prostatic urethra are most commonly involved. The ejaculatory ducts should theoretically be next in line, but they are uncommonly involved in view of the very short segment of the original mesonephric duct which gives rise to this structure. Therefore, the seminal vesicles are next in frequency and the vas deferens follows.

Rectal positioning of the ureter is rare and can be explained embryologically by a very dorsal entry of the original pronephric duct into the cloaca, or by erroneous anterior division of the cloaca by the urorectal septum, so that the division occurs ventral to the point of pronephric duct entry.

Symptoms

Symptoms related to ureteral ectopia are thus dependent upon the site of the ureteral opening and the patient's sex. Inasmuch as the ectopic orifice always opens proximal to the external sphinctor in the male, incontinence should not really ever occur. However, in the female, incontinence is a common complaint since the ureteral orifice is located distal to the sphinctor mechanism in the majority of cases. Ectopic ureters entering the bladder on the lower trigone are usually associated with a ureterocele because of partial obstruction. Furthermore, in either sex, the ectopic ureter, because of obstruction is almost always associated with uretral dilatation which can be so severe that the upper renal segment becomes very hydronephrotic and eventually non-functioning.

Ureteroceles

A ureterocele is a cystic dilation of the ureter into the bladder. Except for the few which would be acquired from injury to the ureteral orifice with subsequent scarring, the majority is, of congenital origin and is thought to be related to incomplete rupture of Chwalla membrane with resultant stenosis of the epithelial lining at the vesical end of the ureter. Urine flow into the bladder is thus obstructed and the pressure produced by the ureteral peristalsis pushes the peri-ureteral vesical mucosa into the bladder.

The resultant dilatation, which is related to the degree of obstruction and the length of the intravesical ureter, produces the characteristic urographic "cobra head" or "spring onion" filling defect. A second classical finding is the halo or negative shadow effect which surrounds the cystic outline of the ureterocele filled with concentrated contrast media (see Figs. 1.8 and 1.9).

In review, as stated previously, ureteroceles are often but not always associated with ureteral duplication. However, if duplication is present, the ureterocele is always associated with the ureter serving the upper segment of a duplicated kidney that is the ureter which enters in the lower and more dense and medial position of the bladder. Furthermore, the ureter from the lower renal segment – that is the ureter which empties into the more cephalad and lateral position of the bladder may be compromised by a ureterocele and thus also be obstructed and may reflux because of its position off the trigone.

A final point. Because ureteral duplication is more common in females than males, ureteroceles are also more common in females and when encountered in children, whether male or

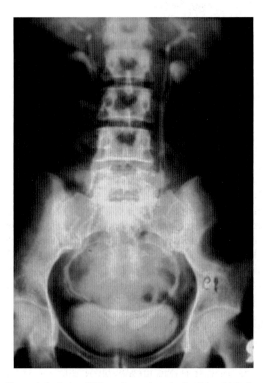

Figure 1.8. X-ray of bilateral complete duplication with "cobra head" filling defect.

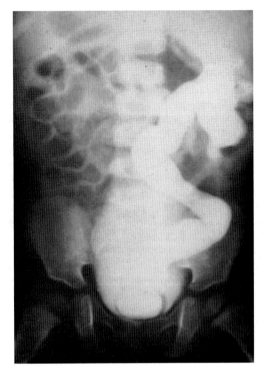

Figure 1.9. X-ray of large ureterocele with halo sign.

Pipestem Ureter

This pipestem megaureter is a dilated ureter without an overt obstructing lesion.(see Fig. 1.10) Two basic types exist. These are the refluxing and non-refluxing types. The refluxing type is associated with gross reflux and is rarely seen. The non-refluxing type is by far the most common type seen and here the functional abnormality appears to be in the terminal ureter. The exact nature of this functional abnormality is not known – but three points are well established. These are:

1. That there is no absence of ganglion cells in the terminal portion of the ureter.
2. The cause is thought to be due to a disproportion of circular and longitudinal muscle fibers in the terminal ureter.
3. That normal peristaltic contraction waves do not pass through this terminal portion of the ureter.

female, may produce extremely difficult diagnostic problems. This is particularly true when they are so large as to almost completely fill the bladder, making cystoscopic observation difficult and confusing. Large ureteroceles may obstruct the vesical neck and even prolapse through the urethra in females. In adults, ureteroceles tend to be bilateral and smaller, thus causing less obstruction and thus fewer symptoms. In males they are often found co-incidentally at time of cystoscopy done prior to transurethral resection of the prostate (TURP) and should be noted so as not to be post operatively related to the resection. The clinical history and clinical findings are related to obstruction and stasis and if symptomatic, the treatment is surgical.

Congenital Ureteral Obstruction

Congenital ureteral obstructions are our next topic of discussion. I will allude to three such types of obstruction and the first of these is the "pipestem" or classic megaureter.

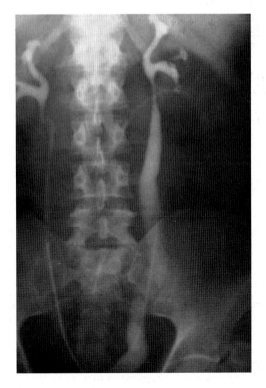

Figure 1.10. Pipestem ureter.

These points are important to consider when surgical correction is planned. The abnormal ureteral segment must be excised and confirmed by pathology to insure that normal ureter is implanted.

Megaureter-Megacystis Syndrome

In contrast to the pipestem ureter, the Megaureter-Megacystis syndrome is characterized by a large capacity bladder with dilated and refluxing ureters in the absence of vesical neck or urethral obstruction. This condition is generally diagnosed during childhood, because of the associated symptoms, has an equal sex incidence, and there is no known cause. The ureter in this syndrome is not only dilated, but also lengthened and tortuous – and although peristalsis is active, the propulsive powers are very limited.

A second significant difference is that the ureteral orifices are widely dilated and permit easy reflux, whereas the orifices in the congenital megaureter are generally normal in appearance. Thirdly, in this syndrome the bladder is characteristically dilated – but without trabeculation or outlet obstruction.

As in congenital megaureter, there appears to be no histological abnormality in the number and distribution of the ganglion cells. The typical clinical history is that of a child which presents with a history of recurrent urinary tract infections, a palpable bladder on physical examination, and evidence of bone changes or manifestations of renal failure if the condition has been present for some time. The diagnosis is made by urography, voiding cystourethrography, and cystoscopy.

In the differential diagnosis we have to consider:

1. Nephrogenic diabetes insipidus.
2. Neurogenic bladder (which is rare in children and seldom has a capacity of over 500 ml).
3. Urethral valves.
4. Prune belly syndrome.

All these possible causes must be excluded and surgical correction usually entails tapering of the ureters prior to re-implantation.

Prune Belly Syndrome

A third type of congenital ureteral dilation is seen in the prune belly syndrome. It is characterized by the congenital absence of abdominal musculature, which generally involves the lower and medial parts of the abdominal wall. The result is a protuberant, thin walled and creased abdomen which gives rise to the classical name.

The condition is seen almost exclusively in males and is associated with serious genitourinary anomalies. These anomalies include a large capacity bladder which may be associated with diverticula or a patent urachus. The ureters are almost always dilated and tortuous with associated reflux and poor contractions. The kidneys are either hydronephrotic or displastic and the urethra may be obstructed. Testicular male-descent is common, penile curvature may occur, and most patients are sterile.

Associated abnormalities include intestinal malrotation, congenital cardiac abnormalities, and talipes. As in Megaurer-Megacystis syndrome the treatment is dependent on the degree of renal deterioration and extent of urological involvement as demonstrated by extensive endoscopic and radiographic evaluation.

Vascular Ureteral Obstructions

The final topic in regard to congenital ureteral obstructions deals with vascular obstruction of the ureter. These may occur at any level, but the most common cause of such obstruction by far is the presence of a residual obstructing lower pole renal vessel at the ureteropelvic junction (UPJ) with secondary hydronephrosis.

Although the presence of a retroiliac ureter is rare, it can occur and when present is seen at the L-5 level. The retrocaval ureter is more common, and both of these are the result of an anomaly of the vena cava rather than the ureter. These anomalies are thought to be due to persistence of the subcardinal vein as the infra-renal segment of the vena cava rather than the supra cardinal vein (see Fig. 1.11).

In this anomalous condition, the ureter abruptly turns medially from a normal position in its upper third and passes behind the vena cava in the region of the third and fourth lumbar vertebra. From there it returns to its normal position lateral to the vena cava after making a

Figure 1.11. Retrocaval ureteral anomaly.

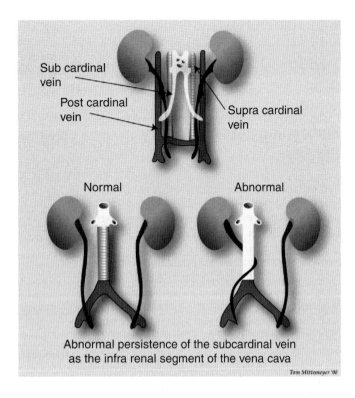

Sub cardinal vein

Post cardinal vein

Supra cardinal vein

Normal

Abnormal

Abnormal persistence of the subcardinal vein as the infra renal segment of the vena cava

Tom Mittemeyer '08

hook or sickle shaped curve. If the obstruction is less than severe it can be missed by radiography since the upper ureter crosses the belly of the psoas muscle where it is often compressed. Obstructive symptoms may vary depending on fluid intake and if a question arises on the basis of symptoms a retrograde ureterogram or intravenous pyelogram (IVP) with abdominal pressure may be necessary (see Fig. 1.12). It is the only anomaly of the genito-urinary tract that is limited to the right side and there are no pathognomonic signs or symptoms. It becomes a clinical problem only because of the hydronephrosis which may result from obstruction of the ureter by the vena cava.

Approximately 25% of the patients have either no symptoms or merely infrequent attacks of colic. For those patients with persistent symptoms of obstruction, or with radiological evidence of renal damage, the treatment includes:

1. Resection of the ureter with re-anastomosis.
2. Resection of the ureter with excision of the postcaval section – which may be stenotic – and re-anastomosis.

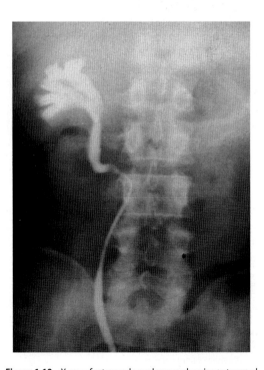

Figure 1.12. X-ray of retrograde pyelogram showing retrocaval ureter.

3. Division of the vena cava with subsequent re-anastomosis after release of the retrocaval ureter.
4. Renal transplantation.

Embryology of the Urinary Bladder

You will recall that the primitive cloaca is formed by the distal portion of the digestive tract – the hindgut. This structure is separated from the fetal exterior by the cloacal membrane and receives the allantois and the paired mesonephric ducts with their ureteral buds. The cloaca is gradually divided by the urorectal septum which grows down to the cloacal membrane and separates the cloaca into two somewhat dilated structures, the posterior rectum and the anterior urogenital sinus. The site of fusion of the urorectal septum with the cloacal membrane becomes the perineal body and this fusion is generally completed by the seventh week of fetal life. The portion of the cloacal membrane anterior to the point of fusion is now known as the urogenital membrane and separates the urogenital sinus from the fetal exterior. The portion posterior to the point of fusion is the anal membrane and separates the rectum from the fetal exterior.

Division of the Urogenital Sinus

Once formed, the urogenital sinus can be divided into an upper and lower segment with Müller's tubercle – which is the point where the fused distal portion of the Müllerian ducts joins the urogenital sinus – serving as the best point of demarcation between them (see Fig. 1.13). This point of demarcation is important because the ventral or pelvic portion forms the bladder and entire urethra in the female and the bladder and prostatic urethra above the verumontanum in the male.

Bladder Development

As the bladder begins to expand about the third month of fetal life, it tapers at its apical end where it is attached to the still patent allantois.

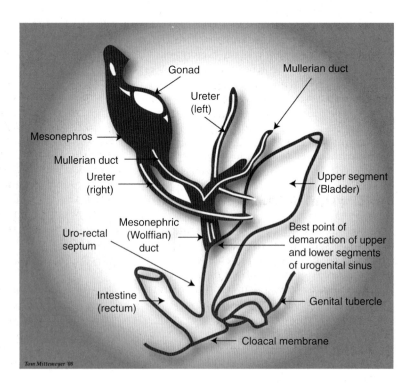

Figure 1.13. Urogenital sinus development – best point of demarcation of upper and lower segments of urogenital sinus.

This apical patent allantois becomes stretched and narrowed as the fetus grows and the bladder descends until the patent allantois is totally obliterated at approximately the fourth month of fetal life. This "tube like" vestigial remnant of the allantois extends extraperitoneally to the umbilicus and is known as the urachus. As the fetus further develops and the bladder continues to descend, the urachus obliterates and forms the urachal ligament.

Urachal Anomalies

Failure of the urachus to obliterate completely results in one of four basic types of anomalies. The most common of these is the completely patent urachus. This condition is commonly associated with bladder outlet obstruction and is generally diagnosed shortly after birth with urinary leakage occurring from the umbilicus. The diagnosis is confirmed by cystogram and/or the use of indigo carmine which confirms the drainage to be of urinary origin. Treatment consists of correcting the lower urinary tract obstruction and excising the fistula if it does not close spontaneously. If the anomaly is that of a partially patent urachus, a mucous fistula is generally seen if the patency is at the umbilical end. If at the bladder end, the apical diverticulum is lined by mucous secreting epithelium that may develop into adenocarcinoma in later life. A urachal cyst results when the umbilical and bladder ends close and a small tube persists centrally. These patients usually present with an infra-umbilical midline suprapubic mass of various sizes and the treatment is surgical excision.

Cloacal Duct Anomalies

Prior to complete division of the cloaca by the urorectal septum, which normally has occurred by the seventh week, a connection remains between the rectum and the urogenital sinus which is known as the cloacal duct. In situations where there is associated anal or rectal maldevelopment such as stenosis, imperforate anus, imperforate anus with blind ending pouch, or normal anus with blind ending rectum, this cloacal duct can fail to close which then leads to a variety of fistulae, the exact type being determined by the sex of the fetus and the stage of development at which time the fistula occurs (see Fig. 1.14).

In the male, such fistulae include: recto-vesical, recto-urethral, and recto-perineal fistulae. Their incidence in the presence of rectal atresia or obstruction is common and occurred in 42% of Gross' series.

In the female, the recto-vesical and recto-urethral fistulae are almost non-existent because of the interposition of the vagina and uterus between the urogenital sinus and rectum (see Fig. 1.15). However, the result is an even higher incidence of recto-vaginal and recto-vestibular fistulae with an incidence of 60% of such cases in Gross' series.

Other Bladder Anomalies

Other congenital bladder anomalies such as agenesis, hypoplasia, duplication, diverticula, and bladder extrophy are in general, rare. Agenesis and hypoplasia are extremely rare and in most cases are associated with either renal agenesis or other anomalies which are incompatible with life. If the latter is not the case, the ureters, generally opens ectopically into a dilated urethral pouch or into the rectum or vagina.

Bladder duplication may be complete in which case two entirely separate bladders lie side by side enclosed within a common sheath. Each has its own ureter and urethra and in the male two penises is generally present. In the female, there may also be duplication of the Müllerian duct derivatives and duplications of the large bowel frequently coexist. In patients with incomplete duplication, the bladders join at the base and have a common urethra. Other bladder divisions include the presence of midline sagittal septums or transverse septums which divide the bladder into an upper and lower half.

Bladder Diverticula

When a bladder diverticulum is thought to be of congenital origin, it is believed to be due to a congenital deficiency in the detrusor muscle. This results in the formation of a diverticulum in face of normal bladder pressures with micturition and no obvious outlet obstruction.

Possible anal and rectal abnormalities:

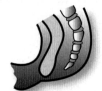
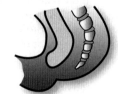
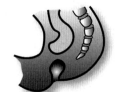

Stenosis at the anus.

Imperforate anus, obstruction by persistant membrane.

Imperforate anus, rectal pouch ends blindly above.

Anus and anal pouch normal. Pouch ends blindly in hollow of sacrum.

Possible fistulae encountered in male patients:

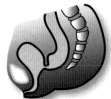
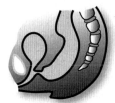
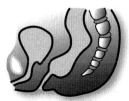

Rectovesical fistula.

Rectaurethral communication.

Rectoperineal fistula.

Possible fistulae encountered in female patients:

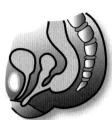
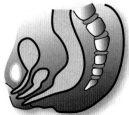
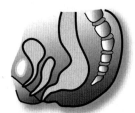

Rectovaginal fistula.

Rectovestibular fistula.

Rectoperineal fistula.

Tom Mittemeyer '08

Figure 1.14. Demonstration of possible anal and rectal abnormalities and associated fistulae encountered in male and female patients.

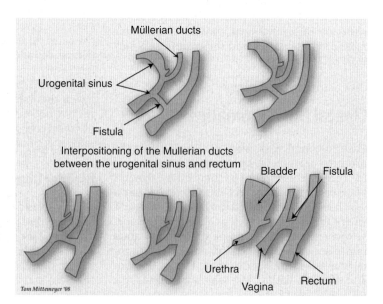

Müllerian ducts

Urogenital sinus

Fistula

Interpositioning of the Mullerian ducts between the urogenital sinus and rectum

Bladder   Fistula

Urethra

Vagina   Rectum

Tom Mittemeyer '08

Figure 1.15. Cloacal duct anomalies in the female – Interpositioning of the Müllerian ducts between the urogenital sinus and rectum.

These diverticula are considered to be congenital in origin.

While bladder diverticula can be congenital, they are generally acquired. The majority of such acquired diverticula are due to some form of outlet obstruction. In children, posterior urethral valves and congenital urethral strictures are the most common cause. In adults, benign prostatic hypertrophy and acquired urethral strictures are the general basis for this problem.

However, the classical distinction, between an acquired and a congenital diverticulum is that the congenital diverticulum displays an adventitial, muscular, and mucosal layer whereas the acquired diverticulum has only an adventitial and mucosal layer. Symptomatology is generally related to stasis with complicating infection, calculus formation or tumor formation. The treatment is surgical if the diverticulum cannot be cystoscoped, does not empty well, or complications exist.

Bladder Extrophy

Extrophy is a severe congenital affliction and is fortunately very rare. It occurs approximately once in 40,000 births and the male is afflicted three times more often than the female. Embryologically, it results from failure of the mesodermal structures of the abdominal wall below the umbilicus to develop normally. Gilles believes that this is due to abnormal forward displacement of the cloacal membrane. On the other hand, Patten believes that it is due to abnormal caudal formation of the paired primordia of the genital tubercle. Other theories exist but whatever the cause, the results are generally devastating.

Varying degrees of bladder extrophy can occur and range from simple epispadias to complete extrophy with epispadias, pubic separation, inguinal hemia, imperforate anus, or persistent cloaca. Testicular maldescent is also frequently associated. In addition, the ureterovesical junction is generally defective with associated reflux.

From a clinical standpoint, it is worthy to note that while urachal remnants can give rise to adenocarcinoma which tends to spread late, bladder extrophy gives rise to adenocarcinoma which spreads early.

Gonadal Development

Sexual differentiation in the fetus is bipotential. This is true not only for the gonad and the external genitalia which are derived from a common primordium but for the ductal structures as well, each sex having its own primordium.

Formation of the undifferentiated gonad begins during the fifth week of fetal life when the proliferation of germinal epithelial cells and the mesenchyme underlying them produce a prominence on the medial side of each mesonephros. This prominence is then known as the gonadal ridge. While the germinal epithelial cells and the underlying mesenchymal tissue continue to proliferate, primordial germ cells migrate into this underlying mesenchyme at about the sixth week of fetal life and the undifferentiated or bipotential gonad is formed (see Fig. 1.16).

Testicular Differentiation

At about the seventh week of fetal life testicular differentiation occurs. Such differentiation of the gonadal primordium occurs through the action of male organizer substance and is thought to be controlled by the Y chromosome. Not until normal testicular development and function has been initiated can development of the male phenotype occur. In the absence of such testicular development, the differentiated gonad will thus develop into an ovary at the 13th to 14th week of fetal life. For normal male fetal development the 7th to 12th week of fetal development are thus essential. If testosterone secretion is delayed for whatever reason, abnormal male development will occur.

When the gonad develops into a testis (see Fig. 1.17)

1. Proliferation of the coelemic epithelium ceases and the sex cords of the undifferentiated stage become the seminiferous tubules. These, with their cellular duality, provide the spermatogonia as well as the Sertoli - or nutritive - support cells.

2. A layer of connective tissue, the tunica albuginea, interposes itself between the coelemic epithelium and the rest of the gland and compartmentalizes the rolled up seminiferous tubules.

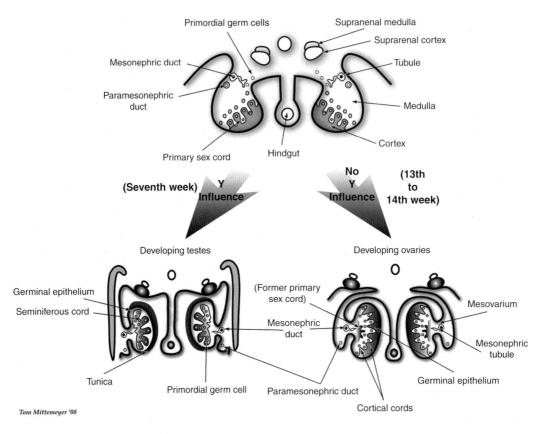

Figure 1.16. Gonad development based on the presence or absence of the Y chromosome.

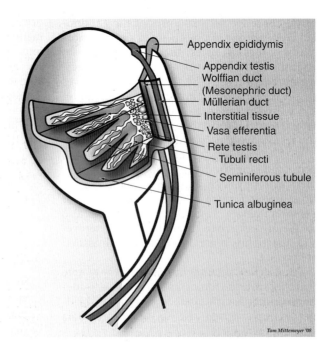

Figure 1.17. Testicular development.

3. The deep portions of the seminiferous tubules narrow to form the tubuli recti, and these converge to form the rete testis. The Sertoli cells, seminiferous tubules, tubuli recti, and rete testis thus all originate from the coelemic epithelium. The Sertoli cells produce Müllerian inhibiting factor (MIF).

4. The interstitial cells of Leydig differentiate between the seminiferous tubules. They produce testosterone, which is the androgenic hormone which influences male genital tract and external genital development and differentiation.

5. As the Wolffian body (Genito-urinary ridge) regresses, the rete testes anastomose with the adjacent mesonephric tubules thus establishing the first genito-urinary connection (GU). These connecting mesonephric tubules are known as the vasa deferentia, and that portion of the mesonephric duct into which they open becomes the epididymis.

As the testicle further develops, it increases in size and shortens into a more compact organ while achieving a more caudal location. Furthermore, its broad attachment to the mesonephros is converted into a gonadal mesentery known as the mesorchium. By the third month of fetal life, the testis has descended and is located retroperitoneally in the false pelvis from where it gradually descends to the abdominal end of the inguinal canal. It remains there until the seventh month of fetal life at which time it passes through the inguinal canal behind the processus vaginalis to enter the scrotum by the end of the eighth month.

Caudal migration of the testes is facilitated by means of the gubenaculum. This fibromuscular band extends from the lower pole of the testis through the developing muscular layers of the anterior abdominal wall to terminate in the subcutaneous tissue of the scrotal swelling. The gubenaculum also has several subsidiary strands that extend to adjacent regions (femoral, interstitial, penile, etc.) and these explain testicular maldescent into these regions.

Ovarian Differentiation

In the absence of male organizer substance, a factor of the XY chromosome the undifferentiated gonad develops into an ovary. Initially, at about the ninth week of fetal life, a primary cortex and medulla form. These structures then give rise to a definitive cortex by the fourteenth week of life. In ovarian development, the coelemic germinal epithelium gives rise to the primary ovarian follicles, the underlying mesenchyme to the stromal cells, and the primordial germ cells to the ova. Like the testis, the ovary also gains a mesentery known as the mesovarium, and settles into a more caudal position as the fetus develops. In addition to this early internal descent, the ovary also becomes attached through the gubernaculum to the tissues of the genital folds, which form the round ligaments of the ovary, as well as to the tissues of the uterovaginal canal which form the broad ligament of the uterus. A small processus vaginalis also forms and passes toward the labial swellings, but this structure is usually obliterated at full term.

Gonadal Anomalies

Gonadal anomalies can simply be broken down into anomalies of development and anomalies of position.

Anomalies of development include anomalies in number such as agenesis or anorchism, hypogenesis, supernumerary gonads or polyorchism, as well as the extremely rare anomaly of gonadal fusion or synorchism.

Anomalies of position include cryptorchidism, or imperfect descent of the testis, which is by far the commonest spermatic tract anomaly. The cause of imperfect testicular descent is unknown, but is usually anatomic or hormonal in origin. Testicular ectopy is due to faulty testicular descent along one of the subsidiary strains of the gubemaculum. In such aberrant descent, the testicle may be interstitial, femoral, penile, perineal, or transverse in its position.

Failure of union between the rete testes and mesonephros, that is, the mesonephric tubules, results in a testis separate from the male genital ducts.

Genital Duct System

Before discussing development of the genital duct system and the external genitalia, it is important to reemphasize that while the Y chromosome and testicular development and function are absolutely essential in the development of the male fetus, neither the 46 XX complement nor the ovaries are necessary, for female fetal development. It has been experimentally shown that if a genetic male fetus is castrated (no testosterone or MIF) before the genitalia differentiate, a female phenotype will develop. Thus while testicular influence is absolutely necessary for male development, ovarian influence is of no significance in female development since the natural tendency of the fetus is to develop into a female.

As alluded to earlier, for normal male phenotype development in utero, the testes must not only differentiate normally but also function normally. Two specific substances which are critical to the development of the male phenotype must be produced by the testes. The first of these is the hormone testosterone which is secreted by the Leydig cells. The second is the Müllerian inhibiting factor (MIF) which is thought to be secreted by the Sertoli cells (see Fig. 1.18).

The Müllerian inhibiting factor is secreted by the Sertoli cells and acts locally (rather than systemically) to suppress the development of the adjacent Müllerian structures in direct contact with the ipsilateral fetal testis. As the testis descends it acts sequentially on the adjacent Müllerian structures with the only remnants being the appendix testis at the superior end and the utricle in the verumontanum at the distal end.

This action cannot be duplicated by androgens since testosterone, which is secreted by the Leydig cells, acts systemically rather than locally and plays the most important role in two other major facets of male phenotype development. First of all, it permits differentiation of the mesonephric tubules and ductal structures into the epididymis, vas deferens, seminal vesicles, and ejaculatory ducts. Secondly, testosterone also acts as a prehormone on the androgen dependent target areas, which include the components of the urogenital tubercle, the urogenital sinus, and that area in the urogenital sinus which will eventually develop into the prostate

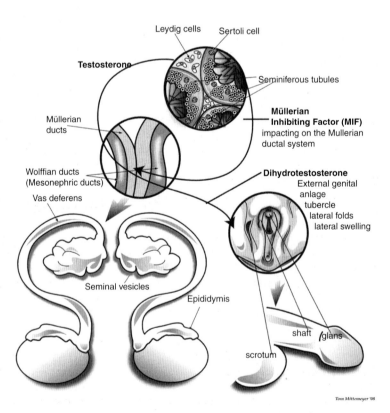

Figure 1.18. Testosterone and Müllerian Inhibition Factor (MIF) influence on gonadal and genital development.

gland. Testosterone enters the cells of these target areas and is converted to dihydrotestosterone by the enzyme 5 A reductase. It is this dihydrotestosterone which permits the differentiation of these structures into the male external genitalia and secondary sex organs.

Disorders of Testicular Function

Disorders of testicular differentiation and development may thus result in the absence or delayed secretion of these two vital testicular substances which are essential for male phenotypic development and müllerian ductal inhibition. The resulting anomalies will vary depending upon on the degree and time of delayed secretion. With this as background, and a clear understanding of the important role which the normally differentiating testis plays on the development of the respective genital ductal system, a closer look at the development of each system is now in order.

Male Ductal System Development

While differentiating, the gonad is situated in close proximity to the mesonephric duct. The mesonephric tubules adjacent to this developing gonad become continuous with the rete testes. These mesonephric tubules, together with that portion of the mesonephric duct into which they drain, will develop into the epididymis on each side and thus establish an actual urogenital connection.

The mesonephric tubules above and below those which were included in the epididymal formation remain as rudimentary structures. Those above the epididymis form the appendix of the epididymis and those below form the paradidymis.

The mesonephric duct distal to that portion forming the epididymis will become the vas deferens. Just proximal to the point where the vas deferens enters the urogenital sinus which forms the urethra, a saccular dilatation evaginates from its wall to form the seminal vesicles. That portion of the mesonephric duct distal to the origin of the seminal vesicles is known as the ejaculatory duct which enters into the urethra.

Development of the Prostate and Urethral Glands

Both above and below that point where the ejaculatory ducts enter the urethra, numerous glandular structures form as out-branchings from the urethral lumen. These are the anterior urethral glands of Littre and Morgagni, as well as the deep urethral (bulbomembranous) glands of Cowper.

At about the eleventh week of fetal life, the prostate (or female homologue) develops both above and below the point of exit of the ejaculatory ducts as multiple outgrowths of endothelium in that portion of the urogenital sinus (urethra) which gives rise to prostatitic urethra in the male and the entire urethra in the female. These tubules form in six groups which ultimately become the definitive prostatic lobes in the male. Eventually, these prostatic buds become surrounded by smooth muscle fibers and connective tissue to form the prostate gland.

In the absence of testosterone, the female homologues of these structures form and are the epoöphoron, (appendix epididymis) paroöphoron (paradidymis), Gartner's duct (vas deferens), Skene's glands (prostate), and Bartholin's glands (Cowper's glands). The Skene and Bartholin glands can become inflamed and symptomatic.

Female Ductal Development

In the developing embryo, the paired Müllerian or paramesonephric ducts are positioned laterally to the mesonephric ducts. At the cephalad end of each duct, an opening with the celomic cavity persists. This is the peritoneal ostium of the uterine tubes which later develop fimbria. The caudal end grows distally as a solid tip and eventually crosses in front of its respective mesonephric duct to meet and fuse with its contralateral mate (see Fig. 1.19).

At first this fusion is partial, with an intermediate septum, but later a single canal develops

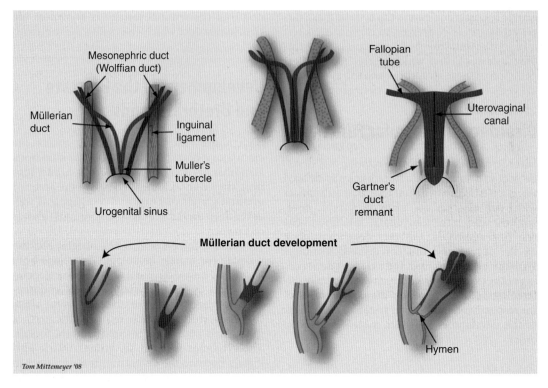

Figure 1.19. Distal Müllerian duct development in the female.

which gives rise to the uterus and the proximal four-fifths of the vagina. Furthermore, it is noteworthy that this eventual canal initially presents as a solid cord which pushes the epithelium of the urogenital sinus outward to become Müller's tubercle (verumontanum) in the male. The two remaining homologues of the Müllerian ductal structures in the male are the appendix testis (fimbriated end of the Müllerian duct) and the utricle (located in the verumontanum), which represent the proximal and terminal ends of the Müllerian ducts.

Although it is somewhat premature to mention it, I will here briefly discuss the development of the distal fifth of the vagina. This distal portion of the vagina develops from that area in the urogenital sinus where the fused müllerian ducts are attached. Through a somewhat complicated growth process, and together with the normal shortening and widening of the urogenital sinus in the female (in the absence of testosterone) the point of union of the fused müllerian and urogenital sinus retracts and is thus pulled upward. This portion of the urogenital sinus then forms the distal fifth of the vagina with the

point of fusion between the urogenital sinus and the fused Müllerian ducts forming the hymen.

Prostatic Urethral Valves

Although the exact cause of prostatic urethral valves in the male remains debated, it is believed that they represent various embryologic remnants of the junction of the sinovaginal bulb and the urogenital sinus (see Fig. 1.20).

Gonadal Duct Anomalies

The probabilities of gonadal duct anomalies are rare indeed. Non-union of the rete testis and the mesonephric ductules can occur and, if bilateral, will result in azospermia and sterility even though a testis and epididymis are present. If the Müllerian ducts do not approximate properly or are incompletely fused, various degrees of female genital duct duplication can occur. Congenital absence of one or both of the Müllerian duct or Wolffian duct structures can

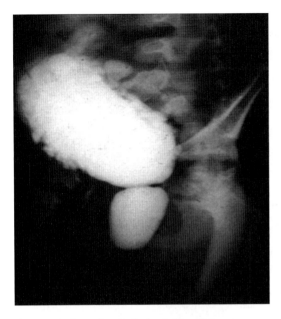

Figure 1.20. X-ray of urethral valves in the male.

occur, although such absence is rare. Finally, if the infratubercular segment of the urogenital sinus does not develop normally, a urogenital sinus will persist with the urethra and vagina having a common external opening.

External Genital Development

A closer look at fetal external genital development reveals that while the fetus is still in the undifferentiated stage, the perineal body becomes surrounded by a mound of tissue known as the genital tubercle. This tissue assumes the form of folds which are known as the urogenital folds which extend along each side of a groove known as the urogenital groove or sulcus, the floor of which is formed by the unruptured urogenital membrane. The remaining major portions of the genital tubercle are the glans proper and the lateral buttresses. More lateral and cephalad to the genital tubercle, two paired elevations, known as the labioscrotal swellings, arise which initially are located on the very lower aspect of the abdominal wall (see Fig. 1.21).

As fetal development continues the genital tubercle gradually elongates into a more or less cylindrical phallus which is the embryological homologue of the penis in the male and the clitoris in the female. At about the seventh week of fetal life, the urogenital membrane in the floor of the urogenital sulcus ruptures providing the urogenital sulcus with an opening to the fetal exterior. This external orifice is now known as the urethral sulcus. It is at this point in fetal development that the presence or absence of testicular hormones impact on further development.

Male External Genital Development

In the presence of normal fetal testicular development and function, the distal urogenital sinus gives rise to the prostatic urethra below the verumontanum and also forms the membranous urethra (see Fig. 1.22). Furthermore, the genital tubercle gradually elongates into a cylindrical phallus to form the penis so that by the third month the bulbar and male penile urethra are formed by fusion of the urogenital folds. These urogenital folds fuse in the midline from behind forward until the entire sulcus to the glans penis is completely closed. The glandular urethra is then formed by canalization of the urethra plate in the glans penis.

The fused edges of these urogenital folds constitute the median raphe and failure of this closure to occur at varying stages of development leads to the varying degrees of hypospadias. The lateral buttresses form the body of the penis and labio scrotal swellings form the scrotum.

Remember that this entire sequence of changes in the male phenotype is directly related to the influence of testosterone on these androgen dependent target areas and must occur and must be completed by the 12th week of male fetal development.

Female External Genital Development

In the female that is in the absence of testicular hormones, the genital tubercle remains rather small and becomes the clitoris (see Fig. 1.23). The urethral sulcus remains short, never extends onto the glans penis as in the male and opens as the vestibule with the urogenital folds becoming the labia minora. The lateral buttresses form the body of the clitoris and the scrotal swellings form the labia majora.

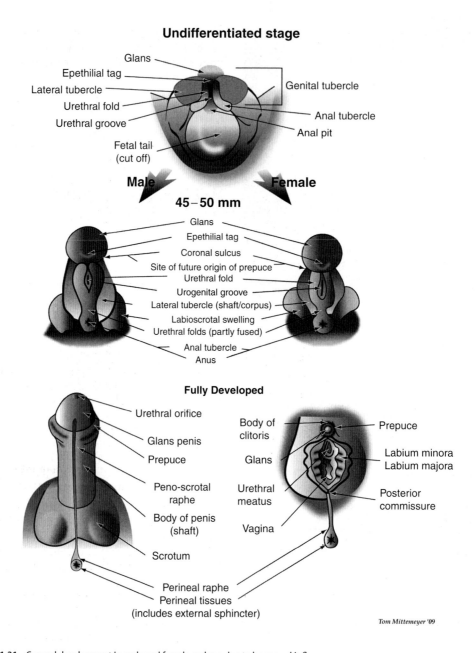

Figure 1.21. General development in male and female embryo due to hormonal influence.

Anomalies of the External Genitalia

Anomalies of the external genitalia are most commonly seen with pseudohermaphrodism. These anomalies are generally related to hormonal aberrations during pregnancy. Although absence or duplication of the penis or clitoris can occur, this anomaly is extremely rare. More commonly, the penis may remain rudimentary or the clitoris may be hypertrophic. Failure or incomplete fusion of the urogenital folds in the male fetus will result in the various degrees of hypospadias. Congenital urethral diverticula are similarly related to abnormal fusion of these folds.

Figure 1.22. Genital tubercle development in the male.

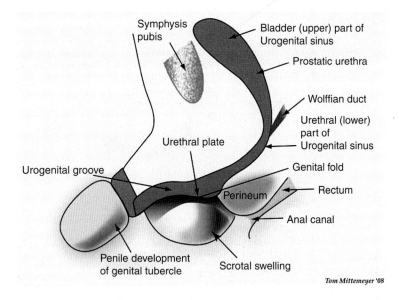

Figure 1.23. Genital tubercle development in the female.

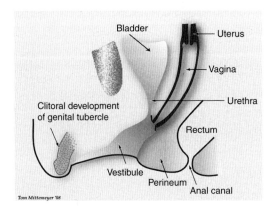

Summary of Genital Development

In summation, sexual differentiation is bipotential with the gonads and the external genitalia developing from common primordia and the ductal structures arising from separate primordia with only one system developing based on the presence or absence of a functioning testis (presence of testosterone and MIF).

Femaleness does not require gonadal influence and the bipotential fetus will develop into a female unless normal testicular influence is present.

Testes must thus be present for:

- Male genital duct development
- Müllerian ductal structure suppression
- Male external genital differentiation

External genital differentiation of the fetus commences during the eighth week of fetal life and is testosterone- and target area- dependent.

The glans of the genital tubercle gives rise to the clitoris in the female and the glans penis in the male.

The lateral buttresses form the body of the penis or clitoris.

The urogenital folds give rise to the labia minora in the female and the median raphe in the male.

The labioscrotal swellings give rise to the labia majora in the female and the scrotum in the male.

Acknowledgment We would like to acknowledge the wonderful illustrations provided by Tom Mittemeyer. The illustrations provided give a visual, graphic picture and they fully illustrate the textual content.

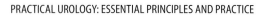
References

1. Netter FH. *CIBA Collection of Medical Illustrations,* The Reproductive System, vol 2. Summit, NJ: Ciba Pharmaceutical Company; 1954

2. Netter FH. *CIBA Collection of Medical Illustrations,* Kidneys, Ureters, and Urinary Bladder, vol 6. Summit, NJ: Ciba Pharmaceutical Company; 1973

3. Patten BM. *Human Embryology.* 3rd ed. New York: The Blakiston Division, McGraw-Hill Book Company; 1968

4. Sadler TW. *Langman's Medical Embryology.* Baltimore: Williams & Wilkins; 1999

5. Schoenwolf GC, Francis-West PH, Brauer PR, Bleyl SB. *Larsen's Human Embryology.* 4th ed. London: Elsevier Health Sciences; 2008

2

Gross and Laparoscopic Anatomy of the Upper Urinary Tract and Retroperitoneum

John N. Kabalin

Overview

The upper urinary tract is contained within the retroperitoneum. The retroperitoneal space is bound by the diaphragm superiorly; posteriorly and laterally by the musculature of the body wall; anteriorly, by the peritoneal envelope; and inferiorly, it is contiguous with the pelvis. The kidneys and ureters lie within the retroperitoneum together with the adrenal glands, as well as significant vascular, lymphatic, and neural structures (see Fig. 2.1). The anterior retroperitoneum also contains the duodenum, pancreas, and portions of the ascending and descending colon, all in close proximity to the upper urinary tract.

The Kidneys

The kidneys are paired, reddish-brown, solid organs that lie deep in the posterior retroperitoneum, on either side of the spine and the great vessels — aorta and inferior vena cava(see Fig. 2.2). An individual normal kidney weighs approximately 150 g in an adult man, approximately 135 g in an adult woman. The normal kidney is 10–12 cm in vertical length, 5–7 cm in transverse width, and approximately 3 cm in anteroposterior thickness. The right kidney tends to be shorter in vertical dimension and sometimes wider than the typically longer, more narrow left kidney. This discrepancy is attributed to the effect of the hepatic mass on the right side, which also tends to push the right kidney to a slightly lower position in the right retroperitoneum, compared to the left kidney on the opposite side.

The kidneys are the organs of urinary excretion, playing a central role in fluid, electrolyte, and acid-base balance; they also have important endocrine functions, including roles in vitamin D metabolism and production of renin and erythropoietin. The kidneys are highly vascular organs, receiving one fifth of the total cardiac output via the renal arteries, which represent major lateral branches from the upper abdominal aorta (see Figs. 2.2 and 2.3).

The substance of each kidney, or renal parenchyma, is friable, but contained by a relatively tough fibroelastic renal capsule. This capsule is capable of holding sutures for renal reconstructive surgery. This capsule can be surgically stripped away from the underlying parenchyma, or elevated by subcapsular hematoma. The renal cortex forms the outer layer of the renal parenchyma, surrounding the central tissue of the renal medulla. The renal medulla does not represent a contiguous layer, but rather consists of multiple conical segments, known as the renal pyramids. The rounded apex of each pyramid is the renal papilla, and points centrally into the renal sinus, where it is cupped by an individual minor calyx of the renal collecting system. The base of each medullary pyramid roughly parallels the external contour of the kidney. The renal cortex extends centrally between individual

C.R. Chapple and W.D. Steers (eds.), *Practical Urology: Essential Principles and Practice*, DOI: 10.1007/978-1-84882-034-0_2, © Springer-Verlag London Limited 2011

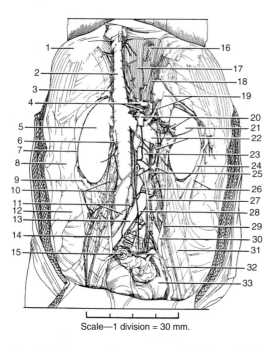

Scale—1 division = 30 mm.

Figure 2.1. The retroperitoneum exposed, with Gerota's fascia removed. *1*, Diaphragm. *2*, Inferior vena cava. *3*, Right adrenal gland. *4*, Celiac artery (upper pointer) and celiac autonomic plexus (lower pointer). *5*, Right kidney. *6*, Right renal vein. *7*, Gerota's fascia. *8*, Pararenal retroperitoneal fat. *9*, Perinephric fat. *10*, Right gonadal vein (*upper pointer*) and right gonadal artery (*lower pointer*). *11*, Lumbar lymph nodes. *12*, Retroperitoneal fat. *13*, Right common iliac artery. *14*, Right ureter. *15*, Sigmoid colon. *16*, Esophagus. *17*, Right crus of diaphragm. *18*, Left inferior phrenic artery. *19*, Left adrenal gland (*upper pointer*) and left adrenal vein (*lower pointer*). *20*, Superior mesenteric artery (*upper pointer*) and left renal artery (*lower pointer*). *21*, Left kidney. *22*, Left renal vein (*upper pointer*) and left gonadal vein (*lower pointer*). *23*, Aorta. *24*, Perinephric fat. *25*, Aortic autonomic plexus. *26*, Gerota's fascia (*upper pointer*) and inferior mesenteric ganglion (*lower pointer*). *27*, Inferior mesenteric artery. *28*, Aortic bifurcation into common iliac arteries. *29*, Left gonadal artery and vein. *30*, Left ureter. *31*, Psoas muscle. *32*, Cut edge of peritoneum. *33*, Pelvic cavity (Reprinted with permission from Kabalin[1] copyright Elsevier 2002).

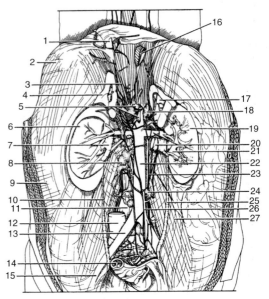

Figure 2.2. The retroperitoneum exposed, with the kidneys and adrenals sectioned and the inferior vena cava removed. *1*, Inferior vena cava. *2*, Diaphragm. *3*, Right inferior phrenic artery. *4*, Right adrenal gland. *5*, Celiac artery (*upper pointer*) and superior mesenteric artery (*lower pointer*). *6*, Right kidney. *7*, Right renal artery (*upper pointer*) and right renal vein (*lower pointer*). *8*, Lumbar lymph node. *9*, Transversus abdominis muscle covered with transversalis fascia. *10*, Right ureter. *11*, Anterior spinous ligament. *12*, Inferior vena cava. *13*, Right common iliac artery. *14*, Sigmoid colon. *15*, Right external iliac artery. *16*, Esophagus. *17*, Left adrenal gland. *18*, Celiac ganglion. *19*, Left kidney. *20*, Left renal artery (*upper pointer*) and left renal vein (*lower pointer*). *21*, Left renal pelvis. *22*, Aorta. *23*, Aortic autonomic nervous plexus. *24*, Inferior mesenteric ganglion. *25*, Left ureter. *26*, Inferior mesenteric artery. *27*, Psoas muscle (Reprinted with permission from Kabalin[1] copyright Elsevier 2002).

pyramids. These interpyramidal cortical extensions are known as the columns of Bertin, and through these pass the smaller branches of the renal arteries and veins as they enter and exit the renal parenchyma. On gross inspection, the renal cortical tissue is lighter in coloration than the medulla, and microscopically most remarkable for the presence of the renal glomeruli. Each glomerulus consists of a complex spherical arrangement of arterial capillaries surrounded by the glomerular (Bowman's) capsule. This is

the microscopic junction where the urinary filtrate leaves the arterial stream and enters the urinary flow. From the glomerulus, the urinary filtrate travels through a lengthy series of microscopic channels, beginning with the proximal convoluted tubule, to the so-called loop of Henle, to the distal convoluted tubule, and finally to the collecting tubules and collecting ducts, traversing the renal medulla to the renal papillae to eventually drain urine into the gross renal collecting system. These multiple tubular channels predominate in microscopic examination of the normal renal parenchyma (see Fig. 2.4).

The renal parenchyma surrounds a central space, the renal sinus, opening anteromedially, and through which the major arterial and venous

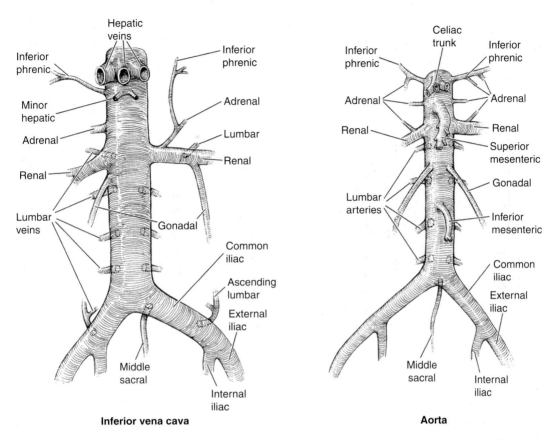

Figure 2.3. The inferior vena cava and abdominal aorta and their branches (Reprinted with permission from Kabalin[1] copyright Elsevier 2002).

vessels to the kidney enter and exit, together with lymphatic channels and nerves. The renal collecting system is largely contained within the renal sinus in most individuals, and exits the kidney through this medial hiatus. All of these structures are surrounded by varying amounts of renal sinus fat. This fat is contiguous with a layer of perinephric fat surrounding each kidney, varying greatly in thickness between individuals. This perinephric fat, the kidneys and ureters, the adrenal glands, and the gonadal blood vessels are all enclosed by an envelope of well-formed perinephric fascia, known as Gerota's fascia (see Fig. 2.5). Gerota's fascia represents an important anatomic barrier. This protective fascial layer typically acts to contain blood or urine or purulent collections emanating from the upper urinary tract, limiting their extension. However, inferiorly, Gerota's fascia opens into the pelvis where larger collections may eventually progress. Gerota's fascia also acts

to contain tumor extension from the kidney or adrenal gland, except in the most advanced stages. Outside of Gerota's fascia is another layer of retroperitoneal fat. Within these layers of retroperitoneal fat and fascia, the kidneys may be remarkably mobile, changing position freely with respiration and movement. This mobility is naturally protective against external trauma, allowing the kidneys to move away from a traumatic blow, but must also be considered in gaining surgical access to the kidneys.

Surgical Anatomy and Approaches to the Kidneys

Posteriorly and superiorly, the diaphragm, pleural reflection, and, especially with full inspiration, the lower lung, overlie the upper pole of each kidney (see Fig. 2.6). Thus, any direct surgical

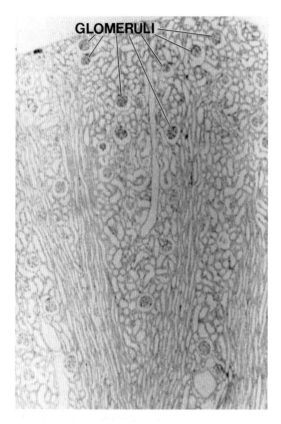

GLOMERULI

Figure 2.4. Microscopic section through the renal cortex, showing array of vessels and uriniferous tubules with interspersed glomeruli (Reprinted with permission from Kabalin[1] copyright Elsevier 2002).

approach to the upper kidney or associated adrenal gland, whether open or endoscopic, risks entering the pleural space. The 12th rib on either side crosses the kidney posteriorly at approximately the lower extent of the diaphragm, and, especially on the left side, the 11th rib may also cross the upper pole kidney. The medial portion of the lower two thirds of both kidneys lies against the psoas muscle. From medial to lateral, the quadratus lumborum muscle and then the aponeurosis of the transversus abdominis muscle or lumbodorsal fascia are encountered posterior to the kidney (see Fig. 2.6). The kidney can be approached directly through this posterior aponeurosis or lumbodorsal fascia without traversing muscle (Fig. 2.7).

In part as a result of the contour of the psoas muscle, the lower pole of both kidneys lies farther from the midline than the upper pole, such that the upper poles tilt inward and medially

(see Fig. 2.8). Similarly, the kidneys do not lie in a simple coronal plane, but the lower pole of each kidney is pushed slightly more anterior than the upper pole. In addition, the medial aspect of each kidney is rotated anteriorly at an angle of about 30° from the true coronal plane (see Fig. 2.8). This rotation tends to displace the posterior renal calyces directly posterior and anterior renal calyces more lateral.

Superior and medial and somewhat posterior to each kidney is an adrenal gland, contained within Gerota's fascia and immediately adjacent to each renal upper pole. On the left side, the adrenal may assume a much more medial and inferior position, often in close proximity to the renal blood vessels (see Figs. 2.2 and 2.6). The right kidney lies behind the liver, and is separated from the liver by peritoneum except for a small area of its upper pole, where Gerota's fascia may come into direct contact with the liver's retroperitoneal bare spot. The duodenum is anterior to the medial aspect of the right kidney, including the right renal pelvis and renal blood vessels. The hepatic flexure of the colon overlies the right lower pole kidney. The spleen, pancreas, stomach and proximal jejunum are all related to the anterior aspect of the left upper pole kidney. The splenic flexure of the colon overlies the left lower pole kidney. All of these structures may be placed at risk during renal surgery.

During open or laparoscopic approaches to the kidneys and upper urinary tract via an anterior, transperitoneal approach, the colon must be carefully reflected on either side to avoid injury. On the right side, the hepatocolic ligamentous attachments must be taken down carefully to avoid traction on the hepatic capsule, tearing, and bleeding as the hepatic flexure is manipulated. The duodenum must then also be carefully reflected ("Kocherized") medially to avoid injury and fully expose the medial aspect of the right kidney. The porta hepatis and common bile duct may be injured during this dissection. Hepatorenal ligamentous attachments, between Gerota's fascia overlying the right upper pole kidney and the liver capsule, must be avoided or divided to prevent traction injury and liver bleeding during either transperitoneal or retroperitoneal approaches to the kidney. On the left side, the splenocolic ligamentous attachments must be taken down carefully to avoid traction on the splenic capsule, tearing, and

GROSS AND LAPAROSCOPIC ANATOMY OF THE UPPER URINARY TRACT AND RETROPERITONEUM

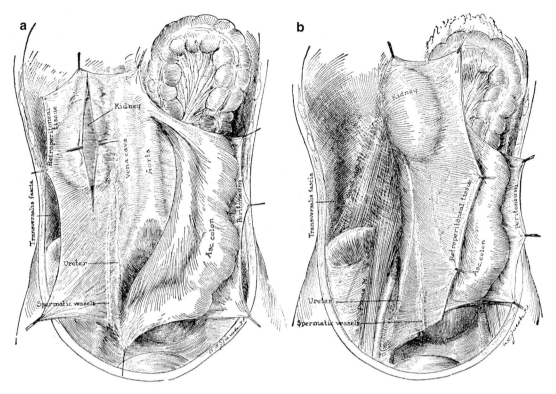

Figure 2.5. (**a**) Anterior view of Gerota's fascia on the right side, split over the right kidney, and showing the inferior extension enveloping the ureter and gonadal vessels. (**b**) Posterior view of Gerota's fascia on the right side, rotated medially with the contained kidney, ureter, and gonadal vessels (Reprinted with permission from Kabalin[1] copyright Elsevier 2002).

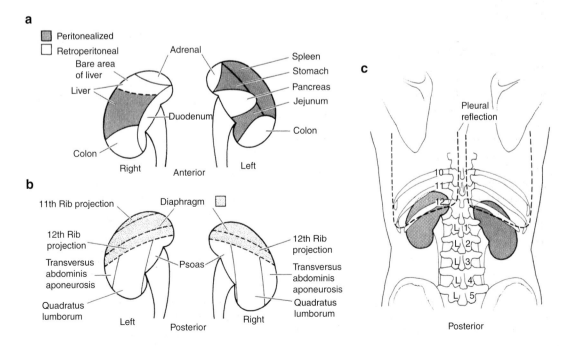

Figure 2.6. Anatomic relations of the kidneys. (**a**) Anterior relations to abdominal viscera. (**b**) Posterior relations to the body wall. (**c**) Posterior relations to the pleural reflections and skeleton (Reprinted with permission from Kabalin[1] copyright Elsevier 2002).

Figure 2.7. Transverse section through the (*right*) kidney and posterior abdominal wall, showing the lumbodorsal fascia incised (Reprinted with permission from Kabalin[1] copyright Elsevier 2002).

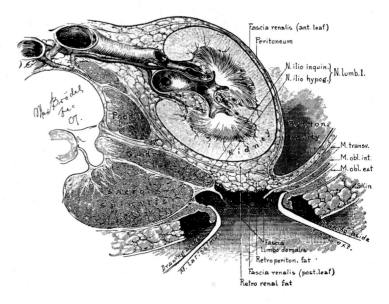

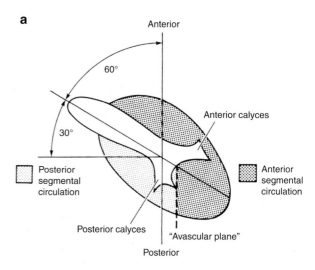

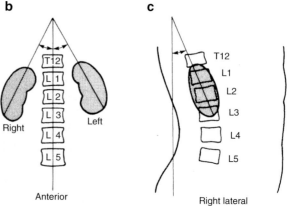

Figure 2.8. Rotational axes of the kidneys. (a) Transverse view showing approximate 30° anterior rotation of the (*left*) kidney from the coronal plane, relative positions of the anterior and posterior rows of calyces, and location of the relatively avascular plane between the anterior and posterior renal segmental circulation. (b) Coronal view showing the inward tilt of the upper poles of the kidneys. (c) Sagittal view showing anterior displacement of the lower pole of the (*right*) kidney (Reprinted with permission from Kabalin[1] copyright Elsevier 2002).

bleeding as the splenic flexure of the colon is manipulated. There are also splenorenal ligamentous attachments between the spleen and Gerota's fascia over the left upper pole kidney, which must be avoided or divided to prevent splenic injury during any left renal operation. The tail of the pancreas lies directly over the left upper pole kidney, and must be manipulated and reflected gently to avoid harm.

The Renal Vasculature

A thorough understanding of the renal vascular anatomy is essential to any surgical approach to the kidneys. The renal arteries and veins typically branch from the aorta and inferior vena cava, respectively, at the level of the second lumbar vertebral body, below the takeoff of the superior mesenteric artery (see Fig. 2.3). The right renal artery typically leaves the aorta at a slightly higher level than the left renal artery, and then must course with a slightly downward trajectory to reach the right kidney, which usually lies lower in the right retroperitoneum than the contralateral left kidney. The right renal artery passes posterior to the inferior vena cava and is considerably longer than the left renal artery. In rare cases, the right renal artery has been observed to cross anterior to the inferior

vena cava. The relatively short left renal artery tends to lie in a horizontal plane or even course slightly superiorly to reach the left kidney. Both renal arteries course somewhat posteriorly from the aorta due to the natural rotation of the kidneys (see Figs. 2.7 and 2.8). The main renal arteries bilaterally typically provide small arterial branches to the renal pelvis and proximal ureter, adrenal gland, renal capsule, and perinephric fat.

As they approach the renal sinus, the main renal arteries divide into four or more segmental renal arteries, with five branches most commonly described (see Fig. 2.9). The first and most constant segmental division is a posterior branch which usually exits the main renal artery outside the renal sinus and proceeds posterior to the renal pelvis to eventually supply a large posterior segment of the renal parenchyma. Four anterior segmental renal arterial branches can be described in most kidneys, proceeding from superior to inferior: the apical, upper, middle, and lower anterior segmental arteries, respectively, each supplying a corresponding segment of renal parenchyma (see Fig. 2.9). The lower anterior segmental artery may cross in close proximity to the ureteropelvic junction, where it may cause compression or, alternatively, be injured during surgery at this location. The posterior segmental artery may be injured during

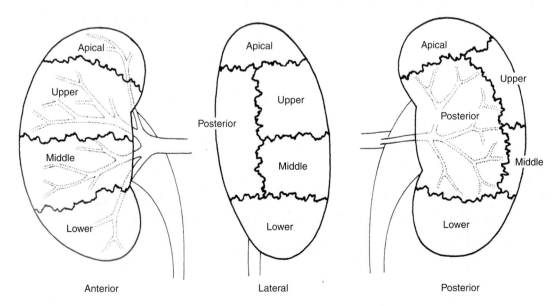

Figure 2.9. Segmental renal arterial circulation (right kidney shown) (Reprinted from Kabalin[1]).

posterior exposure of the renal pelvis. It is important to note that the main renal artery and each succeeding branch artery to the kidney is an end artery, without anastomosis or significant collateral circulation, and thus occlusion or interruption of any of these vessels will produce ischemia and then infarction of the corresponding renal parenchyma which it supplies. This must be taken into account in planning any surgical incision through the renal parenchyma (see Figs. 2.8 and 2.9).

The segmental renal arteries course through the renal sinus and then branch further into lobar arteries, which divide again into interlobar arteries, which then enter the renal parenchyma through the columns of Bertin (see Fig. 2.10). These still large arterial branches often lie in close association with the infundibula of the minor calyces, and may be injured during surgical approaches to the peripheral renal collecting system.[2, 3] The interlobar arteries branch into arcuate arteries at the peripheral bases of the renal medullary pyramids. The arcuate arteries course along the corticomedullary junction, parallel to the renal contour. The arcuate arteries produce multiple radial arterial branches, the interlobular arteries, which extend through the renal cortex, each emitting multiple side branches, which are the afferent arterioles to the glomeruli. From the glomerular capillary network, blood leaves via efferent arterioles, forming additional capillary networks in the renal cortex, or descending into the renal medulla as long straight vascular loops called vasa recta (see Fig. 2.10).

These postglomerular capillary vessels eventually drain into interlobular veins, and then into arcuate, interlobar, lobar, and segmental renal veins, paralleling the arterial anatomy. Typically, three or more large venous segmental trunks will finally coalesce to form the main renal vein. This coalescence usually occurs within the renal sinus, but may extend outside the kidney. Unlike the renal arteries, none of which communicate, the renal veins anastomose freely, especially at the level of the arcuate veins, and may form venous collars around the infundibula of minor calyces. In addition, the interlobular veins communicate via a subcapsular venous plexus of stellate veins with veins in the perinephric fat (see Fig. 2.11). Because of these venous communications, interruption of the main renal vein, especially if this occurs slowly over time (as in the case of growing tumor thrombus), may not result in loss of the kidney, whereas renal artery occlusion will inevitably lead to infarction.

The main renal veins are large caliber vessels, lying anterior to their respective renal arteries. The right renal vein is short and empties directly into the right lateral aspect of the inferior vena cava (see Figs. 2.1 and 2.3). The left renal vein is much longer and courses anterior to the aorta, inferior to the superior mesenteric artery, to empty into the left lateral aspect of the inferior vena cava (see Figs. 2.1 and 2.3). Lateral to the aorta, the left renal vein typically receives the left adrenal vein superiorly, the left gonadal vein along its inferior border, and often a lumbar vein posteriorly. These branches must be accounted for during left kidney operations.

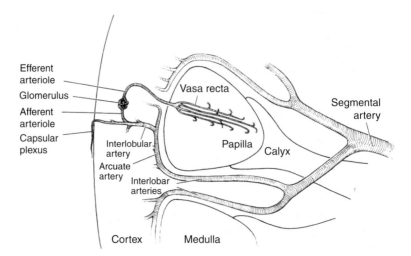

Figure 2.10. Intrarenal arterial anatomy (Reprinted with permission from Kabalin[1] copyright Elsevier 2002).

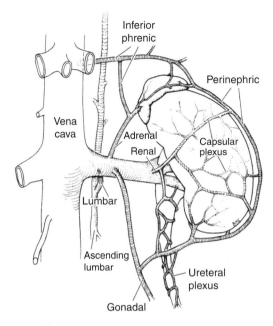

Figure 2.11. Venous drainage of the left kidney, showing extensive venous collateral circulation (Reprinted with permission from Kabalin[1], copyright Elsevier 2002).

Although both main renal veins generally lie directly anterior to their associated main renal arteries, this relationship may vary, and significant separation may occur, especially as one moves more medially away from the renal sinus. While most commonly a single main renal artery and a single main renal vein supplying each kidney are observed, anatomic variations are common, occurring in 25–40% of kidneys. The most common variation is the presence of one or more supernumerary renal arteries, with up to five arteries to a single kidney described. These supernumerary arteries typically arise from the aorta, but may in unusual instances derive from the celiac, superior mesenteric, or iliac arteries. A supernumerary renal artery may enter through the renal sinus, or directly into the parenchyma of the upper or lower pole kidney. Multiple renal veins are a more unusual finding, with two right renal veins draining from the right renal hilum directly into the inferior vena cava the most common venous aberration. On the left side, the main renal vein may divide, sending one limb anterior and one limb posterior to the aorta, and in rare instances only the venous limb posterior to the aorta may be present.

The Renal Collecting System

Each renal medullary papilla extending into the renal sinus is cupped by a corresponding minor calyx of the renal collecting system. The number of papillae and minor calyces is highly variable, but seven to nine are commonly present. There are typically two longitudinal rows of papillae and calyces, roughly perpendicular to one another, extending anteriorly and posteriorly (see Fig. 2.8). Reaching centrally from the papillae, the minor calyces narrow, creating a neck or infundibulum, before joining with other minor calyces to form usually two or three major calyces, which in most cases then coalesce to form a single renal pelvis exiting the renal sinus (see Fig. 2.12).[2] The renal pelvis lies posterior to the main renal vein and artery, respectively. The renal pelvis may be small and completely contained within the renal sinus, or may be quite voluminous and almost entirely extrarenal. The renal pelvis eventually narrows to join with the ureter at the ureteropelvic junction. The entire renal collecting system is one continuous structure from calyces to ureter, and the named anatomic segments, while useful for description, are somewhat artificial. The actual renal collecting system anatomy shows considerable variation between individuals, likened to fingerprints, and these anatomic descriptors may be more or less

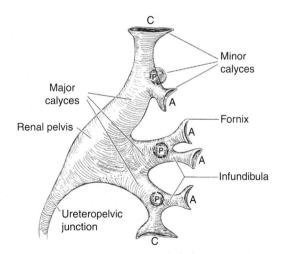

Figure 2.12. Renal collecting system (left kidney shown) (Reprinted with permission from Kabalin[1] copyright Elsevier 2002).

difficult to apply in some cases. Similarly, because of such variation, exact anatomic definitions of pathology versus normal can prove difficult, and often require functional studies to definitively characterize.

Microscopically, the renal collecting system, and subsequently the ureter, consists of layers of smooth muscle which actively propel the urine downward toward the bladder. Externally, these muscular structures are surrounded by a thin layer of adventitial connective tissue which contains blood and lymphatic vessels. Internally, there is a thin connective tissue lamina propria, and then a transitional cell epithelium which lines the collecting system and ureter and is identical to and contiguous with the transitional cell epithelium of the urinary bladder.

The Ureters

Each ureter is the tubular extension of the ipsilateral renal collecting system, coursing downward and medially to connect the kidney to the bladder, providing a pathway for the urinary effluent. The ureter is generally 22–30 cm in total length in the adult, varying with body size. Posteriorly, the ureter is related to the psoas muscle throughout its retroperitoneal course (see Fig. 2.2), crossing the iliac vessels to enter the pelvis at approximately the bifurcation of the common iliac into external and internal iliac arteries. Anteriorly, the right ureter is related to the right colon, cecum, and appendix. Anteriorly, the left ureter is related to the left colon and sigmoid. Either ureter may be injured during operations on these structures. In elevating and reflecting the right or left colon, the ureter may be inadvertently encountered. Within the female pelvis, the ureters are closely related to the uterine cervix and uterine arteries, and may be injured during hysterectomy. Pathologic processes involving the fallopian tubes or ovaries may also impinge upon the ureter at the pelvic brim.

The normal ureters are not of uniform caliber, with three distinct narrowings usually present: at the ureteropelvic junction, at the crossing of the iliac vessels, and distally at the ureterovesical junction. At the ureteropelvic junction, the renal pelvis tapers to become the proximal ureter. As the ureter traverses the iliac vessels, there is some extrinsic compression and also angulation anteriorly, then posteriorly again as the ureter crosses into the pelvis. The most physiologically significant narrowing is at the ureterovesical junction, as the ureter enters the bladder. These three sites of actual or functional ureteral narrowing are clinically significant as common locations for calculi to impact during passage. In addition, the angulation of the ureter, first anteriorly as it passes over the iliac vessels, then posteromedially again as it enters the pelvis, may restrict passage of rigid endoscopes. Appreciation of this normal angulation and the three dimensional course of the ureter is crucial for safe and successful ureteral endoscopy.

The ureters are often arbitrarily divided into segments for purposes of surgical or radiographic description. The abdominal ureter extends from the renal pelvis to the iliac vessels, and the pelvic ureter extends from the iliac vessels to the bladder. The ureter may also be divided into upper, middle, and distal or lower segments, usually for radiographic description. The upper ureter extends from the renal pelvis to the upper border of the sacrum. The middle ureter extends to the lower border of the sacrum, roughly corresponding to the iliac vessels. The distal ureter extends from the lower border of the sacrum to the bladder.

The ureters receive their blood supply from multiple small feeding arterial branches along their course. In the retroperitoneum, the ureters may receive branches from the renal artery, gonadal artery, abdominal aorta, and common iliac artery (see Fig. 2.3). In the pelvis, arterial branches may extend from the internal iliac artery and its branches, including the vesical, uterine, middle rectal, and vaginal arteries. Arterial branches to the upper ureters, above the common iliac vessels, approach from a medial direction. Conversely, within the pelvis, arterial branches approach the distal ureters from a lateral direction. After reaching the ureter, the arteries join a relatively extensive complex of adventitial vessels which anastomose and communicate along the length of each ureter. These longitudinal ureteral arterial communications allow long segments of the ureter to be mobilized surgically, provided that the ureteral adventitia is not stripped away. The venous drainage of the ureter generally parallels the multifocal arterial supply.

Retroperitoneal Lymphatics

The retroperitoneum is rich in lymphatic structures. The lymphatic drainage of the lower extremities, perineum and external genitalia, and pelvic viscera including the lower urinary tract, must course through the retroperitoneum. The lymphatics from these large anatomic distributions eventually coalesce into the common iliac lymphatic vessels and nodes, thereafter forming ascending vertical lumbar lymphatic chains that follow the great vessels, the aorta and inferior vena cava, superiorly (see Fig. 2.1). The ascending lumbar lymphatics are closely applied to the great vessels, with multiple transverse communications between ascending lymphatic channels. It is notable that most of the lateral flow between the ascending lumbar lymphatic trunks moves from right to left. During their retroperitoneal course, these ascending lymphatic trunks are joined by the lymphatic drainage of the gastrointestinal tract, which follows the inferior mesenteric, superior mesenteric, and celiac arteries. Most, if not all, of these ascending lymphatics eventually coalesce to form the thoracic duct. In most cases, the site of this coalescence is marked by a localized dilation of the lymphatic chain which is called the cisterna chyli, usually located in a retrocrural position behind the aorta and anterior to the first or second vertebral body. It is of descriptive and practical use to distinguish three major lumbar nodal areas within the retroperitoneum: (1) the left para-aortic lymph nodes along the left lateral aspect of the aorta, (2) the right paracaval lymph nodes along the right lateral aspect of the inferior vena cava, and (3) the interaortocaval lymph nodes between the great vessels.

The retroperitoneal lymphatics are the secondary or extraregional nodal drainage for the prostate, bladder, and pelvic ureters; and represent the primary or regional nodal drainage for the abdominal ureters, kidneys, adrenal glands, and also the testes whose embryologic origins are from the upper retroperitoneum. The left testis drains primarily to the left para-aortic nodes, with significant drainage to the interaortocaval nodes, but essentially no drainage to right paracaval nodes. The right testis drains primarily to the interaortocaval nodes, with significant drainage to the right paracaval nodes, and also some early nodal metastases found in the left para-aortic nodes. The kidneys have abundant lymphatic drainage, with usually several large lymphatic trunks traversing the renal sinus together with the renal blood vessels, joined by lymphatics from the renal pelvis and proximal ureter. From the left kidney, these lymphatic channels drain primarily into the left lateral para-aortic lymph nodes. From the right kidney these lymphatic channels drain primarily into both interaortocaval and right paracaval lymph nodes. Occasionally, some lymphatics from the right kidney may drain directly into left lateral para-aortic lymph nodes. The lymphatic drainage of the ureters generally parallels their arterial supply. The left para-aortic lymph nodes are the primary site of lymphatic drainage from the abdominal portion of the left ureter. The abdominal portion of the right ureter drains primarily to right paracaval and interaortocaval lymph nodes.

Retroperitoneal Nerves

The paired thoracolumbar symphathetic trunks arise within the chest and course vertically downward along the anterolateral aspect of the spinal column through the retroperitoneum, lying within the groove between the medial aspect of the psoas muscle and the spine bilaterally. The lumbar sympathetic trunks contain variable numbers of ganglia. Sympathetic nerve fibers supplying the abdominal viscera exit the lumbar sympathetic trunks and extend anteriorly over the aorta, forming autonomic nervous plexuses associated with the major branches of the abdominal aorta (see Figs. 2.1 and 2.2). Additional parasympathetic input to these plexuses derives from branches of the vagus nerves. The first and largest of the autonomic nervous plexuses in the abdomen is the celiac plexus on the anterior aorta surrounding the celiac artery. Through this celiac plexus passes most or all of the autonomic innervation to the adrenal, kidney, renal pelvis, and ureter. At the lower extent of the abdominal aorta, the superior hypogastric plexus lies on the aorta anterior to its bifurcation, below the takeoff of the inferior mesenteric artery, and extends inferiorly onto the anterior surface of the fifth lumbar vertebra. Much of the sympathetic input to the pelvic urinary organs and genital tract passes through this plexus. Surgical disruption of the hypogastric plexuses

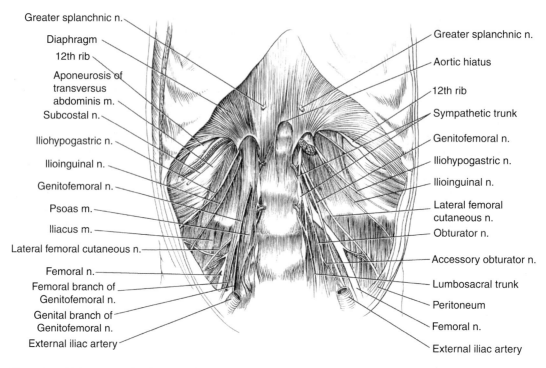

Greater splanchnic n.
Diaphragm
12th rib
Aponeurosis of transversus abdominis m.
Subcostal n.
Iliohypogastric n.
Ilioinguinal n.
Genitofemoral n.
Psoas m.
Iliacus m.
Lateral femoral cutaneous n.
Femoral n.
Femoral branch of Genitofemoral n.
Genital branch of Genitofemoral n.
External iliac artery

Greater splanchnic n.
Aortic hiatus
12th rib
Sympathetic trunk
Genitofemoral n.
Iliohypogastric n.
Ilioinguinal n.
Lateral femoral cutaneous n.
Obturator n.
Accessory obturator n.
Lumbosacral trunk
Peritoneum
Femoral n.
External iliac artery

Figure 2.13. Major nerves within the retroperitoneum (Reprinted with permission from Kabalin[1] copyright Elsevier 2002).

can cause loss of seminal vesicle emission and/ or failure of bladder neck closure that results in retrograde ejaculation.

The somatic sensory and motor innervation to the lower abdomen and lower extremities also traverses the deep retroperitoneum. The lumbosacral plexus is formed from branches of all lumbar and sacral spinal nerves. Nerves from this plexus extend through the psoas muscle (Fig. 2.13). The subcostal nerve is the anterior extension of the 12th thoracic nerve and extends forward, laterally and then anteriorly, from beneath the 12th rib. The iliohypogastric and ilioinguinal nerves originate together from the first lumbar spinal nerve. Together, these three somatic nerves provide multiple motor branches to the abdominal wall musculature, and also cutaneous sensory branches to the lower abdomen and genitalia. The lateral femoral cutaneous nerve and the genitofemoral nerve arise from the first through third lumbar spinal nerves. They provide cutaneous sensory branches to the upper thigh and genitalia. The genital branch of the genitofemoral nerve supplies motor innervation to the cremaster and dartos

muscles in the scrotum. The genitofemoral nerve lies directly on top of the psoas muscle along its retroperitoneal course and can be readily identified in this position. The femoral nerve is a much larger structure, arising from the second through fourth lumbar spinal nerves, and is largely hidden by the body of the psoas muscle in the deep retroperitoneum before exiting the abdomen lateral to the femoral artery in the groin. This important nerve supplies motor innervation of the psoas and iliacus muscles and the large muscle groups of the anterior thigh, as well as sensory branches to anteromedial portions of the lower extremity. The femoral nerve may be compressed by retractor blades placed inferolaterally against the inguinal ligament during operations on the lower abdomen and pelvis, which can produce a significant motor palsy that prevents active extension of the knee. The obturator nerve, an important lateral pelvic landmark, actually arises in the retroperitoneum from the third and fourth lumbar spinal nerves, and eventually provides motor innervation to the adductor muscles of the medial thigh.

The Adrenal Glands

Although not strictly part of the urinary tract, the adrenal glands are intimately related anatomically to the kidneys and much adrenal surgery is performed by urologists. The adrenal glands are paired, yellow-orange, solid endocrine organs that lie within Gerota's fascia superomedial to the kidneys (see Fig. 2.2). The normal adult adrenal gland weighs approximately 5 g and measures 3–5 cm in greatest dimension. The right adrenal gland assumes a pyramidal shape and rests more superior to the upper pole kidney. The left adrenal gland has a more crescentic shape and rests more medial to the upper pole of the left kidney, sometimes directly atop the left renal vein. The right adrenal thus tends to lie more superiorly in the retroperitoneum than the left adrenal, even though the right kidney, in general, lies somewhat more inferiorly than the left kidney. The right adrenal gland may also extend posterior to the inferior vena cava, making surgical access from any anterior approach more difficult.

Each adrenal is a composite of two separate and functionally distinct glandular elements: the peripheral cortex and central medulla. The medulla consists of chromaffin cells derived from the neural crest and is intimately related to the sympathetic nervous system. The adrenal medulla produces neuroactive catecholamines which are released directly into the blood stream via an extensive venous drainage system. The adrenal cortex is mesodermally derived and encases the medulla. Three separate cortical layers can be identified. Outermost is the zona glomerulosa, which produces aldosterone. Next is the zona fasciculata, which produces glucocorticoids. The innermost layer is the zona reticularis, which produces sex steroids. The substance of the adrenal glands is inherently quite delicate and friable, and is enclosed by a collagenous capsule.

The adrenal glands are supplied by multiple small arterial branches which originate from three major arterial sources: (1) superior branches from the inferior phrenic artery on the diaphragm, (2) medial branches directly from the aorta, and (3) inferior branches from the ipsilateral renal artery. In contrast to these multiple small arterial branches, typically a single large adrenal vein drains from each gland along its anteromedial aspect. The right adrenal vein is very short and enters the inferior vena cava on its posterolateral aspect. The left adrenal vein is more elongated and often joined by the left inferior phrenic vein before entering the superior aspect of the main left renal vein. The adrenal lymphatics exit the glands along the course of the venous drainage and empty into para-aortic lymph nodes. The adrenal medulla receives greater autonomic innervation than any other organ in the body. Multiple sympathetic fibers enter each adrenal along the course of the adrenal vein to synapse with chromaffin cells in the medulla.

References

1. Kabalin JN. Surgical anatomy of the retroperitoneum, kidneys, and ureters. In: Walsh PC, Retik AB, Vaughan ED Jr, Wein AJ, eds. *Campbell's Urology*. 8th ed. Philadelphia, PA: Saunders; 2002:3-40
2. Resnick MI, Parker MD. *Surgical Anatomy of the Kidney*. Mount Kisco, NY: Futura; 1982
3. Sampaio FJB. Renal anatomy: endourologic considerations. *Urol Clin North Am*. 2000;27:585-607

3

Gross and Laparoscopic Anatomy of the Lower Urinary Tract and Pelvis

Bastian Amend and Arnulf Stenzl

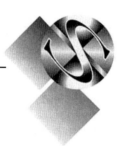

Introduction

An overview of the gross and laparoscopic anatomy of the lower urinary tract should summarize both long-standing anatomic knowledge and current scientific findings. In few fields has the anatomic understanding grown as much as in urology, especially concerning the anatomy of the lower urinary tract. Whereas the gross anatomy is already well known, now research is increasingly contributing to our understanding of the microscopic level. This concerns especially the detailed anatomy and topography of the sphincter mechanism of the urinary bladder, the routing and function of the neural structures in the pelvis and, for example, the anatomic structure of the pelvic floor. The transmission of these new findings in combination with traditional anatomic knowledge into urological practice, including the growing field of laparoscopic surgery, is essential to maintain and improve the success of treatments for our patients. The following chapter gives a clear, detailed and informative summary of the anatomy of the lower urinary tract, especially considering the requirements of laparoscopic and endoscopic surgery.

The History of the Study of the Urological Anatomy

The historiography of urology goes back to 1000 BC in Egypt. The first description of a bladder catheter made of bronze dates to this time, and bladder stone surgery also seems to have been practiced. The prostate was first described by Herophilus of Chalcedon in 300 BC. Human cadaver sections enabled this first glimpse.

After the widespread rejection of anatomical studies up to the Middle Ages, detailed descriptions of human anatomy began to emerge again with the work of Leonardo da Vinci (1452–1519), Andreas Vesalius (1514–1564) from Brussels and their successor Eustachi (1500–1574). The anatomy of the urogenital tract was mainly revealed by Étienne de la Rivière of Paris with the description of the seminal vesicles, Marcellus Malpighi (1628–1694) with the exploration of renal functioning and Lorenzo Bellini (1643–1704) with the identification of the renal tubuli. The progress of microscopic examinations further advanced the basic anatomical knowledge. In 1684, Mery described the existence of the bulbourethral glands, which was later attributed to Cowper.

The founder of the study of the pathology of the urogenital tract was Giovanni Battista Morgagni (1682–1771) with his work "De sedibus et causis morborum". Giovanni Battista Morgagni is considered the first to describe prostatic hyperplasia.

One of the milestones in urology – urological endoscopy – goes back to Phillip Bozzini of Frankfurt who invented the first endoscope using candlelight in 1806. This made possible the exploration of the internal anatomical details of a living individual.[1]

C.R. Chapple and W.D. Steers (eds.), *Practical Urology: Essential Principles and Practice*, DOI: 10.1007/978-1-84882-034-0_3, © Springer-Verlag London Limited 2011

Topographic Anatomy of the Anterior Abdominal Wall

The increasing significance of laparoscopic procedures, especially for intrapelvic and prostate surgery, necessitates a detailed understanding of the topographic anatomy of the anterior abdominal wall. Figure 3.1 illustrates the different structures in addition to a laparoscopic view of the male pelvis (Fig. 3.2) at the beginning of robotic-assisted radical prostatectomy.

Five tissue folds subdivide the anterior abdominal wall. The former embryonic urachus forms the median umbilical ligament between the urinary bladder and the umbilicus. On both sides lateral to the median umbilical ligament, the remnants of the fetal umbilical arteries shape the medial umbilical ligaments/folds – the space in between is called the supravesical fossa. During cystectomy, the medial umbilical ligaments are the main structures to identify and control the superior vesical pedicle including the superior vesical artery. The inferior epigastric vessels underlie the lateral umbilical ligaments/folds. These structures have important significance regarding hernia classification. Medial to the lateral umbilical fold, the medial inguinal fossa represents the passage of direct inguinal hernias. The lateral inguinal fossa corresponds to the deep inguinal ring – the entry to the inguinal canal. An indirect inguinal hernia could accompany the components of the spermatic cord through the inguinal canal. The external iliac vessels and the iliopsoas muscle leave the pelvis below the inguinal ligament, which connects the anterior superior iliac spine to the pubic tubercle. The lacunar ligament is located directly medial to the external iliac vein connecting the inguinal ligament to the superior pubic ramus and represents the caudal extent during lymphadenectomy for prostate or bladder cancer.[2]

Female Pelvis

A plain promontorium and wide-open iliac wings characterize the female pelvic bone. The peritoneal pelvic cavity harbors the urinary bladder, the ureters, the uterus, the vagina, the ovaries, the oviducts and the rectum. The uterus, in between the urinary bladder and the rectum, leads to varying peritoneal conditions, starting from the anterior abdominal wall. The parietal peritoneum covers approximately the upper half of the urinary bladder, the uterus, the adnexa and the anterior wall of the rectum. Thereby the parietal peritoneum forms two parts of the abdominal cavity: the rectouterine excavation (Douglas' fold) and the vesicouterine excavation. The peritoneal fold between the uterus/cervix and the pelvic wall is called the ligamentum latum or broad ligament, although these structures lack some of the typical features of a

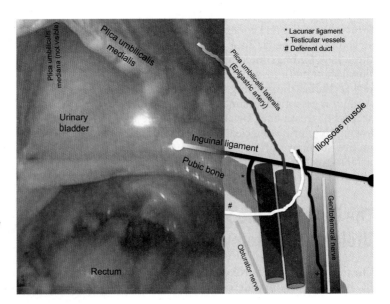

Figure 3.1. Topographic anatomy of the male pelvis. *Left*: laparoscopic view at the beginning of robotic-assisted laparoscopic prostatectomy. *Right*: drawing of the anatomical structures of the inguinal region in addition to the left intraoperative view.

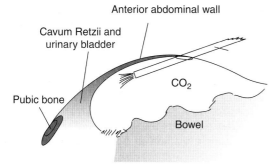

Figure 3.2. The drawing illustrates the laparoscopic line of sight during pelvic or prostate surgery.

ligament in the anatomical sense. The uterine artery, the uterine venous plexus and parts of the distal third of the ureters are included in the broad ligament. Ovaries and the Fallopian tubes are also joined to the broad ligament by a peritoneal duplication. The ovaries receive their blood supply through the suspensory ligament, and they are connected to the uterus by the ovarian ligament. At least, the round ligaments represent connections between the deep inguinal rings and the uterine horns.

The rectouterine folds mark the borders of the rectouterine pouch – they consist of fibrous tissue and smooth muscle fibers, and also include the inferior hypogastric plexus (Fig. 3.3).

The pelvic fascia with its parietal and visceral layer covers the borders of the subperitoneal space; the clinical synonym is "endopelvic fascia". The endopelvic fascia also forms the

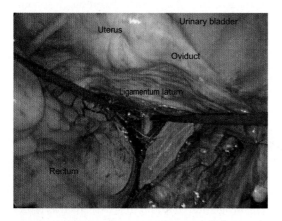

Figure 3.3. Laparoscopic view in the female pelvis. The right rectovaginal fold is marked in *lucent blue*.

superior layer of the fascia of the pelvic and urogenital diaphragm. The urinary bladder is attached to the pubic bone/symphysis pubis via the pubovesical ligaments (analogous to the puboprostatic ligaments in male humans, see also below) with lateral connections to the superior layer of the fascia of the pelvic diaphragm. Between the different subperitoneal organs, connective and fatty tissue fills the resulting spaces (presacral, prevesical paracervical, parametrial). The stability of the uterus and the cervix is guaranteed by the rectouterine (synonym, sacrouterine) ligament and the topography of the other pelvic organs. The cardinal ligaments (synonym, transverse cervical ligaments) on the base of the broad ligament, joining the cervix and the lateral pelvic wall, are not there at birth, but are shaped throughout a lifetime by the increasingly compact and strong connective tissue. They increasingly support the topographical position of the cervix.[2-4]

Male Pelvis

In contrast to the female pelvis, in male humans the pelvic bone is narrower and marked by a more protruding promontorium, resulting in a heart-shaped pelvic entry. The pelvis accommodates the urinary bladder, the ureters, the prostate, the seminal vesicles, the deferent ducts and the rectum. The parietal peritoneum also covers the pelvic organs starting from the anterior abdominal wall to the anterior rectal wall. Between the urinary bladder and the rectum, the deepest point of the abdominal cavity forms the rectovesical excavation. On both sides the rectovesical fold confines the excavation and includes the inferior hypogastric plexus. The deferent ducts shape the paravesical fossa by raising a peritoneal fold.

The subperitoneal space in front of and lateral to the urinary bladder is clinically called the cavum retzii. A look at the existing literature concerning the anatomical conditions of the subperitoneal fascias, especially the prostate-surrounding tissue and the formation of the so-called Denonvilliers' fascia, demonstrates an inconsistent presentation and nomenclature. The following explanations will outline the most usually published anatomical findings and interpretations. The pelvic fascia in males also consists of two parts: a parietal layer, which covers the lateral wall of the pelvis, and a visceral layer covering the pelvic organs. The tendinous arch represents the transition between the parietal and visceral part. Often the visceral layer is clinically indicated as the endopelvic fascia, especially with regard to radical prostatectomy and nerve-sparing procedures. Whether the prostate is actually separated by its own prostatic fascia is under discussion. The absence of the fascia in the apical region of the prostate and the formation of the so-called puboprostatic ligaments[5] by the endopelvic fascia suggest that the visceral layer of the pelvic fascia (= endopelvic fascia) and the fascia of the prostate correlate. The puboprostatic ligaments between the anterior fascia of the prostate and the pubic bone/symphysis pubis do not represent ligamentous structures in the proper sense. In fact the puboprostatic ligaments are characterized by an aggregation of the pelvic fascia. Possibly muscle fibers (smooth or striated) also contribute to the configuration of the so-called puboprostatic ligaments.

Similarly there is a lack of clarity regarding Denonvilliers' fascia. The anatomical nomenclature utilizes the description rectoprostatic fascia or septum. It represents a membranous separation between the rectum and the prostate/urinary bladder. The fascia emerges from two layers of a peritoneal cul-de-sac, ranging from the deepest point of the rectovesical excavation to the pelvic floor. There has been extensive discussion about the possibility of surgical separation of both layers during radical prostatectomy. Currently it is evident that microscopically the rectoprostatic fascia consists of two formerly peritoneal layers, which often cannot be divided bluntly. It is assumed that authors illustrating techniques of fascia separation are referencing the space between Denonvilliers' fascia and the rectal fascia propria (a part of the visceral layer of the pelvic fascia = endopelvic fascia). Periprostatic neural and vascular structures are focused on below.[2,3,5-10]

Pelvic Floor

Two fibromuscular layers are responsible for the closure of the inferior pelvic aperture: the pelvic diaphragm and the urogenital diaphragm. It has to be emphasized at this point that the term urogenital diaphragm is not part of the anatomic nomenclature. Particularly the presence of a deep transverse perineal muscle is under extensive discussion, as demonstrated below.

The pelvic diaphragm consists of the levator ani muscle and the coccygeus muscle (M. ischiococcygeus). The levator ani muscle in turn consists of the following structures, which are named according to their origins and insertions: the pubococcygeus muscle, iliococcygeus muscle and puborectalis muscle. A superior and inferior fascia covers the levator ani muscle, the superior layer being part of the parietal layer of the pelvic fascia as described above. The levator ani muscle forms an archway-shaped opening for the anus and urethra in males, and the anus, vagina and urethra in females. The innervations for the striated muscles derive principally from the sacral plexus (S3 and S4); some nerve fibers reach the puborectal muscle via the pudendal nerve located in the pudendal canal. Even though the contributions of the shape topography and the contraction of the pelvic diaphragm to anal continence seem to be proven, it is still unclear to what extent these anatomical structures also affect urinary continence. Recent publications have reported the muscular independence between the pelvic diaphragm and the striated external urethral sphincter, whereas an association by connective tissue forming a tendinous connection starting from the inferior part of the external urethral sphincter in females could be demonstrated. Especially because of these interactions, the authors suggest the necessity of an intact pelvic diaphragm for urinary continence.

Considering the urogenital diaphragm, the exact anatomical and histomorphological composition is still undefined. Almost all anatomical atlases report that the urogenital diaphragm consists of the deep transverse perineal muscle (less developed in females) with a superior and inferior urogenital fascia. Additionally, the superficial transverse perineal muscle inserting at the perineal body (= central tendon of the perineum), the striated external urethral sphincter and the surrounding connective tissue complete the traditional view of the urogenital diaphragm. Some authors report the existence of a deep transverse perineal muscle, but most recent studies could not verify this conclusion. The urogenital diaphragm is described as layers of connective tissue embedding the external urethral sphincter in conjunction with the perineal body, the structures of the inferior pubic bone and the superficial transverse perineal muscle. Whether these findings about the muscular structures of the urogenital diaphragm are possibly due to age-related fatty degeneration of muscular tissue is under discussion and remains unexplained. The main vascular and neural structures – the internal pudendal artery and the pudendal nerve – are located directly below the urogenital diaphragm. The bulbourethral glands (Cowper's glands) are located laterally to the membranous urethra at the level of the urogenital diaphragm. The urethral sphincter mechanism is described below.[2,11-17]

Urinary Bladder

The urinary bladder is a muscular, distensible organ for urine collection and controlled micturition. Macroscopically the urinary bladder is divided into the apex, corpus, fundus and collum. The average filling volume ranges between 300 and 500 cm^3. The mucosa is only loosely adherent to the subjacent muscular layers, except for the trigone, where a direct adhesion to the submucosal layers can be found. A fold raised between the obliquely passing ureters on both sides forming the ureteral orifices characterizes the trigone.

The urinary bladder wall is structured as followes: mucosa (transitional cells), submucosa, detrusor muscle (three layers), and surrounding adipose and connective tissue. The detrusor muscle is subdivided into an external and internal longitudinal muscle layer, as well as an interjacent circular layer. The bladder neck, including the trigone, consists of two muscular layers. A specialized circular smooth muscle could not be found. The longitudinal muscle fibers in conjunction with the extending longitudinal fibers of both ureters extend below the bladder neck and reach the muscular layers of the urethra. In male humans these structures reach the point of the seminal colliculus.

The blood supply of the urinary bladder generally derives from two main branches of each of the internal iliac arteries: the superior vesical artery and the inferior vesical artery – often named the superior and inferior vesical pedicle during surgery. The superior vesical artery descends from a common branch with the former umbilical artery, which is part of the medial umbilical ligament. The inferior vesical artery arises from a common branch of the middle rectal artery. Prostatic branches generally derive from the inferior vesical artery. Varying distinct venous plexuses on both sides of the vesical base secure the blood drainage of the urinary bladder. These venous vessels communicate extensively with the prostatic venous plexus in male and the vaginal venous plexus in female humans.

Organs of the pelvis, in contrast to other regions, present a widespread field of lymph node drainage. The urinary bladder drains its lymph fluid through external iliac lymph nodes, internal iliac lymph nodes, lymph nodes in the obturator fossa and common iliac lymph nodes (Fig. 3.4).

A complex neural system facilitates the correct functioning of the urinary bladder as a storage and drainage system. Interactions between independent reflex pathways and arbitrary actions are necessary for a precise process. Both the autonomous and the somatic nervous system contribute to carrying out the tasks of bladder filling and emptying.

Anatomic nerve fibers reach the urinary bladder (and adjacent organs) through the inferior hypogastric plexus (= pelvic plexus). The inferior hypogastric plexus thus comprises the parasympathetic and sympathetic nerve tracts. Anatomically the inferior hypogastric plexus derives from the singular superior hypogastric plexus, which reaches the pelvis proximally and

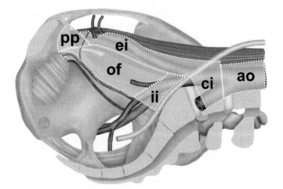

Figure 3.4. Areas of lymphadenectomy for pelvic surgery: post pubic (*pp*), external iliac (*ei*), obturator fossa (*of*), internal iliac (*ii*), common iliac (*ci*), aortal (*ao*). (Reprinted from Schilling et al.[18] with permission from Wiley-Blackwell).

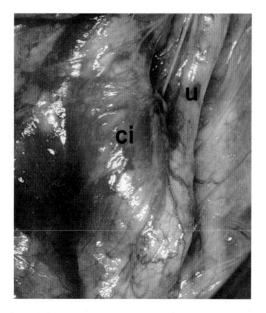

Figure 3.5. Nerve course of the sympathetic fibers deriving from the superior hypogastric plexus (ci: common iliac artery, u: ureter). (Reprinted from Schilling et al.[18] with permission from Wiley-Blackwell).

medial to the crossing of the distal ureter and the common iliac artery on both sides (Fig. 3.5). The plexus is part of the rectouterine or rectovesical fold beside the pouch of Douglas (Fig. 3.3). The plexus extends laterally to the rectum, the vagina (in females), the bladder neck and the seminal vesicles (in males) in a sagittal direction. The continuing course of nerve fibers along the prostate is described in the following chapter. An allocation of nerve fibers within the plexus to innervated targets seems to be possible. Roughly, the anterior part is responsible for urogenital innervations, and the posterior part serves the rectum.

The sympathetic fibers of the hypogastric plexus originate from the superior hypogastric plexus, which is fed by nerve fibers from two superior retroperitoneal sympathetic chains called the sacral splanchnic nerves. Sympathetic excitation generally results in inhibition of the detrusor muscle and stimulation of the smooth muscle sphincter cells, which leads to a filling of the urinary bladder. The parasympathetic fibers derive from the sacral spinal cord (S2–S5) and reach the inferior hypogastric plexus via pelvic splanchnic nerves exiting from the foramina of the sacral bone. Sensory afferent nerve fibers of

the urinary bladder (and most probably of the proximal urethra as well) run along the parasympathetic nerves. Contraction of the detrusor muscle is mediated through the parasympathetic nervous system. The pudendal nerve is part of the somatic nervous system and innervates the striated parts of the external urethral sphincter. The pudendal nerve courses in the pudendal canal at the bottom of the inferior pubic bone after the distribution of the lumbosacral plexus. The variation of an intrapelvic nerve branching off the pudendal nerve prior to entering the pudendal canal and running on the inside of the levator muscle has been described. Stimulation results in increased contraction of the external urethral sphincter and adjacent segments of the levator muscle. Complex interconnections of the different sections of the central nervous system, including Onuf's nucleus (located in the sacral part of the spinal cord), the periaqueductal gray, the pontine micturition center and the frontal lobe of the cerebrum, are involved in the process of filling and emptying. For example, it could be demonstrated that pelvic floor training for stress urinary incontinence not only influences the competence of the sphincteric mechanisms, but the training also results in restructuring of supraspinal central nervous system components.[2,3,18-22]

Prostate, Seminal Vesicles and Deferent Ducts

The prostate is often compared to a chestnut of about 20 g. With the base aligned to the urinary bladder and the apex proximate to the external urinary sphincter, the prostate incorporates the prostatic urethra with a length of about 3 cm.

McNeal defined the different zones of the prostate based on histopathological analysis: the peripheral zone, the central zone, the transitional zone and the anterior fibromuscular zone. This definition has to be separated from the macroscopic classification into lobes. The ejaculatory ducts are paired tubes formed on each side by fusion of the deferent duct and the duct of the seminal vesicle. The orifices of the ejaculatory ducts are located on the seminal colliculus (also called the verumontanum). Fifteen to thirty orifices of ducts of the prostate glands are located beside the seminal colliculus.

The seminal vesicles are located lateral to the deferent ducts. Dorsally and laterally fibers from the inferior hypogastric plexus engulf the vesicles. The space between Dennonvillier's fascia dorsally and the fascia covering the posterior wall of the bladder is called the spatium urovesicale (urovesical space). Branches of the inferior vesical artery, the middle rectal artery and the artery of the vas deferens usually reach the seminal vesicle at its tip.

The deferent duct is characterized by a dilation prior to the confluence with the duct of the seminal vesicle called the ampulla. The deferent duct is accompanied by one or two separate arteries (arteries of the vas deferens), which derive from the inferior vesical artery.

The inferior vesical and the middle rectal artery contribute to the blood supply of the prostate. The main vessels enter the prostate on both sides at the dorsolateral aspect close to the base of the prostate. Smaller vessels perforate the prostate capsule directly. Venous drainage moves from the surrounding prostatic venous plexus.

Accessory pudendal arteries can be found in about 25% of the patient population undergoing radical prostatectomy. An accessory pudendal artery is defined as a vessel starting above the level of the levator ani running down to the penile structures below the symphysis pubis and the pubic bone, respectively. Some authors subdivide the accessory arteries into lateral (alongside the anterolateral aspect of the prostate) and apical (inferior and lateral to the puboprostatic ligaments) accessory pudendal arteries. The extent of their contribution to the erectile function of the penis is still under investigation and discussion.

The puboprostatic complex includes the puboprostatic ligaments, the prostatic venous plexus and their correlation to the prostate and the external urethral sphincter. The puboprostatic ligaments formed by the endopelvic fascia, first described by Young, are described above. The prostatic venous plexus communicates extensively with the distinct venous plexus of the urinary bladder cranially and the superficial/deep dorsal veins of the penis. The proper name (Santorini's plexus) refers to their initial discovery by Giovanni Domenico Santorini in 1724. The venous plexus is imbedded in the fibrous structure of the so-called puboprostatic ligaments. The puboprostatic plexus directly covers the anterior elevated part of the external urethral sphincter (see also Chap. Sphincter Mechanisms).

The description of the anatomic affiliations of pelvic lymph nodes to the drainage field was originally based on lymphographic studies. Recent findings are the results of sentinel lymph node studies. The injection of ^{99m}Tc-labeled nanocolloid into the prostate facilitates the identification of sentinel lymph nodes either by surgery or by radiological imaging (Fig. 3.6). The lymph nodes of the obturator fossa, the external iliac lymph nodes, the internal and finally the common iliac lymph nodes are responsible for the drainage of the prostate gland (Figs. 3.4 and 3.7).

Although oncological aspects are still the main concern of every radical prostatectomy treating prostate cancer, quality of life aspects including erectile function as well as continence have become important. The existence of the endopelvic fascia equipollent to the visceral layer of the pelvic fascia has been outlined above. Most authors would agree that the neurovascular structures are located between the prostate surface with its fibromuscular capsule and the visceral layer of the pelvic fascia, which extends to Denonviellers' fascia at the dorsolateral aspect of the prostate (Fig. 3.8). Some studies describe a merger between these two layers. Whether nervous tissue can also be found in the fold between the visceral and the parietal layer of the pelvic fascia remains unclear. In 1985, Donker, Walsh et al. were the first to extensively describe the neurovascular bundle. The technique of nerve-sparing radical prostatectomy and cystectomy was adapted regarding these anatomical findings. Especially the course of these periprostatic nerves has resurfaced as a focus of academic interest. The entry of the inferior hypogastric plexus into the pelvis and its location lateral to the seminal vesicles, including the convergent fibers of the sacral splanchnic nerves (sympathetic) and pelvic splanchnic nerves (parasympathetic), has been referred to above. In contrast to a separate dorsolateral nerve bundle, several authors reinvestigated the anatomy and described different nerve dispersions. The periprostatic nerves proceed divergently especially in the midpart of the prostate; therefore, a varying amount of nerve tissue can be found also in the anterior and anterolateral aspect of the prostate in addition to the known accumulation in the dorsolateral course (Fig. 3.9). Characteristically, nerve fibers converge towards the apex located at the posterior and posterolateral side of the apex and the urethra, respectively. In addition, parts of the

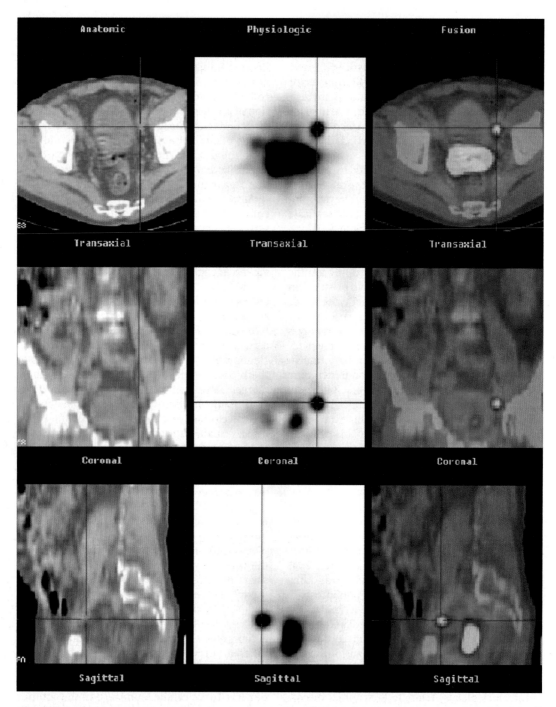

Figure 3.6. Radiological image of sentinel lymph nodes after injection of ^{99m}Tc-labeled nanocolloid into the prostate. *Left column*: CT scan images, *middle column*: SPECT images, *right column*: CT/SPECT fused images. Sentinel lymph node located inside *the red indicator*.

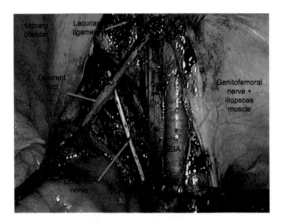

Figure 3.7. Situs after laparoscopic lymphadenectomy for prostate cancer; *EIV*: external iliac vein, *EIA*: external iliac artery. The lacunar ligament as the distal extent of lymphadenectomy.

Urethra

Male Urethra

The urethra is subdivided into four different parts: the intramural part (= pre-prostatic urethra) at the bladder neck, the prostatic urethra, the membranous urethra and the spongy urethra surrounded by the corpus spongiosum. Transitional cells in large sections characterize the mucosa. The distal part near the navicular fossa is marked by a stepwise transition over stratified columnar cells to stratified squamous cells. The muscle layer is divided into an inner longitudinal, a middle circular and an inconsistently described outer longitudinal stratum. The bulbourethral artery, a branch of the internal pudendal artery entering at the level of the penile bulb, supplies the spongy urethra.

Female Urethra

The female urethra is about 3–5 cm long. The histology is equivalent to the male urethra.

Aspects of the urethral closure mechanisms are focused on in the following chapter.

periprostatic nerves leave the craniocaudal course and enter into the prostate for innervations. Initial investigations demonstrated the correlation of neural impulses routed through the nerve fibers on the anterior aspect of the prostate and erectile function. Further investigations are needed to delineate a generally accepted periprostatic anatomy and to map the physical impacts on the different nerve fibers surrounding the prostate. These investigations will lead to a better understanding of which nerve-sparing approach is needed to obtain necessary and sufficient function (Fig. 3.10).[2,3,5-10,14,20,23-37]

Sphincter Mechanisms

Traditional anatomy reports two muscular structures to achieve continence of the lower urinary tract: the voluntary, striated, external

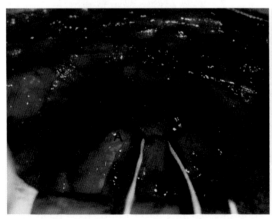

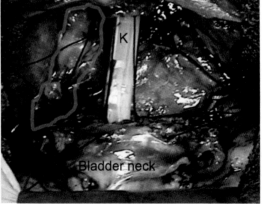

Figure 3.8. Retropubic radical prostatectomy. *Left*: prostate after u-shaped apical (*A*) preparation with isolated urethra (*U*). *Right*: nerve-sparing procedure on left side (*marked in blue*) and partial nerve-sparing procedure on right side before knotting of the anastomosis (*K*: transurethral catheter).

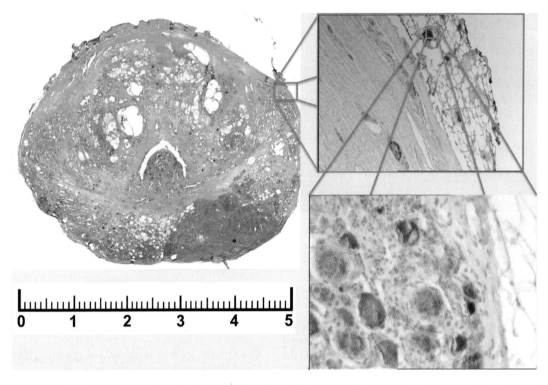

Figure 3.9. Whole mounted horizontal section (*left side*, HE staining) of the prostate (*prostate carcinoma). Staining with protein-gene-product (PGP) 9.5 antibodies (*right side*) illustrates the existence of nerve fibers anterolaterally[23].

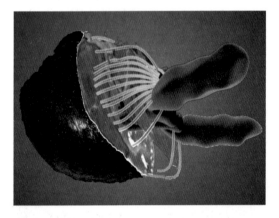

Figure 3.10. Possibility of 3D reconstructions of nerve courses (*right side*: green lines) based on prostate specimens (*left side*) and whole mounted sections (*middle part*).

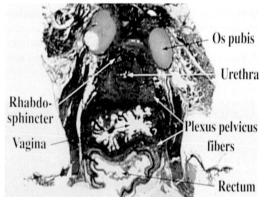

Figure 3.11. Fetal female pelvis illustrating the omega-shaped rhabdosphincter surrounding the urethra and the topographical location of plexus pelvicus fibers. (Reprinted from Colleselli et al.,[38] copyright 1998, with permission from Elsevier).

urethral sphincter (rhabdosphincter) located in the urogenital diaphragm and the autonomous, smooth internal sphincter (lissosphincter) located in the bladder neck. However, the anatomical and functional understanding of the sphincter complex has changed over time

(Fig. 3.11). In comparison to the periprostatic anatomy, various descriptions have been published. The contribution of three different components to the sphincter complex is commonly accepted: the detrusor muscle fibers of the bladder neck including the trigone, the intrinsic smooth muscle fibers of the urethral wall and the external urethral sphincter. The descriptions of the systematic anatomical circumstances and the interaction of the mentioned components varies with different authors.

The Bladder Neck Component

The presence of the circumscribable, circularly oriented smooth muscle sphincter at the outlet of the urinary bladder was denied by different authors 200 years ago. It has been demonstrated both that the detrusor muscle fibers condense especially in the direction of the trigone and that the smooth intrinsic fibers of the urethral wall arrange a complex interacting network of muscle strands at the bladder outlet. In male humans, as reported before, the detrusor fibers reach the point of the seminal colliculus. The bladder neck component is thought to be innervated by the autonomic nervous system.

The Urethral Wall Component

The smooth muscle fibers of the urethral wall do not act as a detached actor. In fact, they can be interpreted as a continuance of the muscular complex of the bladder neck. The urethral muscular layer consists of longitudinally [an inner and (inconsistently described) outer layer] and circularly (middle layer) oriented muscle fibers. Reports of the exact anatomical condition vary. Also these smooth muscle fibers receive autonomic innervations.

The External Urethral Sphincter

Many authors have shaped the anatomical understanding of the external urethral sphincter, but an overall accepted anatomical and functional definition is still lacking. Consensus of opinion exists regarding the three-dimensional profile of the external sphincter. The terms omega-shaped and horseshoe-shaped are most often used to illustrate the external sphincter in male as well as female humans (Fig. 3.12). Muscle fibers are located in the anterior and lateral part of the urethra – only fibrous tissue forms the dorsal interconnection between the dorsolateral

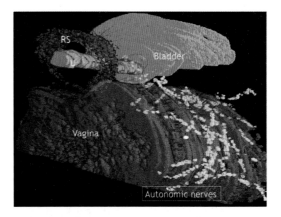

Figure 3.12. 3D reconstruction of the rhabdosphincter (*RS*) and the autonomic nerve supply based on female fetal pelvic studies. U urethra (U). (Reprinted from Colleselli et al.,[38] copyright 1998, with permission from Elsevier).

"ends" of the external sphincter. In the same way, authors concur that the external sphincter is not part of a urogenital diaphragm (deep transverse perineal muscle) and that the external sphincter only has a fibrous connection to the surrounding tissue (including the pelvic diaphragm).

There is extensive discussion about the vertical extent and the histological constitution of the external urethral sphincter.

The participation of striated muscle fibers in the configuration of the external sphincter has long been well known. Essentially the external sphincter has to secure continence continuously as well as during rapid abdominal pressure. Whereas some authors favor the existence of two different striated muscle fibers ("slow twitch fibers" for basic pressure of the external sphincter and "fast twitch fibers" for rapid pressure increases), others report the existence of a smooth muscle component located inside the coat of the striated external sphincter. Therefore, the description internal urethral sphincter (in contrast to the internal vesical sphincter) is used. It is accepted that the pudendal nerve (somatic nervous system) is responsible for the innervations of the voluntary striated external sphincter. Whether autonomous fibers resulting from the inferior hypogastric plexus (routed through the periprostatic plexus) with potential impact after nerve sparing radical prostatectomy are involved in the sphincter innervations is still under investigation.

In male humans it is assumed that the striated muscle fibers of the pronounced anterior part of the sphincter disperse below the puboprostatic ligaments. It is still unclear if striated muscle fibers communicate with the structures of the bladder neck. In females it could be demonstrated that parts of the striated external sphincter could only be found in the two distal thirds of the urethra.[2,3,7,11,13,14,16,17,38-40]

Summary

Knowledge of the anatomy of the lower urinary tract was substantiated by comprehensive investigations long ago. Over time, many consolidated findings have been refuted and then recognized again. Current urological treatments are based on these anatomical conclusions. It has been shown that while some irrevocable facts have been substantiated in several fields of urological anatomy, extensive exploration is still taking place. Especially the complex sphincter mechanism in both females and males as well as the pelvic neuroanatomy are examples of these interesting research subjects. Only functional studies will validate whether these upcoming new aspects of anatomy will also lead to better treatment outcomes for our patients.

References

1. Toellner R. *Illustrated History of Medicine*. Salzburg, Austria: Andreas & Andreas; 1986
2. Benninghoff D. *Anatomy*. München, Germany: Urban & Fischer Verlag; 2003
3. Netter FH. *Atlas of Human Anatomy*. Stuttgart, Germany/ New York: Thieme; 1997
4. Otcenasek M, Baca V, Krofta L, et al. Endopelvic fascia in women: shape and relation to parietal pelvic structures. *Obstet Gynecol*. 2008;111:622-630
5. Shapiro E, Hartanto V, Perlman EJ, et al. Morphometric analysis of pediatric and nonhyperplastic prostate glands: evidence that BPH is not a unique stromal process. *Prostate*. 1997;33:177-182
6. Stolzenburg JU, Rabenalt R, Do M, et al. Intrafascial nerve-sparing endoscopic extraperitoneal radical prostatectomy. *Eur Urol*. 2008;53:931-940
7. Stolzenburg, JU, Schwalenberg T, Horn LC, et al. Anatomical landmarks of radical prostatectomy. *Eur Urol*. 2007;51:629-639
8. Van Ophoven A, Roth S. The anatomy and embryological origins of the fascia of Denonvilliers: a medico-historical debate. *J Urol*. 1997;157:3-9
9. Wimpissinger TF, Tschabitscher M, Feichtinger H, et al. Surgical anatomy of the puboprostatic complex with special reference to radical perineal prostatectomy. *BJU Int*. 2003;92:681-684
10. Young HH. The radical cure of cancer of the prostate. *Surg Gynecol Obstet*. 1937;64:472-484
11. Fritsch H, Lienemann A, Brenner E, et al. Clinical anatomy of the pelvic floor. *Adv Anat Embryol Cell Biol*. 2004;175(III-IX):1-64
12. Nakajima F, Takenaka A, Uchiyama E, et al. Macroscopic and histotopographic study of the deep transverse perineal muscle (musculus transversus perinei profundus) in elderly Japanese. *Ann Anat*. 2007;189:65-74
13. Oelrich TM. The striated urogenital sphincter muscle in the female. *Anat Rec*. 1983;205:223-232
14. Oelrich TM. The urethral sphincter muscle in the male. *Am J Anat*. 1980;158:229-246
15. Shafik A, Sibai OE, Shafik AA, et al. A novel concept for the surgical anatomy of the perineal body. *Dis Colon Rectum*. 2007;50:2120-2125
16. TA S, Delancey JO. Structure of the perineal membrane in females: gross and microscopic anatomy. *Obstet Gynecol*. 2008;111:686-693
17. Wallner C, Dabhoiwala NF, Deruiter MC, et al. The anatomical components of urinary continence. *Eur Urol*. 2009;55(4):932-943
18. Schilling D, Horstmann M, Nagele U, et al. Cystectomy in women. *BJU Int*. 2008;102(9 Pt B):1289-1295
19. Baader B, Baader SL, Herrmann M, et al. Autonomic innervation of the female pelvis. Anatomic basis. *Urologe A*. 2004;43:133-140
20. Baader B, Herrmann M. Topography of the pelvic autonomic nervous system and its potential impact on surgical intervention in the pelvis. *Clin Anat*. 2003;16:119-130
21. Di Gangi Herms AM, Veit R, Reisenauer C, et al. Functional imaging of stress urinary incontinence. *Neuroimage*. 2006;29:267-275
22. Ghoneim MA, Abol-Enein H. Lymphadenectomy with cystectomy: is it necessary and what is its extent? *Eur Urol*. 2004;46:457-461
23. Sievert KD, Hennenlotter J, Laible I, et al. The periprostatic autonomic nerves-bundle or layer? *Eur Urol*. 2008;54(5):1109-1117
24. Corvin S, Schilling D, Eichhorn K, et al. Laparoscopic sentinel lymph node dissection – a novel technique for the staging of prostate cancer. *Eur Urol*. 2006;49: 280-285
25. Dorschner W, Biesold M, Schmidt F, et al. The dispute about the external sphincter and the urogenital diaphragm. *J Urol*. 1999;162:1942-1945
26. Eichelberg C, Erbersdobler A, Michl U, et al. Nerve distribution along the prostatic capsule. *Eur Urol*. 2007;51:105-110; discussion 110-101
27. Ganzer R, Blana A, Gaumann A, et al. Topographical anatomy of periprostatic and capsular nerves: quantification and computerised planimetry. *Eur Urol*. 2008;54:353-361
28. Gil-Vernet JM. Prostate cancer: anatomical and surgical considerations. *Br J Urol*. 1996;78:161-168
29. Heidenreich A, Ohlmann CH, Polyakov S. Anatomical extent of pelvic lymphadenectomy in patients undergoing radical prostatectomy. *Eur Urol*. 2007;52:29-37

30. Kaiho Y, Nakagawa H, Saito H, et al. Nerves at the ventral prostatic capsule contribute to erectile function: initial electrophysiological assessment in humans. *Eur Urol.* 2009;55(1):148-155

31. Karam I, Droupy S, Abd-Alsamad I, et al. The precise location and nature of the nerves to the male human urethra: histological and immunohistochemical studies with three-dimensional reconstruction. *Eur Urol.* 2005; 48:858-864

32. McNeal JE. Regional morphology and pathology of the prostate. *Am J Clin Pathol.* 1968;49:347-357

33. Mulhall JP, Secin FP, Guillonneau B. Artery sparing radical prostatectomy – myth or reality? *J Urol.* 2008; 179: 827-831

34. FP S, Touijer K, Mulhall J, et al. Anatomy and preservation of accessory pudendal arteries in laparoscopic radical prostatectomy. *Eur Urol.* 2007;51: 1229-1235

35. Villers A, Steg A, Boccon-Gibod L. Anatomy of the prostate: review of the different models. *Eur Urol.* 1991;20: 261-268

36. Woods ME, Ouwenga M, Quek ML. The role of pelvic lymphadenectomy in the management of prostate and bladder cancer. *ScientificWorld J.* 2007;7:789-799

37. Yucel S, Baskin LS. An anatomical description of the male and female urethral sphincter complex. *J Urol.* 2004;171:1890-1897

38. Colleselli K, Stenzl A, Eder R, et al. The female urethral sphincter: a morphological and topographical study. *J Urol.* 1998;160(1):49-54

39. Koraitim MM. The male urethral sphincter complex revisited: an anatomical concept and its physiological correlate. *J Urol.* 2008;179:1683-1689

40. Strasser H, Ninkovic M, Hess M, et al. Anatomic and functional studies of the male and female urethral sphincter. *World J Urol.* 2000;18:324-329

4

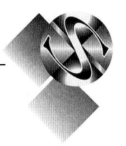

Anatomy of the Male Reproductive System

Klaus Steger and Wolfgang Weidner

Testis, Epididymis, and Ductus Deferens

Testis and Scrotum

Male mammals have two testicles, which are components of both the reproductive and the endocrine system. Therefore, the two main functions of the testicles are producing sperm (approximately one million per hour) and male sex hormones (e.g., testosterone) (Fig. 4.1).

The average testicular volume is 18 cm³ per testis with normal size ranging from 12 to 30 cm³. A testicular volume of both testicles less than 15 mL is associated with infertility. It is most common for one testis to hang lower than the other. In about 85% of men, the lower hanging testis is the right one. This is due to differences in the vascular anatomical structure on the right and left sides (see below).

Testes (and epididymes) are contained within an extension of the abdomen, called scrotum. The scrotum, which is homologous to the labia majora in females, keeps the testis at a temperature of about 34.4°C, as temperatures above 36.7°C are damaging to sperm count. The temperature is regulated by blood flow and positioning of the testes toward and away from the heat of the body by contraction and relaxation of the musculus cremaster and the tunica dartos, a layer of smooth muscles under the skin of the scrotum.

Descensus testis: Many anatomical features of the adult testis reflect its developmental origin in the abdomen (Fig. 4.2). The layers of tissue enclosing each testicle are derived from the layers of the anterior abdominal wall. Parallel to the descensus testis in the embryo, the processus vaginalis peritonei protrude into the scrotum creating the cavitas serosa scroti, which is surrounded by the epiorchium (inner layer, covers the tunica albuginea) and the periorchium (outer layer). Epiorchium and periorchium together form the tunica vaginalis testis. The fascia spermatica interna, following the periorchium, arises from the fascia transversalis. It contains the cremasteric muscle which arises from the internal oblique muscle. The cremasteric muscle is covered by the fascia spermatica externa which arises from the fascia of the body. Testicles and layers of the testicles are covered by the skin of the scrotum. Below the body skin lies the tunica dartos comprizing a fibromuscular layer with hairs and pigments, but no fat (Fig. 4.3 and Table 4.1).

Clinic: Incomplete descensus testis results in cryptorchidism associated with male infertility. In cryptorchidism, in more than 95% of cases, the non-descended testicle is in an inguinal position.[1] Abdominal and ectopic positions are clinically important and need gentle investigation when the inguinal canal seems to be empty (Fig. 4.4). In case of incomplete shut of the processus vaginalis peritonei, part of the intestine might protrude via the canalis inguinalis into the cavitas serosa scroti (indirect inguinal hernia).

C.R. Chapple and W.D. Steers (eds.), *Practical Urology: Essential Principles and Practice,*
DOI: 10.1007/978-1-84882-034-0_4, © Springer-Verlag London Limited 2011

Figure 4.1. Localization of male genital organs.

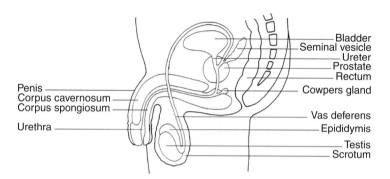

Figure 4.2. Descensus testis.

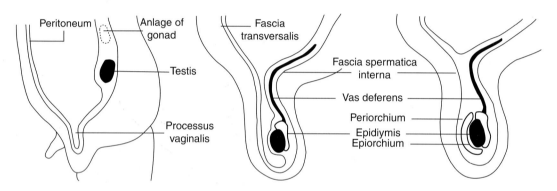

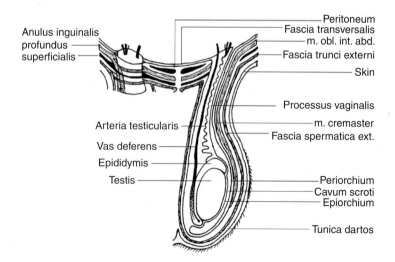

Figure 4.3. Origin of testicle layers from body fasciae.

Table 4.1. Connection between layers of the testis and layers of the ventral body

Layers of testis	Layers of ventral body
Epiorchium and periorchium	Peritoneum
Fascia spermatica interna	Fascia transversalis
M. cremaster	M. obliquus internus abdominis and m. transversus abdominis
Fascia spermatica externa	Fascia superficialis and fascia of m. obliquus externus abdominis
tunica dartos and skin of scrotum	subcutaneous connective tissue and skin

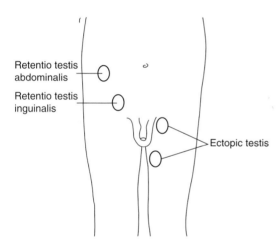

Figure 4.4. Various forms of cryptorchidism.

The testicles are covered by the tunica albuginea consisting of an outer epiorchium and an inner tunica vaginalis. The latter divides the testicular parenchym via septula testis (contain blood and lymph vessels) into lobuli testis. Beneath the tunica albuginea, the testis comprises fine coiled seminiferous tubules (diameter: 180–200 μm) containing the seminiferous epithelium where spermatogenesis takes place. Tubules are surrounded by a lamina propria. Between the tubules, intertubular tissue contains Leydig cells, which produce the male sex hormone testosterone that stimulates spermatogenesis and sperm production.

Within the embryo, gonads are at first capable of becoming either ovaries or testes. Starting at about gestational week 4, gonadal rudiments are present within the intermediate mesoderm adjacent to developing kidneys. At about gestational week 6, sex cords develop within the forming testes comprising early Sertoli cells that surround germ cells which migrate into the gonads shortly before sex determination starts. The sexual differentiation is depicted in Fig. 4.5. The transformation of testosterone to dihydrotestosterone due to the activity of 5α-reductase is the decision step for the formation of the penis, the scrotum, and the prostate. The sex-specific gene SRY that is found on the Y-chromosome initiates sex determination by downstream regulation of sex-determining factors, which leads to the development of the male phenotype including directing development of the early bipotential gonad down the male path of development.[2]

Spermatogenesis

Spermatogenesis occurs within the seminiferous epithelium on the surface of the somatic Sertoli cells (Fig. 4.6a, b). Functional Sertoli cells are required for normal spermatogenic progression resulting in the continuous production of numerous fertile spermatozoa, which in turn is necessary to maintain Sertoli cells in their functional differentiation state. Adjacent Sertoli cells form Sertoli-Sertoli junctional complexes dividing the seminiferous epithelium into a basal and an adluminal compartment. During spermatogenesis, germ cells migrate through the Sertoli-Sertoli junctional complexes successively passing through the following three developmental stages:

1. Mitosis: Following mitosis of a spermatogonial stem cell, one spermatogonium is conserved as a spermatogonial stem cell, while the other spermatogonium undergoes further mitoses and, subsequently, enters meiosis.
2. Meiosis: During the first meiotic division, one primary spermatocyte gives rise to two secondary spermatocytes. During the second meiotic division, each of the two secondary spermatocytes gives rise to two round spermatids. In order to preserve the number of chromosomes in the offspring, each gamete must have half the usual number of chromosomes present in somatic cells. Otherwise,

Figure 4.5. Development of male genital organs.

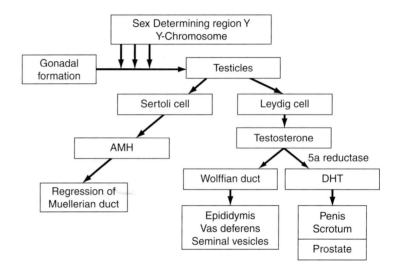

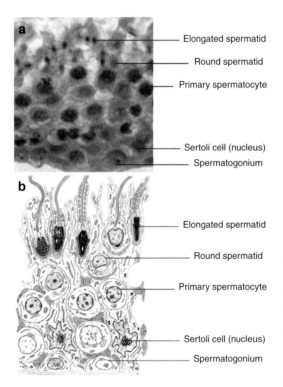

Figure 4.6. Organization of the seminiferous epithelium. (**a**) Histology, H&E. (**b**) Scheme.

the offspring will have twice the normal number of chromosomes resulting in serious abnormalities.

3. Spermiogenesis: Round spermatids do no longer divide, but differentiate into mature spermatozoa undergoing numerous morphological, biochemical, and physiological modifications. Nuclear chromatin condensation, development of the acrosome, and formation of the flagellum occur simultaneously in haploid spermatids.

Each cell division – from spermatogonium to spermatid – is incomplete, as germ cells remain connected to one another by intercellular bridges. This is a prerequisite for synchronous development. Germ cells are subjected to permanent proliferation and differentiation processes resulting in the appearance of various germ cell populations each representing a particular phase of germ cell development. A defined arrangement of germ cell populations is called the stage of the seminiferous epithelium (Fig. 4.7). A complete series of changes in stages arranged in the logical sequence of germ cell maturation is called the cycle of the seminiferous epithelium. In men, the seminiferous epithelial cycle is divided into six stages (I–VI).[3] Due to the nuclear morphology of the spermatids and the reactivity of spermatid nuclei with periodic-acid-Schiff (PAS), spermatid differentiation is further subdivided into eight steps (1–8). Development from spermatogonia to spermatozoa lasts 74 days. As maturation within the epididymis lasts 8–17 days, the generation of a spermatozoon from a stem spermatogonia lasts at least 82 days.

ANATOMY OF THE MALE REPRODUCTIVE SYSTEM

Figure 4.7. Stages of the seminiferous epithelial cycle. *B* spermatogonium type B; *PL* primary spermatocytes in preleptotene; *L* leptotene; *Z* zygotene; *P* pachytene; *SS* secondary spermatocytes; *1-8* spermatids in steps; *RB* residual body.

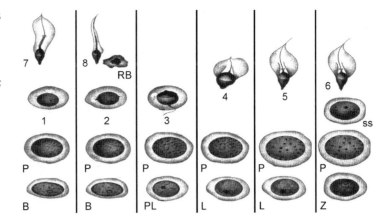

Hormonal Regulation of Spermatogenesis

Spermatogenesis is highly sensitive to fluctuations in hormones. Testosterone is required in high local concentrations to maintain spermatogenesis. This is achieved via binding of testosterone by androgen-binding protein (ABP) present in seminiferous tubules. Hormonal regulation of spermatogenesis is organized as control circuit with a negative feedback mechanism involving hypothalamus, pituitary, and testis (Fig. 4.8). Specific neurons of the hypothalamus synthesize gonadotropin releasing hormone (GnRH), which induces the production of two hormones within the pituitary, luteinizing hormone (LH) and follicle stimulating hormone (FSH). While high pulse rate of GnRH release (1 impulse per 1 h) results in the production of LH, low pulse rate of GnRH release (1 impulse per 2 h) results in the production of FSH. Within the testis, LH causes synthesis of testosterone by intertubular Leydig cells, which negatively influences hormone release in hypothalamus and pituitary. By contrast, FSH acts on intratubular Sertoli cells. It induces the production of ABP by means of which testosterone can pass the Sertoli–Sertoli junctional complexes, as well as the production of activin and inhibin by

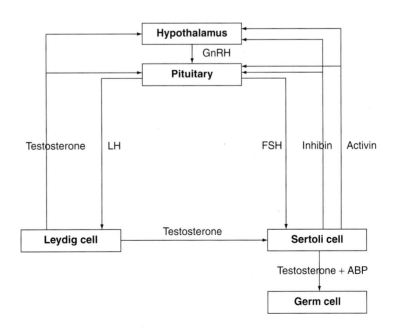

Figure 4.8. Hormonal regulation of spermatogenesis.

Sertoli cells, which influences hormone release both in hypothalamus and pituitary.

Genetic Regulation of Spermatogenesis

The differentiation of spermatogonial stem cells into fertile sperm requires stringent temporal and stage-specific gene expression. This becomes evident when studying the sequential nucleo-protein expression in developing germ cells resulting in histone to protamine exchange in haploid spermatids.[4] Although, in man, replacement of histones is only about 85% complete,[5] protamines represent the predominant nucleo-proteins of elongated spermatids and mature spermatozoa.

Protamines bind lengthwise within the minor groove of the DNA double helix with their central polyarginine segment cross-linking and neutralizing the phosphodiester backbone of the DNA. These DNA-protamine complexes of one DNA strand fit exactly into the major grooves of a parallel DNA strand and are packed side by side in a linear array within the sperm nucleus.[6] In addition to DNA binding, protamine molecules interact with other protamine molecules by forming disulfide bonds between cysteine residues, thereby facilitating DNA compaction. Ward[7] performed a model for the packing of the entire haploid genome into the sperm nucleus in which DNA loop domains are packed as doughnuts attached to the sperm nuclear matrix. Protamine bound DNA is coiled into large concentric circles that collapse into a doughnut in which the DNA-protamine complexes are tightly packed together by van der Waal's forces.

Protamine-DNA interactions result in chromatin condensation causing cessation of transcription in elongating spermatids. This occurs at a time when many proteins need to be synthesized and assembled for the complete condensation of the chromatin, the development of the acrosome, and the formation of the flagellum. Therefore, it is evident that precise temporal regulation of gene expression via transcriptional and translational control mechanisms is of fundamental importance to ensure complete differentiation of round spermatids into mature spermatozoa.[4]

Blood Vessels, Lymphatic Drainage, and Nerves

The testicular artery originates from the abdominal aorta. Due to the descensus testis, the testicular artery is located within the retroperitoneum. It crosses the psoas muscle and the ureter, passes the canalis inguinalis and enters the spermatic cord where it makes anastomoses with the arteria ductus deferentis and the arteria cremasterica. The arteria testicularis passes the testis dorsal and enters the tunica albuginea from ventral basal to ventral apical branching into the septula testis. From the rete testis, arteriae recurrentes supply the tubuli seminiferi (Fig. 4.9). This special schedule of arterial supply is the rationale for the operation approach to retrieve testicular material coming always rom the free rim of the testicle.

The testicular artery is surrounded by the plexus pampiniformis. Veins merge to the vena testicularis dextra which opens into the vena cava inferior and the vena testicularis sinistra which opens into the vena renalis sinistra.

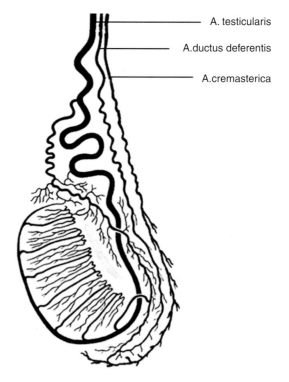

A. testicularis

A. ductus deferentis

A. cremasterica

Figure 4.9. Blood supply of testicle.

Lymphatic drainage starts at the septula testis and occurs via the tunica albuginea and the rete testis. Lymph vessels pass the spermatic cord and the canalis inguinalis and opens into nodi lymphatici lumbales in direct vicinity to the abdominal aorta.

Note that blood supply and lymphatic drainage are distinct between testis and scrotum. The paired testicular arteries arise directly from the abdominal aorta and descend through the inguinal canal, while the scrotum and the rest of the external genitalia is supplied by the internal pudendal artery (itself a branch of the internal iliac artery). Lymphatic drainage of the testes follows the testicular arteries back to the para-aortic lymph nodes, while lymph from the scrotum drains to the inguinal lymph nodes.

Nerves originate from the plexus testicularis, which is located within the retroperitoneum where the testicular artery leaves the aorta. Nerves join the testicular artery on its way to the testis and ramify within the tunica albuginea, but do not enter the seminiferous tubules. Therefore, the seminiferous epithelium is devoid of any nerves. Although crushing of testes (e.g., sport) is extremely painful, only little is known about afferent nerve fibers ending at around the level of thoracal segment 10 of the spinal cord. Sensoric innnervation of the scrotum occurs via the genitofemoralis nerve (ramus genitalis) and the ilioinguinalis nerve. The nervus genitofemoralis, in addition, is responsible for the motoric innervation of the musculus cremaster and the tunica dartos.

The blood–testis barrier: Due to the presence of tight junctions between adjacent Sertoli cells, large molecules cannot pass from the blood into the lumen of the seminiferous tubules. While spermatogonia are located within the basal compartment (deep to the level of the tight junctions), primary and secondary spermatocytes, as well as round and elongated spermatids occur in the adluminal compartment. The blood–testis barrier is thought to prevent an auto-immune reaction, as mature sperm (and their antigens) arise long after immune tolerance is established in infancy. Therefore, as sperm are antigenically different from self-tissue, a male animal can react immunologically to his own sperm. In fact, he is capable of making antibodies against them. Injection of sperm antigens causes inflammation of the testis (autoimmune orchitis).

Clinically, besides vasectomy, induction of anti-sperm antibodies (ASA) is discussed for urogenital infections, genital trauma, and testicular tumors as risk factors determining fertility.[8]

Epididymis and Ductus Deferens

As has already been mentioned, spermatogenesis occurs within the seminiferous epithelium of the seminiferous tubules. Following spermiation, spermatozoa pass the rete testis and enter the ductuli efferentes, 8–12 of which connect the rete testis with the ductus epididymidis.

The columnar epithelium of the ductuli efferentes is underlined by smooth muscles and consists of two cell types: absorptive cells with microvilli and cells with kinocilia responsible for the transport of still immotile spermatozoa. As the height of these two cell types is variable, the lumen shows a characteristic wavy outline (Fig. 4.10).

Spermatozoa enter the epididymis via the head (caput), progress to the body (corpus), and finally reach the tail (cauda), where they are stored. During their passage through the epididymis, spermatozoa undergo maturation to acquire the motility necessary for fertilizing an egg. Note that final maturation is completed within the female reproductive tract (capacitation).

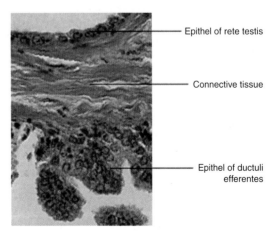

Figure 4.10. Histology of ductuli efferentes, H&E.

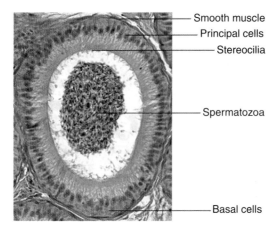

Smooth muscle
Principal cells
Stereocilia

Spermatozoa

Basal cells

Figure 4.11. Histology of epididymis, H&E.

The ductus epididymidis is about 6 m long and is lined by a tall columnar epithelium, which is underlined by smooth muscles and consists of basal cells and principal cells with nonmotile stereocilia. From caput to cauda, the height of the epithelium decreases, while the diameter of the ductus and the lumen increases (Fig. 4.11).

The ductus deferens or vasa deferentia – each about 30 cm long – connect right and left epididymis to the ejaculatory ducts. The ductus deferens can be divided into pars funiculi spermatici, pars inguinalis, pars pelvina, ampulla ductus deferentis, and ductus ejaculatorius, which open into the urethra (colliculus seminalis).

The mucosa forms longitudinal folds and is lined by a columnar epithelium. The muscularis is up to 1.5 mm thick and consists of a thick

circular layer of smooth muscles between inner and outer longitudinal layers. The prominent muscularis, which makes the ductus deferens palpable within the spermatic cord (Fig. 4.12), is covered by an adventitia. During ejaculation, smooth muscles within the wall of the ductus deferens contract and propel the sperm forward into the urethra. This impulse originates from abdominal and pelvic sympathetic noradrenergic nerves and results in the release of norepinephrine that subsequently binds to α1A receptors located on smooth muscles.[9]

Clinic: Vasectomy is the major operation of the vas deferens. Nearly 7% of all married couples choose vasectomy as their form of birth control.[10] The ductus deferens is part of the spermatic cord or funiculus spermaticus. This structure is covered by an external spermatic fascia (a continuation of the fascia from the external oblique muscle), the cremasteric fascia (a continuation of the fascia from the internal oblique muscle) and an internal spermatic fascia (a continuation of the transversalis fascia). It contains the ductus deferens, arteries (testicular artery, deferential artery, and cremasteric artery), the pampiniform plexus, lymphatic vessels, nerves (genitofemoralis nerve and sympathetic nerve), and the processus vaginalis.

The spermatic cord is sensitive to torsion. The most common age at which testicular torsion occurs is during puberty and the second most common is in the newborn. As a consequence, testicles may rotate within its sac and may kick off its own blood supply resulting in irreversible damage to the testicles within hours.

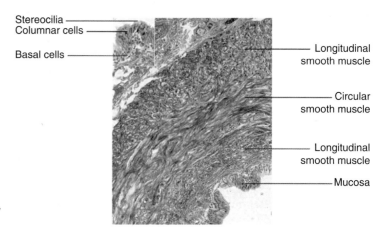

Stereocilia
Columnar cells

Basal cells

Longitudinal smooth muscle

Circular smooth muscle

Longitudinal smooth muscle

Mucosa

Figure 4.12. Histology of vas deferens, H&E.

In addition, some of the contents of the abdominal cavity may protrude into the spermatic cord causing an indirect inguinal hernia.

Accessory Sex Glands

The male reproductive system includes three different accessory sex glands, namely, the prostate, a pair of seminal vesicles, and a pair of bulbourethral glands (Fig. 4.1).

Prostate

The prostate is homologous to Skene´s glands found in many females. It measures approximately 2 × 3 × 4 cm and surrounds the urethra just below the urinary bladder to which it is fixed. Within the prostate, the urethra merges with the ductus ejaculatorii which open into the colliculus seminalis. While the ventral apex of the prostate reaches the diaphragma urogenitale, the ventral part is located at the pubic bone and the dorsal part lies in direct vicinity to the ampulla of the rectum. Therefore, the prostate is palpable during rectal examination approximately 4 cm from the anus.

From inside to outside, according to Mc Neal,[11] the prostate can be divided into three concentric zones (Fig. 4.13). The central zone surrounds the ejaculatory ducts and contains mucosal glands, the transition zone surrounds the proximal part of the urethra and contains submucosal glands, and the peripheral or subcapsular zone surrounds the distal part of the urethra and contains the main glands. The latter comprises 30–50 tubuloalveolar glands that empty into 15–30 independent excretory ducts,

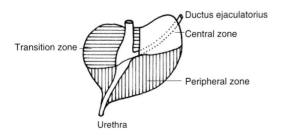

Figure 4.13. Organization of prostate, according to Mc Neal.[11] Sagittal section, from left.

which are lined by a simple columnar epithelium and open into the urethra. The glands are embedded into a fibromuscular stroma and are surrounded by a capsule.

Due to papillary projections of the mucosa into the lumen, secretory alveoli are irregular in shape. Round eosinophilic bodies, called corpora amylacea, represent a characteristic feature of secretory alveoli. These bodies may undergo calcification and may appear in semen. The glandular epithelium is columnar to cuboidal depending on the secretory activity, hormonal situation, and age and contains basal cells, which represent progenitors of the secretory cells (Fig. 4.14).

The secretory cells contain granules, which among other molecules produce prostate-specific acid phosphatase. The secretion, therefore, is acidic (pH 6.4). It constitutes approximately 30% of the seminal fluid and contains many enzymes, as well as citric acid, prostaglandins that stimulate smooth muscles of the female genital tract to enhance the migration of sperm, zinc which is involved in the testosterone metabolism, spermine which accounts for the typical smell of the seminal fluid and fibrinolysin which liquifies the semen. Secretion is regulated by dihydrotestosterone (DHT).

Blood supply via arteria rectalis media and arteria vesicalis inferior (dorsal and lateral) and arteria pudenda interna (ventral). Veins open into the plexus vesicoprostaticus. Lymphatic drainage occurs via nodi lymphatici iliaci interni et externi. Nerves originate from the plexus prostaticus.

Clinic: The anatomical model of Mc Neal[11] is important. Benign prostatic hyperplasia (BPH) is the disease of the periurethral zone, whereas prostatitis and prostate cancer (PCa) are mainly located in the peripheral zone. BPH occurs in older men due to an enlargement of the transition zone. Hyperplastic tissue may constrict the urethra and impede the urine flow. PCa represents the second most malignant tumor in men older than 50 years.

Seminal Vesicles

Seminal vesicles or glandulae vesiculosae are located posterior-inferior to the urinary bladder and lateral to the ampulla of the ductus deferens. Beneath an outer layer of connective tissue lies the muscularis consisting of an outer

Figure 4.14. Histology of prostate, H&E.

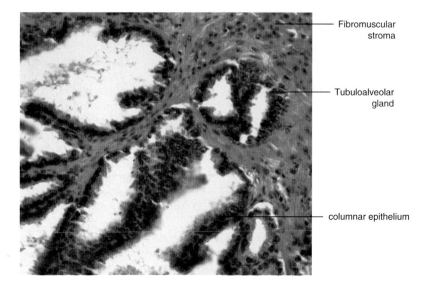

Fibromuscular stroma

Tubuloalveolar gland

columnar epithelium

longitudinal and an inner circular layer of smooth muscles. Close to the lumen lies the mucosa consisting of a columnar epithelium with cuboidal cells along the lamina propria. The height of the cells mirrors their activity depending on the serum testosterone level. Excretory ducts open into the ductus ejaculatorius of the ductus deferens as it enters the prostate.

In former times, seminal vesicles were thought to store semen – hence their name. However, this turned out to be wrong. The secretion is strongly acidophilic and constitutes 60–80% of the ejaculate volume. It contains several proteins and enzymes, as well as mucus and vitamin C. The yellow fluorescing pigment flavin is of use in forensic medicine for the detection of semen stains. Prostaglandins stimulate smooth muscles of the female genital tract to enhance the migration of sperm from the vagina to the uterus. The large amount of fructose serves as an energy source for the sperm.

Blood supply via arteria vesicalis inferior, arteria rectalis media, and arteria ductus deferentis. Veins open into the plexus vesicoprostaticus. Lymphatic drainage occurs via nodi lymphatici iliaci interni et externi et hypogastrici. Nerves originate from plexus hypogastricus superior et inferior.

Clinic: The fructose concentration within the seminal plasma serves as indicator for the function of the seminal vesicles (reference >13 μmol ejaculate[12];), especially in patients with a central

obstruction of the seminal pathways and agenesis of the glands.

Bulbourethral Glands

Bulbourethral glands or Cowper's glands are homologous to Bartholin's glands in the female. They are located posterior-lateral to the membranous portion of the urethra at the base of the penis. Glandular units are surrounded by smooth muscles originating from the musculus transversus perini profundus. Excretory ducts open into the ampulla of the urethra releasing a clear viscous secretion known as pre-ejaculate.

Penis

The human penis is made up of three columns of tissue (Fig. 4.15). Two corpora cavernosa are located next to each other on the dorsal side and one corpus spongiosum lies between them on the ventral side. The end of the corpus spongiosum is enlarged and forms the glans, which supports the foreskin or prepuce, a loose fold of skin that in adults can retract to expose the glans. The area on the underside of the penis, where the foreskin is attached, is called the frenulum. The urethra traverses the corpus spongiosum and its opening lies on the tip of the glans. It is a passage for both urine and semen. The raphe is the visible ridge between

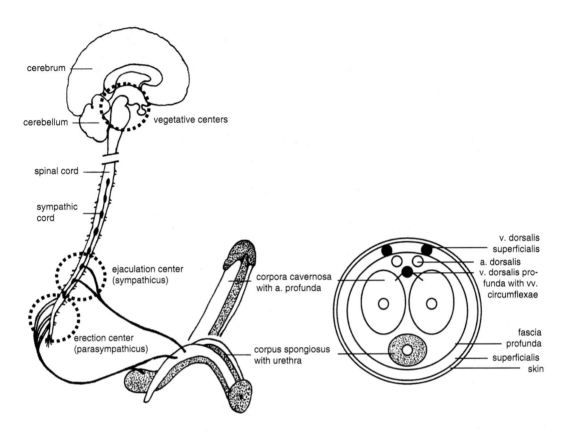

Figure 4.15. Anatomy of penis. *Left*: erection and ejaculation. *Right*: blood supply.

the lateral halves of the penis, found underside of the penis running from the meatus (opening of the urethra) across the scrotum to the perineum (area between scrotum and anus).

The glans penis is homologous to the clitoral glans, the corpora cavernosa are homologous to the body of the clitoris and the corpus spongiosum is homologous to the vestibular bulbs beneath the labia minora. The raphe does not exist in females because there the two halves are not connected.

Blood supply via arteriae pudenda interna dextra et sinistra from which there originate three branches: (1) Arteria dorsalis penis to skin, prepuce and glans; (2) Arteria profunda penis which give rise to several arteriae helicinae that opens into the chambers of the corpora cavernosa; (3) Arteria bulbi penis to urethra and corpus spongiosum. Many venae circumflexae merges to the vena dorsalis penis that opens into the plexus vesicoprostaticus. Lymphatic

drainage occurs via nodi lymphatici inguinales. Sensoric nerves originate from the nervus pudendus. The sympathicus is responsible for vasoconstriction, while the parasympathicus causes vasodilation.

Erection and Ejaculation

Erection is caused by the parasympathic (S3 of spinal cord) dilation of the arteriae helicinae that supply blood to the chambers of the corpora cavernosa. As a consequence, more and more blood fills the chambers causing the penis to lengthen and stiffen. The now engorged erectile tissue presses against and constricts the veins that carry blood away from the penis. As a consequence, more blood enters than leaves the penis until an equilibrium is reached where an equal volume of blood flows into the dilated arteries and out of the constricted veins.

Ejaculation, by contrast, is caused by the sympathetic nervous system (L2/3 of spinal cord) and is usually accompanied by orgasm. A series of contractions of the musculi bulbospongiosus et ischiocavernosus delivers semen from the penis into the vagina. It is usually the result of sexual stimulation, which may include prostate stimulation. Ejaculation may also occur spontaneously during sleep (nocturnal ejaculation).

References

1. Kolon TF, Patel RP, Huff DS. Cryptorchidism: diagnosis, treatment, long-term prognosis. *Urol Clin North Am.* 2004;31:469–480
2. George FN, Wilson JD. Hormonal control of sexual development. Vitam Horm. 1986;43:145–196
3. Clermont Y. The cycle of the seminiferous epithelium in man. *Am J Anat.* 1963;112:35–51
4. Steger K. Transcriptional and translational regulation of gene expression in haploid spermatids. *Anat Embryol.* 1999;199:471–487
5. Tanphaichitr N, Sohbon P, Taluppeth N, Chalermisarachai P. Basic nuclear proteins in testicular cells and ejaculated spermatozoa in man. *Exp Cell Res.* 1978;117:347–350
6. Balhorn R. A model for the structure of chromatin in mammalian sperm. *J Cell Biol.* 1982;93:298–305
7. Ward WS. Deoxyribonucleic acid loop domain tertiary structure in mammalian spermatozoa. *Biol Reprod.* 1993;48:1193–1203
8. Jarow JP, Sanzone JJ. Risk factors for male partners antisperm antibodies. *J Urol.* 1992;148:1805–1807
9. Kihara K. Introduction to innervation of the vas deferens. *Microsc Res Tech.* 1998;42:387–389
10. Schlegel P, Goldstein M. *Survey of Male Infertility.* Philadelphia, PA: Saunders; 1995
11. Mc Neal JE. The prostate gland morphology and pathophysiology. *Renographs Urol.* 1983;9:3–33
12. WHO. *WHO Laboratory Manual for the Examination of Human Sperm and Sperm-Cervial Mucus Interaction.* 4th ed. Cambridge, UK: Cambridge University Press; 1999

5

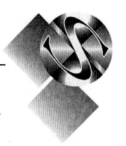

Imaging of the Upper Tracts

Ferekh Salim

Anatomy of the Upper Tracts and Introduction to Imaging Modalities

Introduction

Imaging plays a central role in the diagnosis and management of many urological conditions. The aim of this chapter is to describe the applications and limitations of various imaging modalities in relation to abnormalities of the upper urinary tract. Particular attention will be given to the important imaging features of conditions seen in everyday urological practice.

Renal Upper Tract Basic Anatomy

The kidneys are situated superiorly in the retroperitoneum and lie obliquely along the plane of the psoas muscles. The right kidney lies medial to the ascending colon and is placed slightly lower than the left kidney due to the mass effect of the right liver lobe of liver.

The left kidney lies inferior to the spleen and is situated medial to the descending colon.

Each kidney consists of an outer cortex and an inner medulla, which consists of several cone shaped structures known as the renal pyramids. The pyramids project into the renal sinus, which is comprised of the pelvicalyceal system (or collecting system), fat, renal vessels, and fibrous supportive tissue.

The kidneys are surrounded by fat that is enclosed by a condensation of fibrous tissue (Gerotas fascia), which outlines the perinephric space.

The major renal vessels enter the kidney through a concave recess at its medial border known as the renal hilum. Typically, the vein enters the hilum anterior to the renal artery with the renal pelvis situated behind the vessels.

The renal collecting systems drain into the ureters, which continue retroperitoneally from the pelviureteric junction to the bladder. The ureter measures approximately 20 cm in length and is lined by transitional cell epithelium. Smooth muscle within the ureteric wall allows peristalsis, facilitating urine flow to the bladder. The ureter is narrowed at the pelviureteric junction, at the level where it crosses the common iliac vessels and at the vesicoureteric junction.

Modalities Used for Imaging the Upper Tracts

Several imaging modalities are available for imaging the upper tracts, namely ultrasound, intravenous urography, isotope renography, CT, and MRI.

Ultrasound

Most solid intra-abdominal organs are well shown by ultrasound. The advantages of ultrasound include its ready availability, relative low

C.R. Chapple and W.D. Steers (eds.), *Practical Urology: Essential Principles and Practice*, DOI: 10.1007/978-1-84882-034-0_5, © Springer-Verlag London Limited 2011

cost, and high portability. The absence of any associated ionizing radiation makes it particularly useful in patients where radiation needs to be avoided, for example, in children or pregnant patients. In order to achieve accurate diagnostic results, a high degree of operator expertise is necessary.

The kidneys are usually well imaged by ultrasound making it a valuable first-line test for assessment of suspected renal pathology. Visualization of the ureters by ultrasound is variable and frequently limited as a result of obscuration by overlying bowel gas. Nevertheless, the proximal and terminal segments can be visualized if dilated and are recognizable as tubular anechoic structures. The renal capsule can be identified as a well-defined echogenic line surrounding the kidneys. The cortex appears echopoor; prominent sections of cortex known as Columns of Bertin (Fig. 5.1) can sometimes be seen indenting the renal sinus. The renal pyramids appear echopoor relative to the cortex and can be seen as broad-based triangular structures projecting into the strongly echogenic renal sinus.

IVU

Intravenous urogram or IVU is a study of the renal tract, which involves the acquisition of a series of abdominal radiographs following intravenous injection of iodinated contrast medium. An initial control image is usually obtained, which is used to identify renal tract calcification. A bolus of intravenous contrast medium is subsequently injected, which is rapidly filtered and excreted by the renal tubules resulting in enhancement of the renal outlines and opacification of the pelvicalyceal system, ureters, and bladder.

IVU demonstrates the renal outlines allowing assessment of renal size, position, and morphology. Detailed images of the pelvicalyceal systems obtained by IVU allow assessment of the mucosal surfaces and can highlight suspicious filling defects.

Delayed excretion and dilatation of the collecting system and ureters indicates renal obstruction.[1]

The disadvantages of IVU include the use of ionizing radiation and the associated risks of administration of intravenous contrast, which include the possibility of adverse reaction and contrast-induced nephropathy, the latter is of particular concern in patients with pre existing renal insufficiency. From a technical viewpoint IVU images can be of limited diagnostic value if there is poor renal excretion and concentration, or if there is obscuration of the renal tract by overlying bowel gas shadows. IVU has a low sensitivity for the detection of renal cortical masses and is therefore an inappropriate test if renal carcinoma is suspected. Recent years have seen a decline in the use of IVU in many centers in favor of other imaging techniques such as CT urography and MRI.

CT

CT is the modality of choice for the imaging of many upper tract conditions. For example, CT has in many centers become the first-line test for detection of ureteric calculi in suspected renal colic. In addition CT is widely accepted as the most useful imaging modality for characterization of renal masses and for the staging of renal malignancies. CT urography refers to a study of the renal tract acquired in the excretory phase following iodinated intravenous contrast injection. Enhancement of the renal parenchyma and opacification of the collecting system and ureters allows detailed evaluation of the entire renal tract. Important applications of CT Urography include investigation of hematuria, and evaluation of hydronephrosis.[2]

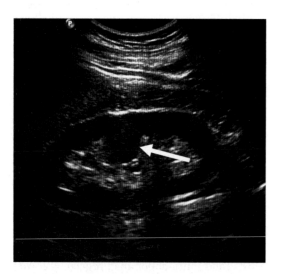

Figure 5.1. Ultrasound of a normal kidney, note prominent cortex (Column of Bertin) indenting the renal sinus (*arrow*).

The past few years have seen rapid advances in CT technology. Multidetector row CT (MDCT) provides high resolution imaging coupled with fast study times; typically the entire renal tract can be imaged in less than 30 s. The images are acquired in the axial plane; however, multiplanar reformatted (MPR) images, which have spatial resolutions similar to the axial images, can be generated. 3-D volume-rendered images (Fig. 5.2) can also be created from the CT data, which may be useful for surgical planning.

MRI is able to provide high contrast resolution detailed images of soft tissue structures and is a useful imaging modality for characterization of renal masses, for the assessment of ureteric obstruction, and for evaluation of the renal vasculature. One of the major advantages of MRI includes the absence of ionizing radiation, which makes it useful for the evaluation of renal tract pathology in younger patients and in pregnancy.

In the context of urological imaging, the main disadvantage of MRI is the poor sensitivity for calcium detection making it unsuitable for the imaging of renal tract calculi. Other disadvantages include long study times making it unsuitable for unstable, confused, or agitated patients. Cardiac pacemakers are an absolute contraindication to MRI as there is a risk of pacemaker malfunction resulting in fatal arrhythmia.

Nuclear medicine can be used to define split renal function or to provide an objective analysis of renal excretory and drainage dynamics.

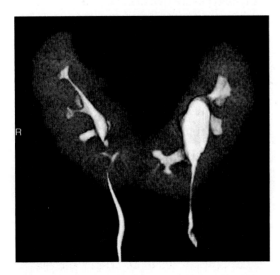

Figure 5.2. CT – volume-rendered image of a horseshoe kidney.

Radiation Issues

The radiation doses associated with imaging investigations are relatively small; however, in order to minimize the potentially harmful effects of radiation exposure (such as genetic mutations and malignancy), tests that utilize ionizing radiation need to be used judiciously.

The radiation dose, measured in millisieverts (mSv) varies widely between different imaging tests. For example, the dose estimate from a chest radiograph is 0.02 mSv whereas the dose estimate from abdominal CT scan is considerably higher at around 10 mSv. To put this into context, a year's natural background radiation from cosmic and terrestrial sources equates to about 2–3 mSv.[3]

In patients where ionizing radiation is of particular concern, for example, pregnant patients and children, imaging modalities such as ultrasound and MRI which do not involve ionizing radiation should be used if possible in preference to high radiation dose tests such as CT.

Contrast Issues

Iodinated contrast medium is the most frequently used drug in medical imaging and is used in a number of important urological imaging tests such as CT and intravenous urography. Although generally considered to be safe, iodine contrast medium can provoke an allergic reaction in a small proportion of patients. The vast majority of adverse reactions are mild and self-limiting with serious reactions occurring in 0.04% of cases. Iodinated contrast is therefore contraindicated in patients with a history of allergy to iodine.

The other main concern in relation to iodinated contrast media is the risk of inducing contrast nephrotoxicity, which can lead to impairment of renal function. Contrast nephrotoxicity can be defined as an increase in serum creatinine by more than 25% or 44 µmol/L (0.5 mg/dL) within 3 days following the intravascular administration of iodinated contrast medium in the absence of an alternative cause.

In the majority of cases, impairment of renal function caused by iodinated contrast is thought to be transient and self-limiting. However, in patients with pre-existing renal

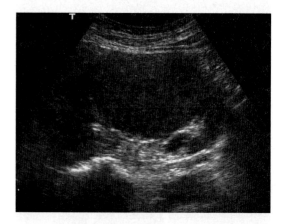

dysfunction, particularly in those with diabetic nephropathy, the administration of iodinated contrast can lead to severe deterioration in renal function. In order to minimize the risk of contrast nephrotoxicity, the serum creatinine should be checked before administration of iodine contrast in patients with suspected renal impairment. Precautions should be taken in high-risk patients to reduce the likelihood of contrast nephropathy. These include ensuring adequate hydration and the cessation of nephrotoxic drugs prior to administration of contrast.[4]

Caution is also advisable in diabetic patients taking Metformin undergoing contrast-enhanced studies. Metformin is excreted by the kidneys and in patients with renal dysfunction the administration of iodinated contrast leads to a small increase in the risk of lactic acidosis. The serum creatinine should therefore be checked in these patients and Metformin should be withdrawn in those with renal impairment prior to the administration of contrast. Careful subsequent monitoring of the renal function should be performed until the administration of Metformin can be recommenced safely.

Gadolinium-based contrast agents are commonly used in MRI examinations. Allergic reactions to Gadolinium are relatively rare however recent reports suggests a link between certain Gadolinium based contrast agents and nephrogenic systemic fibrosis (NSF). Clinical features of NSF include pain, pruritis and erythema later followed by thickening of the skin and subcutaneous tissues as well as life threatening fibrosis of the internal organs. Patients with end stage renal failure (GFR < 30 mL/min) are at higher risk of developing NSF and implicated Gadolinium-based contrast agents should not be used in this patient subgroup.[5]

Renal and Upper Tract Tumors

Renal masses can be benign or malignant. The most commonly encountered malignant renal mass is renal cell carcinoma. Other malignant tumors include transitional cell carcinoma, lymphoma, renal liposarcoma, and metastases. Benign renal tumors include oncocytoma and angiomyolipoma.

RCC

Renal cell carcinoma (RCC) is the most common malignant renal mass and accounts for 2–3% of all human malignancies.

Clinically, RCCs are often silent but may present with hematuria, flank pain, or a loin mass. Increasingly RCCs are being detected as incidental findings during imaging for other reasons.

Renal carcinoma tends to metastasize primarily to regional lymph nodes, lung, and bones. Metastases to liver, pancreas, and brain are less common.

On ultrasound renal cell carcinomas can be echogenic, iso echoic, or echopoor relative to the surrounding renal parenchyma and are usually associated with distortion of the normal renal architecture (Fig. 5.3). Sensitivity for tumor detection is low for tumors less than 2 cm in diameter.

CT is the preferred imaging modality for renal tumor characterization and staging.[6] The TNM staging of renal carcinoma is outlined in Table 5.1. The majority of renal cell carcinomas are well-defined, rounded, or lobulated masses which enhance heterogeneously, following contrast injection (Fig. 5.4). Regional retroperitoneal lymph nodes larger than 8 mm are regarded as suspicious. Tumor growth into the ipsilateral renal vein is a feature of renal cell carcinoma with occasional propagation into the IVC. Pulmonary and skeletal metastases (usually of the lytic type) are well demonstrated by CT.

Figure 5.3. Ultrasound demonstrates a well-circumscribed echopoor mass arising from the midpole of left kidney in keeping with a renal cell carcinoma.

Table 5.1. TNM staging of renal cell carcinoma

Primary tumor (T)	
T1	Tumor < 7 cm mass confined to kidney
T1a	Tumor < 4 cm
T1b	Tumor >4–7 cm
T2	Tumor > 7 cm mass confined to kidney
T3a	Tumor invasion into adrenal gland or perinephric fat but not beyond Gerotas fascia
T3b	Tumor invasion into renal vein or vena cava below diaphragm
T3c	Tumor invasion into vena cava above diaphragm
T4	Tumor Invasion beyond Gerotas fascia
Regional Nodes (N)	
NX	Regional lymph nodes cannot be assessed
N0	No regional node metastasis
N1	Metastasis in a single regional node
N2	Metastases in more than one regional node
Metastases (M)	
MX	Distant metastasis cannot be assessed
M0	No distant metastasis
M1	Distant metastasis

MRI is as sensitive as contrast-enhanced CT for the detection of renal tumors and is useful in the characterization of renal masses in those patients who cannot receive iodinated contrast media. MRI has an important role in the staging of advanced renal malignancy in defining the extent of inferior vena cava tumor thrombus extension associated with T3 disease[6] (Fig. 5.6). MRI is preferable to CT in younger patients requiring repeated studies to follow up renal masses (e.g., patients with Von Hippel Lindau disease) in order to avoid repeated radiation exposure.

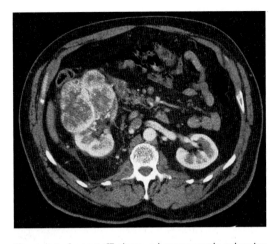

Figure 5.4. Contrast CT shows a heterogenously enhancing lobulated mass arising from the right kidney indicating a renal cell carcinoma.

Benign Renal Tumors

The most frequently occurring benign renal tumors are oncocytoma and angiomyolipoma. Oncocytoma appears as a well defined enhancing mass, the presence of a central 'scar' is a well recognised feature but is not specific enough to allow differentiation from renal cell carcinoma.

Angiomyolipoma (AML) is a benign renal tumor which consists of fat, muscle, and blood vessels. Multiple bilateral AMLs are associated with Tuberose Sclerosis. Angiomyolipomas are frequently seen as incidental lesions on ultrasound appearing as well-defined echogenic lesions. The presence of a fat containing renal mass on CT or MRI is considered diagnostic for AML (Fig. 5.5). Larger AMLs can undergo hemorrhage, and prophylactic embolization is a therapeutic option for lesions greater than 4 cm in diameter.

Transitional Cell Carcinoma

Transitional Cell Carcinomas (TCC) arise from the urothelium of the urinary tract. The commonest site is the urinary bladder, followed by the renal pelvis and ureter.

Clinically the commonest manifestation of TCC is microscopic or macroscopic hematuria. Flank pain may be due to "clot colic." Tumors occurring at or below the level of the renal pelvis may cause hydronephrosis due to renal obstruction.

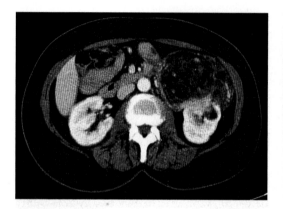

Figure 5.5. CT shows a large mass arising anteriorly from the left kidney. Abundant fat within the mass is consistent with angiomyolipoma.

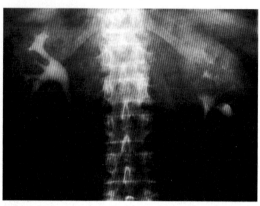

Figure 5.7. IVU demonstrates extensive filling defect within the left pelvicalyceal system in keeping with transitional cell carcinoma.

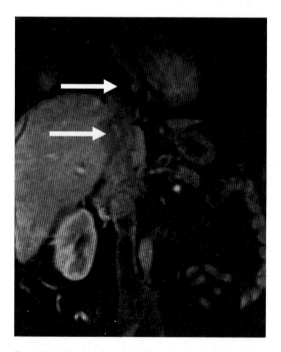

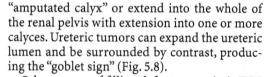

Figure 5.8. IVU demonstrates extensive lobulated filling defect (*arrow*) within the distal right ureter consistent with transitional cell carcinoma.

Figure 5.6. T3c renal tumor: MRI scan demonstrates tumor thrombus in the right renal vein and supra diaphragmatic IVC extension into the right atrium (*arrows*).

Urinary cytology may be positive but is an unreliable method for TCC detection.

TCCs appear as solitary or multifocal filling defects on IVU (Fig. 5.7). The appearances can be subtle with only slight irregularity of the mucosa. Larger tumors can occupy a complete calyx resulting in the appearance of an "amputated calyx" or extend into the whole of the renal pelvis with extension into one or more calyces. Ureteric tumors can expand the ureteric lumen and be surrounded by contrast, producing the "goblet sign" (Fig. 5.8).

Other causes of filling defects can mimic TCC and may therefore lead to diagnostic uncertainty. Commonly encountered causes are listed in Table 5.2, including pyeloureteritis cystica (Fig. 5.9).

Small tumors are not usually detectable on ultrasound. Larger TCCs can be identified as a

Table 5.2. Nonmalignant causes of upper tract filling defects

Thrombus

Sloughed papilla

Radiolucent calculus

Pyeloureteritis cystica

Fungus ball

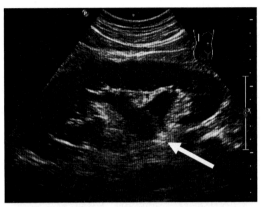

Figure 5.10. Ultrasound demonstrates a mass in the renal pelvis (*arrow*) causing slight hydronephrosis in keeping with transitional cell carcinoma.

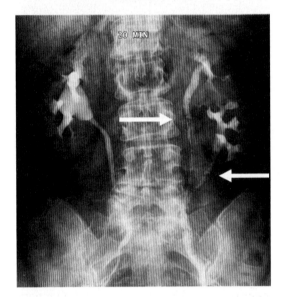

Figure 5.9. Pyeloureteritis cystica, submucosal cyst formation seen in association with chronic urinary tract infections. IVU shows multiple rounded filling defects (*arrows*) within the left renal pelvis and ureters in a duplex collecting system.

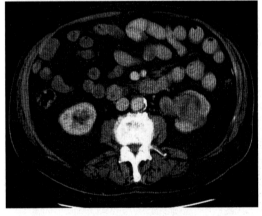

Figure 5.11. CT demonstrates a soft tissue mass on the left renal pelvis. The tumor occupies the renal sinus and is demonstrating to be extending into the renal parenchyma indicating invasive transitional cell carcinoma.

relatively echopoor mass within a calyx or renal pelvis (Fig. 5.10). Associated hydronephrosis may be a feature in obstructing lesions.

On CT, the diagnosis is made by the demonstration of an enhancing soft tissue mass within the renal collecting system or ureteric lumen (Figs.5.11 and 5.12). CT can usually distinguish between TCC and filling defects due to benign causes such as lucent stone and thrombus and is often used to clarify equivocal ultrasound or IVU appearances.

TCCs can enlarge and invade into renal parenchyma. More centrally situated tumors can invade beyond pelvic wall into the peripelvic fat and into adjacent retroperitoneal structures.[7]

Renal and proximal ureteric TCC typically spreads to para-aortic and paracaval lymph nodes whilst distal ureteric tumors spread to iliac and obturator nodes.

Retrograde studies are useful in those patients with suspicion of upper tract TCCs where noninvasive imaging studies have been inconclusive and can be combined with ureteroscopy to evaluate an abnormal ureter or pelvicalyceal system. The technique involves placing a retrograde catheter within the ureter via a cystoscope and subsequently injecting iodinated contrast directly into the ureteric lumen and collecting system (Fig. 5.13). The images thus obtained can be scrutinized to establish whether any mucosal abnormality or filling defect is present.

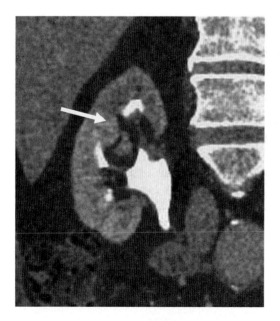

Figure 5.12. Right upper pole TCC identified on CT Urography (*arrow*).

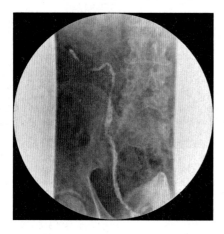

Figure 5.13. Retrograde ureterogram in a patient with severe hydronephrosis and macroscopic hematuria. Multiple irregular filling defects are identified throughout the ureter indicating extensive ureteric TCC.

Renal Mass Biopsy

If there is uncertainty about the nature of a renal mass, percutaneous image-guided biopsy can be performed. Image-guided renal biopsy can be performed under ultrasound, which allows the biopsy needle to be viewed in real time (Fig. 5.14), or under CT guidance. The sensitivity of biopsy for the diagnosis of malignancy is about 80–90%.[8]

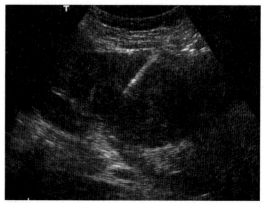

Figure 5.14. Ultrasound guided renal biopsy: Highly reflective biopsy needle can be identified within a renal mass.

A biopsy may be indicated in patients with a known extrarenal malignancy presenting with a renal mass in order to distinguish between a renal metastasis and primary renal tumor. Renal biopsy may also be helpful in the evaluation of an indeterminate renal mass where an inflammatory lesion or lymphoma is suspected.

Renal Stone Disease

Renal calculi are relatively common with an approximate incidence of 10% in the adult population. Recurrent urinary tract infections, renal structural anomalies (Table 5.3), such as medullary sponge kidney (Fig. 5.15), hypercalciuric states and urinary stasis predispose to an increased risk of stone formation.

Renal calculi are often detected in patients undergoing investigations for hematuria or urinary tract infections. Clinically, silent calculi may be detected incidentally during imaging tests for other reasons. Acute ureteric colic is a frequent presentation in patients with renal calculi. Although small calculi usually pass spontaneously, occlusive ureteric calculi left untreated may lead to obstructive nephropathy. Occasionally, obstructing ureteric calculi can lead to

Table 5.3. Upper tract structural abnormalities predisposing to stone formation

Medullary sponge kidney
Calyceal diverticulum
Pelvi-ureteric junction obstruction
Horseshoe kidney

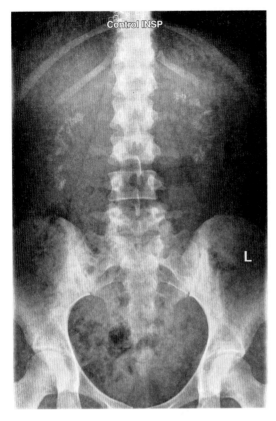

Figure 5.15. Medullary sponge kidney. An autosomal dominant condition in which calcifications develop within dilated ectatic renal collecting ducts. A characteristic appearance is seen on plain radiographs with multiple renal calculi distributed throughout the medulla.

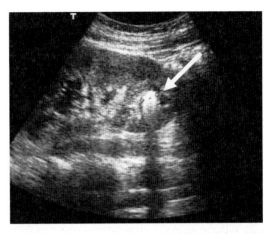

Figure 5.16. Ultrasound image demonstrating a calculus in the lower pole of left kidney (*arrow*) with associated acoustic shadowing.

life-threatening urosepsis. Accurate imaging is therefore essential for appropriate management.

Renal calculi can be imaged by plain radiographs, IVU, ultrasound, or CT. MRI, due to its inability to visualize calcified structures has no clearly defined role in the imaging of renal calculi.

Ultrasound

Renal calculi are often be detectable by ultrasound however visualisation of calculi can be inconsistent and unreliable.[9] Typically, renal calculi are seen as echogenic foci situated in the renal medulla with associated acoustic shadowing (Fig. 5.16).

In acute renal colic, ultrasound may demonstrate features indicating renal obstruction. This is usually suggested by the presence of hydronephrosis. Visualization of ureteric calculi is often problematic as the ureter is often obscured by overlying bowel gas. However, it may be possible to detect calculi at the pelviureteric junction or at the vesico ureteric junction.

Plain Radiographs and IVU

Plain radiographs have a sensitivity of 60% for renal calculus detection and are useful for the follow-up of patients with known radio-opaque calculi (Fig. 5.17). Combined with IVU, they can provide useful information about stone size, configuration, and anatomical position.

Calcium oxalate, calcium phosphate, and cysteine stones are generally visible on plain radiographs, whilst stones composed of uric acid, xanthine, and matrix material are radiolucent.

In acute renal colic, IVU usually demonstrates delayed contrast excretion from the affected kidney with associated hydronephrosis and hydroureter (Fig. 5.18). IVU for ureteric colic has in many centers been replaced by the use of CT-KUB.

CT

Non-contrast CT (NCCT) is the imaging test of choice for detection of renal calculi. With a sensitivity of over 98%, it has in many centers become established as the first-line test for patients with suspected renal colic. CT for ureteric colic does not require the use of intravenous contrast medium, thus avoiding the

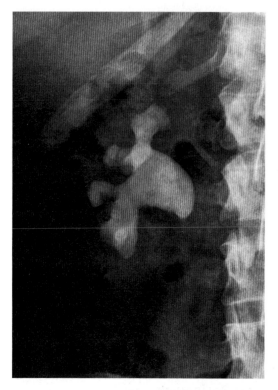

Figure 5.17. Plain radiograph demonstrating a right staghorn calculus.

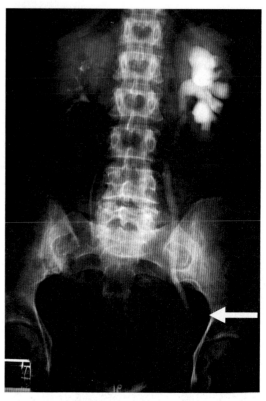

Figure 5.18. IVU image showing left hydronephrosis and hydroureter due to an obstructing distal left ureteric calculus (*arrow*).

potential risks of adverse reaction and contrast nephropathy.

Signs indicating renal colic include demonstration of ureteric calculus, hydronephrosis, hydroureter, renal enlargement, and soft tissue stranding in the perinephric fat[10] (Figs. 5.19 and 5.20). CT accurately demonstrates stone size which is relevant to management as the majority of stones less than 4mm in size will pass spontaneously, conversely calculi greater than 8 mm are unlikely to pass. Peri-ureteric calcifications can cause interpretational difficulties, in particular pelvic phleboliths, calcified concretions within thrombosed veins can lead to diagnostic uncertainty. The presence of a soft tissue rim representing ureteric edema surrounding a ureteric calculus is sometimes a helpful sign in differentiating a ureteric calculus from a phlebolith (Fig. 5.21).

The scout image can be evaluated for stone visibility in cases where ureteric stone is confirmed (Fig. 5.22). Visible stones can be followed up by plain radiographs.

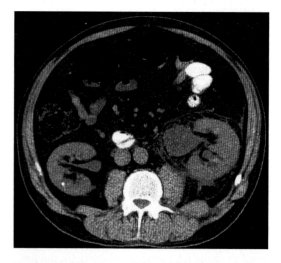

Figure 5.19. Non-contrast CT shows left-sided renal enlargement, hydronephrosis, and soft tissue stranding in the perinephric fat indicating acute renal obstruction. Incidental calculus seen in the right kidney.

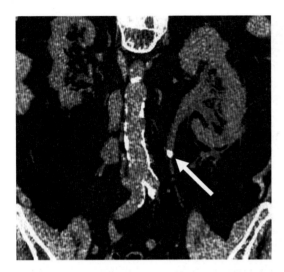

Figure 5.20. Coronal reformat image from a non-contrast CT demonstrates a left proximal mid ureteric calculus (*arrow*) causing renal obstruction.

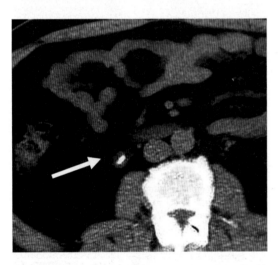

Figure 5.21. Mid-ureteric calculus on a non-contrast CT with associated "soft tissue rim sign" indicating ureteric edema.

CT can identify certain nonobstructive renal conditions and extrarenal pathologies, which can sometimes present with flank pain indistinguishable from ureteric colic (Table 5.4). It may be necessary in these cases to administer intravenous contrast to fully evaluate the underlying abnormality.[11]

For patients with complex stone disease CT urography provides useful information regarding stone morphology and renal anatomy. Postprocessing techniques allow construction of multiplanar reformats (Fig. 5.23) as well as detailed 3-D images. This facility is particularly useful for surgical planning in those patients with complex stone disease being considered for percutaneous nephrolithotomy or ureteroscopy.

Renal Cystic Disease

Benign Renal Cysts

Benign or "simple" renal cysts are common and may be seen in at least 50% of the population over the age of 60. The majority are situated in the renal cortex and are usually asymptomatic although larger cysts can enlarge leading to pressure symptoms. Occasionally, benign cysts become infected resulting in sepsis or undergo hemorrhage giving rise to flank pain. Symptomatic cysts can often be managed by radiologically guided percutaneous drainage.

On ultrasound, simple cysts are unilocular anechoic structures with associated posterior acoustic enhancement (Fig. 5.24). On CT they can be recognized as rounded non-enhancing homogenous fluid density structures. Renal cysts are not usually identifiable IVU, however larger cysts can result in lobulation of the renal outline or distortion the renal collecting system.

Hereditary Renal Cystic Disease

Adult polycystic kidney disease (APCKD) is an autosomal dominant condition, which usually presents in the third or fourth decade of life. Clinical features can include flank pain, hematuria, hypertension, or a palpable loin mass. There is gradual decline in renal function and need for long-term dialysis. Imaging demonstrates parenchymal replacement by numerous bilateral cysts throughout the renal cortex and medulla. The cysts tend to vary in size and content, often containing proteinaceous fluid or blood resulting in high attenuation on CT.

Von Hippel Lindau disease is also an autosomal dominant condition, which is characterized by the presence of retinal angiomas, central nervous system hemangioblastomas, and abdominal lesions. Renal tumors and cysts are important features of this condition. Unlike APCKD, the cysts are associated with increased risk of malignancy.

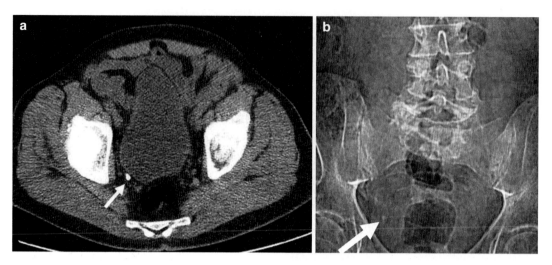

Figure 5.22. Paired images: (**a**) The axial CT image shoes a distal right ureteric calculus (*arrow*), which is clearly visible on the (**b**) accompanying scout image (*arrow*) indicating follow-up imaging by plain radiographs could be carried out if required.

Table 5.4. Nonobstructive renal and nonrenal causes of flank pain

Nonobstructive renal causes of flank pain
• Acute pyelonephritis
• Renal tumor
• Renal hemorrhage
• Renal infarction
• Renal vein thrombosis
Nonrenal causes of flank pain
• Appendicitis
• Diverticulitis
• Pelvic inflammatory disease
• Cholecystitis
• Aortic aneurysm

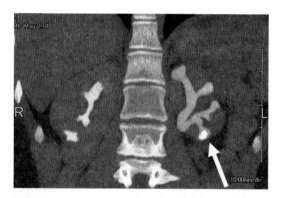

Figure 5.23. Coronal CT urography image demonstrating the presence of renal calculi within the left lower pole calyx. There is generalized left renal cortical atrophy.

Parapelvic renal cysts arise adjacent to the renal pelvis resulting in extrinsic compression of the renal collecting system. They tend to contain lymphatic fluid and are usually asymptomatic. On ultrasound they can be seen as rounded anechoic structures situated in the renal medulla.

Occasionally, parapelvic cysts can give rise to diagnostic confusion on ultrasound and on unenhanced CT as their appearance can be difficult to distinguish from hydronephrosis. On IVP, they may result in distortion and stretching of the pelvicalyceal system. Definitive diagnosis

can be made by CT urography, which opacifies the collecting system and allows the cysts to be identified separately (Fig. 5.25).

Complex Renal Cysts

Complex renal cysts demonstrate atypical features that may warrant follow-up or consideration of surgical removal. Atypical features include, increased wall thickness, nodularity, septations, calcification, or internal contents not typical for simple fluid. Complex renal cysts are usually evaluated by CT. MRI can also help further characterize complex cysts and may be useful as a supplementary test.

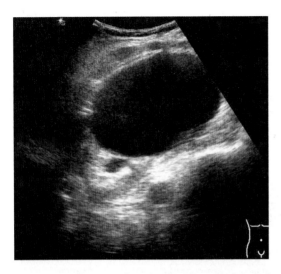

Figure 5.24. Ultrasound image demonstrating a benign renal cyst.

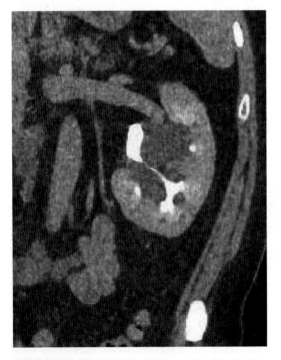

Figure 5.25. CT urography: Para pelvic cysts are seen as homogenous low attenuation structures adjacent to the opacified pelvicalyceal system.

The Bosniak classification, which is based on CT appearances is used to categorize renal cysts in increasing order of complexity and radiological concern (Table 5.5 and Fig. 5.26). Bosniak category 1 cysts are noncomplex renal cysts that can be safely regarded as benign and do not require follow-up. Bosniak category 2 lesions are cysts with subtle atypical features such as fine septations and minor calcification, these are also benign. Hemorrhagic cysts also fall into this category.

Bosniak 3 cysts are lesions which demonstrate prominent atypical features such as wall and septal thickening, nodularity, coarse calcifications and may also demonstrate enhancement. These are potentially malignant lesions that may warrant surgical removal. Bosniak 4 lesions are frankly malignant cystic masses.[12]

Class 2F lesions are cysts that cannot easily be classified as Bosniak 2 or 3 lesions, close follow-up imaging of these lesions is indicated.

Renal cysts may also occur in association with dialysis. These occur in up to 50% of patients on long-term hemodialysis. There is an increased risk of malignant change in these cysts.

Upper Tract Infective and Inflammatory Disease

Most patients with urinary tract infections do not require imaging investigations. However, imaging may be appropriate in those patients with severe recurrent infections to identify any underlying renal tract abnormality. Ultrasound is a useful first-line test to assess renal morphology and is frequently used to investigate patients with recurrent UTIs. IVU or CT urography may also be helpful in identifying any underlying upper tract abnormality.

Chronic pyelonephritis results in renal scarring, atrophy, and distortion of the renal calyces and is readily appreciated on ultrasound or CT.

Urosepsis: In this situation it is important to distinguish between pyelonephritis, which is treated medically from other causes of urosepsis such as, pyonephrosis, renal abscess, and emphysematous pyelonephritis, which may require surgical or radiological intervention.

Acute Pyelonephritis can be diffuse or focal. Characteristic changes on ultrasound include swelling of the kidney, reduced echogenicity as a result of parenchymal edema, and diminished vascularity. However, ultrasound is a relatively insensitive test for the assessment of acute pyelonephritis and may underestimate the severity of the disease.

Table 5.5. Bosniak classification of renal cysts

Category	CT features	Significance
Class 1	Water density, homogenous, noncalcified, smooth margin, no enhancing component	Benign
Class 2	Thin septae (<1 mm) , thin calcification (<1 mm), hemorrhagic cysts	Benign
Class 2F		Likely benign, follow-up imaging indicated
Class 3	Thick septa, thick wall, thick calcification, multilocular +/− enhancement	Approximately 50% malignant
Class 4	Enhancing solid mass component, i.e., cystic carcinomas	Definitely malignant

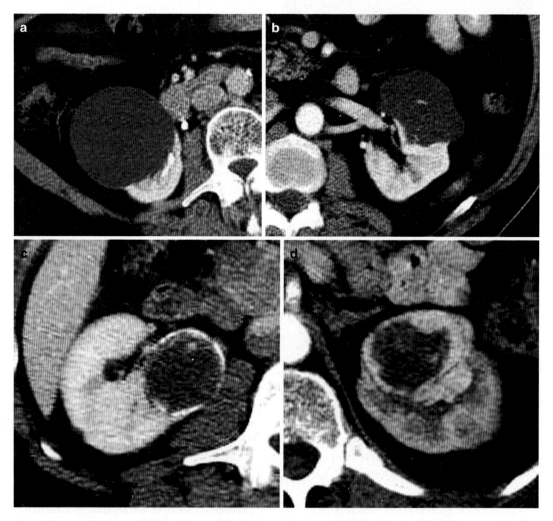

Figure 5.26. (**a–d**) Series of CT images showing various renal cysts. Image (**a**) shows a non-complex homogenous (Bosniak 1) renal cyst. Image (**b**) demonstrates a cyst containing fine septations (Bosniak 2 lesion). Cyst containing coarse calcification and soft tissue component (**c**) in keeping with a Bosniak 3 cyst. Image (**d**) demonstrates a malignant cystic mass (Bosniak 4 lesion).

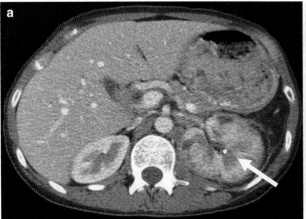
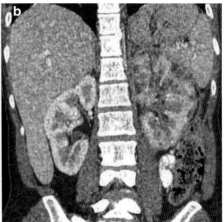

Figure 5.27. (a) Axial and (b) coronal CT images demonstrate diffuse abnormal enhancement and swelling of the left kidney with soft tissue stranding in the perinephric fat. Appearances are in keeping with acute pyelonephritis. Note also the presence of a small left renal calculus (*arrow*).

CT features of acute pyelonephtitis include patchy or wedge shaped low attenuation poorly enhancing areas within the renal parenchyma and swelling of the affected kidney often with inflammatory changes in the perinephric fat[13] (Fig. 5.27).

Renal abscess can arise secondary to severe pyelonephritis or may be associated with underlying stone or cystic disease. On ultrasound renal abscess can be recognized as a thick walled cystic structure, which may contain echogenic fluid indicating internal debris.

CT typically demonstrates a thick walled enhancing fluid containing structure (Fig. 5.28).

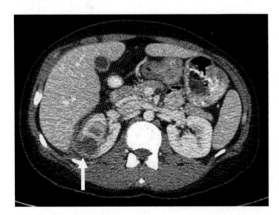

Figure 5.28. Thick walled fluid collection demonstrated in the upper pole of right kidney (*white arrow*) in patient with swinging pyrexia and leucocytosis, appearances indicate renal abscess.

The presence of gas within a renal fluid collection is virtually diagnostic for abscess.

Renal abscesses can be treated with antimicrobial therapy but percutaneous drainage may be necessary if conservative measures fail.

Emphysematous Pyelonephritis is a rare life-threatening condition in which there is severe renal infection resulting in gas formation within the renal parenchyma. The vast majority of cases (90%) are seen in diabetic patients. CT readily demonstrates abnormal renal enhancement and presence of gas in the renal parenchyma which is diagnostic for emphysematous pyelonephritis (Fig. 5.29). Nephrectomy is indicated if conservative measures fail.

Pyonephrosis: Pus in an obstructed renal collecting system can lead to life-threatening sepsis and is a urological emergency. Urgent decompression of the kidney either by nephrostomy drain or ureteric stent is indicated.

Pyonephrosis commonly occurs in kidneys obstructed by ureteric calculi although can occur secondary to any cause of renal obstruction. Ultrasound typically demonstrates hydronephrosis, which in the context of flank pain and pyrexia strongly suggests the diagnosis of pyonephrosis. Echogenic fluid within the collecting system or sedimented debris representing purulent material within the renal pelvis is also sometimes a feature (Fig. 5.30).

Xanthogranulomatous pyelonephritis (XPN) is an inflammatory renal condition associated with chronic urinary tract infection (usually caused

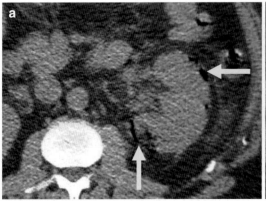

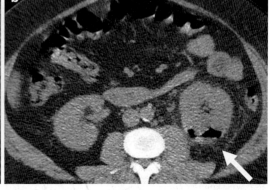

Figure 5.29. (a, b) CT scan images in a patient with poorly controlled diabetes and pyrexia of unknown origin. Pockets of gas are present in the renal parenchyma (*white arrow*) and perinephric space (*yellow arrows*) which confirm the diagnosis of emphysematous pyelonephritis. The patient was successfully treated with antibiotics and ureteric stent insertion. Images courtesy of Mr. Nigel Boucher (Consultant Urological Surgeon, Chesterfield Royal Infirmary).

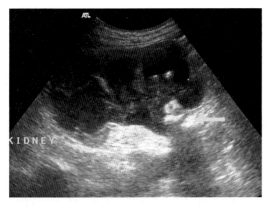

Figure 5.30. Ultrasound in a patient with loin pain and fever shows a severely hydronephrotic kidney with an obstructing calculus at the pelvi-ureteric junction (*yellow arrow*). Echogenic fluid is identified in the collecting system in keeping with pyonephrosis.

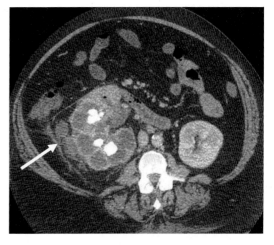

Figure 5.31. Xanthogranulomatous pyelonephritis CT scan demonstrates an enlarged inflamed kidney. Multiple renal calculi and abnormal parenchymal enhancement is shown. Note extension of infection into the perinephric fat (*arrow*).

by E. Coli or Proteus species). Histologically, the kidney is infiltrated by lipid laden macrophages, which destroy the normal renal parenchyma. Clinical features include flank pain and pyrexia. The condition is usually unilateral, more common in women and can be focal or diffuse.

CT usually demonstrates renal enlargement with replacement of normal renal parenchyma by areas of low attenuation of xanthomatous tissue (Fig. 5.31). Associated stone formation, usually of the staghorn type is seen in up to 80% of cases. Extrarenal extension of XPN into the perinephric fat, Gerotas fascia, and adjacent psoas muscle is a common feature.

Imaging of Upper Urinary Tract Obstruction

There are many causes for obstruction of the upper urinary tract, which can occur at any level between the pelvi ureteric junction and bladder. Causes can be divided into intrinsic pathology arising within the renal tract or extrinsic (Table 5.6). Hydronephrosis, dilatation of the pelvicalyceal system is the main imaging feature of renal obstruction. Depending on the

Table 5.6. Intrinsic and extrinsic causes of upper urinary tract obstruction

Intrinsic	Extrinsic
Calculus	Lymphadenopathy
Transitional cell carcinoma	Retroperitoneal fibrosis
PUJ obstruction Congenital megaureter	Pelvic cancer, e.g., prostate, rectosigmioid, cervix
Schistosomiasis, TB	Pregnancy
	Abdominal abscess
Prostatic carcinoma	Crossing vessels
Fungus ball	Endometriosis

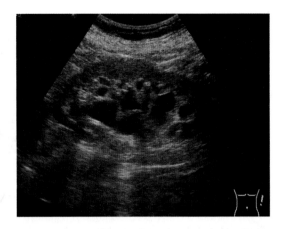

Figure 5.33. Parapelvic cysts: Commonly misinterpreted as hydronephrosis. The presence of noncommunicating anechoic areas with separating septations representing the walls of the cysts helps differentiate this appearance from hydronephrosis.

underlying etiology renal obstruction may lead to a gradual or acute deterioration in renal biochemistry.

Ultrasound has a sensitivity of almost 100% for the detection of hydronephrosis, which is easily appreciated as dilatation of the renal pelvis and calyces (Fig. 5.32) and is commonly performed as a first-line test in suspected renal obstruction.[14] Hydronephrosis, however, does not always indicate obstruction and is sometimes seen in well-hydrated patients and in those with bladder distension. Para pelvic cysts (Fig. 5.33), extra renal pelvis, and prominent renal vasculature can mimic hydronephrosis potentially leading to a false positive diagnosis

of renal obstruction. Cortical atrophy is usually seen in chronic obstructive uropathy.

Obstructing pelvic masses may be visible on ultrasound; however, the retroperitoneal structures are frequently obscured by overlying bowel gas and alternative imaging tests are often necessary to demonstrate the underlying obstructing pathology.

Delayed contrast excretion, a dense nephrogram, and hydronephrosis are the principal IVU features of acute obstruction (Fig. 5.34). Associated hydroureter may also be evident depending on the level of obstruction. Obstructing ureteric calculi and ureteric can often be identified. However, extrinsic causes of renal obstruction cannot in most cases be diagnosed by IVU. Absence of renal excretion is seen in cases of severe acute obstruction or chronic obstructive uropathy.

Unenhanced CT has a high sensitivity for the detection of renal calculi and is the most accurate imaging modality for investigation of suspected obstructing ureteric calculi[10]. CT urography can readily demonstrate obstructing ureteric tumors as well as extrinsic abdominal or pelvic masses. Hydronephrosis with associated reduced parenchymal enhancement and cortical atrophy are features of chronic obstructive uropathy (Fig. 5.35).

MRI is useful for the assessment of patients with renal obstruction in those patients with renal impairment or iodine contrast allergy. MRI is particularly valuable for the diagnosis

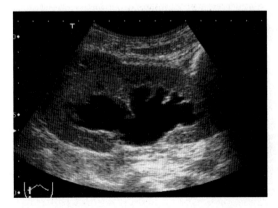

Figure 5.32. Hydronephrotic kidney demonstrated by ultrasound. The renal cortical thickness is preserved in keeping with acute obstruction.

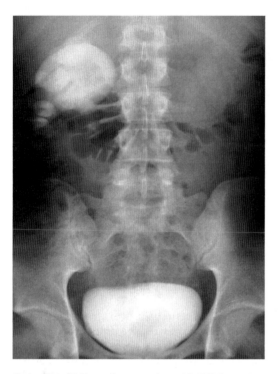

Figure 5.34. IVU image demonstrating a right PUJ obstruction.

and evaluation of pelvic masses and is superior to CT for the local staging of bladder and prostate tumors. Heavily T2-weighted sequences are utilized to demonstrate the degree and level of ureteric obstruction[15] (Fig. 5.36). The main disadvantage of MRI is its inability to adequately demonstrate obstructing ureteric calculi.

Management of Acute Renal Obstruction

Urgent decompression of the upper renal tracts is indicated in patients with renal obstruction resulting in acute renal failure or urosepsis. This can be achieved by percutaneous nephrostomy tube (Fig. 5.37) or ureteric stent insertion.

Percutaneous renal drainage via a nephrostomy tube involves the insertion of a catheter into the kidney under imaging guidance and results in rapid decompression of the collecting system.

Typically the procedure is performed under local anasthesia. Complications are uncommon but include renal hemorrhage, sepsis, and inadvertent damage to surrounding organs. Nephrostomy drains can be left in situ until definitive treatment of the underlying cause of obstruction is dealt with.

Ureteric stents provide internal drainage of the upper tracts and are usually inserted retrogradely via a cystoscope. The main advantages over nephrostomy tubes are patient convenience as external drainage bags are not needed and avoidance of trauma to the renal parenchyma with less risk of hemorrhagic complications. The procedure is usually performed under general anasthesia. Retrograde stent insertion may be difficult or impossible in patients with extensive pelvic malignancy, in these patients antegrade ureteric stent insertion via a nephrostomy track may be feasible.

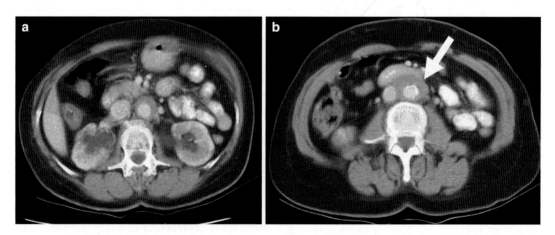

Figure 5.35. (**a, b**) Contrast-enhanced CT demonstrates bilateral hydronephrosis. A para-aortic soft tissue mass is shown (*arrow*) indicating retroperitoneal fibrosis.

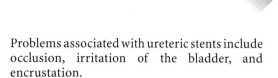

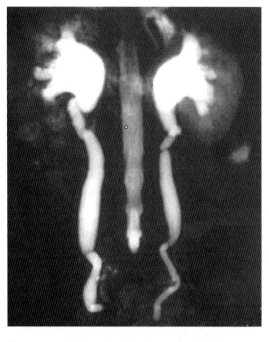

Figure 5.36. MRI T2 maximum intensity projection (MIP) image showing bilateral ureteric obstruction in a patient with underlying locally invasive endometrial carcinoma.

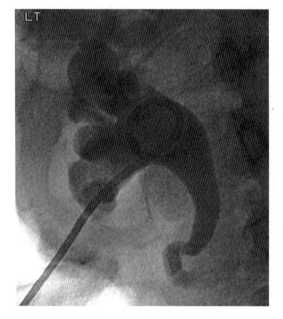

Figure 5.37. Nephrostomy drain: Pigtail lies within the renal pelvis.

Problems associated with ureteric stents include occlusion, irritation of the bladder, and encrustation.

Renal Trauma

Blunt accident-related abdominal trauma accounts for the majority of renal injuries. Penetrating injuries are less common. Renal injury can also occur iatrogenically during percutaneous, endourological, or open surgical procedures.

The kidneys are afforded some protection by the lower most ribs which overlie the posterolateral aspects of the renal upper poles. Ectopic kidneys, such as pelvic or horseshoe kidney and pathologically enlarged kidneys are at greater risk of injury.

Renal injuries vary in severity and can range from relatively minor requiring conservative management only to life-threatening injuries due to hemorrhagic shock (Table 5.7). Hematuria is a common feature of renal trauma but may be absent particularly in cases of ureteropelvic or renovascular injury.

Imaging is indicated following renal injury in the presence of macroscopic hematuria or microscopic hematuria with associated hypotension.

Table 5.7. The American Association for the surgery of trauma classification of renal injury

Grade 1	Cortical contusion, urological studies normal
Grade 2	Non-expanding perirenal hematoma – confined to retroperitoneum. Superficial cortical laceration < 1 cm, without urinary extravasation
Grade 3	Cortical laceration > 1 cm but no urinary extravasation
Grade 4	Cortical lacerations involving the collecting system
	Main renal artery or vein injury with contained hemorrhage
Grade 5	Shattered kidney
	Avulsion of the renal hilum with devascularized kidney

The majority (over 90%) of renal injuries are classified as minor and can be managed conservatively. Open exploration and possible nephrectomy is indicated in patients with persistent life-threatening hemorrhage[16].

Ultrasound can detect renal subcapsular hematomas and has a high sensitivity for demonstration of intraperitoneal blood. However, it is a relatively poor test for detecting renal lacerations and is therefore of limited value for the assessment of patients with suspected renal injury.

IVU can identify injuries involving the renal collecting system by demonstrating contrast extravasation. Renal parenchymal injuries however are not adequately demonstrated by IVU and its role has largely been replaced by CT.

Contrast-enhanced CT is the imaging modality of choice for assessment of renal trauma and can help differentiate between those injuries that can be managed conservatively from those that require surgical intervention.

Major renal trauma is frequently associated with injuries to the chest and other abdominal organs. CT can detect a wide range of intra-abdominal injuries and the study can be extended to include the thorax if required.

Post iv contrast studies are obtained to identify renal cortical laceration, vascular injuries and haematoma formation. These can be supplemented by delayed excretory phase images obtained 5-20 minutes following contrast injection if there is concern regarding injury to the collecting system.

CT accurately demonstrates parenchymal lacerations which are identified as hypoattenuating areas or perfusion defects within the renal cortex (Fig. 5.38). Major lacerations extend into the renal medulla and may involve the collecting system.

Subcapsular and perinephric hematoma can be recognized as a high attenuation collection adjacent to the renal cortex.

Vascular injuries can be serious and life-threatening. Trauma to the renal pedicle can result in renal artery occlusion leading to renal infarction (Fig. 5.39). Contrast-enhanced CT demonstrates abrupt occlusion of the renal artery with non-enhancement of the kidney indicating renal infarction. More serious injuries can result in avulsion of the renal pedicle leading to catastrophic hemorrhage.

AV fistula or pseudoaneurysm formation can occur following penetrating renal trauma (Fig. 5.40). Angiographic studies with a view to therapeutic embolization may be necessary in these types of injury.

Major renal trauma is frequently associated with injuries to the chest and other abdominal organs. CT can detect a wide range of intra-abdominal injuries and the study can be extended to include the thorax if required.

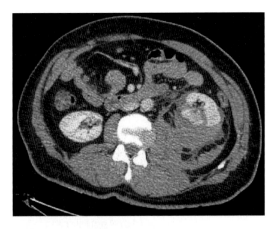

Figure 5.38. Grade 3 injury involving left kidney demonstrating a cortical laceration and retroperitoneal hematoma.

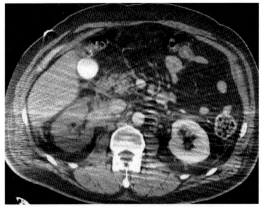

Figure 5.39. Non-enhancing right kidney as a result of traumatic infarction.

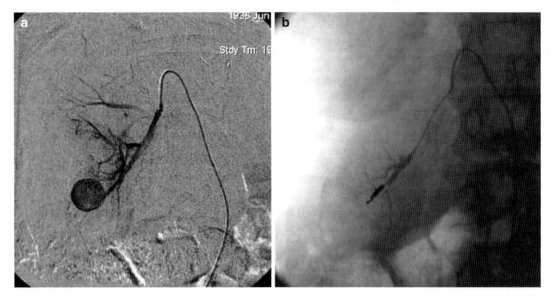

Figure 5.40. Catheter angiography demonstrating renal artery pseudoanurysm (**a**) following penetrating renal injury with subsequent successful therapeutic embolistaion (**b**).

References

1. Dyer RB, Chen MYM, et al. Intravenous urography: technique and interpretation. *RadioGraphics.* 2001;21: 799-824

2. Nolte-Ernsting C, Cowan N. Understanding multislice CT urography techniques – Many roads lead to Rome. *Eur Radiol.* 2006;16:2670-2686

3. Royal College of Radiologists. *Making the Best Use of a Department of Clinical Radiology.* 6th ed. London: RCR; 2007

4. European Society of Urogenital Radiology. Guidelines on Contrast Media. Version 7.0 2008

5. American College of Radiologists. *Manual on Contrast Media.* Version 6. 2008. www.acr.org

6. Coll DM, Smith RC. Update on radiological imaging of renal cell carcinoma. *BJU International.* 2007;99:1217-1222

7. Anderson EM, Murphy R, et al. Multidetector computed tomography urography (MDCTU) for diagnosing urothelial malignancy. *Clin Radiol.* 2007;62:324-332

8. Silverman SG, Gann YU. Renal masses in the adult patient: the role of percutaneous biopsy. *Radiology.* 2006;240(1):6-22

9. Fowler K, Locken J. US for detecting renal calculi with nonenhanced CT as a reference standard. *Radiology.* 2002;222:109-113

10. 10 Smith RC, Coll DM. Helical computed tomography in the diagnosis of ureteric colic. *BJU Int.* 2000;86 (Suppl 1):33-41

11. Talner L, Vaughan M. Nonobstructive renal causes of flank pain: findings on non-contrast helical CT (CT KUB). *Abdom Imaging.* 2003;28(2):210-216

12. Israel GM, Hindman N, Bosniak MA. Evaluation of cystic renal masses: comparison of CT and MR imaging by using the Bosniak classification system. *Radiology.* 2004;231:365-371

13. Stunnell H, Buckley O, et al. Imaging of acute pyelonephritis in the adult. *Eur Radiol.* 2007;17:1820-1828

14. Webb JAW. Ultrasonography and Doppler studies in the diagnosis of renal obstruction. *BJU Int.* 2000;86 (Suppl 1):25-32

15. Leyendecker JR, Barnes CE. MR Urography techniques and clinical applications. *Radiographics.* 2008;28:23-46

16. Heyns CF. Renal Trauma – Indications for imaging and surgical exploration. *BJU Int.* 2004;93:1165-1170

6

Principles of Bacterial Urinary Tract Infections and Antimicrobials

Florian M.E. Wagenlehner, Wolfgang Weidner, and Kurt G. Naber

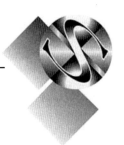

Introduction

Urinary tract infections (UTIs) are among the most prevalent microbial diseases, and their financial burden on society is substantial. A large part of antibiotic treatment is therefore allotted to UTIs. UTIs accounted for more than 100,000 hospital admissions annually in the USA, most often for pyelonephritis.[1,2] They also account for at least 40% of all hospital-acquired infections which are in the majority of cases catheter associated.[3-5]

UTIs can be classified into uncomplicated and complicated UTI. Uncomplicated UTI are those where complicating factors are not present. Complicated UTI in contrast is a very heterogenous entity, with a common pattern of complicating factors:

- Anatomical, structural, or functional alterations of the urinary tract (e.g., stents, urine transport disturbances, instrumentation of the urinary tract, stones, tumors, neurological disorders)
- Impaired renal function, by parenchymal diseases, or pre-, intra, or post-renal nephropathies (e.g., acute, chronic renal insufficiencies, heart insufficiency)
- Accompanying diseases that impair the patient's immune status (e.g., diabetes mellitus, liver insufficiency, immunosuppression, cancer, AIDS, hypothermia)

In uncomplicated UTI the virulence properties of the causative bacteria are the predominant factors leading to the infection, whereas in complicated UTI the host immune deficiency in its various forms is the leading cause.

Pathophysiology

Bacteria can reach the urinary tract by hematogenous or lymphatic spread, but there is abundant clinical and experimental evidence to show that the ascent of microorganisms from the urethra is the most common pathway leading to a UTI, especially organisms of enteric origin (i.e., *Escherichia coli* and other Enterobacteriaceae, enterococci). Therefore, UTI are more frequent in women than in men and there is an increased risk of infection following bladder catheterization or instrumentation. A single insertion of a catheter into the urinary bladder in ambulatory patients, for example, results in urinary infection in 1–2% of cases. It is thought that in those cases bacteria migrate within the mucopurulent space between the urethra and catheter leading to the development of bacteriuria in almost all patients within about 4 weeks.

The concept of bacterial virulence or pathogenicity in the urinary tract infers that not all bacterial species are equally capable of inducing infection. The more compromised the natural defense mechanisms (e.g., obstruction,

C.R. Chapple and W.D. Steers (eds.), *Practical Urology: Essential Principles and Practice*,
DOI: 10.1007/978-1-84882-034-0_6, © Springer-Verlag London Limited 2011

bladder catheterization), the fewer the virulence requirements of any bacterial strain to induce infection. This is supported by the well-documented in vitro observation that bacteria isolated from patients with a complicated UTI frequently fail to express typical virulence factors. The virulence concept also suggests that certain bacterial strains within a species are uniquely equipped with specialized virulence factors, for example, different types of pili, which facilitate the ascent of bacteria from the fecal flora, introitus vaginae or periurethral area up the urethra into the bladder, or less frequently, allow the organisms to reach the kidneys to induce systemic inflammation. In complicated UTI other factors may become more important, such as the ability of the bacteria to form biofilms. Biofilm has been defined as an accumulation of microorganisms and their extracellular products, forming a structured community on a surface. A biofilm infection develops not only around foreign body surfaces, such as urinary catheters or stents, but also in urinary stones, scars or necrotic tissues, obstructive uropathies, or even chronic bacterial prostatitis. In biofilm infection antimicrobial susceptibility of the pathogens is several-fold reduced when compared with planctonic or pure culture cells.[6]

This differentiation into uncomplicated and complicated UTIs is important for therapy. In uncomplicated UTI almost exclusively antibiotic treatment is required, whereas in complicated UTI, in addition to high-dosed antibiotic treatment, the removal of the complicating factor is essential.

Testing of Antimicrobials in the Laboratory

An antimicrobial agent is a drug that acts primarily against infectious organisms. The testing of an antimicrobial in the laboratory evaluates the in vitro interactions between an isolated microbe and antimicrobial agents that would be appropriate for treatment of an infection in vivo. This testing in the laboratory provides data to help the clinician decide whether an antimicrobial would be clinically efficient and the selected doses are adequate.

Susceptibility and Resistance

In the microbiological laboratory, cultured bacteria are usually tested for phenotypic expression of resistance mechanisms to direct the best antimicrobial treatment and to avoid ineffective treatment. The results of these tests are rendered to the practicing physician by categorized terms called susceptible, intermediate, and resistant. This information over the time merges in a local and regional surveillance of resistance and is therefore the guide for empiric antimicrobial treatment.

The cut-off concentrations used for the breakpoints can follow two different principals. The epidemiological breakpoint and the clinical breakpoint[7]:

- The epidemiological breakpoint is the cut-off concentration that delimits the wild-type population of a bacterial species of the non-wild-type population. For example, the antibacterial concentrations needed to inhibit bacterial growth (minimal inhibitory concentrations-MIC) differ in the bacterial populations. The epidemiological breakpoints can be used as the most sensitive measure of resistance development for measuring resistance development in hospitals and the community, for measuring the effect of interventions, and for developing strategies to counteract further resistance development.

- The clinical breakpoint is the cut-off concentration predicting if an antimicrobial treatment in a certain dosage will have clinical success. For example, based on pharmacological data, the predicted likelihood of antimicrobials at certain dosages to achieve clinical success in an individual patient is considered. The clinical breakpoints should be used in everyday clinical laboratory work to advice on therapy in the patient.

The clinical breakpoints have been internationally accepted and adapted. Until recently, however, significantly different standards were used all over the world. Harmonization in Europe was recently achieved by offering uniform standards in the EUCAST (European Committee on Antimicrobial Susceptibility Testing) definitions[7]:

Epidemiological Breakpoints

The epidemiological breakpoints are categorized into wild-type and non-wild-type microorganisms by applying the appropriate cut-off value in a defined phenotypic test system. Wild-type and non-wild type microorganisms may or may not respond clinically to antimicrobial treatment. These cut-off values will not be altered by changing circumstances.

- *Wild-type*: A microorganism is defined as wildtype for a species by the absence of acquired and mutational resistance mechanisms to the drug in question.
- *Microbiological resistance-non-wild type*: A microorganism is defined as non-wild type for a species by the presence of an acquired or mutational resistance mechanism to the drug in question.

Clinical Breakpoints

The clinical breakpoints are categorized into susceptible, intermediate, and resistant by applying the appropriate breakpoint in a defined phenotypic test system. These clinical breakpoints may be altered with legitimate changes in circumstances, such as new pharmacological data on antimicrobial substances.

- *Clinically susceptible* (S): A microorganism is defined as susceptible by a level of antimicrobial activity associated with a high likelihood of therapeutic success.
- *Clinically intermediate* (I): A microorganism is defined as intermediate by a level of antimicrobial agent activity associated with uncertain therapeutic effect. It implies that an infection due to the isolate may be appropriately treated in body sites where the drugs are physically concentrated or when a high dosage of drug can be used; it also indicates a buffer zone that should prevent small, uncontrolled, technical factors from causing major discrepancies in interpretations.
- *Clinically resistant* (R): A microorganism is defined as resistant by a level of antimicrobial activity associated with a high likelihood of therapeutic failure.

The establishment of clinical breakpoints implies the assessment of pharmacodynamic and pharmacokinetic parameters.

Pharmacodynamic Parameters

Pharmacodynamic parameters are those that describe the action of an antimicrobial at the bacterial cell. Several laboratory tests have been implemented to assess phenotypical pharmacodynamic parameters in vitro and thus predict the effectiveness of an antimicrobial therapy in vivo.

The primary aim of laboratory testing with antimicrobials is to predict therapeutic success in the individual patient treated. The most frequently used tests were designed to quantitate the lowest concentration of an antimicrobial that inhibits visible in vitro growth of the microbe, which is called the minimal inhibitory concentration (MIC). The MIC can be assessed by different tests, the most frequently used tests are the broth- and agar dilution tests. The disk diffusion procedure is a simplified method to approximate the MIC. The MIC is a parameter defined to predict therapeutic success, at least in an immunocompetent environment. The factors that determine the outcome of an infection are, however, complex and incompletely addressed by in vitro tests. A variety of factors can influence the efficacy of antimicrobials in vivo: Aminoglycosides or fluoroquinolones lose their activity in acidic pH as frequently found in urine or at sites of purulent infection. The concentrations of certain cations, such as Ca^{2+} or Mg^{2+}, which is extensively varying in urine, also influence the activity of aminoglycosides or fluoroquinolones in UTI. The MIC has therefore to be interpreted with caution.

The minimal bactericidal concentration (MBC) is defined as the lowest concentration of an antimicrobial that kills 99.9% of the inoculum. This test is not used in clinical routine with the exception of certain questions, such as treatment of infections in compartments deprived of the immune system, such as endocarditis, meningitis, or neutropenic situations. The MBC can also be used in situations where the medium to be tested is turbid, such as urine, where the inhibition of growth cannot be assessed.

Because of the worldwide increase of antibiotic resistance, a secondary aim in the treatment of infections has been defined for antimicrobial substances. Especially in the development of new antibiotics, substances with a low potential to cause emergence of antibiotic resistance are selected nowadays. One parameter that describes the probability of an antimicrobial substance is the mutant preventive concentration (MPC). The MPC is defined as the concentration needed to inhibit the emergence of resistant mutants among 10^{10} bacteria. The MPC might be a future parameter to assess antimicrobial substances and dosing.

Pharmacokinetic Parameters

The pharmacokinetic parameters describe the absorption, distribution, and elimination of an antimicrobial substance, which also includes metabolization of a substance. For simplification, the pharmacokinetic parameters are usually assessed in the blood. However, the pivotal target is the effective antibiotic concentration at the site of infection, which in case of urinary tract infections is the urine and the tissues of the urogenital organs (kidney, bladder, prostate). Additionally, modifying factors, such as protein binding, will influence the concentrations at the site of infection. Pharmacokinetics can also vary remarkably within the population and especially between the patients being the targets treated. Therefore, mathematical models such as the Monte-Carlo simulations are nowadays applied to transfer limited pharmacokinetic data from clinical studies to large population collectives and better reflect the interindividual variations.

Pharmacokinetic/Pharmacodynamic Correlations

The effect of an antimicrobial substance over the time at the site of infection is the most important pharmacological parameter reflecting therapeutic success. This aspect can be assessed in an integrated evaluation of the pharmacokinetic and pharmacodynamic parameters. In this regard pharmacokinetic parameters are often correlated with the MIC as the pharmacodynamic parameter (Fig. 6.1). Employing those evaluations it became evident that drug classes behave differently toward the pathogens at which they are directed:

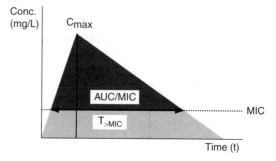

Figure 6.1. Association of pharmacokinetic and pharmacodynamic parameters in serum. C_{max} maximal concentration, *MIC* minimal inhibitory concentration, *AUC/MIC* area under the curve (AUC) over MIC, $T_{>MIC}$ time above MIC.

β-Lactam agents have their rate of killing maximized at a low multiple of the MIC, because the effect of β-lactams is dependent on their binding to the β-lactam-binding protein within the bacterial cell. The antibacterial effect only appears if a substantial portion of the binding proteins is already occupied by the β-lactam agent. At increasing drug concentrations, the effect quickly maximizes. Therefore, achieving higher drug concentrations does not result in greater killing. For β-lactam agents the best therapeutic results are obtained by using smaller doses more frequently during the day.[8]

Other antibiotic substances such as aminoglycosides or fluoroquinolones exhibit a concentration dependent post-antibiotic effect. For example, after the removal of the antibiotic there exists still an inhibitory effect on the bacterial cells. This inhibitory effect is greater the higher the initial concentration is. Therefore, for best therapeutic results those antibiotics are usually administered once or twice per day with high doses in order to achieve high peak concentrations (C_{max}) or a high area under the concentration time curve (AUC).

Bacterial Spectrum and Antimicrobial Resistance Patterns

The above mentioned aspects lead to a selection of antibiotic substances for the individual indication, such as UTI. In the next step a further selection is carried forward based upon the bacterial spectrum and the current antimicrobial resistance patterns. This is modified over the time depending on the development of bacterial resistance.

In uncomplicated UTI *E. coli* is the most common pathogen, typically being isolated from approximately 80% of outpatients with acute uncomplicated cystitis across the various regions of the world.[2,9-11]

A recent surveillance study, the ARESC (Antimicrobial Resistance Epidemiology Survey on Cystitis) project exclusively investigated female patients with uncomplicated cystitis.[12]

The results of this study showed that antibiotic substances classically used for the treatment of uncomplicated cystitis, such as TMP/SMX, fluoroquinolones or aminopenicillins, lose their effectiveness due to increasing resistance. Substances with high susceptibility rates were fosfomycin tromethamine, nitrofurantoin, or pivmecillinam.

In uncomplicated pyelonephritis, the identical resistance developments should be expected. For treatment, fluoroquinolones or group 3a cephalosporines might be suitable substances.

In complicated and nosocomially acquired UTI, Gram-negative species account for approximately 60–80% of the bacterial spectrum and comprises *E. coli*, followed by *Klebsiella* spp., *Pseudomonas* spp., *Proteus* spp., *Enterobacter* spp., and *Citrobacter* spp. The Gram-positive pathogens account for about 20–40% of the spectrum and comprise enterococci and staphylococci.[13-18]

Nosocomial uropathogens are frequently subject to antibiotic pressure and cross-infection. Different species of uropathogens show distinct abilities to develop antibiotic resistance.

Surveillance studies such as the SENTRY-, ESGNI- or PEP study, or a local urological surveillance study revealed that, considering the total bacterial spectrum investigated, in general the aminopenicillins (with β-lactamase inhibitors) showed resistance rates of approximately 60% (respectively 30%). TMP/SMX showed resistance rates between 22% and 45%. Resistance to ciprofloxacin was approximately 20–40%, to gentamicin 18–34%, to ceftazidime 13–28%, to piperacillin/ tazobactam 8–15%, to imipenem 7–14%. Resistance in enterococci to vancomycin was between 0% and 5%.[13-18] In all the studies, increasing rates of antibiotic resistance were found with specific species like *E. coli*,

P. aeruginosa, *Klebsiella spp.*, *Enterobacter spp.*, enterococci, and coagulase negative staphylococci. Extended-spectrum β-lactamase producing *E. coli* and *K. pneumoniae* rapidly increase and may cause significant clinical problems in the treatment of UTI.[19,20] Carbapenems fortunately still retained their activity in most of these uropathogens.

Election of an Antibiotic Treatment

The choice of an antibiotic and its dosage for the treatment of an infection depends on all those described aspects and parameters. Additionally, nowadays the different propensity of the antibiotics to cause so called collateral damages is also considered. Collateral damages are defined as ecological adverse effects of antibiotic therapy, namely, the selection of drug-resistant organisms and the unwanted development of colonization or infection with multidrug-resistant organisms. Different antibiotic classes have significantly different propensities to cause collateral damage. Cephalosporin use, for example, has been linked to subsequent infection with vancomycin-resistant enterococci, extended-spectrum beta-lactamase-producing (ESBL) *Klebsiella pneumoniae*, beta-lactam-resistant *Acinetobacter* species, and *Clostridium difficile*. Quinolone use has been linked to infection with methicillin-resistant *Staphylococcus aureus* (MRSA) and with increasing quinolone resistance in Gram-negative bacilli, such as *Pseudomonas aeruginosa*.[21]

To incorporate these different aspects into a concept of antimicrobial chemotherapy of UTIs, for uncomplicated UTIs and especially uncomplicated cystitis, antimicrobials exclusively used for this indication are recommended. For complicated UTIs antibiotics with optimal activity in the urinary tract and high dosage are recommended.

Uncomplicated, Community Acquired UTI

Ideal substances are those with high susceptibility rates, exclusively used for this indication, such as fosfomycin tromethamine, nitrofurantoin or pivmecillinam for the treatment of uncomplicated cystitis (Table 6.1).

Table 6.1. Groups and dosages of elected antibiotics for the treatment of uncomplicated cystitis

Antibiotic groups[a]	Antimicrobial substance	Dosage/ duration Oral
Fosfomycines		
	Fosfomycin trometamol	3,000 mg/ single dose
Nitrofuranes		
	Nitrofurantoin retard	2 × 100 mg/ 5–7 days
Amidinopenicillins		
	Pivmecillinam	2 × 200 mg/ 7 days

[a]Cotrimoxazole and fluoroquinolones not regarded as first-line agents.

Fosfomycin

Fosfomycin acts as an analogue of phosphoenolpyruvate and forms a covalent bond with the active site cysteine residue (Cys 115) of UDP-*N*-acetylglucosamine enolpyruvyltransferase (MurA), which is a key enzyme of peptidoglycan synthesis.[22] It thus inhibits cell-wall synthesis other than β-lactam antibiotics. Fosfomycine tromethamine has approximately 40% oral bioavailability and is primarily excreted unchanged in the urine (approximately 90%).[23] The substance is active against Gram-positive and Gram-negative bacteria, but shows decreased activity against *M. morganii*, *P. vulgaris*, *P. aeruginosa* and *E. faecium*.

Nitrofurantoin

Nitrofurantoin belongs to the nitroheterocyclic compounds. The nitrogroup coupled onto the heterocyclic furan ring represents the proper site of effect. The nitrogroup is inactive and has to be activated by microbial nitroreductases after penetration into the microbial cell.[24] Nitrofurantoin interferes with the carbohydrate metabolism. The bioavailability is about 90% and the urinary excretion is 40%.[25] Susceptibility against *E. coli* is excellent, against gram-negative pathogens other than *E. coli.*, like *Klebsiella* spp. or *Enterobacter* spp. reduced. There is no activity against *Proteus* spp. or *P. aeruginosa*.[26] Nitrofurantoin is nowadays mainly used in preventing recurrent urinary tract infections in children and women.[27] Potential severe side effects with nitrofurantoin were reported, such as lung- and hepatotoxicity, especially in long-term usage.[28]

Pivmecillinam

Pivmecillinam is a β-lactam antimicrobial that has been used for the treatment of acute uncomplicated urinary infection for more than 20 years. Pivmecillinam is the prodrug (ester) of mecillinam and shows no antibacterial activity until transformed into the active drug after absorption.[29] Mecillinam is an amidine derivative of the penicillin group. The mechanism of action differs slightly from other β-lactams, because it interacts with the penicillin-binding protein 2.[30] With a bioavailability of 60–75% it is well absorbed orally and 45% are excreted in the urine.[29] Mecillinam has high activity against Gram-negative organisms such as *E. coli* and other Enterobacteriaceae. *S. saprophyticus* is considered resistant.

Complicated and Nosocomially Acquired UTI

A wide variety of antibiotic agents is available for the treatment of complicated and nosocomially acquired UTI (Table 6.2). The election of the antibiotics for treatment should follow regional surveillance studies. Additionally, all substances suitable for treatment should be used in order to decrease the antibiotic pressure of individual substances.

β-Lactam-Antibiotics

β-Lactam antibiotics are chemically characterized by the presence of the β-lactam in the molecule, which is a cyclic amide forming a four-atom ring. All β-lactam antibiotics inhibit the bacterial cell wall synthesis by irreversible inhibition of the transpeptidases known as penicillin binding proteins. The β-lactam group includes three important families of antibiotics, which differ in the moiety fused to the β-lactam ring. The penicillins harbor a five-atom ring, a thiazolidine, the cephalosporins have a six-atom ring, a dihydrothiazine, and the carbapenems harbor a five-atom ring, in which the sulfur atom in position 1 of the structure has been replaced with a carbon atom.[31]

PRINCIPLES OF BACTERIAL URINARY TRACT INFECTIONS AND ANTIMICROBIALS

Table 6.2 Groups and dosages of elected antibiotics for the treatment of complicated UTI and uncomplicated pyelonephritis

Antibiotic groups	Antimicrobial substance	Dosage	
		Oral	I.V/I.M
β-Lactams			
Aminopenicillin + BLI	Ampicillin/sulbactam	2 × 750 mg	3 × 0.75–3 g
	Amoxicillin/clavulanic acid	2 × 1 g	3 × 1.2–2.2 g
Acylureidopenicillin + BLI	Piperacillin/tazobactam	–	3 × 2.5–4.5 g
	Piperacillin/combactam	–	3 × 5 g
Cephalosporin Gr. 1	Cephalexin	For prophylaxis only	–
Cephalosporin Gr. 2	Cefuroxime axetil	2 × 250–500 mg	–
	Cefuroxime	–	3 × 0.75–1.5 g
	Cefotiam	–	2–3 × 1–2 g
Cephalosporin Gr. 3	Cefpodoxim proxetile	2 × 200 mg	–
	Ceftibuten	1 × 200-400 mg	–
Cephalosporin Gr. 3a	Cefotaxime	–	2–3 × 1–2 g
	Cetriaxone	–	1 × 1–2 g
Cephalosporin Gr. 3b	Ceftazidime	–	2–3 × 1–2 g
Cephalosporin Gr. 4	Cefepime	–	2 × 2 g
Carbapenem Gr. 1	Imipenem	–	3 × 500 mg
	Meropenem	–	3 × 500 mg
Carbapenem Gr. 2	Ertapenem	–	1 × 400 mg
Fluoroquinolone Gr. 2	Ciprofloxacin	2 × 500–750 mg	2 × 400–600 mg
Fluoroquinolone Gr. 3	Levofloxacin	1-2 × 500 mg	1–2 × 500 mg
Pyrimethamines			
Trimethoprim		2 × 200 mg	
Trimethoprim +		2 × 160 mg+	
Sulfamethoxazole		2 × 800 mg	
Aminoglycoside	Gentamicin	–	1 × 5–7 mg/KG
	Tobramycin	–	1 × 5–7 mg/KG
	Amikacin	–	1 × 15 mg/KG
Oxazolidinones			
Oxazolidinone	Linezolid	2 × 600 mg	2 × 600 mg/kg
Glycopeptides			
Glycopeptide	Vancomycin	–	2 × 1,000 mg
	Teicoplanin	–	1 × 400 mg

BLI beta-lactamase inhibitor; *KG* body weight.

Penicillins

Penicillins are classified mainly according to the different chemical structures of the substituents at position 6 of the β-lactam molecule.

Penicillin G is primarily active against Gram positive pathogens, if no resistance mechanisms have been acquired.[31]

The aminopenicillins ampicillin and amoxicillin feature the amino group, which confers stability against amidase, an enzyme produced by some Gram-negative bacteria that hydrolyzes the penicillin side chain, and stability against gastric acid. Oral absorption of ampicillin is approximately 50%, whereas amoxycillin is absorbed 90%. Urinary excretion of both antibiotics is about 70%. The aminopenicillins ampicillin and amoxycillin are active against *E. coli* and *P. mirabilis*, but almost inactive against other enterobacteria and totally inactive against *Pseudomonas* spp. The aminopenicillins are not stable against the β-lactamases frequently found in *S. aureus* and many enterobacteria. Combination with a β-lactamase-inhibitor such as clavulanic acid or sulbactam enhances Gram-negative activity to a certain extent, but not against bacteria producing AmpC β-lactamases, such as *Enterobacter* spp. or *Citrobacter* spp.[32]

The acylamino (ureido)-penicillins, such as piperacillin, own stronger polar groups on the amino-group. However, the compound is not stable against the β-lactamases of *S. aureus* and some strains of *Enterobacter* spp. and *Serratia* spp. Combination of piperacillin with the β-lactamase inhibitor tazobactam can counteract some of the β-lactamases increasingly produced by Gram-negative bacteria. Urinary excretion of both, piperacillin and tazobactam is approximately 70%. Piperacillin exhibits activity against *Pseudomonas* spp. and *Proteus vulgaris*.[33]

Cephalosporins

The cephalosporins are classified according to their primary route of administration (parenteral vs. oral), and in groups according to their antibacterial spectrum. For structure activity relationships, comparable characteristics can be seen as with penicillins. Substitutions at the side chain mainly influence activity, whereas modifications in position 3 of the nucleus influence mainly pharmacokinetics. The various groups of cephalosporins differ from one another in the spectrum of activity and in potency against Gram-negative bacilli.[34]

The first group cephalosporin cephalexin harbors the phenylglycine side chain that is also encountered in the aminopenicillins. Cephalexin is primarily active against staphylococci, but less active against many Gram-negative bacteria, because it is hydrolyzed by their β-lactamases. The bioavailability of cephalexin is about 90%, and the renal excretion is about 90% either.[35] First group cephalosporins should however not be used for the treatment of UTI, but only for prophylaxis, because of the overall lower activities compared with second group cephalosporins.

Second group cephalosporins such as cefuroxime and cefotiam show an increased β-lactamase stability. This is mainly due to the oxime-group in cefuroxime and the thiazoleamino group in cefotiam. After intravenous injection the renal excretion is 90% in cefuroxime[36] and 70% in cefotiam.[37] In contrast to cefuroxime, the prodrug cefuroxime axetil is resorbed with a total bioavailability of 40% after rapid hydrolysis to the active parent compound, cefuroxime.[38] These cephalosporins show an enhanced activity against some Gram-negative uropathogens. Against susceptible Gram-negative bacteria, second group cephalosporins are four to eight times more potent than first group compounds. There is no activity against *P. vulgaris*, *Morganella* spp., *Serratia* spp., and *P. aeruginosa*. Cefotiam is more active against *E. coli*, *Klebsiella* spp., and *P. mirabilis* than cefuroxime.

Cephalosporins of the group 3a such as cefotaxime and ceftriaxone, and the orally active substances cefpodoxime-proxetil and ceftibuten exhibit a further increased activity against Gram-negative organisms, because the side chain protects the molecule from cephalosporinases by steric hindrance.[39] Cefotaxime is metabolized in about 30% to desacetylcefotaxime, which shows inferiorer antimicrobiological activitiy.[40] Ceftriaxone undergoes a partial biliar excretion of about 45%.[41] The bioavailability of cefpodoxime-proxetil is about 40%,[42] while the bioavailability of ceftibuten is about 90%.[43] The renal excretion rates are about 80%, 55%, 90%, and 90% for cefotaxime, ceftriaxone, cefpodoxime, and ceftibuten, respectively.[40-43] Third group cephalosporins are approximately ten times more active than the second group cephalosporins against Gram-negative pathogens.

Cephalosporins group 3b comprises the intravenously administered ceftazidime. The propylcarboxy moiety at the side chain is responsible for increased affinity to penicillin-binding-proteins of Gram-negative bacilli and a high stability to β-lactamases. The pyridine group is responsible for rapid intrabacterial penetration and favorable pharmacokinetic properties. Ceftazidime underlies no relevant metabolism and the unchanged urinary excretion averages 90%. Compared to cefotaxime, ceftazidime exhibits a tenfold increased activity against *P. aeruginosa*.[44]

Group 4 cephalosporins comprise the intravenously administered cefepime. It contains a thiazole-amino group and an oxime group at position 7 and a quaternary ammonium substituent at position 3. The quaternary nitrogen imparts β-lactamase stability and improves both the cell penetration and the pharmacokinetic properties. The urinary excretion of the unchanged drug accounts for about 85%. Cefepime shows excellent activity against *P. aeruginosa* and good stability against β-lactamases.[45]

Carbapenems

Carbapenems maintain antibacterial efficacy against the vast majority of β-lactamase-producing organisms. This stability against serine-β-lactamases is due to the trans-1-hydroxyethyl substituent and its unique juxtaposition to the β-lactam carbonyl group.[46] The stability encompasses extended spectrum-β-lactamases and AmpC β-lactamases; however, it does not extend to metallo-β-lactamases. The classification of carbapenems can be done by groups and follows the bacterial spectrum as in other antibiotic classes.[47]

According to that, ertapenem is the sole representative of the first group. It contains a 1β-methyl substituent which reduces hydrolysis of the β-lactam group by the renal dihydropeptidase I. It further contains a meta-substituted benzoic acid substituent, which increases the molecular weight and lipophilicity of the substance, and a carboxylic acid moiety resulting in a net negative charge. This results in a high protein binding, which leads to a longer serum half-life.[46] Urinary excretion is 80%. Ertapenem exhibits a broad spectrum activity against Gram-negative and Gram-positive pathogens, with only limited activity against non-fermenting Gram-negative bacteria. It is also not active against *P. aeruginosa*, MRSA, and enterococci.[46,47]

Imipenem and meropenem are the representatives of the second group. Imipenem is hydrolyzed by the renal dihydropeptidase I and is therefore combined with the specific inhibitor cilastatin. Meropenem contains the 1β-methyl-substituent and is therefore stable against the renal dihydropeptidase I. Urinary excretion of imipenem (if combined with cilastatin) and meropenem is 70%. They feature an additional broad-spectrum activity against non-fermenting Gram-negative bacteria. They are active against many Gram-positive and Gram-negative uropathogens excluding MRSA, *E. faecium*, and vancomycin-resistant enterococci (VRE). Compared with imipenem, meropenem is somewhat more active against *P. aeruginosa*, but less active against Gram-positive uropathogens.[48]

Aminoglycosides

Aminoglycosides are multifunctional hydrophilic sugars that possess several amino and hydroxy functionalities. Aminoglycosides act primarily by impairing bacterial protein synthesis through binding to prokaryotic ribosomes.[49] The aminoglycoside antibiotics can be divided according to the nature of the core aminocyclitol ring into streptidine, bluensidine, 2-deoxystreptamine, and actinamine antibiotics. Clinically, the 2-deoxystreptamine-containing aminoglycosides are most important, which are subdivided into the 4,6-disubstituted, and the 4,5-disubstituted deoxystreptamines.[49-51] The 4,6-disubstituted deoxystreptamine group comprises the agents kanamycin, gentamicin, tobramycin, netilmicin, and amikacin. The 4,5-disubstituted deoxystreptamine group comprises agents such as neomycin, which are the more potent antibiotics, but show a high degree of nephrotoxicity and ototoxicity, which almost exclusively prevents their systemic use.[50,51] For treatment of UTI, therefore, only the 4,6-disubstituted deoxystreptamine group is indicated. Antibiotic activity in this group is related to the number and location of amino groups in the hexose moiety linked to the deoxystreptamine as follows in decreasing order: 2′,6′-diamino > 6′-amino > 2′-amino > no amino group. The activity is enhanced if the same primed sugar is not hydroxylated, thus gentamicins are generally more active than kanamycins.[49] In parallel, the more active substances, however, are better substrates for inactivating nucleotidyltransferases. Because of the aminocyclitol ring the aminoglycosides are basic molecules and have a high degree of solubility in water and poor solubility in lipids. They are therefore poorly absorbed and distributed in the tissues and they must be actively transported across the bacterial cell membrane. Aminoglycosides are almost exclusively excreted in the urine by glomerular filtration, but approximately 5% of the administered dose is retained in the epithelial cells lining the S1 and S2 segments of the proximal tubules.[51] The aminoglycosides thus accumulate in the lysosomes of the tubular cells. This accumulation in renal tubular cells renders aminoglycosides suitable for treatment of pyelonephritis, but eventually also causes the lysosomes to rupture above a certain cut-off concentration. The highly concentrated aminoglycoside together with the lysosomal enzymes are then released into the cytosol and eventually lead to cell damage and is the reason for nephrotoxicity.

Fluoroquinolones

Fluoroquinolones can be classified according to antibacterial spectrum and activity and the main indications into four groups.[52] Among the agents frequently used for the treatment of UTI, the first group comprises agents such as norfloxacin, with indications essentially limited to UTI. The second group encompasses agents such as ofloxacin and ciprofloxacin with broad indications for systemic use and predominant Gram-negative activity. The third group comprises agents such as levofloxacin with good Gram-negative activity and, in addition, improved activity against Gram-positive and atypical pathogens, and the fourth group comprises agents with good Gram-negative activity and, in addition, further improved activity against Gram-positive and atypical and anaerobic bacteria, such as moxifloxacin.

Fluoroquinolones form ternary complexes between DNA and the bacterial topoisomerases II and IV, which play a critical role in the organization of the bacterial DNA. Thus the DNA destabilizes and consequently apoptosis of the bacterial cell is induced.[53] The structure-property relationships of the different substituents corresponding to the pharmacophore show the following aspects[53]: Elements that enhance activity and reduce resistance selection include a cyclopropyl at position 1, a methoxy at position 8, a pyrrolidine or substituted piperazine at position 7, and a fluor substituent at position 6.[53] Moieties or elements that enhance the volume of distribution are a cyclopropyl at position 1, and those that enhance half-life and central nervous system penetration are a bulky side chain at position 7.[53] Fluoroquinolones work mainly in a concentration-dependent manner and exert a marked post-antibiotic effect. The antibacterial activity in urine however is reduced, because fluoroquinolones form antibacterially inactive/less active complexes with divalent cations.[54]

Most fluoroquinolones show excellent bioavailability (60–100%) and a high volume of distribution. Penetration into the prostate tissue is better than any other antibiotic substance. The serum levels are usually low.[53] The urinary excretion of fluoroquinolones differs widely between substances. A high urinary excretion (≥75%) can be observed with levofloxacin (84%), lomefloxacin (75%), and ofloxacin (81%). An intermediate excretion rate (40–74%) is seen with ciprofloxacin (43%), enoxacin (53%), fleroxacin (67%), and a low excretion rate (<40%) is seen with moxifloxacin (20%) and norfloxacin (20%).[55]

Trimethoprim, Cotrimoxazole

Cotrimoxazole is the combination of trimethoprim (TMP) and sulfamethoxazole (SMX) in the ratio of 1:5. Both substances inhibit different steps in the folic acid biosynthetic pathway. SMX is a structural analogue of *p*-aminobenzoic acid, the basic building block used by bacteria to synthesize dihydrofolic acid, the first step in the reaction leading to folic acid. SMX competitively inhibits this step. TMP competitively prevents the conversion of dihydrofolic acid to tetrahydrofolic acid, the metabolically active cofactor for synthesis of purines.[56] Of all sulfonamides, SMX was paired with TMP because of similar absorptive and pharmacodynamic properties. Each drug is well absorbed. Approximately 85% of total SMX is recovered in the urine, 30% as free drug and the rest as acetylated metabolite. Similarly, most of TMP is not metabolized and is excreted unchanged in the urine.[56] Many aerobic Gram-positive and Gram-negative bacteria are inhibited or killed including *E. coli, Proteus mirabilis, Klebsiella* spp., and *Enterobacter* spp. There is no effect on *Pseudomonas* spp. In complicated UTIs TMP/SMX should only be used in accordance with sensitivity testing because of the high resistance rates.

Glycopeptides

The glycopeptides (vancomycin, teicoplanin) inhibit the synthesis of cell walls in susceptible microbes by inhibiting peptidoglycan synthesis. Vancomycin and teicoplanin are related substances. Teicoplanin is more lipophilic. Both substances are administered intravenously. Teicoplanin has an increased half-life compared to vancomycin, as well as a better tissue penetration. The urinary excretion of both substances is 90%. They are active exclusively against Gram-positive uropathogens, such as enterococci and methicillin susceptible and resistant staphylococci.[57]

Linezolid

Linezolid is a member of the oxazolidinone class synthetic antibacterial agents that inhibit bacterial protein synthesis through a unique mechanism. In contrast to other inhibitors of protein synthesis, linezolid acts early in translation by preventing the formation of a functional initiation complex.[58] Linezolid is rapidly absorbed after oral dosing with an absolute bioavailability of about 100%. Serum half-life is about 5.5 h, and protein binding approximately 31%.[59,60] Approximately, 35% is excreted in urine as the parent drug and 50% as the two major metabolites. However, linezolid is active exclusively against Gram-positive uropathogens, such as enterococci and methicillin susceptible and resistant staphylococci. Linezolid can be used for the treatment of UTIs caused by multiresistant Gram-positive bacteria like MRSA or VRE.

Conclusion

Development of resistance in the treatment of UTI is dramatically increasing. Therefore, the basis of anti-infective therapy, the action of current available antimicrobial substances and the structure-property relationships have to be understood for the prudent use of antibiotics. Pharmacokinetic and pharmacodynamic parameters should be used to improve dosing. The potential to induce resistance of certain antibiotic substances should be more investigated. Substances with a low potential should be preferred.

Considering this, the management of infectious diseases must be highly responsible.

References

1. Foxman B. Epidemiology of urinary tract infections: incidence, morbidity, and economic costs. *Am J Med.* 2002;113(Suppl 1A):S5-S15
2. Warren JW, Abrutyn E, Hebel JR, Johnson JR, Schaeffer AJ, Stamm WE. Guidelines for antimicrobial treatment of uncomplicated acute bacterial cystitis and acute pyelonephritis in women. Infectious Diseases Society of America (IDSA). *Clin Infect Dis.* 1999;29(4):745-758
3. Gales AC, Jones RN, Gordon KA, et al. Activity and spectrum of 22 antimicrobial agents tested against urinary tract infection pathogens in hospitalized patients in Latin America: report from the second year of the SENTRY antimicrobial surveillance program (1998). *J Antimicrob Chemother.* 2000;45(3): 295-303
4. Ruden H, Gastmeier P, Daschner FD, Schumacher M. Nosocomial and community-acquired infections in germany. Summary of the results of the first national prevalence study (NIDEP). *Infection.* 1997;25(4):199-202
5. Maki DG, Tambyah PA. Engineering out the risk for infection with urinary catheters. *Emerg Infect Dis.* March/April 2001;7(2):342-347
6. Goto T, Nakame Y, Nishida M, Ohi Y. Bacterial biofilms and catheters in experimental urinary tract infection. *Int J Antimicrob Agents.* 1999;11(3–4):227-231. discussion 37–39
7. Kahlmeter, G. The European Committee on antimicrobial susceptibility testing – EUCAST. 2008 18.11.2008. Available from: http://www.escmid.org/research_projects/eucast/. [cited 2008 08.12.2008]
8. Drusano GL. Pharmacokinetics and pharmacodynamics of antimicrobials. *Clin Infect Dis.* 2007;45(suppl 1):S89-S95
9. Gupta K, Hooton TM, Stamm WE. Increasing antimicrobial resistance and the management of uncomplicated community-acquired urinary tract infections. *Ann Intern Med.* 2001;135(1):41-50
10. Hooton TM. The current management strategies for community-acquired urinary tract infection. *Infect Dis Clin North Am.* 2003;17(2):303-332
11. Kahlmeter G. An international survey of the antimicrobial susceptibility of pathogens from uncomplicated

urinary tract infections: the ECO.SENS Project. *J Antimicrob Chemother.* 2003;51(1):69-76

12. Naber KG, Schito G, Botto H, Palou J, Mazzei T. Surveillance study in Europe and Brazil on clinical aspects and antimicrobial resistance epidemiology in females with cystitis (ARESC): implications for empiric therapy. *Eur Urol.* 2008;54(5):1164-1175

13. Jones RN, Kugler KC, Pfaller MA, Winokur PL. Characteristics of pathogens causing urinary tract infections in hospitals in North America: results from the SENTRY Antimicrobial Surveillance Program, 1997. *Diagn Microbiol Infect Dis.* 1999;35(1):55-63

14. Gordon KA, Jones RN. Susceptibility patterns of orally administered antimicrobials among urinary tract infection pathogens from hospitalized patients in North America: comparison report to Europe and Latin America. Results from the SENTRY Antimicrobial Surveillance Program (2000). *Diagn Microbiol Infect Dis.* 2003;45(4):295-301

15. Mathai D, Jones RN, Pfaller MA. Epidemiology and frequency of resistance among pathogens causing urinary tract infections in 1, 510 hospitalized patients: a report from the SENTRY Antimicrobial Surveillance Program (North America). *Diagn Microbiol Infect Dis.* 2001; 40(3):129-136

16. Bouza E, San Juan R, Munoz P, Voss A, Kluytmans JA. European perspective on nosocomial urinary tract infections I. Report on the microbiology workload, etiology and antimicrobial susceptibility (ESGNI-003 study). European Study Group on Nosocomial Infections. *Clin Microbiol Infect.* 2001;10:523-531

17. Wagenlehner FM, Niemetz A, Dalhoff A, Naber KG. Spectrum and antibiotic resistance of uropathogens from hospitalized patients with urinary tract infections: 1994–2000. *Int J Antimicrob Agents.* 2002;19(6):557-564

18. Bjerklund Johansen TE, Cek M, Naber K, Stratchounski L, Svendsen MV, Tenke P. Prevalence of hospital-acquired urinary tract infections in urology departments. *Eur Urol.* 2007;51(4):1100-1111. discussion 12

19. Livermore DM, Woodford N. The beta-lactamase threat in Enterobacteriaceae, Pseudomonas and Acinetobacter. *Trends Microbiol.* 2006;14(9):413-420

20. Ena J, Arjona F, Martinez-Peinado C, Lopez-Perezagua Mdel M, Amador C. Epidemiology of urinary tract infections caused by extended-spectrum beta-lactamase-producing *Escherichia coli. Urology.* 2006;68(6):1169-1174

21. Paterson DL. "Collateral damage" from cephalosporin or quinolone antibiotic therapy. *Clin Infect Dis.* 2004; 38(suppl 4):S341-S355

22. McLuskey K, Cameron S, Hammerschmidt F, Hunter WN. Structure and reactivity of hydroxypropylphosphonic acid epoxidase in fosfomycin biosynthesis by a cation- and flavin-dependent mechanism. *Proc Natl Acad Sci USA.* 2005;102(40):14221-14226

23. Patel SS, Balfour JA, Bryson HM. Fosfomycin tromethamine. A review of its antibacterial activity, pharmacokinetic properties and therapeutic efficacy as a single-dose oral treatment for acute uncomplicated lower urinary tract infections. *Drugs.* 1997;53(4):637-656

24. Hof H. Antimicrobial therapy with nitroheterocyclic compounds, for example, metronidazole and nitrofurantoin. *Immun Infekt.* 1988;16(6):220-225

25. Conklin JD. The pharmacokinetics of nitrofurantoin and its related bioavailability. *Antibiot Chemother.* 1978;25:233-252

26. Mazzulli T, Skulnick M, Small G, et al. Susceptibility of community Gram-negative urinary tract isolates to mecillinam and other oral agents. *Can J Infect Dis.* 2001;12(5):289-292

27. Williams GJ, Wei L, Lee A, Craig JC. Long-term antibiotics for preventing recurrent urinary tract infection in children. *Cochrane Database Syst Rev.* 2006;3: D001534

28. Koulaouzidis A, Bhat S, Moschos J, Tan C, De Ramon A. Nitrofurantoin-induced lung- and hepatotoxicity. *Ann Hepatol.* 2007;6(2):119-121

29. Sjovall J, Huitfeldt B, Magni L, Nord CE. Effect of beta-lactam prodrugs on human intestinal microflora. *Scand J Infect Dis Suppl.* 1986;49:73-84

30. Spratt BG. The mechanism of action of mecillinam. *J Antimicrob Chemother.* 1977;3(suppl B):13-19

31. Donowitz GR, Mandell GL. Beta-Lactam antibiotics (1). *N Engl J Med.* 1988;318(7):419-426

32. Nathwani D, Wood MJ. Penicillins. A current review of their clinical pharmacology and therapeutic use. *Drugs.* 1993;45(6):866-894

33. Drusano GL, Schimpff SC, Hewitt WL. The acylampicillins: mezlocillin, piperacillin, and azlocillin. *Rev Infect Dis.* 1984;6(1):13-32

34. Marshall WF, Blair JE. The cephalosporins. *Mayo Clin Proc.* 1999;74(2):187-195

35. Jones RN, Preston DA. The antimicrobial activity of cephalexin against old and new pathogens. *Postgrad Med J.* 1983;59(suppl 5):9-15

36. Smith BR, LeFrock JL. Cefuroxime: antimicrobial activity, pharmacology, and clinical efficacy. *Ther Drug Monit.* 1983;5(2):149-160

37. Brogard JM, Jehl F, Willemin B, Lamalle AM, Blickle JF, Monteil H. Clinical pharmacokinetics of cefotiam. *Clin Pharmacokinet.* 1989;17(3):163-174

38. Perry CM, Brogden RN. Cefuroxime axetil. A review of its antibacterial activity, pharmacokinetic properties and therapeutic efficacy. *Drugs.* 1996;52(1):125-158

39. Molavi A. Cephalosporins: rational for clinical use – review article. *Am Fam Phys.* 1991;43(3):937-948

40. Dudley MN, Barriere SL. Cefotaxime: microbiology, pharmacology, and clinical use. *Clin Pharm.* 1982; 1(2):114-124

41. Brogden RN, Ward A. Ceftriaxone. A reappraisal of its antibacterial activity and pharmacokinetic properties, and an update on its therapeutic use with particular reference to once-daily administration. *Drugs.* 1988;35 (6):604-645

42. Chocas EC, Paap CM, Godley PJ. Cefpodoxime proxetil: a new, broad-spectrum, oral cephalosporin. *Ann Pharmacother.* 1993;27(11):1369-1377

43. Owens RC Jr, Nightingale CH, Nicolau DP. Ceftibuten: an overview. *Pharmacotherapy.* 1997;17(4):707-720

44. Bergogne-Berezin E. Structure-activity relationship of ceftazidime. Consequences on the bacterial spectrum. *Presse Méd*. 1988;17:1878-1882

45. Wynd MA, Paladino JA. Cefepime: a fourth-generation parenteral cephalosporin. *Ann Pharmacother*. 1996; 30(12):1414-1424

46. Hammond ML. Ertapenem: a Group 1 carbapenem with distinct antibacterial and pharmacological properties. *J Antimicrob Chemother*. 2004;53: ii7-ii9. Suppl 2

47. Shah PM, Isaacs RD. Ertapenem, the first of a new group of carbapenems. *J Antimicrob Chemother*. 2003;52(4): 538-542

48. Hellinger WC, Brewer NS. Carbapenems and monobactams: imipenem, meropenem, and aztreonam. *Mayo Clin Proc*. 1999;74(4):420-434

49. Mingeot-Leclercq MP, Glupczynski Y, Tulkens PM Aminoglycosides: activity and resistance. *Antimicrob Agents Chemother*. 1999;43(4):727-737

50. Benveniste R, Davies J. Structure-activity relationships among the aminoglycoside antibiotics: role of hydroxyl and amino groups. *Antimicrob Agents Chemother*. 1973;4(4):402-409

51. Mingeot-Leclercq MP, Tulkens PM. Aminoglycosides: nephrotoxicity. *Antimicrob Agents Chemother*. 1999; 43(5):1003-1012

52. Naber KG, Adam D. Classification of fluoroquinolones. *Int J Antimicrob Agents*. 1998;10(4):255-257

53. Van Bambeke F, Michot JM, Van Eldere J, Tulkens PM. Quinolones in 2005: an update. *Clin Microbiol Infect*. 2005;11(4):256-280

54. Okhamafe AO, Akerele JO, Chukuka CS. Pharmacokinetic interactions of norfloxacin with some metallic medicinal agents. *Int J Pharm*. 1991;68(1–3):11-18

55. Naber KG. Which fluoroquinolones are suitable for the treatment of urinary tract infections? *Int J Antimicrob Agents*. 2001;17(4):331-341

56. Smilack JD. Trimethoprim-sulfamethoxazole. *Mayo Clin Proc*. 1999;74(7):730-734

57. Hermans PE, Wilhelm MP. Vancomycin. *Mayo Clin Proc*. 1987;62(10):901-905

58. Shinabarger D. Mechanism of action of the oxazolidinone antibacterial agents. *Expert Opin Investig Drugs*. 1999;8(8):1195-1202

59. Conte JE Jr, Golden JA, Kipps J, Zurlinden E. Intrapulmonary pharmacokinetics of linezolid. *Antimicrob Agents Chemother*. 2002;46(5):1475-1480

60. MacGowan AP. Pharmacokinetic and pharmacodynamic profile of linezolid in healthy volunteers and patients with Gram-positive infections. *J Antimicrob Chemother*. 2003;51:(suppl 2):ii17-ii25

7

An Overview of Renal Physiology

Mitchell H. Rosner

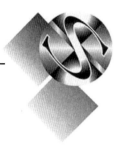

Introduction

The kidney is responsible for varied and critical functions that maintain homeostasis (this can be seen in Table 7.1, which demonstrates the excretory capacity of the kidney). These functions include maintaining the volume and composition of the extracellular fluid (despite drastic and variable difference in daily intake), removal of toxic waste products (such as the end-products of metabolism such as urea, phosphates, sulfates, and uric acid), the conservation of essential nutrients (glucose, amino acids, electrolytes), regulation of acid–base balance, production of hormones (active 1,25-vitamin D and erythropoietin), regulation of blood pressure, and the excretion of drugs that are metabolized. In order to achieve these functions, the kidney acts as an integrative organ of its constitutive parts: the nephrons. There are approximately 1.2 million nephrons per kidney at birth and it is the function of these units that controls homeostasis.

The nephron consists of a series of specialized segments each with a specific function that impacts the final composition of the urine. Furthermore, hormonal influences affect the functions of these segments in order to control the final urine composition. Sequentially, the nephron includes the afferent and efferent arterioles which bring blood to and away (respectively) from the tubules, the glomerulus which is responsible for producing an ultrafiltrate of blood that will enter the tubules through Bowman's capsule, and then specialized tubular subsegments (the proximal tubule, loop of Henle, distal tubule, and cortical collecting duct). Within the tubule, each specialized portion consists of tubular cells with specific transport proteins that are responsible for the excretion and reabsorption of specific electrolytes and nutrients. For example, in the proximal tubule, specialized transport proteins are responsible for the reabsorption of glucose and amino acids and secretion of hydrogen ions (H^+) (Fig. 7.1). Furthermore, specific disease processes, both genetically and acquired, target specific tubular subsegments and processes. The Fanconi syndrome, which can be either genetic or acquired (due to multiple myeloma or drugs such as ifosfamide), results from disruption of proximal tubular function. This leads to wasting of glucose, amino acid, and bicarbonate in the urine.

Glomerular Structure and Function

The formation of urine begins with the filtration of plasma water and its nonprotein constituents for the glomerular capillaries into Bowman's space (termed ultrafiltration). The forces involved in glomerular ultrafiltration are the Starling forces (intravascular hydrostatic pressure, plasma oncotic pressure, hydrostatic pressure, and

C.R. Chapple and W.D. Steers (eds.), *Practical Urology: Essential Principles and Practice*,
DOI: 10.1007/978-1-84882-034-0_7, © Springer-Verlag London Limited 2011

Table 7.1. Daily renal turnover

	Filtered	Excreted	Reabsorbed	Percentage of reabsorbed
Water (L/day)	180	1.5	178.5	99.2
Na$^+$(mmol/day)	25,000	150	24,850	99.4
HCO$_3^-$ (mmol/day)	4,500	2	4,498	99.9+
Cl$^-$ (mmol/day)	18,000	150	17,850	99.2
Glucose (mmol/day)	800	0.5	799.5	99.9+
Calcium (mmol/day)	540	10	530	98.1
Potassium (mmol/day)	720	100	620	86.1
Urea (mmol/day)	920	460	460	50

Note: A patient's serum electrolytes remain remarkably constant despite wide variations in intake.

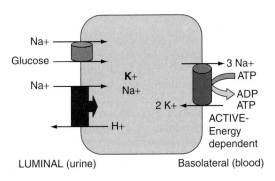

Figure 7.1. Schematic representation of transport processes occurring in the proximal tubule. Sodium (Na$^+$) and glucose are absorbed from the luminal (urine) side of the proximal tubule through a specialized cotransporter. Hydrogen (H$^+$) ions are excreted by a specific Na$^+$/H$^+$anti-porter. The energy for these processes is derived from the basolateral (blood) side Na$^+$/ potassium (K$^+$) ATPase. This protein uses the energy from ATP (adenosine tri-phosphate) breakdown to pump K$^+$ into cells and Na$^+$ out of cells against their concentration gradients. In doing so, the intracellular K$^+$ concentration is very high and the intracellular Na$^+$ concentration is very low. This allows Na$^+$ from the luminal side to flow down its concentration gradient into cells. In doing so, either cations (such as H$^+$) can be secreted or other substances (glucose, amino acids) can be absorbed utilizing the movement of Na$^+$ down its concentration gradient.

oncotic pressure within Bowman's space). The net result of the interplay of these forces is that there is net ultrafiltration into Bowman's space from the capillary beds (termed glomerular filtration rate (GFR)). This filtrate is generally free of significant quantities of plasma proteins.

The glomerular capillary wall consists of three layers: (1) endothelial cells, (2) glomerular basement membrane, and (3) epithelial cells (podocytes with foot processes). The endothelium is thought to be freely permeable to even large molecules but does exclude blood cells. The basement membrane consists of three filamentous layers (lamina rara interna, lamina densa, and lamina rara externa). Many consider the basement membrane to be the most important restrictive filtration barrier. The epithelium consists of highly specialized cells called podocytes that are attached to the basement membrane by foot processes (pedicels), which are separated by filtration slits bridged by thin diaphragms. These epithelial cells also have the ability to phagocytize macromolecules that have leaked through the basement membrane. Adding to the selective permeability characteristics of the glomerular filtration barrier is the presence of negatively charged glycosialoproteins, which tend to repel negatively charged plasma proteins such as albumin.

GFR is tightly regulated. Over a range of arterial pressures between 80 and 180 mmHg, total resistance varies in direct proportion to arterial pressure and the flow remains approximately unchanged. This phenomenon whereby renal blood flow (RBF) and glomerular filtration rate (GFT) are maintained constant is called *autoregulation*. Auto-regulation is achieved by changes within the kidney to affect renal blood flow and GFR. There are two factors which are responsible for autoregulation of renal blood flow and glomerular filtration rate, (1) *myogenic mechanism*, this is a pressure sensitive mechanism in which there is an intrinsic tendency of vascular smooth muscle to contract when it is stretched. As arterial pressure increases, the afferent arteriole is stretched and the smooth muscle contracts, (2) *tubuloglomerular feedback*: this mechanism involves a feedback loop in which the macula densa of the distal tubule cells senses some component of the distal tubule fluid (likely chloride concentration), which then affects GFR. For example, when GFR increases, distal tubule flow rate increases sending a signal that causes RBF and GFR to return to normal levels. Other factors that alter renal blood flow and GFR include, (1) *sympathetic control*: sympathetic neurons that release norepinephrine innervate both the afferent and efferent arterioles. Norepinephrine produces vasoconstriction by binding to alpha 1-adrenoceptors, thereby decreasing renal blood flow and glomerular filtration rate; (2) *hormones*: there are various vasoconstrictor hormones including epinephrine, norepinephrine, angiotensin II, thromboxane, and parathyroid hormone. Vasodilator hormones include PGE_2, PGI_2, bradykinin, histamine, and atrial natriuretic peptide; (3) *protein intake*: high protein intake increases both GFR and renal blood flow.

The GFR is equal to the sum of the filtration rates of all the functioning nephrons and thus is an important index of kidney function and it is used clinically as a global marker of kidney function. A decreasing GFR is a sensitive and vitally important marker of worsening kidney function. While there are many methods for determining the GFR, two are used most commonly in the clinical setting: (1) creatinine clearance determination from a 24-h urine collection or (2) use of regression formulas to determine GFR based upon serum creatinine measurements. Creatinine clearance is determined by the collection of a 24-h urine specimen and a plasma sample, both of which are measured for creatinine concentration. Given that, in the steady state, creatinine excretion is equal to the creatinine filtration rate, clearance can be determined as the urine concentration of creatinine multiplied by the urine volume divided by the plasma concentration of creatinine. In should be noted that this relationship holds true only for an ideal molecule that only appears in the urine via glomerular filtration and then is not secreted, metabolized, or absorbed by the tubules. While creatinine is freely filtered and does not undergo either tubular reabsorption, it can undergo tubular secretion. Thus, a GFR calculated using a creatinine clearance tends to overestimate the true GFR by the amount that is secreted into the urine.

Given that creatinine clearance is only an estimate of GFR and in some cases creatinine secretion by the tubules can be increased (such as with chronic kidney disease), there is a need for a more precise and more easily obtained measure of GFR. Furthermore, collection of 24 h urine is difficult and unreliable. Using data from thousands of patients in the Modification of Diet in Renal Disease (MDRD) trial where sensitive GFR was measured, a regression equation was developed that allows a serum creatinine value to be converted into an estimated GFR with a high degree of correlation to a measured GFR. The equation requires only a measurement of serum creatinine: GFR = 175 × serum creatinine – 1.154 × age – 0.203 × 1.212 [if black] × 0.742 [if female]. Use of this equation has gained widespread acceptance as a method for determining and following GFR.

Body Fluid Compartments

The amount of the body that is composed of water is variable and dependent upon the amount of fat. Thus, patients with higher body fat percentages will have lower water content. For this reason, women tend to have about 5% less total body water than men. Total body water constitutes approximately 60% of body weight (or 42 L for a 70 kg male). This is further divided into an intracellular compartment (40% of body weight) and an extracellular compartment (20% of body weight). The extracellular compartment is further divided into an intravascular (5% of body weight) and interstitial compartments (15% of body weight).

The major solute constituents are electrolytes with a smaller proportion of proteins, nutrients, and waste products. Sodium is by far the most abundant extracellular cation, while chloride and bicarbonate are the most abundant extracellular anions. Potassium is the most abundant intracellular cation and organic phosphates and proteins are the most abundant intracellular anions. In order to maintain the unequal distribution of solutes across body compartments, several mechanisms are operative: (1) semipermeable cell membranes, and (2) the existence of cellular channels and pumps (transporters) that use energy to maintain a difference in solute concentrations across the membranes.

The osmolality of interstitial fluid is equal to that of intracellular fluid, and changes in osmolality between these compartments govern fluid movement. For instance, if the osmolality of the extracellular compartment was acutely increased (for instance, with mannitol) this would cause water movement out of cells down the osmotic gradient into the extracellular compartment.

The volume of the extracellular compartment is dependent upon the amount of body sodium (since this is the major extracellular cation). Within the extracellular compartment, hydrostatic and oncotic pressures (Starling forces) determine the movement of fluid and volume between the plasma and interstitial spaces.

Regulation of Sodium, Chloride, and Water Reabsorption by the Proximal Tubule

Important factors regulating the movement of solute and water from proximal tubule lumen into the peritubular capillaries are the Starling forces which include capillary oncotic pressure (π_{cap}), the hydrostatic pressure in the intercellular space (P_{is}), the interstitial oncotic pressure (π_{is}), and the capillary hydrostatic pressure (P_{cap}). Peritubular capillary pressure can be altered by the vascular tone of the efferent arteriole. An increase in efferent arteriole tone will reduce peritubular capillary pressure (providing less hindrance to solute reabsorption). On the other hand, a decrease in efferent arteriole tone will increase peritubular capillary pressure and increase hindrance to solute reabsorption. Furthermore, the peritubular oncotic pressure can be altered by the efferent arteriole as well. Efferent arteriole constriction can increase the filtration fraction (FF = GFR/RPF), which will increase peritubular oncotic pressure. An increase in peritubular oncotic pressure will increase solute and water reabsorption by the proximal tubule. These forces are involved in a phenomenon known as *glomerulotubular balance* (G-T balance). The operation of G-T balance enables a constant fraction of filtered sodium and water to be reabsorbed by the proximal tubule despite variations in GFR. For example, when GFR decreases by 25% the rate of proximal sodium reabsorption also decreases by 25%. Thus the net effect of GT-balance is to minimize the ability of changes in GFR to produce large changes in sodium excretion.

Control of Body Osmolality and Body Fluid Volume

The osmolality of the extracellular fluid (ECF) is tightly regulated with variations of only 1–2% in normal circumstances. This need for tight control is due to the important effect of osmolality on cellular volume. For example, if the osmolality of the ECF falls, it creates a disequilibrium favoring movement of water into the intracellular compartment with resultant cellular swelling. In the central nervous system, this can lead to intracranial hypertension and mental status changes that in the extreme can lead to cerebellar herniation and death. This contrasts with the volume of the ECF fluid, which is not as tightly regulated and can vary by a much larger percentage. Body osmolality is regulated by renal handling of water and is under the control of arginine vasopressin (AVP, or antidiuretic hormone (ADH)). Body volume is regulated by renal handling of sodium and the major mediators are the renin-angiotensin-aldosterone system (RAAS) and the sympathetic nervous system (SNS).

In response to water deprivation (or sodium ingestion), plasma osmolality is increased. This is sensed by osmoreceptors in the supraoptic and paraventricular nuclei in the hypothalamus and leads to the release of AVP. AVP is released in response to either increased osmolality (less than 1% change) or decreased volume (greater than 10% change) of the ECF. Note that secretion of AVP in response to increased osmolality has a lower threshold and a higher sensitivity (slope) than the response to decreased ECF volume. The hypothalamic receptors also increase thirst. AVP then acts to increase the water permeability of the collecting duct in the distal tubule resulting in free water retention, decreased urine volume, and increased urine osmolality. The combination of thirst and increased free water reabsorption by the kidney restores plasma osmolality to normal.

In contrast, in the setting of excess water ingestion, plasma osmolality is decreased and this results in the suppression of both thirst and AVP release. This leads to decreased permeability of the collecting duct to water, excretion of dilute urine, and the return of plasma osmolality to normal.

AVP acts through a specific vasopressin type-2 receptor on the basolateral side of the collecting duct. This leads to an increase in intracellular cyclic AMP, activation of protein kinase A, and increased trafficking of aquaporin (water channels) proteins to the luminal membrane to increase water permeability of the cell. The greatest stimulus to AVP release is an increase of plasma osmolality. AVP can also be stimulated by ECF volume depletion (7–10%). Volume depletion also causes the sensitivity of AVP release to increase and thus a lower plasma osmolality is tolerated in states of volume depletion. Outside of these physiological stimuli for AVP release, several non-physiological (but clinical important) stimuli exist. These include medications (selective serotonin release inhibitors, narcotic and chemotherapeutic drug), nausea and vomiting, carcinomas, pulmonary and CNS disorders. These non-physiological stimuli for AVP release can result in hyponatremia and hypo-osmolality (the syndrome of inappropriate ADH release (SIADH)). Conversely, either the inability of the hypothalamus to produce or secrete AVP or the ability of the collecting duct to respond to AVP lead to the conditions of central or nephrogenic (respectively) diabetes insipidus (DI). In this state, the kidney continues to excrete a large volume of dilute urine and patients need to either take synthetic AVP (for the central form of DI) or increase their intake of water to keep pace with the renal losses. If this does not occur, then increasing urine water losses will lead to hypernatremia and hyperosmolality.

Regulation of Potassium Balance

Potassium is abundant in the body totaling about 3,500 mEq for a 70 kg individual. Ninety-eight percent of potassium is located within the cell where the concentration averages between 100 and 150 mEq/L. Potassium is important for: (1) volume regulation, (2) chemical reactions, (3) cell division and growth, (4) acid–base status, (5) glucose uptake and glycogen synthesis, and (6) excitability and contractility of neuromuscular cells.

Distribution of Potassium (internal potassium balance): Potassium homeostasis involves the following processes: (1) gastrointestinal intake, (2) internal distribution, and (3) excretion. There appears to be little regulation of potassium uptake by the gastrointestinal tract so that virtually all the ingested potassium is transferred into the extracellular fluid. The distribution of potassium within the body is critical for maintaining normal serum potassium following normal dietary intake. For example, if one ingests 50 mEq of potassium (three to four glasses of orange juice) a rise in serum potassium of 3.6 mEq/L would occur if all the ingested potassium remained in the extracellular fluid. However, because of rapid redistribution into the intracellular compartment, the rise in plasma potassium is attenuated. To maintain potassium balance, however, all the ingested potassium must eventually be excreted by the kidneys. There are several factors which affect potassium distribution between intracellular and extracellular compartments.

1. *Epinephrine*: adrenergic receptors are involved in the distribution of potassium. Stimulation of alpha adrenergic receptors increases plasma potassium while stimulation of beta 2 receptors decreases plasma potassium concentration. The use of beta blockers such as propranolol can produce a significant increase in serum potassium concentration under certain circumstances.

2. *Insulin*: stimulates potassium uptake into the cells by activating the Na, K-ATPase.

3. *Aldosterone*: similar to insulin, aldosterone secretion is stimulated by high plasma potassium concentration and acts to promote potassium uptake into muscle cells. This action of aldosterone (to promote potassium uptake into muscle) is not as important as the effect of insulin on potassium uptake by muscle, or as important as the action of aldosterone on potassium transport by renal epithelial cells (see below).

4. *Acid–base balance*: Changes in the pH of the extracellular fluid alter intracellular pH and redistributes potassium. In acidemia, plasma potassium concentration increases because potassium moves out of the cells. In alkalemia, plasma potassium concentration falls because potassium moves into cells.

5. *Exercise*: During exercise skeletal muscle cells release potassium and produces variable degrees of hyperkalemia. Usually, these changes produce no symptoms and are reversed after several minutes of rest. However, under certain circumstances a significant increase in plasma potassium concentration can occur such as the individuals who are using beta blockers during exercise.

Excretion of potassium by the kidneys: Approximately 92% of ingested potassium is excreted by the kidney. The remaining 8% is excreted by the gastrointestinal tract. Potassium is freely filtered by the glomerulus and normally the urinary potassium excretion is 15% of the amount filtered. The proximal tubule reabsorbs about 67% of the filtered load of potassium, whereas the loop of Henle reabsorbs 20%. It is in the distal tubule and the collecting duct where regulation of potassium secretion occurs. When dietary intake is normal, potassium is secreted by these distal nephron segments, however, when potassium intake is below normal potassium reabsorption occurs.

The mechanism by which potassium is secreted by the principal cells of the collecting duct is provided by an electrochemical gradient. The uptake of potassium via the Na, K-ATPase in the basolateral membrane increases the potassium concentration within the cell, and provides a (1) chemical gradient for potassium to exit across the apical membrane through potassium channels. Sodium conductance at the apical membrane depolarizes the apical membrane relative to the basolateral membrane and thus provides an (2) electrical gradient (lumen negative charge favoring potassium excretion).

There are various factors which regulate potassium secretion by the principal cells.

1. *Plasma potassium concentration*: Plasma potassium concentration is an important determinant of potassium secretion by the distal tubule and collecting duct. An increase in the plasma potassium concentration stimulates the Na, K-ATPase, thereby raising intracellular potassium concentration and increasing the chemical gradient for potassium secretion.

2. *Aldosterone*: Aldosterone stimulates sodium reabsorption by the distal tubule and collecting duct, and enhances potassium secretion by increasing activity of the Na, K-ATPase.

3. *Flow rate of tubule fluid*: An increase in tubule fluid flow rate increases potassium secretion.

4. *Plasma flow rate*: Flow rate influences potassium secretion by the distal tubule and collecting duct.

5. *Plasma pH*: Alkalemia increases potassium secretion and acidemia decreases potassium secretion.

6. *Sodium concentration of the tubule fluid*: An increase in the sodium concentration in the distal tubule fluid stimulates potassium secretion, whereas a fall has the opposite effect.

Regulation of Acid–Base Balance

The body maintains the systemic pH in a narrow range to permit normal metabolic functions. The CO_2/HCO_3 buffer system is the most important buffer system in the body because it is under the regulation of both the lungs and the kidney. The relationship is characterized by the Henderson–Hasselbalch equation.

$$pH = \frac{6.1 + \log\left[HCO_3\right]}{0.03\left(PCO_2\right)}$$

In the normal individual, metabolism of carbohydrates and fats produce large quantities of CO_2. CO_2 is in equilibrium with H_2CO_3, a volatile acid. In addition to volatile acids, metabolism of amino acids produces nonvolatile acids. The metabolism of cysteine and methionine yields sulfuric acid, whereas lysine, arginine, and histidine produce hydrochloric acid. A normal diet produces about 70–100 mmol/day of nonvolatile acid. These acids then consume bicarbonate from the ECF, and must be replenished in order to maintain acid–base balance.

The kidney has a major role in replenishing bicarbonate loss. There are essentially two components to renal bicarbonate generation. The first involves the reabsorption of filtered bicarbonate, and the second involves synthesis of new bicarbonate.

Reabsorption of Filtered Bicarbonate: Of the filtered load of bicarbonate (4,500 mEq/day), approximately 85% is reabsorbed by the proximal tubule and most of the rest is reabsorbed by the loop of Henle and collecting duct less than 1% is lost in the urine.

Synthesis of New Bicarbonate: As discussed above, because dietary intake involves the consumption of volatile acids, which amounts to about 70–100 mmol/day, we must excrete this amount of acid daily to stay in acid–base balance. This is achieved primarily by the secretion of titratable acids (H_2PO_4, and NH_4^+). In states of acidemia, the filtered load of phosphate is not regulated and therefore has a limited capacity to excrete extra acid (30–50 mmol/day). However, NH_3 production in response to acidemia increases dramatically, therefore, becomes the dominant pathway for acid excretion (NH_4^+). Urine NH_4^+ excretion begins with glutamine metabolism in the proximal tubule forming NH_3. NH_3/NH_4^+ enters the lumen of the proximal tubule and, through a convoluted process, enters the collecting duct as NH_3 and traps H^+ secreted by the H^+-ATPase in the collecting duct. It is the presence of NH_3 which permits the H^+ to continue to be secreted by the collecting duct. Without NH_3 the lumen PH would decrease to a point where limiting gradient would exit and prevent further excretion of H^+.

A defect in renal excretion of H^+ or in reclamation of bicarbonate leads to a group of disorders termed renal tubular acidosis. These disorders result in a metabolic acidosis as well as, in some cases, a propensity to nephrolithiasis.

Regulation of Calcium and Phosphate Balance

Calcium: Calcium is importantly involved in bone formation, subdivision and growth, blood coagulation, intracellular signaling, and excitation concentration coupling. The following will be limited to the renal handling of calcium. In the blood, approximately 50% of the calcium in plasma is present in a free ionized form. The majority of ionized calcium is bound to plasma proteins, primarily albumin, and a very small percent is complexed through several anions, including HCO_3, PO_4, and SO_4. The free ionized

calcium concentration in blood is dependent upon the plasma pH as hydrogen ions compete with calcium ions for binding by plasma proteins. In states of acidemia, hydrogen ions displace calcium from proteins, thereby increasing the plasma concentration of free ionized calcium. In contrast, in states of alkalemia, hydrogen ions are displaced from plasma protein binding sites and replaced by calcium ions, thereby decreasing the plasma free ionized calcium concentration.

Of the filtered load of calcium, approximately 99% of the free ionized calcium is reabsorbed by the nephron, the majority of which is reabsorbed by the proximal tubule (70%). The thick ascending limb is responsible for the reabsorption of 20% of the filtered load of calcium, and the distal tubule and collecting ducts combine to reabsorb approximately 10% of the filtered load of calcium. The net result is that approximately 1% of the filter load is excreted into the urine. Calcium reabsorption occurs through a transcellular or a paracellular pathway. In the proximal tubule and in the thick ascending limb, changes in sodium reabsorption alter calcium reabsorption in parallel. In contrast, in the distal tubule and collecting duct it appears that calcium and sodium transport are independently regulated. Therefore, changes in urinary calcium and sodium excretion do not always occur in parallel. For example, thiazide diuretics inhibit NaCl transport by the distal tubule increasing sodium excretion but decreasing calcium excretion. Factors that are associated with an increase in calcium excretion includes: A decrease in parathyroid hormone (PTH) levels, ECF volume expansion, phosphate depletion, and metabolic acidosis. Factors which are associated with a decrease in calcium excretion include: An increase in PTH, ECF volume concentration, phosphate loading metabolic alkalosis, and 1,25 $(OH)_2 D_3$ (vitamin D).

Phosphate: The kidney is an important organ in the maintenance of phosphate homeostasis. Phosphate is an important component in nucleotides, ATP, and it is an important component of bone. The proximal tubule reabsorbs approximately 80% of the phosphate filtered load, and the distal tubule reabsorbs approximately 10%. The loop of Henle and the collecting duct have an insignificant contribution to phosphate reabsorption. Phosphate reabsorption across the apical membrane of the proximal tubule occurs by sodium phosphate cotransport mechanism. PTH is an important regulator of phosphate excretion. PTH increases cyclic AMP production and inhibits phosphate reabsorption by the proximal tubule. Other factors which increase phosphate excretion include phosphate loading, ECF volume expansion, glucocorticoids, and acidosis. Other factors which are important in decreasing phosphate excretion include phosphate depletion, ECF volume contraction, and alkalosis.

Diuretics

Diuretics produce an increase in urine output by increasing sodium excretion (natriuresis). Various classes of diuretics affect specific nephron segments. The site of action determines the magnitude of natriuresis. For example, in general, proximal acting diuretics such as carbonic anhydrase inhibitors, or osmotic diuretics are weak diuretics because the more distal nephron segments reabsorb the increase in sodium and chloride delivered to it. On the other hand, the more distal acting diuretics like loop diuretics are potent diuretics. Diuretics gain access to the tubule fluid by glomerular filtration, secretion by organic anions and cationic secretory mechanism located in the proximal tubule. By gaining access through the tubule fluid they can exert their action by interacting with transport mechanism located in the apical membrane of nephron segments.

Osmotic Diuretics: Osmotic diuretics such as mannitol or glucose inhibit reabsorption of solute and water by altering osmotic forces along the nephron. In addition, inhibition of sodium reabsorption by the more proximal nephron, allows more sodium to be delivered to and absorbed by the thick ascending limb. This reabsorptive response by the distal segments limits the degree of natriuresis seen with osmotic diuretics. *Mannitol* is usually the drug of choice among osmotic agents. It is a common clinical impression that mannitol improves renal hemodynamics in a variety of situations of impending or incipient acute renal failure (rapid reduction in glomerular filtration rate). The incidence of acute renal failure in hospitalized patients is significant and associated with an increase in morbidity and mortality. Thus its prevention has been the focus of much research. Although mannitol has been tested in animal models of acute renal failure, its efficacy in human acute renal failure is controversial and it cannot be recommended for this purpose. Infusions of mannitol are used to lower the elevated intracranial pressure of cerebral edema associated with tumors, neurosurgical procedures, or other conditions. Osmotic agents cause the redistribution of body fluid, increase urine flow rate, and accelerate the renal elimination of filtered solutes.

Carbonic Anhydrase Inhibitors: Carbonic anhydrase facilitates the reabsorption of sodium bicarbonate. This enzyme is located primarily in the proximal tubule and represents the major site of action. The degree of natriuresis is not as great as expected for the same reason as discussed with osmotic diuretics (i.e., distal reabsorption of sodium delivered). *Acetazolamide* is used effectively to treat chronic open-angle glaucoma. Since the aqueous humor has a high bicarbonate concentration, these drugs can be used to reduce aqueous humor formation. Acetazolamide is also used to prevent and treat acute mountain sickness, to alkalinize the urine, and to treat metabolic alkalosis.

Loop Diuretics: Loop diuretics primarily inhibits sodium reabsorption by the thick ascending limb by blocking the Na-2Cl-1K cotransport mechanism located in the apical membrane of these cells. This class of diuretics exert a potent inhibition of sodium reabsorption by the thick ascending limb because it not only inhibits sodium transport by the thick ascending limb, but it also impairs dilution and concentrating ability (one function of the thick ascending limb is to produce a hypertonic medullary interstitium). Inhibition of transport by furosemide decreases tonicity of the interstitium. *Furosemide, torasemide ethacrynic acid* may increase renal blood flow for brief intervals during which urinary excretion of prostaglandin E is elevated. Intravenous injections of furosemide reduce pulmonary arterial pressure and peripheral venous compliance. Indomethacin, an inhibitor of prostaglandin synthesis, interferes with all these actions. Vascular phenomena of this sort occurring in the kidney and elsewhere precede the onset of diuresis. The therapeutic value of loop diuretics in pulmonary edema may be attributable in part to stimulation of prostaglandin synthesis in the lung. The greater efficacy of loop agents often enables their successful use in evoking diuresis in edematous patients with disturbances of cardiovascular, renal, or hepatic origin. For example, an oliguric patient whose GFR is only 10% of normal derives no benefit from a thiazide but may respond well to a large dose of a loop diuretic. In addition, furosemide is an important adjunct in the treatment of acute pulmonary edema. The drug increases pulmonary and peripheral venous compliance, thereby affording rapid relief, and then maintains these beneficial effects by reducing the plasma volume. The initial vascular effects are not linked to actions on the renal tubule (venodilatation occurs in anephric patients). Because of the effect of loop diuretics in inducing an increase in calcium excretion, they are used to lower serum calcium concentrations in patients with hypercalcemia. Isotonic saline is often coadministered to maintain the glomerular filtration rate. Loop diuretics increase K^+ excretion and thus are useful in the treatment of acute and chronic hyperkalemia.

Thiazide Diuretics: Thiazide diuretics are organic anions which are filtered and secreted by the proximal tubule. They inhibit sodium transport by the distal convoluted tubule, or that portion of the distal tubule just beyond the thick ascending limb. These diuretics block a sodium chloride cotransport mechanism located in the apical or luminal membranes of these cells. All of the thiazides act in the same way, with the differences among them attributable largely to pharmacokinetic characteristics and inherent carbonic anhydrase inhibitory activity. In general, these agents are used in the treatment of hypertension, CHF and in other conditions when reduction of ECF volume is beneficial. Reduction of blood pressure in patients with hypertension results, in part, from contraction of ECF volume. This occurs acutely, leading to a decrease in cardiac output with compensatory elevation of peripheral resistance. Vasoconstriction then subsides enabling cardiac output to return to normal values. Augmented synthesis of vasodilator prostaglandins is reported and may be a crucial factor for long-term maintenance of a lower pressure, even though ECF volume tends to return toward normal. In addition to treatment of edematous disorders and hypertension, thiazide diuretics have been found effective in the treatment of other disorders. Because thiazide diuretics decrease renal calcium excretion, they are used in the treatment of calcium nephrolithiaisis and osteoporosis. Thiazide diuretics are also used to in the treatment of patients with nephrogenic diabetes insipidus. In this disorder, the tubules are unresponsive to vasopressin and therefore these patients undergo a water diuresis. Often the volume of dilute urine excreted is large enough to lead to intravascular volume depletion if the excreted volume is not matched by adequate intake of fluid. Chronic administration of thiazides increases the urine osmolality and reduces urine flow in this condition. The mechanism hinges on the excretion of sodium and hence removal of sodium from the ECF, an action that inevitably contracts ECF volume. The proximal tubule then avidly reabsorbs sodium. Urine flow rate diminishes and urine osmolality rises when sodium transport in the distal convoluted tubule is inhibited by the diuretic. Drug therapy in this instance is most effective in combination with dietary salt restriction.

Potassium-Sparing Diuretics: In this group are two types of diuretics which inhibit potassium secretion. *Spironolactone* acts by antagonizing aldosterone action on the principal cell of the collecting duct. Aldosterone increases sodium absorption and potassium secretion by increasing the number of functional sodium and potassium channels in the apical membrane, as well as increasing the number of basolateral Na, K-ATPase pumps. Aldosterone blocks this effect and prevents sodium absorption and potassium secretion. *Amiloride* and *triamterene* are compounds which represent a second class of diuretics which antagonize potassium secretion. The mechanism by which these diuretics inhibit potassium secretion is through inhibition of sodium channels located in the apical membranes of principal cells. By blocking these channels they block the electrical gradient for potassium secretion. Depletion of body potassium with or without significant lowering of serum potassium concentration (only 2% of total body potassium is present in ECF) is probably the most common side effect of diuretic therapy. Hypokalemia of sufficient magnitude creates many problems and may be life threatening. These problems may include impairment of neuromuscular function, cardiac arrhythmia, intestinal disturbances, and partial loss of the ability to concentrate urine. Predisposition of diuretics to potassium wasting is especially worrisome during the treatment of congestive heart failure. In patients receiving digitalis preparations and a diuretic, diuretic-induced hypokalemia can ensue and sensitize the heart to the toxic effects of the cardiac glycoside. Measures to elude the hazards of potassium deficit or to correct an established deficit are plentiful, but success is not guaranteed. The first steps are precautionary: dietary intake of large amounts of potassium, avoidance of excessive NaCl intake, and monitoring of serum potassium concentrations. If serum potassium concentrations do not stabilize at an acceptable value, supplements of potassium chloride may be prescribed; however, compliance may be a problem.

Spironolactone is most effective in patients with primary (adrenal adenoma or bilateral adrenal hyperplasia) or secondary hyperaldosteronism (congestive heart failure, cirrhosis, nephrotic syndrome) and is ineffective in patients with nonfunctional adrenal glands. The drug prevents binding of aldosterone to a cytosolic receptor in principal cells of the collecting tubule. Consequently, the hormonal stimulus to formation of aldosterone-induced proteins ceases. In the absence or reduction in the amount of this protein, the permeability of the luminal membrane to sodium and potassium decreases, with the result that sodium excretion is enhanced and potassium secretion is diminished. Cellular entry of potassium across the basolateral membrane also abates. Because spironolactone diminishes the lumen negative potential in the collecting tubule, proton secretion decreases. Spironolactone is used for correction of hypokalemia. The drug is also administered alone, with thiazides, or a loop diuretic, to reduce the ECF volume without causing potassium depletion or hypokalemia. The drug is especially appropriate for the treatment of cirrhosis with ascites, a condition invariably associated with secondary hyperaldosteronism. In comparison to loop or thiazide diuretics, spironolactone is equivalent or more effective. The reason for this observation could be related to the differences in the mechanism of drug action. Thiazides and loop are highly protein bound and enter the tubule fluid primarily by proximal tubule secretion and not by glomerular filtration. In patients with cirrhosis and ascites, tubular secretion of these agents decreases as a consequence of competition with accumulated toxic organic metabolites. Because thiazide and loop diuretics are lumenally acting agents, decreased tubule secretion reduces their effectiveness. In contrast, the activity of spironolactone does not depend on filtration or secretion as they gain access to their receptors from the blood side. Thus in patients with cirrhosis and ascites, the effectiveness of spironolactone is unimpaired. A combination of loop diuretic in addition to spironolactone can be used to boost natriuresis when the diuretic effect of spironolactone alone is inadequate. Although its natriuretic action is weak, spironolactone lowers blood pressure in patients with mild or moderate hypertension and is frequently prescribed for this purpose.

Triamterene or amiloride is generally used in combination with potassium-wasting diuretics, especially when maintenance of normal serum potassium concentrations is clinically important (e.g., patients with dysrhythmias, receiving a cardiac glycoside, or with low serum potassium concentrations). Fixed-combination preparations are generally not appropriate for initial therapy but may be more expedient when the dosage schedule is demonstrated to be correct. Because these drugs possess a different site and mechanism of action from those of thiazides or loop agents, they are sometimes administered together to increase the response in patients who are refractory to a single agent.

Suggested Reading

Brenner B, ed. *The Kidney*. 8th ed. Philadelphia, PA: W.B. Saunders Co; 2007

Giebisch G, Seldin D, eds. *Diuretic Agents: Clinical Physiology and Pharmacology*. San Diego, CA: Academic Press; 1997

Koeppen BM, Stanton BA, eds. *Renal Physiology*. 2nd ed. St. Louis, MO: Mosby Year Book; 1996

Rose BD, Post TW. *Clinical Physiology of Acid-Base and Electrolyte Disorders*. New York, NY: Mc Graw Hill, Inc.; 2001. ISBN 5

Valtin H, Schafe JA, eds. *Renal Function*. 3rd ed. Boston, MA: Little, Brown & Company; 1995

Vander AJ et al., eds. *Renal Physiology*. 5th ed. New York, NY: McGraw-Hill, Inc.; 1995

8

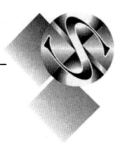

Ureteral Physiology and Pharmacology

Daniel M. Kaplon and Stephen Y. Nakada

Ureteral Anatomy

The ureters are retroperitoneal structures responsible for urine transport between the kidneys and the bladder. They are typically 22–30 cm in length and are composed of four layers. The inner layer is transitional epithelium, over which lies the lamina propria. The lamina propria is invested with a muscle layer that is composed of inner longitudinal and outer circular muscle fibers. Overlying the muscle is the adventitia, which contains the blood vessels and lymphatics coursing with the ureter.[1]

The urothelium is composed of seven layers of cells, which not only serve as protective barrier but are critical to function.[2] Serving as the first line of contact with the urinary environment, the urothelium is able to sense chemical and mechanical changes within the lumen and then signal smooth muscle, neurons, and capillaries via the release of prostaglandins, catecholemines, and cytokines.[2]

The smooth muscle layer of the ureter accounts for ureteral peristalsis as well as structural support.[3] It is divided into an inner helical layer and an outer mesh-like arrangement.[3] The inner helical layer is responsible for peristalsis while the outer mesh-like layer offers structural support.[3]

Blood supply to the ureter above the pelvic brim arises medially from the renal artery, abdominal aorta, gonadal artery, and common iliac artery. Below the pelvic brim, arterial inflow arises laterally from the internal iliac arteries and its branches.[4]

Umbrella cells form the urine plasma barrier and are found in the ureter as well as the bladder. They are unique in that they have the ability to increase and decrease size considerably in response to intraluminal pressure[5] (Fig. 8.1).

Initiation and Modulation of Peristalsis

Precise coordination between ureteral smooth muscle and neurotransmission is required for downstream propagation of urine between the kidneys and bladder. As with all smooth muscle, contraction of the ureter is the result of depolarization of the cell membrane. In the resting smooth muscle cell, the membrane potential is −50 to −80 mV.[6] When stimulated by a chemical signal or direct signaling, sodium and potassium conductance increases the membrane potential to 50 mV, generating an action potential. The effect is an increase in permeability to calcium and subsequent calcium influx into cells.[1] Intracellular calcium then activates calmodulin, which binds myosin light chain kinase and leads to myosin phosphorylation. Phosphorylated myosin then migrates up actin filaments, resulting in smooth muscle contraction.[1]

Mediators that increase intracellular calcium cause ureteral contraction. Interactions with

C.R. Chapple and W.D. Steers (eds.), *Practical Urology: Essential Principles and Practice*, DOI: 10.1007/978-1-84882-034-0_8, © Springer-Verlag London Limited 2011

Figure 8.1. Summary of cell types mediating ureteral contraction.

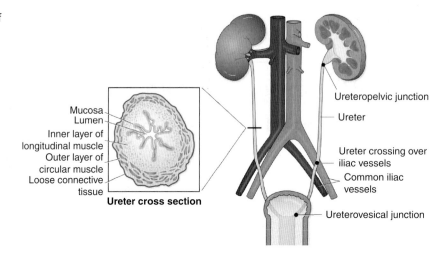

Mucosa
Lumen
Inner layer of longitudinal muscle
Outer layer of circular muscle
Loose connective tissue

Ureter cross section

Ureteropelvic junction
Ureter
Ureter crossing over iliac vessels
Common iliac vessels
Ureterovesical junction

1,4,5-triphosphate and diacylglycerol cause increased contraction, whereas mediation of G-protein coupled receptor complexes via cAMP and cGMP reduce contraction by lowering calcium levels.[6]

Urinary tract pacemaking originates in the pelvicalyceal junctions. This is known from experiments demonstrating aperistalsis of human preparations with only the renal pelvis and major calyx, and peristalsis when the specimen includes the minor calyx.[7]

It has become clear that peristalsis is initiated not by neurons, but rather by smooth muscle itself, as experiments using tetrodoxin or autonomic nerve blockers fail to block ureteral contractions.[8] In addition, denervated transplant ureters are able to maintain contractility.[9]

Ureteral pacemaking involves three types of cells: typical, atypical, and renal interstitial cells.[10] Signaling initiates within the atypical cells and ultimately passes to typical cells, but receives modulatory influence from the renal interstitial cells. Renal interstitial cells demonstrate c-kit receptor positivity.[11] Such receptors can be influenced by outside influences such as the nervous system, prostaglandins, and other hormones, causing changes in contractility in different situations.[12] Renal interstitial cells with c-kit positivity are more numerous in the upper ureter, explaining the higher rate of contractility in this area[11] (Fig. 8.2).

Modulation of Peristalsis

While initiation of ureteral contraction is to some degree independent from the nervous

system, modulation of peristalsis relies heavily on the autonomic and sensory nervous system, as well as prostaglandins. Ureteral contraction can vary with regard to *rate* and *contractility*.

The autonomic nervous system influences ureteral contraction through both parasympathetic and sympathetic fibers. The parasympathic nervous system acts via muscarinic receptors with acetylcholine as its major neurotransmitter. Significant evidence indicates that the effect of such cholinergic stimulation varies by species. For example, in anesthetized dogs with obstructed ureters, parasympathic stimulation results a decrease in peristaltic rate and contractility.[13] In a pig model, however, muscarinic stimulation causes an increase in rate and contractility, although only in the proximal ureter.[14] In humans, it is generally believed that cholinergic stimulation results in an increase in the rate and force of ureteral contractions, although these effects are much more subtle than in the bladder.[1] The sympathetic nervous system affects ureteral function in three ways:

1. Directly modulating ureteral contraction
2. Influencing pacemaking
3. Mediating ureteral contraction.

It has been shown that administration of norepinephrine in an obstructed ureter results in increased spasm and decreased flow at the area of obstruction.[14] This can be reversed with the alpha-blocker phentolamine.[15] Beta agonists, however, clearly cause ureteral relaxation. This effect has been demonstrated in pigs as well as humans.[16]

Sensory nerves are able to modulate peristalsis via capsaicin-sensitive fibers. The sensory

Figure 8.2. Summary of ureteral anatomy.

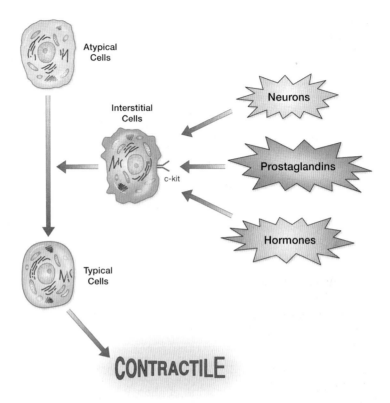

nerves found in the ureter are unmyelinated C fibers and poorly myelinated A-delta fibers.[12] Sensory afferent nerve fibers release several molecules which influence peristalsis. Among these are tachykinins, calcitonin gene-related-peptides (CGRP), and prostaglandins. Examples of tachykinins are neurokinins and substance P.[17] Tachykinins are released in response to painful stimuli and cause smooth muscle contraction via G-protein coupled receptors. Hence, the presence of neurokinin A and substance P is associated with increase contraction in the proximal and distal ureter.[18] Neurokinin A has been shown to be the most potent of the tachykinins, and treatment of ureters in vitro with a neurokinin antagonist decreased ureteral contraction by 80%.[19]

In addition to the nervous system, prostaglandins have been shown to play a role in ureteral contractility. Prostaglandins originate from arachadonic acid as a result of cyclooxygenase (COX) activity. COX exists in two isoforms: COX-1 and COX-2. The expression of COX-1 is relatively consistent, whereas COX-2 expression is heavily influenced by outside stimuli such as inflammation and obstruction. The effect of prostaglandin release varies between obstructed and non-obstructed ureters. COX-2 expression is up-regulated in obstructed ureters as compared to non-obstructed ureters.[20]

There are several subtypes of prostaglandins (PGs), and each has been studied independently regarding their effect on ureteral contraction. It has been shown in vitro that $F_{2\alpha}$, PGD_2, and TXA_2 increase ureteral contraction. PGE_2 is unique in that it has been shown to have a condition-dependent effect on ureteral contractility, namely, inducing contractility in the obstructed porcine and human ureter while relaxing normal ureter.[21]

Structural changes in the ureter may also influence changes in peristalsis. Chronically obstructed ureters possess decreased amounts of interstitial smooth muscle cells, suggesting that a lack of peristaltic integration may contribute to ureteral obstruction.[22] Moreover, abnormalities of innervation and collagen expression have also been identified in obstructed segments[23] (Table 8.1).

Table 8.1. Various substances and their effect on ureteral contraction

Substance	Effect
Acetylcholine	Contraction
α-Agonists	Contraction
β-Agonists	Relaxation
Neurokinin A and B	Contraction
$PGF_{2\alpha}$	Contraction
PGD_2	Contraction
TXA_2	Contraction
PGE_2	[21]Contraction in obstruction, relaxation in normal
PGE_1	Relaxation

Physiologic Implications of Ureteral Obstruction

Ureteral obstruction has profound effects on the ureter. Obstruction, whether from a stone or other source, results in stimulation of afferent sensory neurons reacting to stretch and distention of the ureter. Along with pain, the stretch causes an increase in the rate and amplitude of contractions. It has been shown in rats that partial ureteral obstruction causes a 500% increase in the amplitude of ureteral contractions in a rat model.[24] Ureteral obstruction also affects renal function and blood flow. It has been shown in animal models that unilateral complete obstruction result in complete loss of function in the renal unit if the obstruction lasts more than 6 weeks.[25]

Ureteral stents provide drainage of the upper tracts in cases of obstruction. Studies of ureteral stents have broadened our understanding of the physiology of ureteral obstruction. In a porcine model of the stented ureter, normal peristalsis disappeared for days 1 and 2, then became irregular after day 5.[26] In general, ureteral peristalsis is increased initially in response to stent placement but ultimately is largely reduced or completely eliminated.[27]

There have been multiple studies investigating flow patterns in the stented ureter. Mardis et al. observed that stents with larger luminal diameter and side holes provided better drainage.[28]

Ramsey et al., however, demonstrated in vitro that urine tends to drain around stents rather than through them, suggesting that luminal size is less of a clinical concern.[29] Clayman examined both standard double pigtail as well as specialty stents, and determined that only standard stent configurations flow based on luminal diameter.[30]

Ureteral stents have been shown to decrease ureteral peristalsis. As such, ureteral calculi are less likely to pass while in the stented ureter.[31] Notably, Stoller et al. demonstrated an increased stone passage rate using spiral-ridged stents as compared to traditional double pigtail stents.[31] In general, ureteral stents are placed often to allow gradual passage of stones to avoid Steinstrausse formation.

Ureteral Pharmacology

Ureteral pharmacology has been studied since 1970. The long accepted premise that ureteral spasm and increased contractility cause pain was demonstrated by Laird et al. in 1997.[32] This leads to efforts to achieve targeted therapy to reduce ureteral spasm via the known physiologic pathways of ureteral contraction.

Opioids have traditionally been utilized to control the symptoms associated with ureteral obstruction. They work by activating *mu* receptors and thus blocking the afferent pain pathways caused by ureteral obstruction. Interestingly, however, some studies have revealed a spasmogenic effect of opioids on the ureter,[33] so clearly their effect on pain relief is not related to ureteral relaxation.

Prostaglandins are generally potent contractants of smooth muscle. As such, agents such as nonsteroidal anti-inflammatories (NSAIDS) have been successful in inhibiting ureteral contractility in multiple studies.[34] Both nonselective COX inhibitors and selective COX-2 inhibitors have been shown to decrease ureteral contraction.[35] Because COX-2 expression is up regulated in inflammation and obstruction, inhibition of COX-2 is successful in relaxing the ureter in these circumstances. In addition, celecoxib as well as indomethacin have been shown to inhibit prostaglandin release in the ureter, even when

COX-2 was upregulated.[20] Despite the clear effect on ureteral contractility, the clinical use of NSAIDS may be limited due to their effect on renal function. Because prostacyclin-driven contralateral renal vasodilation in cases of obstruction is dependent on COX-2, blocking this pathway has the potential to lead to a high rate of renal insufficiency.[14]

Phosphodiesterase (PDE) inhibitors produce significant effects on ureteral contractility.[36] PDE enzymes degrade cAMP and cGMP, and blocking this process leads to accumulation of these nucleotides and subsequent smooth muscle relaxation by activation of protein kinase A and phosphorylation of myosin light chain kinase. There are seven isoforms of PDE, but inhibition of PDE-IV has been shown to have the greatest effect on ureteral relaxation.[37]

Calcium channel blockers have been proposed as a method for inhibiting ureteral contraction and thus reducing pain in situations of obstruction. Nifedipine and verapamil have been studied and interestingly found to inhibit fast phasic contractions while preserving slow phasic contractions,[38] thus preventing spasm while maintaining normal peristalsis. For this reason, nifedipine has been investigated as a stone expulsive agent. In one study, nifedipine was shown to increase stone passage rate from 65% to 87%.[39] In another series, 96 patients with distal ureteral stones received either deflazacort and nifedipine or conservative management. Stone expulsion rate in the nifedipine group was 79% compared to 35% in the conservatively managed group. Mean time to stone passage was 7 days in the nifedipine groups versus 20 days in the conservative group.[40] Despite the clear increase in stone passage rate, there is no evidence that calcium channel blockers contribute to pain control from obstruction. One study evaluated nifedipine versus placebo in 30 patients with renal colic and found no significant difference in pain control.[41]

There is a significant body of literature to support alpha antagonists as expulsive agents for stones. Alpha antagonists can be broadly grouped into either selective or nonselective, depending on their affinity for alpha 1A and 1D receptors, which are abundant in the ureter. Both nonselective and selective alpha antagonists have been shown to effectively reduce ureteral spasm. Yilmaz et al. studied tamsulosin, terazosin, and doxazosin and found that they increased stone passage rate from 52% to 79%, 78%, and 75%, respectively.[42]

Numerous randomized studies have examined tamsulosin compared to either nifedipine or placebo for expulsive therapy. In these studies the stone passage rate was 97–100% compared to 64–70% in the placebo groups.[43,44] Tamsulosin offered a 20% increase in passage rate when compared to nifedipine.[45] In general, studies thus far favor the use of alpha blockers over calcium channel blockers due to efficacy and a low side effect profile. In 2006, Hollingsworth and colleagues published a meta-analysis of nine randomized controlled trials investigating the use calcium channel blockers and alpha blockers. Compared with the control group, patients treated with nifedipene or tamsulosin had an overall 65% greater likelihood of stone passage.[46] A subsequent meta-analysis from the combined AUA/EUA ureteral stone guidelines demonstrated an increase in passage rate for nifedipine of 9% which was not statistically significant. Meta-analysis of tamsulosin versus control demonstrated an absolute increase in passage rate of 29% which was significant.[47]

Most alpha blocker studies have included the use of steroids in their study groups. A randomized trial of 60 patients to either alpha blockers and steroids or steroids alone found no difference in overall passage rate, but a more rapid rate of passage in the steroid group (72 vs 120 h).[48] In general, steroids provide some benefit as expulsive therapy when combined with other agents, but not alone.[46] Moreover, there is even evidence to suggest that alpha blockers contribute to analgesia in cases of obstruction. Tamsulosin has been shown to decrease discomfort associated with shockwave lithotripsy as well as steinstrasse which develops following shockwave lithotripsy.[49,50]

An important finding is that alpha antagonists cause complete relaxation of the ureter only in the presence of epinephrine (the endogenous ligand of beta and alpha receptors).[51] This phenomenon suggests a role of beta adrenergic receptors in ureteral relaxation, as unopposed beta stimulation seems to have an effect on ureteral relaxation. For this reason, future studies of expulsive therapy will likely include beta agonists.

Neurokinin receptor antagonists have been studied in vitro as alternative agents to modulate ureteral contractility. The three neurokinin receptors, NK1, NK2, and NK-3 have affinity for substance P, neurokinin A and neurokinin B, respectively.[52] Blockage of these receptors prevents phospholipase C synthesis and ultimately calcium influx into the smooth muscle cell. The result is ureteral relaxation.[52] NK-2 is the predominant receptor in the human ureter, and its inhibition in vitro prevents ureteral contractility.[52] NK-2 blockade has yet to be studied clinically, but if safe may decrease obstruction-related pain and increase stone passage rates.

Nitric oxide (NO) is a major inhibitory neurotransmitter in the ureter. Based on axons that stain positive for nitric oxide synthase in the human ureter, it has been suggested that nitric oxide may play a role in ureteral relaxation.[53] In vitro, it has been shown that NO inhibits ureteral contractility in rats.[54] Interestingly, NO seems to play a specific role at the ureterovesical junction, where it has been postulated to regulate the valve-like effect in this area.[55]

Other pharmacological agents being studied in vitro include histamine antagonists, 5-HT receptor antagonists, neuropeptides, Vasoactive intestinal polypeptide, Calcitonin Gene-related Peptide, Neuropeptide Y, and agents which effect the Rho Kinase pathway. Each of these agents has the common endpoint of a decrease in ureteral contractility. Multiple experimental models have been created to measure ureteral contractility and thus aid our understanding of these myriad agents[56] (Table 8.2).

Table 8.2. Experimental agents for medical expulsive therapy

Beta agonists
Neurokinin receptor antagonists
Nitric oxide
Histamine antagonists
5-HT receptor antagonists
Neuropeptides
Vasoactive intestinal peptide
Calcitonin gene-related peptide

Special Situations in Ureteral Physiology

Infection of the upper tract has been shown in vitro and in vivo to impair ureteral contraction. As early as 1913, Primbs demonstrated that toxins released by *E. coli* and staphylococcus had the ability to inhibit contractions in the guinea pig ureter.[57] In humans, decreased peristalsis and even absence of peristalsis has been documented in the ureter in cases of infection, and can be a radiographic disease hallmark.[58]

Not surprisingly, ureteral contractility and ureter response to various stimuli changes with age. In vitro studies have observed that an intraluminal pressure load will cause more deformation in a neonatal rabbit ureter than in an adult.[59] In addition, there seems to be a decrease in the response of the ureter to Beta adrenergic agents with age, an event likely mediated by decreased cAMP levels.[60]

Pregnancy has been known to cause varying degrees of hydroureteronephrosis, although the mechanism of this phenomenon has been debated over time. Likely, a combination of obstruction and hormonal changes are responsible. Evidence for obstructive hydronephrosis includes the fact that pregnant women demonstrate elevated resting pressures in the ureter above the pelvic brim, which can be reversed with positional changes. In addition, hydronephrosis of pregnancy does not occur in quadriplegic patients, whose uterus hangs away from the ureters.[61] Evidence for hormonal effects on the ureter is conflicting. Although some studies have demonstrated increased ureteral dilatation due to progesterone, others have failed to show any correlation.[61] In general, obstruction appears to be the primary factor in hydronephrosis of pregnancy, although hormones may play a secondary role.[61]

Conclusion

Ureteral physiology involves a complex interplay between various tissues, cells, receptors, and proteins. Clinical modulation of ureteral contraction has great promise for managing ureteral colic as well as expanding our understanding of medical expulsive therapy. To date, the most promising agents remain NSAIDS, alpha blockers, PDE-IV inhibitors, and NK antagonists. More work on the subject is necessary to determine the optimal agent or combination of agents to treat the human ureter.

References

1. Weiss RM. Physiology and pharmacology of the renal pelvis and ureter. In: Walsh PC, Retik AB, Vaughan ED, Wein A, eds. *Campbell's Urology*. Philadelphia, PA: WB Saunders; 1998:839-869.

2. Birder L. Role of the urothelium in bladder function. *Scand Urol J*. 2004;215:48-53.

3. Morita T, Ando M, Kihara K, Oshima H. Function and distribution of autonomic receptors in canine ureteral smooth muscle. *Urol Int*. 1995;55:123-127.

4. Kabalin JN. Surgical anatomy of the retroperitoneum, kidneys, and ureters. In: Walsh PC, Retik AB, Vaughan ED, Wein A, eds. *Campbell's Urology*. Philadelphia, PA: WB Saunders; 1998:49.

5. Yoshimura N, Chancellor M. Physiology and pharmacology of the bladder and urethra. In: Walsh PC, Retik AB, Vaughan ED, Wein A, eds. *Campbell's Urology*. Philadelphia, PA: WB Saunders; 2008:1923-1926.

6. Andersson R, Nilsson K. Cyclic AMP and calcium in relaxation in intestinal smooth muscle. *Nat New Biol*. 1972;238:119.

7. Longrigg N. Minor calyces as primary pacemaker sites for ureteral activity in man. *Lancet*. 1975;1:253.

8. Davidson ME, Lang RJ. Effects of selective inhibitors of cyclooxygenase-1 (COX-1) and cyclooxygenase-2 (COX-2) on the spontaneous myogenic contractions in the upper urinary tract of the guinea-pig and rat. *Br J Pharmacol*. 2000;129(4):661-670.

9. O'Conor VJ Jr, Dawson-Edwards P. Role of the ureter in renal transplantation I: studies of denervated ureter with particular reference to ureteroueretal anastomosis. *J Urol*. 1959;82:566.

10. Lang RJ, Exintaris B, Teele ME, et al. Electrical basis of peristalsis in the mammalian upper urinary tract. *Clin Exp Pharmacol Physiol*. 1998;25:310.

11. David SG, Cebrian C, Vaughan ED Jr, et al. c-kit and ureteral peristalsis. *J Urol*. 2005;173:292.

12. Lang RJ, Davidson ME, Exintaris B. Pyeloureteral motility and ureteral peristalsis: essential role of sensory nerves and endogenous prostaglandins. *Exp Physiol*. 2002;87:129.

13. Tomiyama Y, Wanajo I, Tamazaki Y, et al. Effects of cholinergic drugs on ureteral function in anesthetized dogs. *J Urol*. 2004;172:1520.

14. Hernandez M, Prieto D, Simonsen U, et al. Noradrenaline modulates smooth muscle activity of the isolated intravesical ureter of the pig through different types of adrenoceptors. *Br J Pharmacol*. 1992;107:924.

15. Peters HJ, Eckstein W. Possible pharmacological means of treating renal colic. *Urol Res*. 1975;3:55.

16. Wanajo I, Tomiyama Y, Yamazaki Y, et al. Pharmacological characterization of beta-adrenoceptor subtypes mediating relaxation in porcine isolated ureteral smooth muscle. *J Urol*. 2004;172:1155.

17. Martin TV, Wheeler MA, Weiss RM. Neurokinin induced inositol phosphate production in guinea pig bladder. *J Urol*. 1997;157:1098.

18. Jerde TJ, Saban R, Bjorling DE, et al. Distribution of neuropeptides, histamine content, and inflammatory cells in the ureter. *Urology*. 2000;56:173.

19. Nakada SY, Jerde TJ, Bjorling DE, et al. In vitro contractile effects of neurokinin receptor blockade in the human ureter. *J Urol*. 2001;166:1534.

20. Jerde TJ, Calamon-Dixon JL, Bjorling DE, et al. Celecoxib inhibits ureteral contractility and prostanoid release. *Urology*. 2005;65:185.

21. Ankem MK, Jerde TJ, Wilkinson ER, Nakada SY. Third prize: prostaglandin E(2)-3 receptor is involved in ureteral contractility in obstruction. *J Endourol*. 2005;19:1088-1091.

22. Solari V, Piotrowska AP, Puri P. Altered expression of interstitial cells of Cajal in congenital ureteropelvic junction obstruction. *J Urol*. 2003;170:2420.

23. Murakumo M, Nonomura K, Yamashita T, et al. Structural changes of collagen components and diminution of nerves in congenital ureteropelvic junction obstruction. *J Urol*. 1997;157:1963.

24. Laird JM, Roza C, Cervero F. Effects of artificial calculosis on rat ureter motility: peripheral contribution to the pain of ureteric colic. *Am J Physiol*. 1997; 272(R):1409.

25. Vaughan ED Jr, Shenasky JHI, Gillenwater JY. Mechanism of acute hemodynamic response to ureteral occlusion. *Invest Urol*. 1971;9:109.

26. Roshani H, Dabhoiwala NF, Dijkhus T, et al. Pharmacological modulation of ureteral peristalsis in a chronically instrumented conscious pig model. I: Effect of cholinergic stimulation and inhibition. *J Urol*. 2003;170:264.

27. Venkatesh R, Landman J, Minor SD, et al. Impact of a double-pigtail stent on ureteral peristalsis in the porcine model: initial studies using a novel implantable magnetic sensor. *J Endourol*. 2005;19:170.

28. Mardis HK, Kroeger RM, Hepperlen TW, Mazer MJ, Kammandel H. Polyethelene double-pigtail ureteral stents. *Urol Clin N Am*. 1982;9:95-101.

29. Payne SR, Ramsay JW. The effects of double J stent of renal pelvic dynamics in the pig. *J Urol*. 1988;140:637-641.

30. Olweny EO, Portis AJ, Afane JS, et al. Flow characteristics of 3 unique ureteral stents: investigation of a Poiseuille flow pattern. *J Urol*. 2000;164:2099-2103.

31. Stoller ML, Schwartz BF, Frigstad JR, et al. An in vitro assessment of the flow characteristics of spiral-ridged and smooth-walled JJ ureteric stents. *BJU Int*. 2000;85:628-631.

32. Laird JM, Roza C, Cervero F. Effects of artificial calculosis on rat ureter motility: peripheral contribution to the pain of ureteric colic. *Am J Physiol*. 1997;272: R1409-R1414.

33. Kaplan N, Elkin M, Sharkey J. Ureteral peristalsia and the autonomic nervous system. *Investig Urol*. 1968;5:468-482.

34. Cole RS, Fry CH, Shuttleworth KE. The action of prostaglandins on isolated human ureteric smooth muscle. *Br J Urol*. 1988;61:19-26.

35. Mastrangelo D, Wisard M, Rohner S, Leisinger H, Iselin CE. Diclofenac and NS-398, a selective cyclooxygenase-2 inhibitor, decrease agonist-induced contractions of the pig isolated ureter. *Urol Res.* 2000;28:376-382.

36. Stief CG, Taher A, Truss M, Becker AJ, Schulz-Knapp P, et al. Phosphodiesterase isoenzymes in human ureteral smooth muscle: identification, characterization, and functional effects of various phosphodiesterase inhibitors in vitro. *Urol Int.* 1995;55:183-189.

37. Becker AJ, Stief CG, Meyer M, Truss M, Forssman WG. The effect of the specific phosphodiesterase-IV-inhibitor rolipram on the ureteral peristalsis of the rabbit in vitro and in vivo. *J Urol.* 1998;160:920-925.

38. Hertle L, Nawrath H. Calcium channel blockade in smooth muscle of the human upper urinary tract. II. Effects on norephinephrine-induced activation. *J Urol.* 1984;132:1270.

39. Hertle L, Nawrath H. Calcium channel blockade in smooth muscle of the human upper urinary tract. I. Effects on depolarization-induced activation. *J Urol.* 1984;132:1265.

40. Porpiglia F, Destenanis P, Fiori C, et al. Effectiveness of nifedipine and deflazacort in the management of distal ureter stones. *Urology.* 2000;56:579.

41. Caravati EM, Runge JW, Bossart RJ, et al. Nifedipine for the relief of renal colic: a double blind, placebo-controlled clinical trial. *Ann Emerg Med.* 1989; 18:352.

42. Yilmaz E, Batislam E, Bassar MM, Tuglu D, Ferhat M, et al. The comparison and efficacy of 3 different alpha1-adrenergic blockers for distal ureteral stones. *J Urol.* 1005;173:2010-2012.

43. Dellabella M, Milanese G, Muzzonigro G. Efficacy of tamsulosin in the medical management of juxtavesical ureteral stones. *J Urol.* 2003;170:2202.

44. Dellabella M, Milanese G, Muzzonigro G. Randomized trial of the efficacy of tamsulosin, nifedipine and phloroglucinol in medical expulsive therapy for distal ureteral calculi. *J Urol.* 2005;174:167.

45. Dellabella M, Milanese G, Muzzonigro G. Medical-expulsive therapy for distal ureterolithiasisi: randomized prospective study on role of corticosteroids used in compination with tamsulosin-simplified treatment regimen and health-related quality of life. *Urology.* 2005;666:712.

46. Hollingsworth JM, Rogers MA, Kaufman SR, Bradford TJ, Saint S. Medical therapy to facilitate urinary stone passage: a meta-analysis. *Lancet.* 2006;368: 1171-1179.

47. Preminger GM, Tiselius HG, Assimos DG, Alken P, Buck C, Gallucci M. 2007 guideline for the management of ureteral calculi. *J Urol.* 2007;178:2418-2434.

48. Dellabella M, Milanese G, Muzzonigro G. Medical-expulsive therapy for distal ureterolithiasis: randomized

prospective study on role of corticosteroids used in combination with tamsulosin-simplified treatment regimen and health-related quality of life. *Urology.* 2005;66:712-715.

49. Gravina GL, Costa AM, Ronchi P, Galatioto GP, Angelucci A, et al. Tamsulosin treatment increases clinical success rate of single extracorporeal shock wave lithotripsy of renal stones. *Urology.* 2005;66:24.

50. Resim S, Ekerbicer HC, CIftci A. Role of tamsulosin in treatment of patients with steinstrasse developing after extracorporeal shock wave lithotripsy. *Urology.* 2005;66:945.

51. Nakada SY, Hedican SP, Moon TD, Jerde TJ. Doxazosin relaxes ureteral smooth muscle and reverses epinephrine-induced ureteral contractility. *J Urol.* 2005;173(suppl):299. Abstract 1104.

52. Regoli D, Nguyen K, Calo G. Neurokinin receptors. Comparison of data from classical pharmacology, binding, and molecular biology. *Ann NY Acad Sci.* 1997;812:144-146.

53. Stief CG, Uckert S, Truss MC, Becker AJ, Machtens S, Jonas U. A possible role for nitric oxide in the regulation of human ureteral smooth muscle tone in vitro. *Urol Res.* 1996;24:333-337.

54. Iselin CE, Alm P, Schaad NC, Larsson B, Graber P, Anderson KE. Localization of nitric oxide synthase and haemoxygenase, and functional effects of nitric oxide and carbon monoxide in the pig and human intravesical ureter. *Neurol Urodyn.* 1997;16:209-227.

55. Yucel S, Baskin LS. Neuroanatomy of the ureterovesical junction: clinical implications. *J Urol.* 2003;170:945-948.

56. Venkatesh R, Landman J, Minor SD, Lee DI, Rehman J. Impact of a double-pigtail stent on ureteral peristalsis in the porcine model: initial studies using a novel implantable magnetic sensor. *J Endourol.* 2005;19:170-176.

57. Primbs K. Untersuchungen uber die Einwirkung von Bakterientoxinen auf der uberlebenden Meerschweinchenureter. *Z Urol Chir.* 1913;1:600.

58. Ross JA, Edmond P, Kirkland IS. *Behavior of the Human Ureter in Health and Disease.* Edinburgh, Scotland: Churchill Livingstone; 1972.

59. Akimoto M, Biancani P, Weiss RM. Comparative pressure-length-diameter relationships of neonatoal and adult rabbit ureters. *Invest Urol.* 1977;14:297.

60. Wheeler MA, Housman A, Cho YH, Weiss RM. Age dependence of adenylate cyclase activity in guinea pig ureter homogenate. *J Pharmacol Exp Ther.* 1986; 239:99.

61. Weiss RM. Physiology and pharmacology of the renal pelvis and ureter. In: Walsh PC, Retik AB, Vaughan ED, Wein A, eds. *Campbell's Urology.* Philadelphia, PA: WB Saunders; 2008:1916-1917.

9

Physiology and Pharmacology of the Bladder

Karl-Erik Andersson

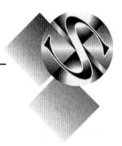

Introduction

The functions of the lower urinary tract (LUT) are to store and periodically release urine. These functions are dependent upon a complex interplay between the central and peripheral nervous systems and local regulatory factors.[1] The neural circuitry that controls these interactions is complex and involves pathways at many levels of the brain, the spinal cord, and the peripheral nervous system, and it is mediated by multiple neurotransmitters. Micturition is under voluntary control and depends on learned behavior that develops during maturation of the nervous system. Normal micturition requires coordination of the activity of the bladder and urethra with that of urethral striated muscle, and depends on the integration of pontine centers and autonomic and somatic efferent mechanisms within the lumbosacral spinal cord (see Fowler et al.[2]).

Malfunction at various levels may result in micturition disorders, which roughly can be classified as disturbances of storage or emptying. Failure to store urine may lead to various forms of incontinence (mainly urgency and stress incontinence). Pharmacologic treatment of urinary incontinence is a main option, and several drugs with different modes and sites of action have been tried.[3,4] To be able to optimize treatment, knowledge about the mechanisms of micturition and of the targets for treatment is necessary.

Nervous Control of Bladder Function

The nervous mechanisms for bladder emptying and urine storage involve a complex pattern of afferent and efferent signaling in *parasympathetic*, *sympathetic*, and *somatic* nerves. These nerves constitute reflex pathways, which either maintain the bladder in a relaxed state, enabling urine storage at low intravesical pressure, or which initiate micturition by relaxing the outflow region and contracting the bladder smooth muscle. Under normal conditions, there is a reciprocal relationship between the activity in the detrusor and the activity in the outlet region. During voiding, contraction of the detrusor muscle is preceded by a relaxation of the outlet region, thereby facilitating the bladder emptying.[1] On the contrary, during the storage phase, the detrusor muscle is relaxed, and the outlet region is contracted to maintain continence.

Afferent Signaling Pathways

The parasympathetic, sympathetic, and somatic nerves all contain *sensory* fibers conveying afferent information from the LUT. Most of the sensory nerves to the LUT originate in the dorsal root ganglia at the lumbosacral level of the spinal cord and travel via the pelvic nerve to the periphery. These fibers serve not only to initiate the micturition reflex, but also to monitor the

C.R. Chapple and W.D. Steers (eds.), *Practical Urology: Essential Principles and Practice*,
DOI: 10.1007/978-1-84882-034-0_9, © Springer-Verlag London Limited 2011

bladder volume during the filling phase. In addition, some afferents originate in dorsal root ganglia at the thoracolumbar level and travel in the hypogastric nerve. The sensory nerves to the striated muscle of the external urethral sphincter travel in the pudendal nerve to the sacral region of the spinal cord.[5] After entering the spinal cord, the primary afferent fibers of the pelvic and pudendal nerves travel rostrally in Lissauer's tract, and are connected to second order neurons.

The most important afferents for the micturition process are myelinated Aδ-fibers and unmyelinated C-fibers travelling in the pelvic nerve to the sacral spinal cord,[6,7] conveying information from receptors in the bladder wall. The Aδ-fibers respond to passive distension and active contraction, thus conveying information about bladder filling.[8,9] The activation threshold, i.e., the intravesical pressure at which humans report the first sensation of bladder filling, is for Aδ-fibers 5–15 cm H_2O.[10] C-fibers have a high mechanical threshold and respond primarily to chemical irritation of the bladder urothelium/suburothelium[11] or cold.[12] Following chemical irritation, the C-fiber afferents exhibit spontaneous firing when the bladder is empty and increased firing during bladder distension. These fibers are normally inactive and are therefore termed "silent fibers."

Efferent Signaling

Parasympathetic Nerves

Contraction of the detrusor smooth muscle and relaxation of the outflow region result from activation of *parasympathetic* neurones located in the sacral parasympathetic nucleus (SPN) in the sacral spinal cord at the level of S2–S4.[5] The axons pass through the pelvic nerve and synapse with the postganglionic nerves either in the pelvic plexus, in ganglia on the surface of the bladder (vesical ganglia), or within the walls of the bladder and urethra (intramural ganglia). The preganglionic neurotransmission is predominantly mediated by acetylcholine (ACh) acting on nicotinic receptors, although the transmission can be modulated by adrenergic, muscarinic, purinergic, and peptidergic presynaptic receptors.[10] The postganglionic neurones in the pelvic nerve mediate the excitatory input to the normal human detrusor smooth muscle by releasing ACh acting on muscarinic receptors. However, an atropine-resistant (non-adrenergic, non-cholinergic: NANC) contractile component is regularly found in the bladders of most animal species.[1] Such a component can also be demonstrated in functionally and morphologically altered human bladder tissue, but contributes only up to a few percent to normal detrusor contraction.[13] ATP is one important mediator of the NANC contraction,[14] although the involvement of other transmitters cannot be ruled out.[13] The pelvic nerve also conveys parasympathetic nerves to the outflow region and the urethra. These nerves exert an inhibitory effect on the smooth muscle, by releasing nitric oxide (NO), and other transmitters.[13]

Sympathetic Nerves

Most of the *sympathetic* innervation of the bladder and urethra originates from the intermediolateral nuclei in the thoraco-lumbar region (T10-L2) of the spinal cord. The axons leave the spinal cord via the splanchnic nerves and travel either through the inferior mesenteric ganglia (IMF) and the hypogastric nerve, or pass through the paravertebral chain to the lumbosacral sympathetic chain ganglia and enter the pelvic nerve. Thus, sympathetic signals are conveyed in both the hypogastric nerve and the pelvic nerve.[5] The preganglionic sympathetic transmission is, like the parasympathetic preganglionic transmission, predominantly mediated by ACh acting on nicotinic receptors. Some preganglionic terminals synapse with the postganglionic cells in the paravertebral ganglia or in the IMF, while other synapse closer to the pelvic organs, and short postganglionic neurones innervate the target organs. Thus, the hypogastric and pelvic nerves contain both pre- and postganglionic fibers.[5] The predominant effect of the sympathetic innervation is to contract the bladder base and the urethra. In addition, the sympathetic innervation inhibits the parasympathetic pathways at spinal and ganglionic levels too. In humans, noradrenaline is released in response to electrical stimulation in vitro, and the normal response to released noradrenaline is relaxation.[1] However, the importance of the sympathetic innervation for relaxation of the human detrusor has never been established. In contrast, in several animal species, the adrenergic innervation has been demonstrated to mediate relaxation of the detrusor during filling.

Somatic Nerves

The *somatic* innervation of the urethral striated muscles (rhabdosphincter) and of some perineal muscles (for example compressor urethrae and urethrovaginal sphincter), is provided by the pudendal nerve. These fibers originate from sphincter motor neurons located in the ventral horn of the sacral spinal cord (levels S2–S4) in a region called Onuf's (Onufrowicz's) nucleus.[15] They release ACh, which activates the muscles via nicotinic receptors, both during the bladder storage phase as well as under stress conditions (the guarding reflex, see below).

The Storage Phase

During the storage phase the bladder has to relax in order to maintain a low intravesical pressure. Urine storage is regulated by two separate storage reflexes, of which one is sympathetic (autonomic) and the other is somatic.[15] The sympathetic storage reflex (pelvic-to-hypogastric reflex) is initiated as the bladder distends (myelinated Aδ-fibers) and the generated afferent activity travels in the pelvic nerves to the spinal cord. Within the spinal cord, sympathetic firing from the lumbar region (L1–L3) is initiated, which, by effects at the ganglionic level decreases excitatory parasympathetic inputs to the bladder, but also through postganglionic neurons releases noradrenaline, which facilitates urine storage by stimulating β-adrenoceptors (ARs) in the detrusor smooth muscle (see below). As mentioned previously, there is little evidence for a functionally important sympathetic innervation of the human detrusor, which is in contrast to what has been found in several animal species. The sympathetic innervation of the human bladder is found mainly in the outlet region, where it mediates contraction. During micturition, this sympathetic reflex pathway is markedly inhibited via supraspinal mechanisms to allow the bladder to contract and the urethra to relax. Thus, the Aδ afferents and the sympathetic efferent fibers constitute a vesico-spinal-vesical storage reflex which maintains the bladder in a relaxed mode while the proximal urethra and bladder neck are contracted.

In response to a sudden increase in bladder pressure, such as during a cough, laugh or sneeze, a more rapid somatic storage reflex (pelvic-to-pudendal reflex), also called the guarding or continence reflex, is initiated. The evoked afferent activity travels along myelinated Aδ afferent nerve fibers in the pelvic nerve to the sacral spinal cord, where efferent somatic urethral motor neurons, located in the nucleus of Onuf, are activated. Afferent information is also conveyed to the periaqueductal grey (PAG) and to the pontine storage center (the L-region). Axons from these motor neurons of the nucleus of Onuf travel in the pudendal nerve and release ACh, which activates nicotinic cholinergic receptors on rhabdosphincter, which contracts. This pathway is tonically active during urine storage. During sudden abdominal pressure increases, however, it becomes dynamically active to contract the rhabdosphincter. During micturition this reflex is strongly inhibited via spinal and supraspinal mechanisms to allow the rhabdosphincter to relax and permit urine passage through the urethra. In addition to this spinal somatic storage reflex, there is also supraspinal input from the pons, which projects directly to the nucleus of Onuf and is importance for volitional control of the rhabdosphincter.

The Emptying Phase

Vesico-Bulbo-Vesical Micturition Reflex

Electrophysiological experiments in cats and rats provide evidence for a voiding reflex mediated through a vesico-bulbo-vesical pathway involving neural circuits in the pons, which constitute the pontine micturition centre (PMC). Other regions in the brain, important for micturition, include the hypothalamus and cerebral cortex.[2,10] Bladder filling leads to increased activation of tension receptors within the bladder wall and to increased afferent activity in Aδ-fibers. These fibers project on spinal tract neurones mediating increased sympathetic firing to maintain continence as discussed above (storage reflex). In addition, the spinal tract neurones convey the afferent activity to more rostral areas of the spinal cord and the brain. One important receiver of the afferent information from the bladder is the PAG in the rostral brainstem. The PAG receives information from both afferent neurones in the bladder and from more rostral areas in the brain, i.e., cerebral cortex and hypothalamus. This information is integrated in the

PAG and the medial part of the PMC (the M-region), which also control the descending pathways in the micturition reflex. Thus, PMC can be seen as a switch in the micturition reflex, inhibiting parasympathetic activity in the descending pathways when there is low activity in the afferent fibers, and activating the parasympathetic pathways when the afferent activity reaches a certain threshold.[10] The threshold is believed to be set by the inputs from more rostral regions in the brain. In cats, lesioning of regions above the inferior colliculus usually facilitates micturition by elimination of inhibitory inputs from more rostral areas of the brain. On the other hand, transactions at a lower level inhibit micturition. Thus, the PMC seems to be under a tonic inhibitory control. A variation of the inhibitory input to PMC results in a variation of bladder capacity. Experiments on rats have shown that the micturition threshold is regulated by, e.g., GABA-ergic inhibitory mechanisms in the PMC neurones.

Vesico-Spinal-Vesical Micturition Reflex

Spinal lesion rostral to the lumbo-sacral level interrupt the vesico-bulbo-vesical pathway and abolish the supraspinal and voluntary control of micturition. This results initially in an areflexic bladder accompanied by urinary retention.[10] An automatic vesico-spinal-vesical micturition reflex develops slowly, although voiding is generally insufficient due to bladder-sphincter dyssynergia, i.e., simultaneous contraction of bladder and urethra. It has been demonstrated in chronic spinal cats that the afferent limb of this reflex is conveyed through unmyelinated C-fibers which usually do not respond to bladder distension,[11] suggesting changed properties of the afferent receptors in the bladder. Accordingly, the micturition reflex in chronic spinal cats is blocked by capsaicin, a neurotoxin which blocks C-fiber mediated neurotransmission (see below).

Targets for Pharmacologic Intervention

Peripheral Targets

Although there are many drugs acting on peripheral targets involved in micturition control many of them are less useful in the clinical situation due to the lack of selectivity for the LUT, which may result in intolerable side effects. For example, calcium antagonists and potassium channel openers should theoretically be good targets for drugs aimed for bladder control. However, no such drugs have been developed with sufficient selectivity for the LUT.

Detailed discussions of possible targets and of the basis for therapeutic interventions, as well as assessments of current therapeutic principles can be found in recent comprehensive reviews.[4,13,16]

Afferent Signaling Mechanisms

Urothelium

Recent evidence suggests that the urothelium may serve as a mechanosensor which, by producing NO, ATP, ACh and other mediators, can control the activity in afferent nerves, and thereby the initiation of the micturition reflex.[17] Low pH, high K^+, increased osmolality, and low temperatures can all influence afferent nerves, possibly via effects on the "vanilloid" (TRPV1) receptor, which is expressed both in afferent nerve terminals and in the epithelial cells that line the bladder lumen.[18,19] A network of interstitial cells (Interstitial Cells of Cajal; ICC), extensively linked by Cx43-containing gap junctions, was found to be located beneath the urothelium in the human bladder.[20,21] This interstitial cellular network was suggested to operate as a functional syncytium, integrating signals and responses in the bladder wall. The firing of suburothelial afferent nerves and the threshold for bladder activation may be modified by both inhibitory (e.g., NO) and stimulatory (e.g., ATP, ACh, tachykinins, prostanoids) mediators. ATP, generated by the urothelium, has been suggested as an important mediator of urothelial signaling.[22] Supporting such a view, intravesical ATP induces detrusor overactivity in conscious rats.[23] Furthermore, mice lacking the $P2X_3$ receptor were shown to have hypoactive bladders.[24,25]

There seem to be other, thus far unidentified, factors in the urothelium that could influence bladder function.[13] Fovaeus et al.[26] found a previously unrecognized nonadrenergic, non-nitrergic, non-prostanoid inhibitory mediator is released from the rat urinary bladder by muscarinic receptor stimulation. However, it was not clear whether this factor came from the detrusor muscle or from both the bladder and the urothelium. Hawthorn et al.[27] presented data suggesting the presence of a diffusable, urothelium-derived inhibitory factor, which could not be identified, but appeared to be neither nitric oxide, a cyclooxygenase product, a catecholamine, adenosine, γ-aminobutyric acid (GABA) nor any substance sensitive to apamin. The identity and possible physiologic role of the unknown factor remains to be established and should offer an interesting field for further research. These mechanisms can be involved in the pathophysiology of the overactive bladder syndrome (OAB) and detrusor overactivity (DO) and thus seem to be interesting targets for pharmacologic intervention.

Myocytes

Myogenic activity can be defined as the ability of a smooth muscle cell to generate mechanical activity independent of external stimuli.[1] In the individual myocyte, contractile activity is preceded and initiated by an action potential, which is calcium driven.[28] It has been suggested that the detrusor muscle is arranged into units (modules), which are circumscribed areas of muscle.[29] These modules show contractile activity during the filling phase of the micturition cycle and might be controlled by several factors including a peripheral myovesical plexus, consisting of intramural ganglia and ICC[30]. Intercellular connections may contribute to module control, but also locally generated mediators. Kinder and Mundy[31] found that spontaneous contractile activity developed more often in muscle strips from overactive than normal bladders, a finding underlined by Brading,[32] and confirmed by Mills et al.[33] Turner and Brading[34] discussed the occurrence of "patchy denervation" in cases of DO with subsequent changes of the smooth muscle cells, e.g., supersensitivity to ACh. Such an increased sensitivity has been demonstrated in smooth muscle preparations from patients with idiopathic and neurogenic DO.[35] It has been reported that suburothelial ICC respond to purinergic stimulation by firing Ca^{2+} transients.[36] Interestingly, these suburothelial ICC may be able to affect the activity of the detrusor myocytes.[37-39] The frequency of the spontaneous rhythmic contractions of isolated detrusor

smooth muscle preparations seems to vary between species, and is probably also dependent on experimental factors (see, Andersson and Arner[1]).[30] Characteristically, these contractions are resistant to the Na-channel blocker (TTX) and cannot be blocked by hexamethonium, atropine, α-AR blockers, β-AR blockers, or suramin, apparently excluding direct involvement of nerves and nerve – released transmitters.[1] Contractions can be effectively inhibited by L-type Ca^{2+} channel blockers and K^+ channel openers, supporting the important role of L-type Ca^{2+} channels for the activity. It cannot be excluded that these spontaneous contractions generates part of the afferent activity ("afferent noise") during filling of the bladder.[40]

Cholinergic Receptors

Muscarinic Receptors

Muscarinic receptors comprise five subtypes, encoded by five distinct genes.[41] The five gene products correspond to pharmacologically defined receptors, and $M_1 - M_5$ is used to describe both the molecular and pharmacological subtypes. In the human bladder, the mRNAs for all muscarinic receptor subtypes have been demonstrated,[42,43] with a predominance of mRNAs encoding M_2 and M_3 receptors.[42,44] These receptors are also functionally coupled to G-proteins, but the signal transduction systems vary.[45-48]

Detrusor smooth muscle contains muscarinic receptors of mainly the M_2 and M_3 subtypes.[45-49] The M_3 receptors in the human bladder are believed to be the most important for detrusor contraction. Jezior et al.[50] suggested that muscarinic receptor activation of detrusor muscle includes both non-selective cation channels and activation of Rho-kinase. Supporting a role of Rho-kinase in the regulation of rat detrusor contraction and tone, Wibberley et al.[51] found that Rho-kinase inhibitors (Y-27632, HA 1077) inhibited contractions evoked by carbachol without affecting the contraction response to KCl. They also demonstrated high levels of Rho-kinase isoforms (I and II) in the bladder. Schneider et al.[49] concluded that carbachol-induced contraction of human urinary bladder is mediated via M_3 receptors and largely depends on Ca^{2+} entry through nifedipine-sensitive channels and activation of the Rho-kinase pathway Thus, the main pathway for muscarinic receptor activation of the detrusor via M_3 receptors may be calcium influx via L-type calcium channels, and increased sensitivity to calcium of the contractile machinery produced via inhibition of myosin light chain phosphatase through activation of Rho-kinase.[52]

The functional role for the M_2 receptors has not been clarified, but it has been suggested that M_2 receptors may oppose sympathetically mediated smooth muscle relaxation, mediated by β-ARs.[53] M_2 receptor stimulation may also activate non-specific cation channels[54] and inhibit K_{ATP} channels through activation of protein kinase C[55,56]. In certain disease states, M_2 receptors may contribute to contraction of the bladder. Thus, in the denervated rat bladder, M_2 receptors, or a combination of M_2 and M_3, mediated contractile responses and the two types of receptor seemed to act in a facilitatory manner to mediate contraction.[57–59] In obstructed, hypertrophied rat bladders, there was an increase in total and M_2 receptor density, whereas there was a reduction in M_3 receptor density.[60] The functional significance of this change for voiding function has not been established. Pontari et al.[61] analyzed bladder muscle specimens from patients with neurogenic bladder dysfunction to determine whether the muscarinic receptor subtype mediating contraction shifts from M_3 to the M_2 receptor subtype, as found in the denervated, hypertrophied rat bladder. They concluded that whereas normal detrusor contractions are mediated by the M_3 receptor subtype, in patients with neurogenic bladder dysfunction, contractions can be mediated by the M_2 receptors.

Muscarinic receptors may also be located on the pre-synaptic nerve terminals and participate in the regulation of transmitter release. The inhibitory pre-junctional muscarinic receptors have been classified as M_4 in the human bladder.[62] Pre-junctional facilitatory muscarinic receptors appear to be of the M_1.[63] The muscarinic facilitatory mechanism seems to be upregulated in hyperactive bladders from chronic spinal cord transected rats. The facilitation in these preparations is primarily mediated by M_3 muscarinic receptors.[63,64]

Muscarinic receptors have also been demonstrated on the urothelium/suburothelium. The porcine urothelium was found to expresses a high density of muscarinic receptors, even higher than the bladder smooth muscle,[27] and, in the rat and human urothelium, the receptor proteins and mRNAs, respectively, for all muscarinic receptor subtypes (M_1–M_5) were demonstrated.[65] However, the expression pattern of the different subtypes in the human urothelium was reported to differ: the M_1 receptors on basal cells, M_2 on umbrella cells, M_3 and M_4 homogenously, and M_5 with a decreasing gradient from luminal to basal cells.[43] Mansfield et al.[66] found, using RT-PCR analysis, an abundant expression of muscarinic M_2 receptors in the human bladder mucosa. These receptors may occur at other locations than the urothelium, e.g., on suburothelial interstitial cells.[67,68]

The suburothelial nerve plexus is close to the urothelium.[69–71] The urothelium, as mentioned previously, has been suggested to work as a mechanosensory conductor, and in response to, e.g., distension, it releases ATP affecting underlying afferent nerve fibers via purinoceptors.[25,72] This may consequently modify the afferent response of the bladder.[73,74] ACh is produced in the urothelium, but the mechanism behind its release does not seem to involve vesicular exocytosis.[75,76] The organic cation transporter 3 subtype has been demonstrated in and suggested to be involved in the non-neuronal release from rat urothelium.[76]

Nicotinic Receptors

Although nicotinic ACh receptors in both the central and peripheral nervous systems play a prominent role in the control of urinary bladder function, little is known regarding expression or function of nicotinic receptors in the bladder urothelium. Beckel et al.[77] examined the expression and functionality of nicotinic receptors in the urothelium, as well as the effects of stimulation of nicotinic receptors on the micturition reflex. mRNA for the α3, α5, α7, β3, and β4 nicotinic subunits was identified in rat urothelial cells using RT-PCR. Western blotting also confirmed urothelial expression of the α3- and α7-subunits. Application of nicotine to cultured rat urothelial cells elicited an increase in intracellular Ca^{2+} concentration, indicating that at least some of the subunits form functional channels. These effects were blocked by the application of the nicotinic antagonist hexamethonium.

More investigations are needed to establish the functional role of urothelial nicotinic receptors, normally and in bladder disorders.

Adrenergic Receptors (ARs)

α-Adrenoceptors

α-ARs may have effects on different locations in the bladder: the detrusor smooth muscle, the detrusor vasculature, the afferent and efferent nerve terminal and intramural ganglia. For some of these possible sites only fragmentary information is available.

Most investigators agree on that there is a low expression of these receptors in the derusor muscle.[78-80] In the human bladder studies Malloy et al.[78] found that two-thirds of the α-AR mRNA expressed was α_{1D}, there was no α_{1B}, and one-third was α_{1A}.

Nomiya and Yamaguchi[81] confirmed the low expression of α-AR mRNA in normal human bladder, and further demonstrated that there was no upregulation of any of the adrenergic receptors with obstruction. In addition, in functional experiments they found a small response to phenylephrine at high drug concentrations with no difference between normal and obstructed bladders. Thus, in the obstructed human bladder, there seemed to be no evidence for α-AR upregulation. This finding was challenged by Bouchelouche et al.[82] who found an increased response to α_1-AR stimulation in obstructed human bladders. If there is a change of sensitivity to α-AR stimulation in the obstructed bladder of clinical importance (influencing the response to α-AR blockers) remains to be established.

All subtypes of α-ARs can be found in different parts of the human vascular tree, and they all mediate contraction. The expression varies with vessel bed and increases with age. In the bladder, the function of the detrusor muscle is dependent on the vasculature and the perfusion. Hypoxia induced by partial outlet obstruction is believed to play a major role in both the hypertrophic and degenerative effects of partial outlet obstruction. Das et al.[83] investigated in rats whether doxazosin affected blood flow to the bladder and reduced the level of bladder dysfunction induced by partial outlet obstruction. They found that 4 weeks treatment with doxazosin increased bladder blood flow in both control and obstructed rats. Furthermore doxazosin treatment reduced the severity of the detrusor response to partial outlet obstruction. Thus, doxazosin could reduce the increase in bladder weight in obstructed animals which could be one of the mechanisms that contributed to a positive effect on DO caused by the obstruction.

β-Adrenoceptors

It has been known for a long time that isoprenaline, a non subtype selective β-AR agonist, can relax bladder smooth muscle.[84] Even if the importance of β-ARs for human bladder function still remains to be established,[1] this does not exclude that they can be useful therapeutic targets. All three subtypes of β-ARs (β_1, β_2, and β_3) can be found in the detrusor muscle of most species, including humans,[1,79] and also in the human urothelium.[85] However, the expression of β_3-AR mRNA[79,81] and functional evidence indicate a predominant role for this receptor in both normal and neurogenic bladders.[79,86,87] The human detrusor also contains β_2-ARs, and most probably both receptors are involved in the physiological effects (relaxation) of noradrenaline in the bladder.[1,79] β_3-AR agonists have a pronounced effect on spontaneous contractions of isolated detrusor muscle,[88] which may be the basis for their therapeutic effects in OAB/DO.

It is generally accepted that β-AR-induced detrusor relaxation is mediated by activation of adenylyl cyclase with the subsequent formation of cAMP.[89] However, there is evidence suggesting that in the bladder K+ channels, particularly BK_{ca} channels, may be involved in β-AR mediated relaxation independent of cAMP.[90-93]

The in vivo effects of β_3-AR agonists on bladder function have been studied in several animal models. It has been shown that β_3-AR agonists increase bladder capacity with no change in micturition pressure and residual volume.[94-97] For example, Hicks et al.[98] studied the effects of the selective β_3-AR agonist, GW427353, in the anesthetized dog and found that the drug evoked an increase in bladder capacity under conditions of acid evoked bladder hyperactivity, without affecting voiding.

β_3-AR selective agonists are currently being evaluated as potential treatment for OAB/DO in humans.[99] One of these, mirabegron (YM187), which mediated muscle relaxation in human bladder strips,[100] was given to patients with OAB in a controlled clinical trial.[101] The primary efficacy analysis showed a statistically significant reduction in mean micturition frequency, compared to placebo, and with respect to secondary variables, mirabegron was significantly superior to placebo concerning mean volume voided per micturition, mean number of incontinence episodes, nocturia episodes, urgency incontinence episodes, and urgency episodes per 24 h. The drug was well tolerated, and the most commonly reported side effects were headache and gastrointestinal adverse effects. The results of this proof of concept study showed that the principle of β_3-AR agonism may be useful for treatment of patients with OAB/DO.

Transient Receptor Potential (TRP) Receptors

Appropriate bladder function is dependent on an intact afferent signaling from the bladder to the CNS. This signaling conveys information about bladder filling and the status of the tissue, e.g., presence of infectious agents etc. As mentioned previously, the afferent nerves comprise small, slowly conducting myelinated Aδ-fibers and slowly conducting, unmyelinated C-fibers. The former are excited by mechanoreceptors and convey information about bladder filling, while C-fibers mediate painful sensations recognized by chemoreceptors. Among these are the TRP receptors.[102,103] The mammalian TRP family consists of 28 channels that can be subdivided into six different classes. TRP channels are activated by a diversity of physical (voltage, heat, cold, mechanical stress) or chemical (pH, osmolality) stimuli and by binding of specific ligands, enabling them to act as multifunctional sensors at the cellular level.

Among the many TRP channels demonstrated in the LUT, so far only the TRPV1 channel has been the target of clinical interventions. By means of capsaicin, a subpopulation of primary afferent neurons innervating the bladder and urethra, the "capsaicin-sensitive nerves," has been identified. It is believed that capsaicin exerts its effects by binding to and activating TRPV1 receptors on these nerves. Capsaicin exerts a biphasic effect: initial excitation is followed by a long-lasting blockade, which renders sensitive primary afferents (C-fibers) resistant to activation by natural stimuli. In sufficiently high concentrations, capsaicin is believed to cause "desensitization" initially by releasing and emptying the stores of neuropeptides, and then by blocking further release. Resiniferatoxin is an analogue of capsaicin, approximately 1,000 times more potent for desensitization than capsaicin,[104,105] but only a few hundred times more potent for excitation.[106] Possibly, both capsaicin and RTX can have effects on Aδ-fibers. It is also possible that capsaicin at high concentrations (mM) has additional, non-specific effects.[107]

Experimental and clinical evidence suggest that capsaicin-sensitive afferents can be involved in a number of urological disorders, including neurogenic and idiopathic DO, painful bladder syndrome/interstitial cystitis, and hemorrhagic cystitis.[102] Both capsaicin and resiniferatoxin have been used successfully to treat bladder function disturbances.[4] However, the difficulties with the handling of resiniferatoxin (e.g., the drug may adhere to the administration device), has limit the use of this therapeutic approach.

Phosphodiesterases (PDEs)

Drugs stimulating the generation of cAMP are known to relax smooth muscles, including the detrusor.[1,89] It is also well established that drugs acting through the NO/cGMP system can relax the smooth muscle of the bladder outflow region.[1] Use of PDE inhibitors to enhance the cAMP- and cGMP-mediated relaxation of LUT smooth muscles (detrusor prostate, urethra) should then be a logical approach to treat OAB/DO.[108]

Studies with the PDE1 inhibitor, vinpocetine (reducing the break-down of cAMP), showed relaxant effects in vitro, but poor clinical efficacy in OAB/DO patients.[109] PDE 4 (which also preferably hydrolyses cAMP) has been implicated in the control of bladder smooth muscle tone. PDE 4 inhibitors reduced the in vitro contractile responses of guinea pig[110] and rat[111,112]; bladder strips, and also suppressed rhythmic bladder contractions of the isolated guinea pig bladder.[30] There seems to be no published experience of the effects of PDE 4 inhibition in the treatment of OAB/DO. However, previous experiences with selective PDE 4 inhibitors, used for other indications, showed emesis to be a dose-limiting effect.[113] If this adverse effect can be avoided, the preclinical information suggests that PDE 4 inhibition may be a promising approach.

Treatment with sildenafil (PDE 5 inhibitor, preventing break-down of cGMP) improved urinary symptom scores in men with erectile dysfunction and LUT symptoms (LUTS[114]), and this observation has been confirmed in randomized, controlled clinical trials.[115–117]

The mechanism(s) behind the beneficial effect of the PDE 5 inhibitors on LUTS/OAB and their site(s) of action largely remain to be elucidated.

CNS Targets

Anatomically, several CNS regions may be involved in micturition control: supraspinal structures, such as the cortex and diencephalon, midbrain, and medulla, but also spinal structures (see, Fowler et al.[2]). Several transmitters and their receptors are involved in the reflexes and sites described above and may be targets for drugs aimed for control of micturition.[13] Although few drugs with a CNS site of action have been developed, several agents acting on the CNS may have effects on micturition.

Opioid Receptors

Endogenous opioid peptides and corresponding receptors are widely distributed in many regions in the CNS of importance for micturition control, e.g., the PAG, the PMC, the spinal parasympathetic nucleus, and the nucleus of Onuf.[117]

It has been well established that morphine, given by various routes of administration to animals and humans, can increase bladder capacity and eventually cause urinary retention. Given intrathecally (i.t.) to anesthetized rats and intravenously (i.v.) to humans, the μ-opioid receptor antagonist, naloxone, has been shown to stimulate micturition,[119,120] suggesting that a tonic activation of μ-opioid receptors has a depressant effect on the micturition reflex.

Morphine given i.t. was effective in patients with DO due to spinal cord lesions,[121] but was associated with side-effects, such as nausea and pruritus. Further side-effects of opioid receptor agonists comprise respiratory depression, constipation and abuse. Attempts have been made to reduce these side effects by increasing selectivity towards one of the different opioid receptor types.[122] At least three different opioid receptors – μ, δ, and κ – bind stereospecifically with morphine, and have been shown to interfere with voiding mechanisms. Theoretically, selective receptor actions, or modifications of effects mediated by specific opioid receptors, may have useful therapeutic effects for micturition control.

Tramadol is a well-known analgesic drug, which by itself, it is a very week μ receptor agonist. However, it is metabolized to several different compounds, some of them almost as effective as morphine at the μ receptor. The drug also inhibits serotonin (5-HT) and noradrenaline reuptake.[123] This profile is of particular interest, since both μ-receptor agonism and amine reuptake inhibition may be useful principles for treatment of OAB/DO.

When tramadol is given to a normal, awake rat, the most conspicuous changes in the cystometrogram are increases in threshold pressure and bladder capacity. Naloxone can more or less completely inhibit these effects.[124] There is a small difference between the doses of morphine that cause inhibition of micturition and those increasing bladder capacity and evoking urinary retention. Tramadol has effects over a much wider range of doses, which means that it could be therapeutically more useful for micturition control. It may be speculated that the difference is dependent on tramadol also inhibiting the 5-HT and noradrenaline reuptake.[124] Clinically, tramadol seems to be as effective as antimuscarinics in the treatment of idiopathic OAB, as shown in a double-blind, placebo-controlled, randomized study.[125] However, considering its adverse effect potential, it may not be an ideal agent for OAB treatment.

Serotonin (5-HT) Mechanisms

It is well established that the lumbosacral autonomic, as well as the somatic motor nuclei (Onuf's nuclei), receive a dense serotonergic input from the raphe nuclei, an innervation which is not subjected to the general decline in lumbosacral spinal innervation found with increasing age.[126] Multiple 5-HT receptors have been found at sites where processing of afferent and efferent impulses from and to the LUT take place.[127] Although, as pointed out by de Groat,[128] there is some evidence in the rat for serotonergic facilitation of voiding, the descending pathway is essentially an inhibitory circuit, with 5-HT as a key neurotransmitter. Thus, electrical stimulation of 5-HT-containing neurons in the caudal raphe nucleus causes inhibition of bladder contractions.[129,130] Most experiments in rats and cats indicate that activation of the central serotonergic system by 5-HT reuptake inhibitors, as well as by 5-HT$_{1A}$ and 5-HT$_2$ receptor agonists, depresses reflex bladder contractions and increases the bladder volume threshold for inducing micturition.[128] 5-HT$_{1A}$ receptors are involved in multiple inhibitory mechanisms controlling the spinobulbospinal micturition reflex pathway. The regulation of the frequency of bladder reflexes is presumably mediated by a suppression of afferent input to the micturition switching circuitry in the pons, whereas the regulation of bladder contraction amplitude may be related to an inhibition of the output from the pons to the parasympathetic nuclei in the spinal cord.

Duloxetine is a combined noradrenaline and serotonin reuptake inhibitor, which has been shown to significantly increase sphincteric muscle activity during the filling/storage phase of micturition in the cat acetic acid model of irritated bladder function.[131,132] Bladder capacity was also increased in this model, both effects mediated centrally through both motor efferent and sensory afferent modulation.[133] The effects of duloxetine was studied in a placebo-controlled study comprising women with OAB[134] and was, compared to placebo, shown to cause significant improvements or decreases in voiding and incontinence episodes, for increases in the daytime voiding intervals, and for improvements in quality of life (I-QoL) scores. Urodynamic studies showed no significant increases in maximum cystometric capacity or in the volume threshold for DO. However, adverse effects were common with nausea, dry mouth, dizziness, constipation, insomnia, and fatigue, limiting its tolerability.

γ-Amino Butyric Acid (GABA) Mechanisms

GABA has been identified as a main inhibitory transmitter in the brain and spinal cord. GABA functions appear to be triggered by binding of GABA to its ionotropic receptors, GABA$_A$ and GABA$_C$, which are ligand-gated chloride channels, and its metabotropic receptor, GABA$_B$.[135] Since blockade of GABA$_A$ and GABA$_B$ receptors in the spinal cord[136,137] and brain[137,138] stimulated rat micturition, an endogenous activation of GABA$_{A+B}$ receptors may be responsible for continuous inhibition of the micturition reflex within the CNS. In the spinal cord GABA$_A$ receptors are more numerous than GABA$_B$ receptors, except for the dorsal horn where GABA$_B$ receptors predominate.[139,140]

Experiments using conscious and anesthetized rats demonstrated that exogenous GABA, muscimol (GABA$_A$ receptor agonist) and *baclofen* (GABA$_B$ receptor agonist) given i.v., i.t. or intracerebroventricularly (i.c.v.) inhibit micturition.[137,138] Baclofen given i.t. attenuated oxyhemoglobin induced DO in rats, suggesting that the inhibitory actions of GABA$_B$ receptor agonists in the spinal cord may be useful for controlling micturition disorders caused by C-fiber activation in the urothelium and/or suburothelium.[137] Beneficial effects of baclofen have also been documented in humans with DO.[141]

Gabapentin

Gabapentin was originally designed as an anticonvulsant GABA mimetic capable of crossing the blood-brain barrier.[142] However, its effects do not appear to be mediated through interaction with GABA receptors, and its mechanism of action is still controversial.[142] Gabapentin is also widely used not only for seizures and neuropathic pain, but for many other indications such as anxiety and sleep disorders due to its apparent lack of toxicity.

In a pilot study, Carbone et al.[143] reported on the effect of gabapentin on neurogenic detrusor activity. They found a positive effect on symptoms and a significant improvement of urodynamic parameters after treatment, and suggested that the effects of the drug should be explored in further controlled studies in both neurogenic and non-neurogenic DO. Kim et al.[144] found that 14 of 31 patients with OAB and nocturia, refractory to antimuscarinic treatment, improved with oral gabapentin. The drug was generally well tolerated and was considered to be an option in selective patients when conventional treatment modalities have failed.

Neurokinin and Neurokinin Receptors

The main endogenous tachykinins, substance P (SP), neurokinin A (NKA) and neurokinin B (NKB), and their preferred receptors, NK1, NK2, and NK3, respectively, have been demonstrated in various CNS regions, including those involved in micturition control.[145–147] NK1 receptor expressing neurons in the dorsal horn of the spinal cord may play an important role in DO, and tachykinin involvement via NK1 receptors in the micturition reflex induced by bladder filling has been demonstrated[148] in normal, and more clearly, rats with bladder hypertrophy secondary to BOO. Capsaicin-induced DO was reduced by blocking NK1 receptor-expressing neurons in the spinal cord, using intrathecally administered substance P-saponin conjugate.[149] Furthermore, blockade of spinal NK1 receptor could suppress detrusor activity induced by dopamine receptor (L-DOPA) stimulation.[104,105]

Aprepitant, an NK-1 receptor antagonist used for treatment of chemotherapy-induced nausea and vomiting,[150] significantly improved symptoms of OAB in postmenopausal women with a history of urgency incontinence or mixed incontinence (with predominantly urgency urinary incontinence), as shown in pilot randomized, placebo-controlled trial.[151] Aprepitant significantly decreased the average daily number of micturitions compared with placebo at 8 weeks. The average daily number of urgency episodes was also significantly reduced compared to placebo, and so were the average daily number of urgency incontinence and total urinary incontinence episodes, although the difference was not statistically significant. Aprepitant was generally well tolerated and the incidence of side effects, including dry mouth, was low. The results of this initial proof of concept study suggest that NK-1 receptor antagonism holds promise as a potential treatment approach for OAB/DO.

Summary

To effectively control bladder activity, and to treat urinary incontinence, identification of suitable targets for pharmacological intervention is necessary. Such targets may be found in the central nervous system (CNS) or peripherally. Drugs, specifically directed for control of bladder activity are under development and will hopefully lead to improved treatment of urinary incontinence.

References

1. Andersson KE, Arner A. Urinary bladder contraction and relaxation: physiology and pathophysiology. *Physiol Rev.* 2004;84(3):935-986
2. Fowler CJ, Griffiths D, de Groat WC. The neural control of micturition. *Nat Rev Neurosci.* 2008;9(6): 453-466
3. Zinner NR, Koke SC, Viktrup L. Pharmacotherapy for stress urinary incontinence: present and future options. *Drugs.* 2004;64(14):1503-1516
4. Andersson K-E, Chapple CR, Cardozo L, Cruz F, Hashim H, Michel MC, Tannenbaum C, Wein AJ. Pharmacological treatment of urinary incontinence. In: Abrams P, Cardozo L, Khoury S, Wein A eds. *Incontinence.* 4th International Consultation on Incontinence. Plymouth: Plymbridge Distributors; 2009
5. Lincoln J, Burnstock, G. Autonomic innervation of the urinary bladder and urethra. In: Maggi CA, ed. *The Autonomic Nervous System.* Vol. 6, *Nervous Control of the Urogenital System.* London: Harwood Academic Publisher; 1993:33–68, chap. 2
6. Zagorodnyuk VP, Costa M, Brookes SJ. Major classes of sensory neurons to the urinary bladder. *Auton Neurosci.* 2006;126–127:390-397
7. Zagorodnyuk VP, Gibbins IL, Costa M, Brookes SJ, Gregory SJ. Properties of the major classes of mechanoreceptors in the guinea pig bladder. *J Physiol.* 2007; 585:147-163
8. Iggo A. Tension receptors in the stomach and the urinary bladder. *J Physiol.* 1955;128:593-607
9. Kuru M. Nervous control of micturition. *Physiol Rev.* 1965;45:425-494
10. de Groat WC, Booth AM, Yoshimura N. Neurophysiology of micturition and its modification in animal models of human disease. In: Maggi CA, ed. *Nervous Control of the Urogenital System.* London: Harwood Academic; 1993:227-290
11. Häbler HJ, Jänig W, Koltzenburg M. Activation of unmyelinated afferent fibres by mechanical stimuli and inflammation of the urinary bladder in the cat. *J Physiol.* 1990;425:545-562
12. Fall M, Lindstrom S, Mazieres L. A bladder-to-bladder cooling reflex in the cat. *J Physiol.* 1990;427:281-300
13. Andersson KE, Wein AJ. Pharmacology of the lower urinary tract: basis for current and future treatments of urinary incontinence. *Pharmacol Rev.* December 2004; 56(4):581-631
14. Burnstock G. Purinergic signalling in lower urinary tract. In: Abbracchio MP, Williams MP, eds. *Purinergic and Pyrimidinergic Signalling I Molecular, Nervous and Urogenitary System Function.* Berlin: Springer; 2001:151, 423–515
15. Thor KB, Donatucci C. Central nervous system control of the lower urinary tract: new pharmacological approaches to stress urinary incontinence in women. *J Urol.* 2004;172(1):27-33
16. Yoshimura N, Kaiho Y, Miyazato M, et al. Therapeutic receptor targets for lower urinary tract dysfunction. *Naunyn Schmiedebergs Arch Pharmacol.* 2008; 377(4–6): 437-448
17. Andersson K-E. Bladder activation: afferent mechanisms. *Urology.* 2002;59(5 Suppl 1):43-50
18. Birder LA, Kanai AJ, de Groat WC, et al. Vanilloid receptor expression suggests a sensory role for urinary bladder epithelial cells. *Proc Natl Acad Sci USA.* 6, 2001;98(23):13396-13401
19. Birder LA, Nakamura Y, Kiss S, et al. Altered urinary bladder function in mice lacking the vanilloid receptor TRPV1. *Nat Neurosci.* 2002;5(9):856-860

20. Sui GP, Rothery S, Dupont E, Fry CH, Severs NJ. Gap junctions and connexin expression in human suburothelial interstitial cells. *BJU Int.* 2002;90(1):118-129

21. Sui GP, Wu C, Fry CH. Electrical characteristics of suburothelial cells isolated from the human bladder. *J Urol.* 2004;171(2 Pt 1):938-943

22. Birder and de Groat, 2007 (Birder LA, de Groat WC. Mechanisms of disease: involvement of the urothelium in bladder dysfunction., Nat Clin Pract Urol. 2007 Jan;4(1):46-54)

23. Pandita RK, Andersson KE. Intravesical adenosine triphosphate stimulates the micturition reflex in awake, freely moving rats. *J Urol.* 2002;168(3):1230-1234

24. Cockayne DA, Hamilton SG, Zhu QM, et al. Urinary bladder hyporeflexia and reduced pain-related behaviour in P2X3-deficient mice. *Nature.* 2000;407(6807): 1011-1015

25. Vlaskovska M, Kasakov L, Rong W, et al. P2X3 knock-out mice reveal a major sensory role for urothelially released ATP. *J Neurosci.* 2001;21(15):5670-5677

26. Fovaeus M, Fujiwara M, Hogestatt ED, Persson K, Andersson KE. A non-nitrergic smooth muscle relaxant factor released from rat urinary bladder by muscarinic receptor stimulation. *J Urol.* 1999;161(2): 649-653

27. Hawthorn MH, Chapple CR, Cock M, Chess-Williams R. Urothelium-derived inhibitory factor(s) influences on detrusor muscle contractility in vitro. *Br J Pharmacol.* 2000;129(3):416-419

28. Hashitani H, Brading AF, Suzuki H. Correlation between spontaneous electrical, calcium and mechanical activity in detrusor smooth muscle of the guinea-pig bladder. *Br J Pharmacol.* 2004;141(1):183-193

29. Drake MJ, Mills IW, Gillespie JI. Model of peripheral autonomous modules and a myovesical plexus in normal and overactive bladder function. *Lancet.* 2001; 358(9279):401-403

30. Gillespie JI. A developing view of the origins of urgency: the importance of animal models. *BJU Int.* 2005;96 (Suppl 1):22-28

31. Kinder RB, Mundy AR. Pathophysiology of idiopathic detrusor instability and detrusor hyper-reflexia. An in vitro study of human detrusor muscle. *Br J Urol.* 1987;60(6):509-515

32. Brading AF. A myogenic basis for the overactive bladder. *Urology.* 1997;50(6A Suppl):57-67; discussion 68-73

33. Mills IW, Greenland JE, McMurray G, et al. Studies of the pathophysiology of idiopathic detrusor instability: the physiological properties of the detrusor smooth muscle and its pattern of innervation. *J Urol.* 2000; 163:646-651

34. Turner WH, Brading AF. Smooth muscle of the bladder in the normal and the diseased state: pathophysiology, diagnosis and treatment. *Pharmacol Ther.* 1997; 75(2):77-110

35. Stevens LA, Chapple CR, Chess-Williams R. Human idiopathic and neurogenic overactive bladders and the role of M2 muscarinic receptors in contraction. *Eur Urol.* 2007;52(2):531-538

36. Wu C, Sui GP, Fry CH. Purinergic regulation of guinea pig suburothelial myofibroblasts. *J Physiol.* 2004;559 (Pt 1):231-243

37. Fry CH, Sui GP, Kanai AJ, Wu C. The function of suburothelial myofibroblasts in the bladder. *Neurourol Urodyn.* 2007;26(6 Suppl):914-919

38. Ikeda Y, Kanai A. Urotheliogenic modulation of intrinsic activity in spinal cord-transected rat bladders: role of mucosal muscarinic receptors. *Am J Physiol Ren Physiol.* 2008;295(2):F454-F461

39. Sui GP, Wu C, Roosen A, Ikeda Y, Kanai AJ, Fry CH. Modulation of bladder myofibroblast activity: implications for bladder function. *Am J Physiol Ren Physiol.* 2008;295(3):F688-F697

40. Gillespie JI, van Koeveringe GA, de Wachter SG, de Vente J. On the origins of the sensory output from the bladder: the concept of afferent noise. *BJU Int.* 2009;103(10): 1324-1333

41. Caulfield MP, Birdsall NJM. International Union of Pharmacology: XVII. Classification of muscarinic acetylcholine receptors. *Pharmacol Rev.* 1998;50: 279-290

42. Sigala S, Mirabella G, Peroni A, et al. Differential gene expression of cholinergic muscarinic receptor subtypes in male and female normal human urinary bladder. *Urology.* 2002;60(4):719-725

43. Bschleipfer T, Schukowski K, Weidner W, et al. Expression and distribution of cholinergic receptors in the human urothelium. *Life Sci.* 2007;80(24–25):2303-2307

44. Yamaguchi O, Shishido K, Tamura K, et al. Evaluation of mRNAs encoding muscarinicreceptor subtypes in human detrusor muscle. *J Urol.* 1996;156:1208-1213

45. Eglen RM, Hegde SS, Watson N. Muscarinic receptor subtypes and smooth muscle function. *Pharmacol Rev.* 1996;48:531-565

46. Hegde SS, Eglen RM. Muscarinic receptor subtypes modulating smooth muscle contractility in the urinary bladder. *Life Sci.* 1999;64(6–7):419-428

47. Chess-Williams R. Muscarinic receptors of the urinary bladder: detrusor, urothelial and prejunctional. *Auton Autacoid Pharmacol.* 2002;22(3):133-145

48. Giglio D, Tobin G. Muscarinic receptor subtypes in the lower urinary tract. *Pharmacology.* 2009;83(5): 259-269

49. Schneider T, Fetscher C, Krege S, Michel MC. Signal transduction underlying carbachol-induced contraction of human urinary bladder. *J Pharmacol Exp Ther.* June 2004;309(3):1148-1153

50. Jezior JR, Brady JD, Rosenstein DI, McCammon KA, Miner AS, Ratz PH. Dependency of detrusor contractions on calcium sensitization and calcium entry through LOE-908-sensitive channels. *Br J Pharmacol.* 2001;134(1):78-87

51. Wibberley A, Chen Z, Hu E, Hieble JP, Westfall TD. Expression and functional role of Rho-kinase in rat urinary bladder smooth muscle. *Br J Pharmacol.* 2003; 138(5):757-766

52. Andersson K-E. Detrusor contraction – focus on muscarinic receptors. *Scand J Urol Nephrol Suppl.* 2004;215: 54-57

53. Hegde SS, Choppin A, Bonhaus D, et al. Functional role of M-2 and M-3 muscarinic receptors in the urinary bladder of rats in vitro and in vivo. *Br J Pharmacol.* 1997;120:1409-1418

54. Kotlikoff MI, Dhulipala P, Wang YX. M2 signaling in smooth muscle cells. *Life Sci.* 1999;64(6–7):437-442

55. Nakamura T, Kimura J, Yamaguchi O. Muscarinic M2 receptors inhibit Ca^{2+}-activated K+ channels in rat bladder smooth muscle. *Int J Urol.* 2002;9(12):689-696

56. Bonev AD, Nelson MT. Muscarinic inhibition of ATP-sensitive K+ channels by protein kinase C in urinary bladder smooth muscle. *Am J Physiol*. 1993;265 (6 Pt 1):C1723-C1728

57. Braverman AS, Luthin GR, Ruggieri MR. M2 muscarinic receptor contributes to contraction of the denervated rat urinary bladder. *Am J Physiol*. 1998;275: R1654-R1660

58. Braverman A, Legos J, Young W, Luthin G, Ruggieri M. M2 receptors in genito-urinary smooth muscle pathology. *Life Sci*. 1999;64:429-436

59. Braverman AS, Tallarida RJ, Ruggieri MR Sr. Interaction between muscarinic receptor subtype signal transduction pathways mediating bladder contraction. *Am J Physiol Regul Integr Comp Physiol*. September 2002; 283(3):R663-R668

60. Braverman AS, Ruggieri MR Sr. Hypertrophy changes the muscarinic receptor subtype mediating bladder contraction from M3 toward M2. *Am J Physiol Regul Integr Comp Physiol*. 2003;285(3):R701-R708

61. Pontari MA, Braverman AS, Ruggieri MR Sr. The M2 muscarinic receptor mediates in vitro bladder contractions from patients with neurogenic bladder dysfunction. *Am J Physiol Regul Integr Comp Physiol*. 2004;286(5):R874-R880

62. D'Agostino G, Bolognesi ML, Lucchelli A, et al. Prejunctional muscarinic inhibitory control of acetylcholine release in the human isolated detrusor: involvement of the M4 receptor subtype. *Br J Pharmacol*. 2000;129(3):493-500

63. Somogyi GT, de Groat WC. Function, signal transduction mechanisms and plasticity of presynaptic muscarinic receptors in the urinary bladder. *Life Sci*. 1999; 64(6–7):411-418

64. Somogyi GT, Zernova GV, Yoshiyama M, Rocha JN, Smith CP, de Groat WC. Change in muscarinic modulation of transmitter release in the rat urinary bladder after spinal cord injury. *Neurochem Int*. 2003;43(1):73-77

65. Tyagi S, Tyagi P, Van-le S, Yoshimura N, Chancellor MB, de Miguel F. Qualitative and quantitative expression profile of muscarinic receptors in human urothelium and detrusor. *J Urol*. 2006;176(4 Pt 1):1673-1678

66. Mansfield KJ, Liu L, Mitchelson FJ, Moore KH, Millard RJ, Burcher E. Muscarinic receptor subtypes in human bladder detrusor and mucosa, studied by radiolig-and binding and quantitative competitive RT-PCR: changes in ageing. *Br J Pharmacol*. 2005;144(8):1089-1099

67. Mukerji G, Yiangou Y, Grogono J, et al. Localization of M2 and M3 muscarinic receptors in human bladder disorders and their clinical correlations. *J Urol*. 2006; 176(1):367-373

68. Grol S, Essers PB, van Koeveringe GA, Martinez-Martinez P, de Vente J, Gillespie JI. M(3) muscarinic receptor expression on suburothelial interstitial cells. *BJU Int*. 11, 2009 [Epub ahead of print]

69. Wakabayashi Y, Tomoyoshi T, Fujimiya M, Arai R, Maeda T. Substance P-containing axon terminals in the mucosa of the human urinary bladder: pre-embedding immunohistochemistry using cryostat sections for electron microscopy. *Histochemistry*. 1993;100(6):401-407

70. Persson K, Alm P, Johansson K, Larsson B, Andersson KE. Co-existence of nitrergic, peptidergic and acetylcholine esterase-positive nerves in the pig lower urinary tract. *J Auton Nerv Syst*. 1995;52(2–3):225-236

71. Gabella G, Davis C. Distribution of afferent axons in the bladder of rats. *J Neurocytol*. 1998;27(3):141-155

72. Ferguson DR, Kennedy I, Burton TJ. ATP is released from rabbit urinary bladder epithelial cells by hydrostatic pressure changes–a possible sensory mechanism? *J Physiol*. 1997;505(Pt 2):503-511

73. Birder LA, Barrick SR, Roppolo JR, et al. Feline interstitial cystitis results in mechanical hypersensitivity and altered ATP release from bladder urothelium. *Am J Physiol Ren Physiol*. 2003;285(3):F423-F429

74. Kullmann FA, Artim DE, Birder LA, de Groat WC. Activation of muscarinic receptors in rat bladder sensory pathways alters reflex bladder activity. *J Neurosci*. 2008;28(8):1977-1987

75. Yoshida M, Inadome A, Maeda Y, et al. Non-neuronal cholinergic system in human bladder urothelium. *Urology*. 2006;67(2):425-430

76. Hanna-Mitchell AT, Beckel JM, Barbadora S, Kanai AJ, de Groat WC, Birder LA. Non-neuronal acetylcholine and urinary bladder urothelium. *Life Sci*. 2007;80(24–25): 2298-2302

77. Beckel JM, Kanai A, Lee SJ, de Groat WC, Birder LA. Expression of functional nicotinic acetylcholine receptors in rat urinary bladder epithelial cells. *Am J Physiol Ren Physiol*. 2006;290(1):F103-F110

78. Malloy BJ, Price DT, Price RR, et al. Alpha1-adrenergic receptor subtypes in human detrusor. *J Urol*. 1998; 160:937-943

79. Michel MC, Vrydag W. Alpha1-, alpha2- and beta-adrenoceptors in the urinary bladder, urethra and prostate. *Br J Pharmacol*. 2006;147(Suppl 2):S88-S119

80. Andersson KE, Gratzke C. Pharmacology of alpha1-adrenoceptor antagonists in the lower urinary tract and central nervous system. *Nat Clin Pract Urol*. 2007; 4(7):368-378

81. Nomiya M, Yamaguchi O. A quantitative analysis of mRNA expression of alpha 1 and beta-adrenoceptor subtypes and their functional roles in human normal and obstructed bladders. *J Urol*. 2003;170(2 Pt 1):649-653

82. Bouchelouche K, Andersen L, Alvarez S, Nordling J, Bouchelouche P. Increased contractile response to phenylephrine in detrusor of patients with bladder outlet obstruction: effect of the alpha1A and alpha1D-adrenergic receptor antagonist tamsulosin. *J Urol*. 2005;173(2): 657-661

83. Das AK, Leggett RE, Whitbeck C, et al. Effect of doxazosin on rat urinary bladder function after partial outlet obstruction. *Neurourol Urodyn*. 2002;21:160-166

84. Andersson K-E. Pharmacology of lower urinary tract smooth muscles and penile erectile tissues. *Pharmacol Rev*. 1993;45:253-308

85. Otsuka A, Shinbo H, Matsumoto R, Kurita Y, Ozono S. Expression and functional role of beta-adrenoceptors in the human urinary bladder urothelium. *Naunyn Schmiedebergs Arch Pharmacol*. 2008;377(4–6):473-481

86. Badawi JK, Seja T, Uecelehan H, et al. Relaxation of human detrusor muscle by selective beta-2 and beta-3 agonists and endogenous catecholamines. *Urology*. 2007;69(4):785-790

87. Leon LA, Hoffman BE, Gardner SD, et al. Effects of the beta 3-adrenergic receptor agonist disodium 5-[(2R)-2-[[(2R)-2- (3-chlorophenyl)-2-hydroxyethyl]amino]pro-pyl]-1, 3-benzodioxole-2, 2-dicarboxylate (CL-316243) on bladder micturition reflex in spontaneously hypertensive rats. *J Pharmacol Exp Ther*. 2008;326(1):178-185

88. Biers SM, Reynard JM, Brading AF. The effects of a new selective beta3-adrenoceptor agonist (GW427353) on spontaneous activity and detrusor relaxation in human bladder. *BJU Int*. 2006;98(6):1310-1314

89. Andersson K-E. Pathways for relaxation of detrusor smooth muscle. In: Baskin LS, Hayward SW, eds. *Advances in Bladder Research*. New York: Kluwer Academic/Plenum; 1999:241-252

90. Uchida H, Shishido K, Nomiya M, Yamaguchi O. Involvement of cyclic AMP-dependent and -independent mechanisms in the relaxation of rat detrusor muscle via beta-adrenoceptors. *Eur J Pharmacol*. 22, 2005;518 (2–3):195-202

91. Frazier EP, Peters SL, Braverman AS, Ruggieri MR Sr, Michel MC. Signal transduction underlying the control of urinary bladder smooth muscle tone by muscarinic receptors and beta-adrenoceptors. *Naunyn Schmiedebergs Arch Pharmacol*. 2008; 377(4–6):449-462

92. Takemoto J, Masumiya H, Nunoki K, et al. Potentiation of potassium currents by beta-adrenoceptor agonists in human urinary bladder smooth muscle cells: a possible electrical mechanism of relaxation. *Pharmacology*. 2008;81(3):251-258

93. Hristov KL, Cui X, Brown SM, Liu L, Kellett WF, Petkov GV. Stimulation of beta3-adrenoceptors relaxes rat urinary bladder smooth muscle via activation of the large-conductance Ca^{2+}-activated K+ channels. *Am J Physiol Cell Physiol*. 2008;295(5):C1344-C1353 [Epub September 17, 2008]

94. Fujimura T, Tamura K, Tsutsumi T, et al. Expression and possible functional role of the beta3-adrenoceptor in human and rat detrusor muscle. *J Urol*. 1999;161(2): 680-685

95. Woods M, Carson N, Norton NW, Sheldon JH, Argentieri TM. Efficacy of the beta3-adrenergic receptor agonist CL-316243 on experimental bladder hyperreflexia and detrusor instability in the rat. *J Urol*. 2001;166(3): 1142-1147

96. Takeda H, Yamazaki Y, Igawa Y, et al. Effects of beta(3)-adrenoceptor stimulation on prostaglandin E(2)-induced bladder hyperactivity and on the cardiovascular system in conscious rats. *Neurourol Urodyn*. 2002; 21(6):558-565

97. Kaidoh K, Igawa Y, Takeda H, et al. Effects of selective beta2 and beta3-adrenoceptor agonists on detrusor hyperreflexia in conscious cerebral infarcted rats. *J Urol*. 2002;168(3):1247-1252

98. Hicks A, McCafferty GP, Riedel E, et al. GW427353 (sol-abegron), a novel, selective beta3-adrenergic receptor agonist, evokes bladder relaxation and increases micturition reflex threshold in the dog. *J Pharmacol Exp Ther*. 2007;323(1):202-209

99. Colli E, Digesu GA, Olivieri L. Overactive bladder treatments in early phase clinical trials. *Expert Opin Investig Drugs*. 2007;16(7):999-1007

100. Takasu T, Ukai M, Sato S, et al. Effect of (R)-2- (2-amin-othiazol-4-yl)-4'- {2-[(2-hydroxy-2-phenylethyl)amino] ethyl} acetanilide (YM178), a novel selective beta3-adrenoceptor agonist, on bladder function. *J Pharmacol Exp Ther*. 2007;321(2):642-647 [Epub February 9, 2007]

101. Chapple CR, Yamaguchi O, Ridder A, et al. Clinical proof of concept study (Blossom) shows novel B3 adrenocep-tor agonist YM178 is effective and well tolerated in the treatment of symptoms of overactive bladder. *Eur Urol Suppl*. 2008;7(3):239. abstract 674

102. Everaerts W, Gevaert T, Nilius B, De Ridder D. On the origin of bladder sensing: Tr(i)ps in urology. *Neurourol Urodyn*. 2008;27(4):264-273

103. Birder LA, de Groat WC. Mechanisms of disease: involvement of the urothelium in bladder dysfunction. *Nat Clin Pract Urol*. 2007;4(1):46-54

104. Ishizuka O, Mattiasson A, Andersson K-E. Urodynamic effects of intravesical resiniferatoxin and capsaicin in conscious rats with and without outflow obstruction. *J Urol*. 1995;154:611-616

105. Ishizuka O, Mattiasson A, Andersson KE. Effects of neurokinin receptor antagonists on L-dopa induced bladder hyperactivity in normal conscious rats. *J Urol*. 1995;154(4):1548-1551

106. Szallazi A, Blumberg PM. Vanilloid receptors: new insights enhance potential as a therapeutic target. *Pain*. 1996;68(2–3):195-208

107. Kuo H-C. Inhibitory effect of capsaicin on detrusor contractility: further study in the presence of ganglionic blocker and neurokinin receptor antagonist in the rat urinary bladder. *Urol Int*. 1997;59:95-101

108. Andersson KE, Uckert S, Stief C, Hedlund P. Phosphodiesterases (PDEs) and PDE inhibitors for treatment of LUTS. *Neurourol Urodyn*. 2007;26(6 Suppl): 928-933

109. Truss MC, Stief CG, Uckert S, et al. Phosphodiesterase 1 inhibition in the treatment of lower urinary tract dysfunction: from bench to bedside. *World J Urol*. 2001; 19:344-350

110. Longhurst PA, Briscoe JA, Rosenberg DJ, Leggett RE. The role of cyclic nucleotides in guinea-pig bladder contractility. *Br J Pharmacol*. 1997;121(8):1665-1672

111. Kaiho Y, Nishiguchi J, Kwon DD, et al. The effects of a type 4 phosphodiesterase inhibitor and the muscarinic cholinergic antagonist tolterodine tartrate on detrusor overactivity in female rats with bladder outlet obstruction. *BJU Int*. 2008;101(5):615-620

112. Nishiguchi J, Kwon DD, Kaiho Y, et al. Suppression of detrusor overactivity in rats with bladder outlet obstruction by a type 4 phosphodiesterase inhibitor. *BJU Int*. 2007;99(3):680-686

113. Giembycz MA. Life after PDE4: overcoming adverse events with dual-specificity phosphodiesterase inhibitors. *Curr Opin Pharmacol*. 2005;5(3):238-244

114. Sairam K, Kulinskaya E, McNicholas TA, Boustead GB, Hanbury DC. Sildenafil influences lower urinary tract symptoms. *BJU Int*. 2002;90(9):836-839

115. McVary KT, Roehrborn CG, Kaminetsky JC, et al. Tadalafil relieves lower urinary tract symptoms secondary to benign prostatic hyperplasia. *J Urol*. 2007; 177(4):1401-1407

116. McVary KT, Monnig W, Camps JL Jr, Young JM, Tseng LJ, van den Ende G. Sildenafil citrate improves erectile function and urinary symptoms in men with erectile dysfunction and lower urinary tract symptoms associated with benign prostatic hyperplasia: a randomized, double-blind trial. *J Urol.* 2007;177(3):1071-1077

117. Stief CG, Porst H, Neuser D, Beneke M, Ulbrich E. A randomised, placebo-controlled study to assess the efficacy of twice-daily vardenafil in the treatment of lower urinary tract symptoms secondary to benign prostatic hyperplasia. *Eur Urol.* 2008;53(6):1236-1244

118. de Groat WC, Yoshimura N. Pharmacology of the lower urinary tract. *Annu Rev Pharmacol Toxicol.* 2001;41: 691-721

119. Murray KH, Feneley RC. Endorphins-a role in lower urinary tract function? The effect of opioid blockade on the detrusor and urethral sphincter mechanisms. *Br J Urol.* 1982;54(6):638-640

120. Dray A, Nunan L, Wire W. Naloxonazine and opioid-induced inhibition of reflex urinary bladder contractions. *Neuropharmacology.* 1987;26(1):67-74

121. Herman RM, Wainberg MC, delGiudice PF, Willscher MK. The effect of a low dose of intrathecal morphine on impaired micturition reflexes in human subjects with spinal cord lesions. *Anesthesiology.* 1988; 69(3):313-318

122. Kieffer BL. Opioids: first lessons from knockout mice. *Trends Pharmacol Sci.* 1999;20(1):19-26

123. Raffa RB, Friderichs E. The basic science aspect on tramadol hydrochloride. *Pain Rev.* 1996;3:249-271

124. Pandita RK, Pehrson R, Christoph T, Friderichs E, Andersson KE. Actions of tramadol on micturition in awake, freely moving rats. *Br J Pharmacol.* 2003; 139(4):741-748

125. Safarinejad MR, Hosseini SY. Safety and efficacy of tramadol in the treatment of idiopathic detrusor overactivity: a double-blind, placebo-controlled, randomized study. *Br J Clin Pharmacol.* 2006;61(4): 456-463

126. Ranson RN, Dodds AL, Smith MJ, Santer RM, Watson AH. Age-associated changes in the monoaminergic innervation of rat lumbosacral spinal cord. *Brain Res.* 16, 2003;972(1–2):149-158

127. Thor KB, Blitz-Siebert A, Helke CJ. Autoradiographic localization of 5hydroxytryptamine1A, 5-hydroxytryptamine1B and 5-hydroxytryptamine1C/2 binding sites in the rat spinal cord. *Neuroscience.* 1993;5(1): 235-252

128. de Groat WC. Influence of central serotonergic mechanisms on lower urinary tract function. *Urology.* 2002;59(5 Suppl 1):30-36

129. McMahon SB, Spillane K. Brain stem influences on the parasympathetic supply to the urinary bladder of the cat. *Brain Res.* 25, 1982;234(2):237-249

130. Sugaya K, Ogawa Y, Hatano T, Koyama Y, Miyazato T, Oda M. Evidence for involvement of the subcoeruleus nucleus and nucleus raphe magnus in urine storage and penile erection in decerebrate rats. *J Urol.* 1998;159(6):2172-2176

131. Katofiasc MA, Nissen J, Audia JE, et al. Comparison of the effects of serotonin selective norepinephrine selective, and dual serotonin and norepinephrine reuptake inhibitors on lower urinary tract function in cats. *Life Sci.* 2002;71(11):1227

132. Thor K, Katofiasc MA. Effects of duloxetine, a combined serotonin and norepinephrine reuptake inhibitor, on central neural control of lower urinary tract function in the chloralose-anesthetized female cat. *J Pharmacol Exp Ther.* 1995;274(2):1014

133. Fraser MO, Chancellor MB. Neural control of the urethra and development of pharmacotherapy for stress urinary incontinence. *BJU Int.* 2003;91(8):743

134. Steers WD, Herschorn S, Kreder KJ, et al. Duloxetine compared with placebo for treating women with symptoms of overactive bladder. *BJU Int.* 2007;100(2):337

135. Chebib M, Johnston GAR. The 'ABC' of GABA receptors: a brief review. *Clin Exp Pharmacol Physiol.* 1999;26(11):937-940

136. Igawa Y, Mattiasson A, Andersson KE. Effects of GABA-receptor stimulation and blockade on micturition in normal rats and rats with bladder outflow obstruction. *J Urol.* 1993;150(2 Pt 1):537-542

137. Pehrson R, Lehmann A, Andersson KE. Effects of gamma-aminobutyrate B receptor modulation on normal micturition and oxyhemoglobin induced detrusor overactivity in female rats. *J Urol.* 2002; 168(6):2700-2705

138. Maggi CA, Santicioli P, Giuliani S, et al. The effects of baclofen on spinal and supraspinal micturition reflexes in rats. *Naunyn Schmiedebergs Arch Pharmacol.* 1987;336(2):197-203

139. Malcangio M, Bowery NG. GABA and its receptors in the spinal cord. *Trends Pharm Sci.* 1996;17(12):457-462

140. Coggeshall RE, Carlton SM. Receptor localization in the mammalian dorsal horn and primary afferent neurons. *Brain Res Brain Res Rev.* 1997;24(1):28-66

141. Taylor MC, Bates CP. A double-blind crossover trial of baclofen-a new treatment for the unstable bladder syndrome. *Br J Urol.* 1979;51(6):504-505

142. Maneuf YP, Gonzalez MI, Sutton KS, Chung FZ, Pinnock RD, Lee K. Cellular and molecular action of the putative GABA-mimetic, gabapentin. *Cell Mol Life Sci.* 2003;60(4):742-750

143. Carbone A, Palleschi G, Conte A, Bova G, Iacovelli E, Bettolo RM. Gabapentin treatment of neurogenic overactive bladder. *Clin Neuropharmacol.* 2006;29(4):206-214.

144. Kim YT, Kwon DD, Kim J, Kim DK, Lee JY, Chancellor MB. Gabapentin for overactive bladder and nocturia after anticholinergic failure. *Int Braz J Urol.* 2004; 30(4):275-278

145. Lecci A, Maggi CA. Tachykinins as modulators of the micturition reflex in the central and peripheral nervous system. *Regul Pept.* 15, 2001;101(1–3):1-18

146. Saffroy M, Torrens Y, Glowinski J, Beaujouan JC. Autoradiographic distribution of tachykinin NK2 binding sites in the rat brain: comparison with NK1 and NK3 binding sites. *Neuroscience.* 2003;116(3):761-773

147. Covenas R, Martin F, Belda M, et al. Mapping of neurokinin-like immunoreactivity in the human brainstem. *BMC Neurosci.* 2003;4(1):3

148. Ishizuka O, Igawa Y, Lecci A, Maggi CA, Mattiasson A, Andersson KE. Role of intrathecal tachykinins for micturition in unanaesthetized rats with and without bladder outlet obstruction. *Br J Pharmacol.* 1994;113(1):111-116

149. Seki S, Erickson KA, Seki M, et al. Elimination of rat spinal neurons expressing neurokinin 1 receptors reduces bladder overactivity and spinal c-fos expression induced by bladder irritation. *Am J Physiol Ren Physiol*. March 2005;288(3):F466-F473

150. Massaro AM, Lenz KL. Aprepitant: a novel antiemetic for chemotherapy-induced nausea and vomiting. *Ann Pharmacother*. 2005;39(1):77-85

151. Green SA, Alon A, Ianus J, McNaughton KS, Tozzi CA, Reiss TF. Efficacy and safety of a neurokinin-1 receptor antagonist in postmenopausal women with overactive bladder with urge urinary incontinence. *J Urol*. 2006;176(6 Pt 1):2535-2540

152. Gillespie JI. The autonomous bladder: a view of the origin of bladder overactivity and sensory urge. *BJU Int*. 2004;93(4):478-483

153. Gillespie JI. Phosphodiesterase-linked inhibition of nonmicturition activity in the isolated bladder. *BJU Int*. 2004;93(9):1325-1332

10

Pharmacology of Sexual Function

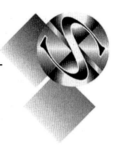

Andreas Meissner and Martin C. Michel

Introduction

Human sexual function involves a complex interaction between the central nervous system (CNS) and peripheral organs. The CNS receives and integrates tactile, olfactory, auditory, visual, and mental stimuli to regulate various domains of sexual function. This chapter will focus on three aspects of sexual function, that is, sexual desire/arousal and, in males, erection and ejaculation. While the manipulation of desire by definition requires drug effects on central nervous function, disorders of erection and ejaculation can potentially be addressed by both centrally and peripherally acting drugs. Our emphasis will be on drug mechanisms, which already are available clinically and/or are currently in clinical development. Potential issues related to ovulation and spermatogenesis will not be discussed.

Sexual Desire/Arousal

In humans there has been described a sexual response cycle by Masters and Johnson in 1966,[1] which is nearly the same for men and women and consists of four phases: the excitement, plateau, orgasmic, and resolution phase. The first phase is also called arousal phase and has, by definition, to be seen as a complex genital response of a human being[2] awaiting the experience of sexual pleasure and possibly orgasm,

which is much more than only getting an erection. It is an integration of physiological and psychological processes. In contrast to this "state," "sexual arousability" means the extent a human being can experience, varying not only between individuals, but also in time in the same individual. In order to experience sexual desire and arousal, an intact interaction of the endocrine and central nervous system is important.[3] The following part consists of the most important hormones, neurotransmitters, and drugs involved in the process of sexual arousal, which is still far away from being fully understood. This, however, would be crucial for causal treatment of sexual dysfunction.

Endocrinology

Steroid hormones are important regulators of the sexual behavior. They are acting slowly via genomic alteration. In case of copulation, they can increase the synthesis of neurotransmitter receptors or of enzymes that regulate neurotransmitter synthesis or release.[4-6]

Steroids in the Male

Testosterone is urgently needed for normal sexual interest and arousability. Replacement therapy can restore symptoms of deficiency. But the impact is still not very well understood. Main effects of testosterone aim on central arousal

C.R. Chapple and W.D. Steers (eds.), *Practical Urology: Essential Principles and Practice,*
DOI: 10.1007/978-1-84882-034-0_10, © Springer-Verlag London Limited 2011

mechanisms. But in eugonadal men the amount of circulating testosterone exceeds the necessary to maintain sexual arousability in the brain. This can lead to the assumption that for peripheral effects of testosterone higher levels are needed. Centrally, it has positive influence on the NO release synthase in the medial preoptic area whereby NO release and consecutively dopamine release is stimulated. To allow the dopamine release, testosterone has to be, at least previously to this, present.[7] Estrogens seem to play an important role too as they are involved in control of gonadotropin secretion, fertility, and psychosexual behavior.[8] The different relation of androgens and estrogens in males compared to females could help to elucidate the distinctions in sexual arousal and the response cycle between both genders.[9]

Hypogonadism has severe impact on the quality of life of an (aging) male and also on his morbidity and mortality. The ESPRIT study (Energy, Sexual desire, and body PropoRtions wIth AndroGel, Testosterone 1% gel therapy), a 6-month, multinational, open label, observational study in hypogonadal men being treated with transdermal AndroGel, tries to search for the effects and safety of replacement therapy.[10] Treatment with Tamoxifen, an estrogen blocker, can decrease libido, whereas estrogens increase libido and frequency of sexual acting.[11]

Steroids in the Female

In the female, the situation is much more complex, which can be explained by their reproductive endocrine system. To obtain sexual arousal the presence of estrogen is necessary, but also testosterone seems to play an important role. Wallen suggests a synergistic effect.[12] In the follicular phase, testosterone levels typically rise to a maximum in the middle third of the cycle. Afterwards there is a decline in the final third to a minimum in the beginning of the follicular phase of the next cycle.

What complicates the situation is the fact that not only testosterone is high in the mid-cycle but also estradiol, which makes it difficult to differentiate the effects of the two hormones.

General agreement exists upon the lowest sexual activity during menstruation period. But then there are also nonhormonal explanations for the drop in sexual activity.

Most studies describe a periovulatory increase in sexual desire or activity whereas during pregnancy a significant lowering in sexual function with progression of pregnancy is stated. Studies observing sexual function under oral contraceptives are not conclusive but hinting at inducing no negative effect.

The impact of endogenous androgens on sexuality is also not clear by now: one large cross-sectional study showed no correlation, whereas some case-control studies did let see that low androgens in women were associated with sexual dysfunction. Even worse is the situation in case of testosterone therapy in premenopausal women: no clear dose-response effect was detected. An important impact on this may be the great difficulty of the measurement of the testosterone level in women. Sex hormones for sure showed a modifying effect on sexual function but also social influences and learned responses. The conclusion of all this is that further studies are urgently required.[13] This is supported by the APHRODITE and other studies, where in postmenopausal women, treated with testosterone patches, at least a modest improvement of sexual function could be detected but with uncertain long-term effects.[14,15]

Neurohormones

This group includes the peptide hormones oxytocin, ß-endorphin, vasopressin, and prolactin. Their role in sexual arousal is complex and still unclear originating from sometimes contrary functions in different places. Bancroft et al. described excitatory and inhibitory effects for oxytocin and β-endorphin whereas prolactin was thought to work as a direct inhibitor of dopaminergic activity, but with inconclusive evidence.[16] Westheide et al. showed that the sexual dysfunction caused by antipsychotics cannot be explained by heightened prolactin levels alone.[17] On the other hand, it has been proven that continuously high prolactin levels are of negative influence of sexual behavior. Because prolactin significantly decreases after orgasm, Krüger et al. proposed that prolactin could function as a neuroendocrine reproductive reflex to the periphery or feedback to dopaminergic neurons in the central nervous system.[18]

Neurotransmitters

Mainly the neurotransmitters dopamine and serotonin play an important role.

Dopamine

Generally speaking, dopamine and dopamine receptor agonists increase, whereas antagonists decrease libido.[19] In three central areas dopamine is released before and/or during intercourse due to sexual stimulation: in the nigrostriatal system, the mesolimbic tract and the medial preoptic area. In the first one it facilitates somatomotor activity; in the mesolimbic tract it is beneficial for different types of motivation, and in the medial preoptic area it centers the motivation of the individual to sexual practice and controls frequency, sexual techniques, and genital reflexes.[6] By increasing NO synthase in the medial preoptic area testosterone can stimulate production of NO, which results in heightened dopamine release. But also glutamate uses the same pathway to increase dopamine and is extracellularly increased during copulation. This means that this interaction together with previous sexual experience is crucial to optimize intercourse and enhance future sexual responsiveness.[5]

Serotonin

Whereas dopamine enhances copulation facilities, serotonin acts chiefly inhibitory in respect of sexual interest. Animal experiments with microinjections of selective serotonin reuptake inhibitors showed a clear delay in beginning of the copulation,[6] a finding possibly related to the use of SSRIs in the treatment of premature ejaculation (see below).

Pharmacological Strategies

CNS Drugs

Sexual function can be hampered by adverse effects of antidepressants, antipsychotics, mood stabilizers, and anxiolytics, or patients can experience worsening of preexistent sexual dysfunction by psychotropics leading to increased psychological difficulties culminating in discontinuation of the medication. Antipsychotics are known to primarily affect desire, whereas the situation remains unclear for anxiolytics or mood stabilizers.[20]

Treatment of sexual dysfunction, and mainly the loss of sexual desire, is difficult, particularly that associated with the use of antidepressants. Popular management strategies, because they are considered most effective and most frequently followed by experts, are dose reduction, antidepressant rotation, and co-medication with phosphodiesterase-5 inhibitors or testosterone replacement in selected cases.[21]

SSRIs affect sexual functioning apparently in a dose-related manner, also varying between different members of the group. This may involve possible accumulation together with inhibition of NO synthase, anticholinergic effects, modification of serotonin and dopamine reuptake, and the amount of prolactin release induced. Common policy is dosage reduction, drug holidays, antidepressant rotation, waiting for development of tolerance, and therapy enhancement with certain serotonin antagonists and α_2-adrenoceptor antagonists, 5-HT$_{1A}$ and dopamine receptor agonists, and also PDE5 inhibitors.[22] Flibanserin, a 5-HT$_{1A}$ receptor agonist and 5-HT$_{2A}$ receptor antagonist, is currently in late stage clinical development for the treatment of hypoactive sexual desire disorder (HHSD) in women.[23] However, very recently its approval has been denied by the FDA.

Enzyme-inducing Antiepileptic Drugs

Many antiepileptic drugs are inducers of the cytochrome P450 enzymes (mostly CYP 3A4), which metabolize testosterone. Moreover, sexual quality of life was observed to decline in men with epilepsy, and that was related not only to duration of epilepsy but also to an increase of sex hormone-binding globulin levels. Both enhanced testosterone metabolism and sequestration by sex hormone-binding globulin could contribute to lower levels of free testosterone. A connection could be drawn between the sex hormone-binding globulin levels in those men, the enzyme-inducing capacity of the antiepileptic drugs, and age of the patient. Surprisingly, in women this was not the case. Therefore, the need for enzyme-inducing antiepileptic drugs should be carefully weighed against their adverse effects on the sexual quality of life in men with epilepsy.[24]

Erectile Function

Erection requires relaxation of penile smooth muscle to allow accumulation of blood within the corpora cavernosa and hence tumescence. The smooth muscle relaxation is brought about by a range of mediators, which is at least partly regulated by the CNS. Some endogenous mediators have complex effects on erectile function as reviewed comprehensively elsewhere.[25] Nevertheless, these mediators can roughly be divided into pro- and anti-erectile agents as well as into centrally and peripherally acting agents (Table 10.1). The most important pro-erectile stimulus is NO, which has both central and, perhaps more importantly, peripheral effects. Other centrally acting pro-erectile stimuli include dopamine, excitatory amino acids, oxytocin, adrenocorticotropin, and related peptides, whereas other peripherally acting pro-erectile stimuli include acetylcholine and prostaglandin E_2. Of note the pro-erectile effects of at least some of these stimuli depend on the presence of androgens. The most relevant endogenous anti-erectile mediator probably is noradrenaline, acting both centrally and, perhaps even more importantly, peripherally by stimulating α_1-adrenoceptors. Other centrally acting anti-erectile transmitters and mediators include serotonin, γ-amino butyric acid, and opioid peptides, whereas peripherally acting anti-erectile mediators include the endothelins, angiotensin II, and ATP, the latter, possibly in part, working via its metabolite adenosine.

While several neurotransmitters are involved in the central promotion of erectile function, only dopamine receptors have evolved into a potential drug target. The pro-erectile mechanisms of dopamine are largely mediated by D_2-like receptors. Apomorphine, an agonist of all dopamine receptor subtypes, has consistently shown pro-erectile effects in animal models, although in some cases this was limited to low doses, whereas high doses had anti-erectile effects. Apomorphine has also shown some degree of efficacy in clinical studies in patients with ED, but the extent of these effects as well as apomorphine-induced nausea have limited its clinical use.[26,27]

NO, which is formed by NO synthases in nerves and in the endothelium of the penis, has pro-erectile effects both at the central and peripheral level. At least in the periphery NO acts by diffusing into smooth muscle cells and activating a soluble guanylyl cyclase to promote

Table 10.1. Pro- and anti-erectile endogenous neurotransmitters and modulators

	Central nervous system	Periphery (penis)
Pro-erectile transmitters and mediators		
NO	+	+
Acetylcholine	Unclear	+
Dopamine	+	−
Excitatory amino acids	+	−
Oxytocin	+	−
Adrenocorticotropin	+	
Prostaglandin E_2	−	+
Anti-erectile transmitters and mediators		
Noradrenaline	+	+
Serotonin	+	
γ-Amino butyric acid	+	−
Opioid peptides	+	
Endothelins	−	+
Angiotensin II	−	+
ATP and adenosine	−	+

Note that this table provides a rather simplified description and that some of the agents listed have complex effects
+ works at the indicated level; − does not work at the indicated level or insufficient evidence. For details see text or Andersson.[25]

the formation of cyclic GMP (cGMP). This may lead to the opening of K^+ channels, which cause cellular hyperpolarization and hence smooth muscle relaxation. The action of cGMP is terminated by phosphodiesterases (PDEs), specifically PDE5. Accordingly, PDE5 inhibitors have become the most effective form of medical treatment of erectile dysfunction.[26] However, it has to be noted that PDE5 inhibition is a mechanism of amplifying endogenous signals of cGMP, implying that it works only in the presence of exogenous pro-erectile stimuli and an at least partly intact innervation of the penis still able to release at least some amount of NO.

An alternative mechanism to induce penile smooth muscle relaxation is stimulation of prostanoid receptors by prostaglandin E_2 or its analogs such as alprostacil.[26] This leads to elevation of intracellular cyclic AMP, which acts similar to cGMP and also at least partly via opening of K^+ channels, but does not require input from endogenous nerves. Even further down-stream, and also independent of endogenous nerves and NO, would be somatic gene therapy to enhance expression of relevant K^+ channels.[28]

While all of the above mechanisms are based on the enhancement or mimicking of endogenous pro-erectile signals, at least theoretically it would also be possible to act by inhibition of endogenous anti-erectile mechanisms. This would make a case for the use of α_1-adrenoceptor antagonists. Despite limited evidence for a moderate efficacy of yohimbine (probably acting centrally) and phentolamine (probably acting centrally and peripherally), selective α_1-adrenoceptor antagonists have proven to be too weak to provide effective treatment of erectile dysfunction.[29]

Ejaculatory Function

Ejaculation is a necessary step to allow semen to reach female oocytes and hence to allow fertilization. However, disorders of ejaculation can not only affect reproductive function but can also lead to psychologically less fulfilling sexual experiences. Two main ejaculatory disorders exist, premature ejaculation and abnormal ejaculation, the latter often being a side effect of drug treatment or surgery.

Premature Ejaculation

The International Society for Sexual Medicine has defined premature ejaculation in 2007 as "a male sexual dysfunction which is characterised by ejaculation which occurs or nearly always occurs prior to or within about a minute of vaginal penetration, and the inability to delay ejaculation on all or nearly all vaginal penetrations and negative personal consequences, such as distress, bother, frustration and/or the avoidance of sexual intimacy," It is considered to involve psychological, environmental, endocrine, neurobiological, and perhaps even genetic factors.[30] Of note, premature ejaculation often coexists with erectile dysfunction.

Behavioral treatment is generally considered to be an important part of treatment approa-

ches of premature ejaculation,[31] but medical treatments have received increasing attention in the past decade. Knowledge on the neurobiology of premature ejaculation is limited and largely has been derived by indirect conclusions from clinical data. The central neurotransmitter serotonin appears to play a key role as it is released in the anterior lateral hypothalamus at the time of ejaculation, where it apparently reduces dopamine release.[6,32] This conclusion is largely based on the observation that various drugs enhancing serotonin concentrations in the synaptic cleft, that is, selective serotonin reuptake inhibitors (SSRI) such as paroxetine or citalopram but also tricyclic antidepressants, have repeatedly been shown to be effective in its treatment. While the clinical effectiveness of SSRI in the treatment of depressive disorders, their primary indication, requires their use over several weeks, they can be effective in treating premature ejaculation upon on-demand administration. Based on such findings a short-acting SSRI, dapoxetine, has been developed specifically for the on-demand treatment of premature ejaculation, and it has been registered for this indication in several European countries but not the USA.[32] The opioid receptor agonist tramadolol, the PDE5 inhibitor sildenafil, and the α_1-adrenoceptor antagonist terazosin have also shown promising results in some studies, implying opiod and α_1-adrenergic receptors as well as cGMP in the pathophysiology of premature ejaculation. However, in general, premature ejaculation is a research field where (often inconsistent) clinical data have advanced more than the pathophysiological understanding of the condition.

Abnormal Ejaculation

Retrograde ejaculation has long been known as a possible adverse result of, for example, a transurethral resection of the prostate. When similar effects were observed upon treatment with α_1-adrenoceptor antagonists, it was first assumed that this was also due to retrograde ejaculation, and many clinical studies code this adverse event as "retrograde ejaculation," However, more recent studies have demonstrated that this actually is a relative anejaculation,[29] most likely due to relaxation of vas deferens smooth muscle.[33] While abnormal ejaculation can occur with each α_1-adrenoceptor antagonist, it is mostly seen with tamsulosin[29] and even more often with the even more α_{1A}-selective silodosin.[34] Interestingly, abnormal ejaculation occurs mostly in younger patients, and when occurring in the context of treatment of lower urinary function suggestive of benign prostatic hyperplasia, it apparently is associated with greater therapeutic efficacy. This may also be the reason why abnormal ejaculation rarely has been a cause for premature study discontinuation, even with tamsulosin or silodosin.

Conclusions

The various aspects of human sexual function are regulated in the central nervous system and also in the periphery. This regulation involves a complex neural and endocrine network, which makes extrapolation from animal models to humans difficult. Moreover, sexual dysfunction is not a life-threatening disorder which implies very high safety thresholds for drugs used in its treatment. Therefore, it is not surprising that only few drugs have been approved for sexual dysfunction treatment. On the other hand, several important drug classes, for example, antidepressants, may have important adverse effects on sexual function. Disorders of sexual arousal remain difficult to treat.

References

1. Masters WH, Johnson VE. *Human Sexual Response*. New York: Bantam; 1981.
2. Bancroft J. Sexual arousal. In: Nadel L, ed. *Encyclopedia of Cognitive Science*. London: Wiley; 2002:1165-1168.
3. Meston CM, Frohlich PR. The neurobiology of sexual function. *Arch Gen Psychiatry*. 2000;57:1012-1030.
4. Halaris A. Neurochemical aspects of the sexual response cycle. *CNS Spectr*. 2003;8:211-216.
5. Hull EM, Dominguez JM. Getting his act together: roles of glutamate, nitric oxide, and dopamine in the medial preoptic area. *Brain Res*. 2006;1126:66-75.
6. Hull EM, Muschamp JW, Sato S. Dopamine and serotonin: influences on male sexual behavior. *Physiol Behav*. 2004;83:291-307.
7. Hull EM, Lorrain DS, Du J, et al. Hormone-neurotransmitter interactions in the control of sexual behavior. *Behav Brain Res*. 1999;105:105-116.
8. Rochira V, Balestrieri A, Madeo B, et al. Congenital estrogen deficiency: in search of the estrogen role in human male reproduction. *Mol Cell Endocrinol*. 2001; 178:107-115.
9. Motofei IG, Rowland DL. The physiological basis of human sexual arousal: neuroendocrine sexual asymmetry. *Int J Androl*. 2005;28:78-87.
10. Behre HM, Heinemann L, Morales A, et al. Rationale, design and methods of the ESPRIT study: energy, sexual desire and body PropoRtions wIth AndroGel®, testosterone 1% gel therapy, in hypogonadal men. *Aging Male*. 2008;11:101-106.
11. Rochira V, Balestrieri A, Madeo B, et al. Congenital estrogen deficiency in men: a new syndrome with different phenotypes; clinical and therapeutic implications in men. *Mol Cell Endocrinol*. 2002;193:19-28.
12. Wallen K. Sex and context: hormones and primate sexual motivation. *Horm Behav*. 2001;40:339-357.
13. Stuckey BG. Female sexual function and dysfunction in the reproductive years: the influence of endogenous and exogenous sex hormones. *J Sex Med*. 2008;5:2282-2290.
14. Davis SR, Moreau M, Kroll R, et al. Testosterone for low libido in postmenopausal women not taking estrogen. *N Engl J Med*. 2008;359:2005-2017.
15. Schover LR. Androgen therapy for loss of desire in women: is the benefit worth the breast cancer risk? *Fertil Steril*. 2008;90:129-140.
16. Bancroft J. The endocrinology of sexual arousal. *J Endocrinol*. 2005;186:411-427.
17. Westheide J, Cvetanovska G, Albrecht C, et al. Prolactin, subjective well-being and sexual dysfunction: an open label observational study comparing quetiapine with risperidone. *J Sex Med*. 2008;5:2816-2826.
18. Krüger THC, Hartmann U, Schedlowski M. Prolactinergic and dopaminergic mechanisms underlying sexual arousal and orgasm in humans. *World J Urol*. 2005;23:130-138.
19. Stimmel GL, Gutierrez MA. Sexual dysfunction and psychotropic medications. *CNS Spectr*. 2006;11 (8 Suppl 9): 24-30.
20. Labbate LA. Psychotropics and sexual dysfunction: the evidence and treatments. *Adv Psychosom Med*. 2008;29: 107-130.
21. Balon R, Segraves RT. Survey of treatment practices for sexual dysfunction(s) associated with anti-depressants. *J Sex Marital Ther*. 2008;34:353-365.
22. Rosen RC, Lance RM, Menza M. Effects of SSRIs on sexual function: a critical review. *J Clin Psychopharmacol*. 1999;19:67-85.
23. Ferger B, Shimasaki M, Ceci A, et al. Flibanserin, a drug intended for treatment of hypoactive sexual desire disorder in pre-menopausal women, affects spontaneous motor activity and brain neurochemistry in female rats. *Naunyn Schmiedeberg's Arch Pharmacol*. 2010; 381:573-579.
24. Mölleken D, Richter-Appelt H, Stodieck S, et al. Sexual quality of life in epilepsy: correlations with sex hormone blood levels. *Epilepsy Behav*. 2009;14:226-231.
25. Andersson K-E. Pharmacology of penile erection. *Pharmacol Rev*. 2001;53:417-450.
26. Hatzimouratidis K, Hatzichristou D. A comparative review of the options for treatment of erectile dysfunction: which treatment for which patient? *Drugs*. 2005; 65:1621-1650.

27. Miner MM, Settel AD. Centrally acting mechanisms for the treatment of male sexual dysfunction. *Urol Clin North Am*. 2007;34:483-496.

28. Melman A, Rojas L, Christ G. Gene transfer for erectile dysfunction: will this novel therapy be accepted by urologists? *Curr Opin Urol*. 2009;19:595-600.

29. van Dijk MM, de la Rosette JJMCH, Michel MC. Effects of a_1-adrenoceptor antagonists on male sexual function. *Drugs*. 2006;66:287-301.

30. McCarty EJ, Dinsmore WW. Premature ejaculation: treatment update. *Int J STD AIDS*. 2010;21:77-81.

31. Melnik T, Glina S, OMjr R. Psychological intervention for premature ejaculation. *Nat Rev Urol*. 2009;6:501-508.

32. Patel K, Hellstrom WJ. Central regulation of ejaculation and the therapeutic role of serotonergic agents in premature ejaculation. *Curr Opin Investig Drugs*. 2009;10: 681-690.

33. Sanbe A, Tanaka Y, Fujiwara Y, et al. a_1-Adrenoceptors are required for normal male sexual function. *Br J Pharmacol*. 2007;152:332-340.

34. Michel MC. The pharmacological profile of the a_{1A}-adrenoceptor antagonist silodosin. *Eur Urol Suppl*. 2010;9: 486-490.

11

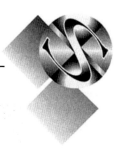

Metabolic Evaluation and Medical Management of Stone Disease

Dorit E. Zilberman, Michael N. Ferrandino, and Glenn M. Preminger

Epidemiology

Renal stone disease continues to be considerable medical problem, often causing significant patient morbidity. The lifetime risk for stone formation has been reported to be as high as 12% for men and 6% for women.[1] However, the rate of female stone formation is insidiously increasing, probably as a result of diet changes and lifestyle associated risk factors such as obesity.[2] Recent studies suggest the current male to female ratio of stone formation is now 1.3:1 (M:F).[2,3]

Moreover, the overall incidence of stone disease is increasing in the USA as stone disease prevalence increased from 3.8% to 5.2% between 1976 and 1994.[2-4] Similar increases have been reported by authors from Japan[5] and Germany.[6] Again, this upsurge is partly attributed to changes in diet and lifestyle and some have suggested that global warming could be augmenting stone formation risk.[7]

As of 2000, the estimated annual cost attributed to urolithiasis was $2.1 billion dollars representing a 50% increase since 1994. This cost estimation includes initial diagnosis, emergent and surgical intervention, and metabolic evaluation.[3] As a consequence of an increased stone disease burden, it is predicted that the overall expenses related to nephrolithiasis will increase by 25% over current expenditures.[7]

Stone Types and Associated Diseases/Metabolic Conditions

Traditionally, stone classification is divided into two main groups: Calcium-based and non-calcium-based stones (Table 11.1). Calcium-based stones, which are the largest group, consist of calcium oxalate monohydrate and calcium oxalate dehydrate, each of which accounts for 40–60%, and less frequently calcium phosphate, which accounts for 2–4% of stones analyzed.[8]

The second group of non-calcium stones consists of (from most to least common): Struvite (infection) stones, uric acid stones, cystine, urate-contained stones, xanthine, and drug-induced stones (indinavir, ephedrine, triamterene, probenecid, sulfinpyrazole, chemotherapy). Table 11.2 summarizes stone composition and their associated metabolic disorders.

Calcium-Based Urolithiasis

Stones with calcium components develop as a result of the greatest variety of metabolic derangements and oftentimes patients present with a combination of stone forming risk factors. The most prevalent diagnoses in calcium stone formers are absorptive hypercalciuria (type I and II), hypocitraturia, hypomagnesiuria, renal leak hypercalciuria,

C.R. Chapple and W.D. Steers (eds.), *Practical Urology: Essential Principles and Practice*,
DOI: 10.1007/978-1-84882-034-0_11, © Springer-Verlag London Limited 2011

Table 11.1. Types of urolithiasis based on stone composition

	Percentage
Calcium based	
Calcium oxalate monohydrate	40-60
Calcium oxalate dihydrate	40-60
Calcium phosphate	20-60
Non-calcium based	
Struvite	5–15
Uric acid	5–10
Cystine	1–2.5
Ammonium acid urate	<1
Sodium urate	<1
Dihydroadenine	<1
Xanthine	<1
Drug-induced (indinavir, ephedrine, triamterene probenecid, sulfinpyrazole, chemotherapy)	<1

Table 11.2. Stone composition and possible clinical associations

Stone analysis	Possible associations
Calcium oxalate	Hypercalciuria
	Hypercalcemia
	Hyperoxaluria
	Hypocitraturia
	Gouty diathesis
	Low urine volumes
Ca Phos	Distal renal tubular acidosis
	Hyperparathyroidism
	Low urine volumes
	UTI
Uric acid	Gouty diathesis
Ammonium acid	Gouty arthritis
Urate	Gouty nephropathy
Sodium urate	Gouty tophi
Dihydroadenine	Hyperuricosuria
Xanthine	Hyperuricosemia
	Inborn errors of metabolism (e.g., Lesch-nyhan disease)
	Myeloproliferative disorder
	Tumor lysis syndrome
	EtOH abuse
Cystine	Cystinuria
Struvite	Urinary tract infection

primary hyperparathyroidism, hyperoxaluria, gouty diathesis, and low urinary volumes. It should be noted that gouty diathesis may also predispose patients to uric acid stone formation, while low urinary volumes may contribute to all causes of calcium stone formation in addition to patients with uric acid stones, cystinuria, and infectious stones.

Uric Acid Urolithiasis

Patients with pure uric acid urolithiasis generally have a low urinary pH (<5.5) and are therefore defined as having gouty diathesis. As previously mentioned, patients with the diagnosis of gouty diathesis (urine pH < 5.5) may form either calcium or uric acid stones.

Infectious Urolithiasis

High urinary pH (>7.5) is associated with the presence of urinary tract infection and the formation of infectious urolithiasis. The presence of urea splitting organisms leads to an increase in the ammonia concentration, which further promotes struvite stone formation.[9,10]

Struvite stones compose the majority of staghorn calculi.

Cystine-Based Urolithiasis

Cystine urolithiasis is the result of an autosomal recessive trait, which disrupts the transepithelial transport of cystine, ornithine, lysine, and arginine. The concentration of cystine rises to levels above the saturation point, and as a consequence, cystine crystals precipitate.[11,12] Of note, even though cystine stone formers all have definitive genetic derangements, they have been found to have a number of other metabolic risk factors, which can contribute to their stone formation.[13]

Metabolic Evaluation of Stone Disease

Aims

The main goal of metabolic evaluation is to prevent recurrent stone formation in high-risk stone producers, as well as to prevent further growth of any existing stones, to help limit the need for surgical intervention. Stone recurrence rate among first time stone formers is as high as 50% in a period of 5–10 years, while remission rates under appropriate treatment can reach as high as 80–90% with appropriate medical stone management.[14-17]

Who Deserves Metabolic Evaluation?

As a rule, any patient with a history of stone disease will benefit from a metabolic evaluation.[18] However, two studies suggest that medical management, which includes metabolic evaluation, may not be cost-effective in the first time stone formers. One study determined that only at a recurrence rate of 0.3–4 stones per year does medical evaluation and treatment become equivalent to management of recurrent episodes.[19]

The same conclusion was reached by a second study group that performed an international cost comparison analysis utilizing urologic literature to support their assumptions.[20] For first time stone formers, the recurrence rate on conservative therapy was determined to be 0.07 stones/patient/year. Conservative therapy was also found to be the least costly for recurrent stone formers but was associated with the highest rate of recurrence (0.3 stones/patient/year) compared to empiric and directed medical therapy (0.06 and 0.084 stones/patient/year, respectively). These authors suggest that first time stone formers should initially be treated conservatively.

Additional studies also support the role of conservative measures to manage initial stone-formers. Dietary modification alone has been shown to decrease the overall rate of recurrence in 58% of patients with a variety of metabolic risk factors.[21] More specifically, a 71% and 47% reduction was demonstrated in stone formation for patients with hypercalciuria and hyperuricosuria, while on high fluid intake and avoidance of dietary excesses, respectively.

There are, however, two studies which support the role of metabolic evaluation in first time stone formers. Both groups found that the incidence and severity of stone formation, including the number of underlying metabolic abnormalities, was identical in recurrent and solitary stone formers.[22,23]

Most would also agree that another group that should undergo a thorough metabolic evaluation is the first time stone producers, who are at a high risk for recurrence. This includes those patients with a family history of stones, intestinal disease/chronic diarrhea, urinary tract infections, history of gout, osteoporosis or skeletal fractures.

Some authors argue that patients with stones composed of uric acid, cystine, and struvite should undergo metabolic evaluation as well.[18,24] However, this same subset of stone compositions has been used to identify patients which may not benefit from further evaluation.[25] Additionally, it is recommended that metabolic evaluation of calcium stone formers should be performed in patients with difficult to treat stones, patients with stones in a solitary kidney, or those individuals with nephrocalcinosis.[18]

Children with nephrolithiasis would clearly benefit from a metabolic evaluation. Young patients with urolithiasis are at similar risk of metabolic disturbances as adults.[26] The increased risk of detrimental effects of repeated episodes of obstruction, urinary tract infections, and the need for surgical intervention strengthen the recommendation for metabolic evaluation and management of children with nephrolithiasis.

When Should Metabolic Evaluation Be Performed?

The first obligation in managing of urolithiasis is treating the offending stone. Apart from relieving obstruction and alleviating accompanying symptoms, stone retrieval enables chemical analysis that by itself provides clues for the underlying pathology that originally caused the problem. Moreover, most suggest that one should wait at least 1 month after stone passage or stone removal, allowing the patient to return to their normal routine, before a metabolic evaluation is initiated. Obtaining urine or blood collections while a patient is obstructed, infected, or suffering from renal colic yields unhelpful information.

Metabolic Workup for Stone Producers

Medical History and Physical Examination

The basic metabolic evaluation begins as any physician–patient interaction should, with a thorough history and physical exam. Key points in the history should include: medical illnesses and surgical procedures, which may contribute to stone formation, family history of nephrolithiasis, evaluation of medications and dietary supplements, as well as dietary habits. Evaluation of general hydration and activity levels are important to consider.

Stone Analysis

The ability to analyze urinary stones is an integral part of the metabolic evaluation. The most common outcome of an acute stone episode is spontaneous passage and patients do not always collect these stones for future chemical analysis.

The operating theater is the most reliable venue for stone collection. Despite the fact that stones or fragments are not always collected, valuable information can be gained from analysis of stone composition. In fact, a further simplification of the metabolic evaluation has been proposed based on stone composition.[25]

For patients with less common stone compositions – cystine, pure struvite, and pure uric acid – minimal to no further evaluation was required and treatment regimens could begin immediately.[25,27,28] Patients with calcium phosphate stones are known to be at increased risk from renal tubular acidosis and primary hyperparathyroidism, while patients with calcium oxalate stone formation have a mixture of metabolic diagnoses.

Serum Chemistry

Serum chemistry consists of basic metabolic panel (e.g., sodium, potassium, chloride, carbon dioxide, blood urea nitrogen, creatinine) as well as calcium and uric acid. This blood panel should be performed in an attempt to identify hypercalcemia, hypokalemia, metabolic acidosis, and hyperuricemia. Hypercalcemia may be indicative of hyperparathyroidism and would warrant further evaluation with a parathyroid hormone assay. The presence of hypokalemia and hyperchloremia is strongly suggestive of metabolic acidosis and is highly associated with distal renal tubular acidosis. Finally, if clinical history suggests possible derangement of purine metabolism serum uric acid may be confirmatory.

Urine Evaluation

Urine Cultures

Urine cultures are valuable if the patient demonstrates signs and symptoms of infection. Cultures positive for Klebsiella pneumonia, Proteus mirabilis, Pseudomonas aeruginosa, or other urea-splitting organisms may indicate the presence of struvite stone. Additionally, clinical and surgical management will vary depending upon the presence or absence of infection.

Urinalysis

Urinalysis should include pH and a review of urinary sediment, as these results may provide a clue to stone composition. A variation in pH may point to particular diagnoses, with a pH between 6.8 and 7.2 suggestive of RTA, a pH greater than 7.5 correlated with urinary tract infection whereas a pH less than 5.5 defines the diagnosis of gouty diathesis. Care should be taken, however, not to rely too heavily on a single urine pH as the patient's dietary may be reflected instead of the underlying metabolic disorders.[29]

Twenty-Four Hour Urine Collections

The urine constituents most commonly assayed include: total volume, pH, calcium, phosphorus, oxalate, citrate, sodium, magnesium, potassium, uric acid, and sulfate. Whereas most of these parameters are self-evident, sulfate is added to the list to assess the volume of animal protein ingested, which may increase the risk of certain stones. Creatinine is measured to evaluate the adequacy of urine collection. Values lower than 500 mg/day should rather be considered as either incomplete collection or dilution with fluid whereas creatinine values >3,000 mg/day in normal-sized individuals suggest an "over collection" of urine. Cystine values should be requested when cystinuria is suspect. It is our routine to have the patient collect two 24 h urine samples on two different days (either consecutive or separate) with the patient on their "normal routine" (normal diet, fluid intake, medications, physical exercise, etc) .

In the past, a third 24 h urine collection was performed to differentiate between the various causes of hypercalciuria–Absorptive hypercalciuria Type I, Type II, and renal leak hypercalciuria. However, discrimination of specific causes of hypercalciuria, while important for physiologic discrimination, has little importance presently, as thiazide diuretics are the only medications available to treat patients with either absorptive or renal leak hypercalciuria.

Radiologic Imaging

Radiologic imaging should be considered part of the basic metabolic evaluation which should not be overlooked. While the utility of imaging is greater as a clinical management tool, there are insights which can be gleaned from plain films, an intravenous pyelogram, or computed tomography (CT). In addition to assessing residual stone burden, radio-opacity/radiolucency of stones on plain films as compared to CT may indicate presence of uric acid, xanthine, and triamterene calculi. Intravenous pyelograms permit appraisal of anatomic anomalies and filling defects. CT scanning is currently the gold standard for the diagnosis of urolithiaisis and will identify stones of all compositions, except for indinavir calculi.[30,31]

Multiple researchers have reported the use of CT to ascertain stone composition based on measurement of Hounsfield units.[32-38] In fact, the use of dual energy CT may further improve the diagnostic capabilities of CT.[39] Additional studies are warranted to further define the use of CT imaging to better predict stone composition.

Medical Management

The primary goal of medical stone management is to prevent urine crystallization and hence the formation or growth of stones. This goal can be achieved either by conservative or by medical management.

Conservative Management

As already mentioned, conservative therapy may be effective as first-line treatment for first time stone formers and for those patients without significant risk factors for recurrent stone formation.[21]

Increased Fluid Intake

The first recommendation for all stone producers would be increased fluid intake as increased urine volume prevents urine stagnation and reduces crystallization of stone-forming salts. Recommended fluid intake is 2–3 L of liquids, preferably water, however, most beverages can be included in the total amount.

Citrus Juices

Especially in cases of hypocitraturia, the addition of citrus juices to fluid intake not only increases urine output but also contributes to the increase of urinary citrate levels, thereby increasing the inhibitory activity against stone formation. Both lemon and orange juices have been sown to reduce the risk of stone formation in certain patients, and can be used to supplement fluid intake in almost all individuals.[40-42] Other studies have assessed the citrate concentrations of various citrate juices and drinks.[42,43] In one study, the highest citrate concentrations were found in grapefruit juice (64.7 mmol/L), lemon juice (47.66 mmol/L), orange juice (47.36 mmol/L), pineapple juice (41.57 mmol/L), reconstituted lemonade (38.65 mmol/L), and lemonade flavored Crystal Light (38.39 mmol/L).

Controversy still exists in the literature with regard to the potential harm of grapefruit juice consumed in excessive amounts; therefore further studies are warranted to evaluate the clinical significance of other citrate-containing juices.[44,45]

Dietary Restrictions

General dietary advice refers to a low sodium and low animal protein diet. Previous studies have suggested that excessive sodium intake increases urinary calcium and decreases urinary citrate probably by producing mild metabolic acidosis and have demonstrated the different physiological effects of sodium and potassium cations by showing that potassium alkali reduces urinary calcium while sodium alkali does not.[46,47] Therefore, it is advisable to generally recommend dietary salt reduction especially among calcium stone producers.

Similarly, we recommend restriction of animal protein intake in stone-forming patients. Studies conducted under controlled clinical laboratory settings have demonstrated the risk of hypercalciuria and hyperuricosuria as a result of diet high in animal protein.[48-50] These findings were further supported by epidemiologic studies that found a positive correlation between diets rich in protein and the high prevalence of stone disease.[51,52]

Later studies have shown the effect of dietary protein restriction on decreasing the levels of calcium, phosphate, oxalate, and uric acid while increasing the levels of urinary citrate.[53,54]

Restricted Oxalate Diet

Although this recommendation may be provided to all stone patients, it is most useful for patients with enteric hyperoxaluria or underlying bowel abnormalities.[55] Traditional foods rich in oxalate includes: black tea, cocoa, spinach, mustard greens, pokeweed, swiss chard, beets, rhubarb, okra, chocolate, nuts, wheat germ, soy crackers, pepper.

Conservative Measures

Under conservative management, the patient should be followed within 3–4 months with current imaging, a basic metabolic panel, and 24 h urine sample collection as described above. Provided the baseline abnormalities have been corrected, an appointment should be re-scheduled in 6–12 months with repeated 24 h urine testing.

Selective Medical Therapy

This entity is kept for persistent metabolic disorders despite proper conservative management. Various regimens currently exist in the market for treating resistant metabolic disturbances and are given in Table 11.3. Drug efficacy and dosage modifications should be monitored via the 24 h urine collection.

Absorptive Hypercalciuria

There is currently no treatment program which is capable of correcting the basic abnormality of absorptive hypercalciuria Type I (AHI). Although sodium cellulose phosphate had been used in the past as a nonabsorbable ion exchange resin to bind calcium and inhibits its absorption, this medication is no longer available.

Thiazide

Thiazide is not considered a selective therapy for absorptive hypercalciuria, since it does not decrease intestinal calcium absorption in this condition. However, this drug has been widely used to treat absorptive hypercalciuria.

Potassium supplementation should be employed when using thiazide therapy in order to prevent hypokalemia and a decrease in urinary citrate excretion. A typical treatment program might include chlorthalidone 25 mg/day with potassium citrate 20 mEq twice/day.

In absorptive hypercalciuria Type II, no specific drug treatment may be necessary since the physiologic defect is not as severe as in absorptive hypercalciuria Type I. A low calcium intake (400–600 mg/day) and high fluid intake (sufficient to achieve a minimum urine output of greater than 2 L/day) would seem ideally indicated.

Orthophosphate

Orthophosphate (neutral or alkaline salt of sodium and/or potassium, 0.5 g phosphorus three to four times/day) has been shown to inhibit $1,25\text{-}(OH)_2D$ synthesis and reduce urinary calcium excretion. Moreover, there is some preliminary evidence that this treatment restores normal intestinal calcium absorption. This medication may be particularly indicated in absorptive hypercalciuria Type III; however, it is contraindicated in nephrolithiasis complicated by urinary tract infection.

Renal Hypercalciuria

Thiazide is ideally indicated for the treatment of renal hypercalciuria. This diuretic has been shown to correct the renal leak of calcium by augmenting calcium reabsorption in the distal tubule and by causing extracellular volume

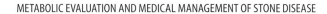

Table 11.3. Stone management – medication summary

Medication	Indications	Side effects	Dose	Other notes
Thiazide	Hypercalciuria (Absorptive Type I, II; renal)	Hypokalemia	Chlorthalidone 25–50 mg PO qd	High sodium intake will offset effect of thiazide
	Hyperoxaluria (primary, idiopathic)		Indapamide: 1.25 mg PO qd	Often administered with K-citrate or amiloride to counter hypo-kalemic effects
				Often administered with K-citrate to counter acidotic effects
Orthophosphate	Hypercalciuria (absorptive)	GI intolerance	Each tab has 250 mg Phos 1–2 tabs PO QID	Side effect profile makes this second line if thiazides are ineffective
Bisphosphonate	Hypercalciuria (resorptive)	Hypocalcemia Rash GI intolerance	Alendronate 5–10 mg PO qd Risendronate 5 mg PO qd	Ensure PTH normal before starting medical therapy
Potassium citrate	Hypercalciuria Hyperoxaluria Gouty diathesis Cystinuria Hypocitraturia	GI intolerance Hyperkalemia	40–90 mEq PO divided BID/TID	Take with meals to avoid GI upset
Sodium bicarbonate	Hyperoxaluria (enteric) Gouty diathesis Distal tubular renal Acidosis Cystinuria	GI intolerance Alkalosis	650–1,300 mg PO up to QID	
Allopurinol	Hyperuricosuria Hyperuricosemia	Rash Xanthine urolithiasis	300–600 mg PO qd	Wait until after acute gouty arthritis attack subsides before starting
D-penicillamine	Cystinuria	Pyridoxine deficiency Rash Agranulocytosis Leukopenia Nephrotic syndrome Arthralgia	500–1,000 mg PO QID	Side effect profile makes this more of a second-line agent Cheaper than thiola

(*continued*)

Table 11.3. (continued)

Medication	Indications	Side effects	Dose	Other notes
Thiola	Cystinuria	Similar to penicillamine but less common and less severe	200–1,200 mg PO divided BID - QID	First- line agent
Captopril	Cystinuria	Cough Renal insufficiency	75–150 mg PO qd	Usually third- line agent
Acetohydroxamic acid	Infection-based nephrolithiasis	Anemia Rash Hepatotoxicity GI upset DVT	250 mg PO TID/ QID	F/U q 3–4 months required on this medication to monitor for side effects
Pyridoxine	Hyperoxaluria (primary) Cystinuria (if penicillamine being used)		Primary: 200–400 PO qd Adjunct: 50 mg PO qd	
Ca supplementation	Hyperoxaluria (enteric)	Constipation	1–4 g PO TID with meals	Follow-up urine collections to avoid hypercalcuria
Mg gluconate	Hyperoxaluria (primary)	GI Intolerance Hyporeflexia Hypotonia/Muscle Paralysis Hypotension Cardiac arrhythmia	Start at 400 or 420 mg PO qd and tailor to response	Side effects usually seen at very high doses
Bile salt resin	Hyperoxaluria (enteric)	GI intolerance	Cholestyramine 1–4 g PO TID with meals	

depletion and stimulating proximal tubular reabsorption of calcium. These effects are shared by hydrochlorothiazide 50 mg twice/day, chlorthalidone 25 mg/day, or trichlormethiazide 4 mg/day. Potassium citrate supplementation (40–60 mEq/day) is advised, since it has been shown to be effective in averting hypokalemia and in increasing urinary citrate, when administered to patients with calcium nephrolithiasis taking thiazide. Thiazide is contraindicated in primary hyperparathyroidism because of potential aggravation of hypercalcemia.

Primary Hyperparathyroidism

Parathyroidectomy is the optimum treatment for nephrolithiasis of primary hyperparathyroidism. Following removal of abnormal parathyroid tissue, urinary calcium is restored to normal commensurate with a decline in serum concentration of calcium and intestinal absorption. There is no established medical treatment for the nephrolithiasis of primary hyperparathyroidism. Although orthophosphates have been recommended for the disease of mild-to-moderate severity, their safety or efficacy has not yet been proven. They should be used only when parathyroid surgery cannot be undertaken. Estrogen has been reported to be useful in reducing serum and urinary calcium in postmenopausal women with primary hyperparathyroidism.

Hyperuricosuric Calcium Oxalate Nephrolithiasis

Allopurinol (300 mg/day) is the physiologically meaningful drug of choice in hyperuricosuric calcium oxalate nephrolithiasis resulting from uric acid over production because of its ability to reduce uric acid synthesis and lower urinary uric acid. Its use in hyperuricosuria associated with dietary purine overindulgence is also reasonable since dietary purine restriction is often impractical. Potassium citrate represents an alternative to allopurinol in the treatment of this condition. Treatment with potassium citrate (at a dose of 30–60 mEq/day in divided doses) may reduce the urinary saturation of calcium oxalate (by complexing calcium), and inhibit urate-induced crystallization of calcium oxalate.

Enteric Hyperoxaluria

Oral administration of large amounts of calcium (0.25–1.0 g four times/day) or magnesium has been recommended for the control of calcium nephrolithiasis of ileal disease. The replacement of dietary fat with medium chain triglycerides may be helpful in those patients who also have malabsorption. Patients may exhibit hypomagnesiuria due to impaired intestinal absorption of magnesium. Oral magnesium supplements, such as magnesium gluconate (0.5–1.0 g three times/day), may correct hypomagnesiuria.

A high fluid intake is recommended to assure adequate urine volume. Since excessive fluid loss may be present, an antidiarrheal agent may be necessary before sufficient urine output can be achieved.

Hypocitraturic Calcium Oxalate Nephrolithiasis

In patients with hypocitraturic calcium oxalate nephrolithiasis, potassium citrate treatment is capable of restoring normal urinary citrate, lowering the urinary saturation and inhibiting crystallization of calcium salts. Since hypocitraturia is found in a number of different conditions, each will be addressed individually.

Distal Renal Tubular Acidosis

Potassium citrate therapy is able to correct the metabolic acidosis and hypokalemia found in patients with distal renal tubular acidosis. In addition, it is capable of restoring normal urinary citrate although large doses (up to 120 mEq/day) may be required in severe acidotic states.

Chronic Diarrheal States

Potassium citrate therapy is indicated for patients with hypocitraturia secondary to chronic diarrheal states. The dose of potassium citrate will be dependent on the severity of hypocitraturia in these patients. The dosages range from 60 to 120 mEq in three to four divided doses. It is recommended that a liquid preparation of potassium citrate be used rather than the slow-release tablet preparation since the slow-release medication may be poorly absorbed due to rapid intestinal transit time. In addition, frequent dose schedules (three to four times/day) for the liquid preparation are necessary since this form of the medication has a relatively short duration of biological action.

Thiazide-Induced Hypocitraturia

Thiazide therapy may induce hypocitraturia due to hypokalemia with resultant intracellular acidosis. Therefore, it should be a common practice to administer potassium supplementation, preferably in the form of potassium citrate, to patients receiving thiazide for treatment of hypercalciuria.

Idiopathic Hypocitraturic Calcium Oxalate Nephrolithiasis

This entity includes hypocitraturia occurring alone, as well as in conjunction with other abnormalities (e.g., hypercalciuria or hyperuricosuria). Stones formed in this condition are predominantly composed of calcium oxalate. Potassium citrate therapy may produce a sustained increase in urinary citrate and a decline in the urinary saturation of the calcium oxalate.

A liquid preparation of potassium citrate with a frequent dosage schedule (three to four times/day) is recommended in chronic diarrheal states. In other conditions, a solid preparation given on a twice daily schedule is generally well tolerated.

Hypomagnesiuric Calcium Nephrolithiasis

Hypomagnesiuric calcium nephrolithiasis is characterized by low urinary magnesium, hypocitraturia, and low urine volume. Therefore, management might include restoration of urinary magnesium levels with either magnesium oxide or magnesium hydroxide as well as correction of the hypocitraturia with potassium citrate.

Gouty Diathesis

The major goal in the management of gouty diathesis is to increase the urinary pH above pH 5.5., preferably between 6.5 and 7.0. In the past, urine alkalinization has been accomplished with either sodium bicarbonate or various combinations of sodium and potassium alkali therapy. While sodium alkali may enhance dissociation of uric acid and inhibit uric stone acid formation by raising urinary pH, this medication may be complicated by the development of calcium-containing stones (calcium phosphate and/or calcium oxalate). Potassium citrate is advantageous because it is not only a good alkalinizing agent, but it appears to be devoid of complication of calcium stones. It should be given at dose sufficient to maintain urinary pH at approximately 6.5 (30–60 mEq/day in 2–3 divided doses). Attempts at alkalinizing the urine to a pH of greater than 7.0 should be avoided. At a higher pH, there is a danger of increasing the risk of calcium stone formation. If the urinary uric acid excretion is elevated or hyperuricemia exists, allopurinol (300 mg/day) is recommended.

Cystinuria

The object of treatment for cystinuria is to reduce the urinary concentration of cystine to below its solubility limit (200–300 mg/L). The initial treatment program includes a high fluid intake and oral administration of soluble alkali (potassium citrate) at a dose sufficient to raise the urinary pH to 6.5–7.0. When this conservative program is ineffective d-penicillamine or alpha-mercaptopropionylglycine (approximately 1–2 g/day in divided doses) has been used. Penicillamine has been associated with frequent side effects including nephrotic syndrome, dermatitis, and pancytopenia. This side effect profile appears to be less marked with alpha-mercaptopropionylglycine.

Infection Lithiasis

If long-standing effective control of infection with urea-splitting organisms can be achieved, new stone formation may be averted and some dissolution of existing stones may be achieved. Unfortunately, such control is difficult to obtain with antibiotic therapy. If there is an existing struvite stone, it is often difficult to completely eradicate the infection because the stone often harbors the organism within its interstices. For this reason, surgical removal of struvite stones is usually recommended.

Acetohydroxamic acid (AHA), a urease inhibitor, may reduce the urinary saturation of struvite and to retard stone formation. When given at a dose of 250 mg three times/day, AHA has been shown to prevent recurrence of new stones and inhibit the growth of stones in patients with chronic urea-splitting infections. In addition, in a limited number of patients, AHA has caused dissolution of existing struvite calculi. However, 30% of patients receiving chronic AHA therapy have experienced minor side effects and 15% developed deep venous thrombosis.

Summary

Stone disease appears to be an increasing problem as a consequence of climate and dietary changes, as well as lifestyle associated risk factors. The key role for proper management of stone disease is obtaining control of its underlying source. This goal can be easily achieved provided there is good patient-physician communication and both sides adhere to simple rules. Only in selected cases should further regimens be added to the equation, while assuring patient tolerance and compliance (see Fig. 11.1).

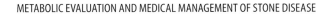

Who?	When?

1. Patient with stone who wishes to undergo metabolic evaluation
2. Single stone with risk factors:
    a. Family history
    b. Intestinal disease
    c. Chronic diarrhea
    d. UTI
    e. Gouty
    f. Osteoporosis
    g. Skeletal fractures
3. Recurrent stone formers
4. Children
5. Controversial: uric acid/struvite/cystine stones
	Following surgical treatment

Workup				
Medical history and physical examination	Stone analysis	Serum chemistry	Urine evaluation	Radiologic imaging
Medical illnesses Medications Social history	Cystine,pure struvite, pure uric acid: No further evaluation required – Start regimens immediately	Sodium, potassium, chloride, carbon dioxide, blood urea nitrogen, creatinine, calcium, uric acid (PTH – optional)	Urine cultures Urine analysis: pH, sediment 2 samples/24 h urine collection: volume, pH, calcium, phosphor, oxalate, citrate, sodium, magnesium, potassium, uric acid, sulfate, creatinine, (cystine)	Renal stone protocol CT KUB IVP

Medical management	
Conservative	Medical – selective
Increase fluid intake: 2–3 L/day to maintain urine output > 2L/day	Potassium citrate
Citrus juices: lemonade, orange	Chlorthalidone

Dietary restrictions
  1. Low sodium
  2. Low animal protein
  3. Restricted oxalate: decrease black tea, spinach, chocolate, nuts
	Allopurinol
	
	(see Table 11.3 for further regimens)

First follow up in 3–4 months period with current imaging, basic metabolic panel and 24 h urine sample collection.

Baseline abnormalities had been corrected – schedule an appointment in 6–12 months with repeated 24 h urine testing.

Figure 11.1. Metabolic evaluation and medical management of stone disease – the essentials.

References

1. Curhan GC. Epidemiology of stone disease. *Urol Clin North Am.* 2007;34(3):287-293

2. Scales CD Jr, Curtis LH, Norris RD, et al. Changing gender prevalence of stone disease. *J Urol.* 2007;177(3):979-982

3. Pearle MS, Calhoun EA, Curhan GC. Urologic diseases in America project: urolithiasis. *J Urol.* 2005;173(3):848-857

4. Stamatelou KK, Francis ME, Jones CA, Nyberg LM, Curhan GC. Time trends in reported prevalence of kidney stones in the United States: 1976–1994. *Kidney Int.* 2003;63(5):1817-1823

5. Yoshida O, Terai A, Ohkawa T, Okada Y. National trend of the incidence of urolithiasis in Japan from 1965 to 1995. *Kidney Int.* 1999;56(5):1899-1904

6. Hesse A, Brandle E, Wilbert D, Kohrmann KU, Alken P. Study on the prevalence and incidence of urolithiasis in Germany comparing the years 1979 vs. 2000. *Eur Urol.* 2003;44(6):709-713

7. Brikowski TH, Lotan Y, Pearle MS. Climate-related increase in the prevalence of urolithiasis in the United States. *Proc Natl Acad Sci USA.* 2008;105(28):9841-9846

8. Moe OW. Kidney stones: pathophysiology and medical management. *Lancet.* 2006;367(9507):333-344

9. Nemoy NJ, Staney TA. Surgical, bacteriological, and biochemical management of "infection stones". *JAMA.* 1971;215(9):1470-1476

10. Healy KA, Ogan K. Pathophysiology and management of infectious staghorn calculi. *Urol Clin North Am.* 2007;34(3):363-374

11. Thier SO, Segal S, Fox M, Blair A, Rosenberg LE. Cystinuria: defective intestinal transport of dibasic amino acids and cystine. *J Clin Invest.* 1965;44:442-448

12. Pak CY, Fuller CJ. Assessment of cystine solubility in urine and of heterogeneous nucleation. *J Urol.* 1983;129(5):1066-1070

13. Sakhaee K, Poindexter JR, Pak CY. The spectrum of metabolic abnormalities in patients with cystine nephrolithiasis. *J Urol.* 1989;141(4):819-821

14. Uribarri J, Oh MS, Carroll HJ. The first kidney stone. *Ann Intern Med.* 1989;111(12):1006-1009

15. Ljunghall S, Danielson BG. A prospective study of renal stone recurrences. *Br J Urol.* 1984;56(2):122-124

16. Ljunghall S. Incidence of upper urinary tract stones. *Miner Electrolyte Metab.* 1987;13(4):220-227

17. Delvecchio FC, Preminger GM. Medical management of stone disease. *Curr Opin Urol.* 2003;13(3):229-233

18. Chandhoke PS. Evaluation of the recurrent stone former. *Urol Clin North Am.* 2007;34(3):315-322

19. Chandhoke PS. When is medical prophylaxis cost-effective for recurrent calcium stones? *J Urol.* 2002;168(3):937-940

20. Lotan Y, Cadeddu JA, Pearle MS. International comparison of cost effectiveness of medical management strategies for nephrolithiasis. *Urol Res.* June 2005;33(3):223-230

21. Hosking DH, Erickson SB, Van den Berg CJ, Wilson DM, Smith LH. The stone clinic effect in patients with idiopathic calcium urolithiasis. *J Urol.* 1983;130(6):1115-1118

22. Pak CY. Should patients with single renal stone occurrence undergo diagnostic evaluation? *J Urol.* 1982;127(5):855-858

23. Coe FL, Keck J, Norton ER. The natural history of calcium urolithiasis. *JAMA.* 1977;238(14):1519-1523

24. Pietrow PK, Preminger GM. Evaluation and medical management of urinary lithiasis. In: Wein AJ, Kavoussi LR, Novick AC, Partin AW, Peters CA, eds. *Campbell-Walsh Urology.* 9th ed. Philadelphia: Sounders Elsevier; 2007:1409

25. Kourambas J, Aslan P, Teh CL, Mathias BJ, Preminger GM. Role of stone analysis in metabolic evaluation and medical treatment of nephrolithiasis. *J Endourol.* 2001;15(2):181-186

26. Bartosh SM. Medical management of pediatric stone disease. *Urol Clin North Am.* 2004;31(3):575-587. x–xi

27. Lingeman JE, Siegel YI, Steele B. Metabolic evaluation of infected renal lithiasis: clinical relevance. *J Endourol.* 1995;9(1):51-54

28. Pak CY, Poindexter JR, Adams-Huet B, Pearle MS. Predictive value of kidney stone composition in the detection of metabolic abnormalities. *Am J Med.* 2003;115(1):26-32

29. Reddy ST, Wang CY, Sakhaee K, Brinkley L, Pak CY. Effect of low-carbohydrate high-protein diets on acid-base balance, stone-forming propensity, and calcium metabolism. *Am J Kidney Dis.* 2002;40(2):265-274

30. Yilmaz S, Sindel T, Arslan G, et al. Renal colic: comparison of spiral CT, US and IVU in the detection of ureteral calculi. *Eur Radiol.* 1998;8(2):212-217.

31. Teichman JM. Clinical practice. Acute renal colic from ureteral calculus. *N Engl J Med.* 2004;350(7):684-693

32. Bellin MF, Renard-Penna R, Conort P, et al. Helical CT evaluation of the chemical composition of urinary tract calculi with a discriminant analysis of CT-attenuation values and density. *Eur Radiol.* 2004;14(11):2134-2140

33. Deveci S, Coskun M, Tekin MI, Peskircioglu L, Tarhan NC, Ozkardes H. Spiral computed tomography: role in determination of chemical compositions of pure and mixed urinary stones – an in vitro study. *Urology.* 2004;64(2):237-240

34. Mitcheson HD, Zamenhof RG, Bankoff MS, Prien EL. Determination of the chemical composition of urinary calculi by computerized tomography. *J Urol.* 1983;130(4):814-819

35. Mostafavi MR, Ernst RD, Saltzman B. Accurate determination of chemical composition of urinary calculi by spiral computerized tomography. *J Urol.* 1998;159(3):673-675

36. Motley G, Dalrymple N, Keesling C, Fischer J, Harmon W. Hounsfield unit density in the determination of urinary stone composition. *Urology.* 2001;58(2):170-173

37. Nakada SY, Hoff DG, Attai S, Heisey D, Blankenbaker D, Pozniak M. Determination of stone composition by noncontrast spiral computed tomography in the clinical setting. *Urology.* 2000;55(6):816-819

38. Zarse CA, McAteer JA, Tann M, et al. Helical computed tomography accurately reports urinary stone composition using attenuation values: in vitro verification using high-resolution micro-computed tom ography calibrated to fourier transform infrared microspectroscopy. *Urology.* 2004;63(5):828-833

39. Graser A, Johnson TR, Bader M, et al. Dual energy CT characterization of urinary calculi: initial in vitro and clinical experience. *Invest Radiol.* 2008;43(2):112-119

40. Seltzer MA, Low RK, McDonald M, Shami GS, Stoller ML. Dietary manipulation with lemonade to treat hypocitraturic calcium nephrolithiasis. *J Urol.* 1996;156(3): 907-909

41. Kang DE, Sur RL, Haleblian GE, Fitzsimons NJ, Borawski KM, Preminger GM. Long-term lemonade based dietary manipulation in patients with hypocitraturic nephrolithiasis. *J Urol.* 2007;177(4):1358-1362. discussion 1362; quiz 1591

42. Haleblian GE, Leitao VA, Pierre SA, et al. Assessment of citrate concentrations in citrus fruit-based juices and beverages: implications for management of hypocitraturic nephrolithiasis. *J Endourol.* 2008;22(6):1359-1366

43. Penniston KL, Nakada SY, Holmes RP, Assimos DG. Quantitative assessment of citric acid in lemon juice, lime juice, and commercially-available fruit juice products. *J Endourol.* 2008;22(3):567-570

44. Goldfarb DS, Asplin JR. Effect of grapefruit juice on urinary lithogenicity. *J Urol.* 2001;166(1):263-267

45. Ameer B, Weintraub RA. Drug interactions with grapefruit juice. *Clin Pharmacokinet.* 1997;33(2):103-121

46. Sakhaee K, Harvey JA, Padalino PK, Whitson P, Pak CY. The potential role of salt abuse on the risk for kidney stone formation. *J Urol.* 1993;150 (2 Pt 1):310-312

47. Preminger GM, Sakhaee K, Pak CY. Alkali action on the urinary crystallization of calcium salts: contrasting responses to sodium citrate and potassium citrate. *J Urol.* 1988;139(2):240-242

48. Pak CY, Barilla DE, Holt K, Brinkley L, Tolentino R, Zerwekh JE. Effect of oral purine load and allopurinol on the crystallization of calcium salts in urine of patients with hyperuricosuric calcium urolithiasis. *Am J Med.* 1978;65(4):593-599

49. Fellstrom B, Danielson BG, Karlstrom B, Lithell H, Ljunghall S, Vessby B. The influence of a high dietary intake of purine-rich animal protein on urinary urate excretion and supersaturation in renal stone disease. *Clin Sci (Lond).* 1983;64(4):399-405

50. Breslau NA, Brinkley L, Hill KD, Pak CY. Relationship of animal protein-rich diet to kidney stone formation and calcium metabolism. *J Clin Endocrinol Metab.* 1988;66(1):140-146

51. Robertson WG, Peacock M, Hodgkinson A. Dietary changes and the incidence of urinary calculi in the U.K. between 1958 and 1976. *J Chron Dis.* 1979;32(6):469-476

52. Robertson WG, Peacock M, Marshall DH. Prevalence of urinary stone disease in vegetarians. *Eur Urol.* 1982; 8(6):334-339

53. Liatsikos EN, Barbalias GA. The influence of a low protein diet in idiopathic hypercalciuria. *Int Urol Nephrol.* 1999;31(3):271-276

54. Giannini S, Nobile M, Sartori L, et al. Acute effects of moderate dietary protein restriction in patients with idiopathic hypercalciuria and calcium nephrolithiasis. *Am J Clin Nutr.* 1999;69(2):267-271

55. Holmes RP, Assimos DG. The impact of dietary oxalate on kidney stone formation. *Urol Res.* 2004;32(5):311-316

12

Molecular Biology for Urologists

Peter E. Clark

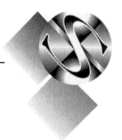

Introduction

The last several decades have seen an explosion of science and technology across all walks of life, and medicine is no exception. Improvements in engineering, optics, laser technology, pharmacology, and molecular biology have radically changed how we take care of patients on a daily basis. The development of the "Targeted Therapies" for advanced renal cell carcinoma (RCC) is just an one example of how discoveries in the basic biology of a disease have contributed to the development of novel therapeutics, thus markedly altering the standard of care for this disease. The field of urology has traditionally been at the forefront of these discoveries, as evidenced by the Nobel Prize winning work of Huggins and Hodges during the last century. As we move through the twenty-first century, a fundamental understanding of molecular biology will be increasingly important to understand the basis for the therapies we prescribe. The purpose of this chapter is to introduce the practicing urologist to the basics of molecular biology and its relevance to our field. It is impossible to relate all of molecular biology, in all its rich, intricate detail, in this short chapter. Therefore, the goal will be to illustrate some basic principles utilizing one of the most prominent examples relevant to urology today. The approach will be to introduce the basic principles of molecular biology using the biology of RCC as an example. The implications and how modern, targeted therapies fit into this biology will be emphasized.

The hope is that by learning the basic principles as they relate to one disease, the interested reader can go on to learn about the relevant pathways in other diseases as well using the same principles. Since it is impossible to give proper attention to every pathway and every disease, and the field changes so rapidly (indeed the pace of change is accelerating), the interested reader is encouraged to pursue specific interests in other pathways/disease via the many recent reviews cited throughout this chapter and elsewhere to explore these concepts in greater depth. Note that many of the terms introduced in this chapter (those that are in bold type and underlined) are listed in Table 12.1 with a brief definition.

Tumor Suppressor Genes and *VHL*

One of the basic principles of molecular biology as it relates to the development of neoplasms (oncogenesis) is the concept of a *tumor suppressor gene*. These genes are important in regulating a variety of cellular processes, but their unifying theme is that when these genes' (or their protein) function is lost in a cell, that cell becomes prone to malignant transformation. This fundamental concept grew out of the development of the tumor suppressor gene theory and the two-hit hypothesis as described by Knudson.[1,2] Under this hypothesis, both copies of a tumor suppressor gene must be disabled in

C.R. Chapple and W.D. Steers (eds.), *Practical Urology: Essential Principles and Practice*,
DOI: 10.1007/978-1-84882-034-0_12, © Springer-Verlag London Limited 2011

Table 12.1. Important definitions and concepts in molecular biology

Term	Section	Definition
Tumor suppressor gene	A	A gene encoding a protein which when lost tends to result in the formation of a neoplasm
Genome	A	All the genes found within a given organism
Somatic cell	A	The cells within a multicellular organism that do not produce gametes (oocyte or sperm). These represent the vast majority of cells in an organism
Germ line mutations	A	A permanent, heritable change in the DNA sequence within the genome of a gamete (oocyte or sperm). As a result, it is present in every cell of any organism which develops from that cell
Chromosome	A	The structure within the cell nucleus that stores the DNA in linear strands associated with a variety of proteins such as histones
Genetic changes	B	Direct mutations or alterations in the DNA sequence that are passed on from parent to progeny cells
Epigenetic changes	B	Heritable changes in the expression of genes which do not involve a direct DNA mutation. An example is DNA methylation
Codon	B	A sequence of three adjacent nucleotides that codes for a particular amino acid. The sequence of these successive codons specifies the amino acid sequence of the resulting protein
Frame shift mutation	B	A mutation (or change in DNA) in which nucleotides are inserted or deleted such that the downstream sequence of codons is scrambled. Since DNA is read three nucleotides at a time (see codon above) a shift in the nucleotide sequence puts the entire remaining sequence out of frame, resulting in a scrambled and nonfunctional protein
Nonsense mutation	B	A mutation (or change in DNA) in which an early or premature stop codon is created, resulting in a truncated protein that is typically nonfunctional.
Missense mutation	B	A mutation (or change in DNA) in which single nucleotide within a codon is changed resulting in a single amino acid change in a protein. This may or may not result in altered function
DNA methylation	B	Modification of DNA in which a methyl group (CH_3) is added to a cytosine that immediately precedes a quanine (CpG island). This is carried out by enzymes called DNA methyl transferases (DNMT)
Promoter	B	The site in the DNA associated with a particular gene where the proteins responsible for transcription bind to initiate mRNA expression. As a result, this site is where the expression of that particular gene is controlled
Response element	C	The DNA nucleotide sequence in the promoter of a gene that is recognized by a regulatory protein that controls transcription, such as the HIFα/β heterodimer. Binding of the regulatory protein to its response element within a particular gene will either up- or downregulate expression of that gene
Messenger RNA (mRNA)	C	A single stranded RNA molecule, coded for by the DNA of a gene, which specifies the subsequent amino acid sequence of a protein during protein synthesis
Transcription	C	The process by which the genetic code in DNA is transcribed into a complementary, single stranded mRNA molecule for subsequent protein synthesis
Translation	C	The process whereby the genetic code stored in the transcribed mRNA molecule is now translated into a sequence of amino acids to form a protein. This is accomplished by the cooperative work of the ribosomes and tRNA that is associated with specific amino acids

Table 12.1. (continued)

Term	Section	Definition
Oncogene	C	A gene that is mutated or overexpressed in a cell, allowing it to become neoplastic or malignant
Polymerase chain reaction (PCR)	C	A technique to significantly amplify a specific stretch of DNA using a set of DNA primers designed to specify an area of interest
RT-PCR	C	A variation of PCR in which mRNA is reverse transcribed into DNA and then PCR is done on a gene of interest. This allows the scientist to measure gene expression at the mRNA level
Genomics	C	A large-scale, rapid screen of gene expression across the entirety of the cell's DNA, that is, its genome
Proteomics	C	A large-scale, rapid screen of the level of all the proteins within a cell at a given time
Angiogenesis	D	The process by which new blood vessels are formed
Ligand	D	A molecule, typically a soluble one such as a hormone, which binds to another molecule to initiate a subsequent downstream effect
Receptor	D	A molecule within or on the surface of a cell that when it binds its specific ligand (see above) it results in specific, downstream effects important to cellular function.
Kinase	D	A frequently used abbreviation for a phosphokinase. These are enzymes which transfer a phosphate group from ATP to another molecule
Cytoplasm	D	The portion of a eukaryotic cell that lies between the outer cellular surface membrane and the inner nucleus. It houses much of the cell's physiologic machinery and organelles, such as the mitochondria, ribosomes, golgi apparatus, and endoplasmic reticulum
Nucleus	D	The large organelle that houses the genomic DNA in eukaryotic cells within chromosomes
Phosphorylation	D	The process whereby phosphate bonds are created between two substrates. In cells this is accomplished usually by kinases
Tyrosine kinase	D	An enzyme that transfers a phosphate group from ATP to a tyrosine residue, either within its own structure or another molecule
Targeted therapy	E	A form of therapy that is designed to specifically target molecules important to the growth of cancer cells, rather than just target rapidly dividing cells such as cytotoxic therapy (i.e., traditional chemotherapy). Examples include antibodies to specific molecules and small molecule kinase inhibitors
Monoclonal antibody	E	An antibody that can be produced in large quantities in a pure form from a single cell clone. Each antibody molecule is identical with respect to its structure and specificity for a particular target (termed an antigen)
Tyrosine kinase inhibitor	F	A small molecule that interferes with the tyrosine kinase activity of enzymes in cells. This is a prototypical example of a targeted therapy
Cell cycle	G	The regulated sequence by which cells undergo the process of growth and cell division/replication
Apoptosis		Also termed programmed cell death, it is the active, regulated process by which cells die in response to external or internal stimuli
Heterodimer		The association between two different proteins to form a complex. An example is the association between HIFα and HIFβ in response to hypoxia or loss of VHL protein
Homodimer		The association between two identical proteins to form a complex. An example is the association between two androgen receptor molecules within a cell

order for a cancer to develop. In a sporadic, non-inherited form of cancer, this means that for any given cell in the body, a mutation is needed in both copies of the same gene. This is because any mutation or change in the *genome* would be in a *somatic cell*, and so, only that particular cell and its progeny would have that change, whereas the remaining cells in the body would not. It would be a rare event that each copy of a particular gene would acquire a mutation in the same cell; so in sporadic, nonfamilial cancers, the tumors generally occur later in life and are usually unifocal. On the other hand, in inherited familial tumor syndromes, there is a *germ line mutation* in one tumor suppressor gene. Thus, every cell in the body has inherited a nonfunctional copy of the gene (the first hit). As a consequence, now it only takes one additional mutation of the same gene (the second hit) in one cell in order for a cancer to develop. Since every cell already has the first hit, having a second hit would be more common. Patients suffering from such inherited tumor syndromes would, therefore, develop cancers in the affected organs at a younger age and tend to have multifocal disease. The basic tenets of this hypothesis were developed in the 1980s for familial tumor syndromes such as retinoblastoma and the *Rb* gene and neurofibromatosis and the *NF-1* and *NF-2* genes.[3–7] In urology, the classic example of this is von Hippel-Lindau disease, the *VHL* gene, and the development of clear cell RCC.

The discovery of the *VHL* gene and its relevance to clear cell RCC grew at first from the observation that the RCC in von Hippel-Lindau disease was identical to its sporadic, nonfamilial counterpart in every respect except it occurred earlier in life and tended to be multifocal. It therefore fit the profile of a familial tumor syndrome characterized by the loss/mutation of a tumor suppressor gene. Careful studies of three different families (kindreds) with a familial tendency toward the development of clear cell RCC had consistently showed aberrations of the short arm of *chromosome* 3 (termed 3p).[8–10] This was followed by a series of studies of clear cell RCC tumors and cell lines that also showed abnormalities of chromosome 3p as a unifying theme.[11–15] The changes noted in chromosome 3 were not present in normal tissues in these sporadic clear cell RCC tumors and were not present in other histologic RCC variants (such as papillary RCC).[16,17]

What followed was based on the recognition that these sporadic clear cell RCCs were also seen in von Hippel-Lindau disease and the abnormality on chromosome 3p fit the profile of a putative tumor suppressor gene. In a series of elegant and groundbreaking studies of multiple different families with von Hippel-Lindau disease, the localization of the *VHL* gene was mapped to a relatively small region on chromosome 3p,[18–20] which was then followed by the identification of the *VHL* gene in a seminal article by Latif et al. in 1993.[21] Since that time, it has been demonstrated that the majority of sporadic clear cell RCC tumors harbor aberrations of *VHL*, strongly suggesting that the same gene was responsible for both the inherited and non-inherited forms of the disease.[1,2,22–26] Indeed, even in cases where mutations of *VHL* were not identified, most often other aberrations were noted such as abnormal hypermethylation of the promoter region of *VHL*, leading to low or absent protein levels (see below).[27]

Since the discovery of *VHL*, its role in the normal function of the cell and how it can act as a tumor suppressor gene has been carefully studied. The principles illustrated here are applicable to a host of other disease processes and serve as an excellent example of how the discoveries at the bench have been translated to the bedside in the form of new targeted agents for advanced RCC. It is instructive, therefore, to describe this in some detail, though the interested reader is encouraged to read any one of the many in-depth reviews on this topic.

Inherited Changes in Cancer Cells

It is worth pausing for a moment to review various ways in which a gene, such as *VHL*, can become aberrantly regulated. A critical element for all of these mechanisms is that they can be inherited or passed on to any progeny cells. Thus, once a "parent" or originating cancer cell acquires one of these changes, those changes are passed on to all its progeny resulting in the growth of a tumor. The two fundamental forms of such changes are *genetic changes*, such as direct mutations of DNA, and *epigenetic changes*, inherited alterations in how genes are expressed (such as DNA methylation). Both of these mechanisms can be demonstrated in the *VHL* gene and clear cell RCC.

Genetic changes (mutations of the DNA in the genome) are inherited from one cell and passed on to all its progeny. If that cell is a gamete, such as an egg or sperm, then this mutation will be found in every cell in the new organism. These are the types of mutations found in familial tumor syndromes such as von Hippel-Lindau Disease. If a mutation occurs in a non-gamete cell (i.e., any cell after conception), then this somatic mutation is passed on only to that cell's progeny. Furthermore, such a somatic mutation will not be passed on from generation to generation. These are the mutations found in sporadic cancers. The types of mutations that can occur in the DNA include insertions or deletions of small or large portions of the DNA. Since every three DNA nucleotides represents one *codon* (coding element for one amino acid), if the insertion or deletion occurs in a multiple of three, the overall protein function may or may not be disrupted depending on what amino acid(s) is inserted/deleted. If the number of nucleotides inserted/deleted is not a multiple of three, then the entire sequence of nucleotide codons and resulting amino acids will be altered resulting in a *frame shift mutation*. This will, in effect, result in a scrambled series of amino acids and a nonfunctional protein. Roughly, half the *VHL* mutations found in sporadic clear RCC are of this type.[22] This will result in a completely nonfunctional protein. In some cases, the nucleotide may be mutated in a way that places a premature stop codon, so a portion of the protein is truncated. These are referred to as *nonsense mutations*. In other cases, one nucleotide is mutated/changed such that only one amino acid is altered. This is termed a *missense mutation* and represents the majority of the remaining *VHL* mutations in sporadic, clear cell RCCs.[22] A more in-depth analysis of the specific *VHL* mutations and their potential relationship to disease biology has been reviewed previously.[28,29]

The expression of genes can also be altered via mechanisms that do not involve a mutation in DNA. If these alterations are heritable, then these are termed epigenetic changes.[30–32] The ability to silence genes is critical to the normal development of an organism. There are a number of mechanisms by which this can be accomplished. This includes modifications of the proteins that are involved in packaging DNA within the nucleus of cells called histones. These histones can have acetyl groups removed from them (de-acetylated via enzymes called histone de-acetylases or HDACs) or methyl groups added (methylated via enzymes called histone methyltransferases, HMTs). In both cases, these can cause gene expression to be silenced. Perhaps the most intensely studies form of epigenetic change as it relates to cancer is the silencing of gene expression via *DNA methylation*. This involves the covalent bonding of a methyl group to a cytosine in areas where there is a cytosine immediately followed by a guanine, a sequence known as a CpG island. This is carried out by a class of enzymes called DNA methyltransferases (DNMTs). When these CpG islands are methylated in the *promoter* of a gene, the gene's expression is often shut down. This mechanism is relevant to clear cell renal cell carcinoma, in that a significant fraction of sporadic RCCs have been shown to lose VHL protein through DNA methylation and gene silencing, an epigenetic change, rather than by a mutation.[27] There is ongoing and intensive interest in the therapeutic potential of HDAC and DNMT inhibitors across a variety of tumor types, though their direct clinical utility in RCC remains to proven.

The Tumor Suppressor VHL, Oncogene HIF, and Gene Regulation

In a normal cell, the VHL protein acts predominantly to regulate the cell's response to the local availability of oxygen.[33–38] When local oxygen levels are normal, there is another regulatory protein, termed hypoxia inducible factor alpha (HIFα), which is hydroxylated permitting it to bind to the VHL protein (see Fig. 12.1).[39,40] The VHL protein is actually part of an enzyme complex (called an E3 ligase) that joins a series of molecules to HIFα called ubiquitin, which in turn marks HIFα for degradation.[41–46] In the normal circumstance, then, HIFα levels are low in the cell. During hypoxia when oxygen levels in the cell are low, HIFα is not hydroxylated, so it does not bind to VHL protein, and consequently is not degraded. The levels of HIFα in the cell rise, allowing it to bind with a similar molecule, HIF-β, that exists at high levels in the cell at all times (see Fig. 12.2). This complex can then bind to specific regions in the cell's nuclear DNA called hypoxia *response elements* (HRE).

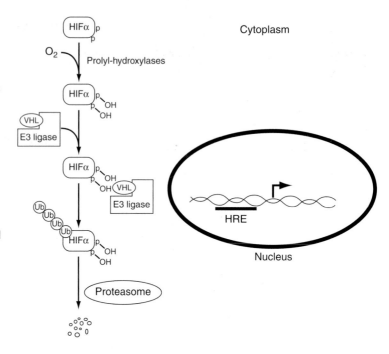

Figure 12.1. Normal regulation of HIFα: under normal conditions, with normal levels of tissue oxygenation, HIFα is hydroxylated through the action of enzymes termed prolyl-hyroxylases. This hydroxylation allows it to associate with an E3 Ligase complex that includes the VHL protein. The VHL protein in particular is critical to this association. The E3 Ligase then enzymatically tags HIFα with a series of molecules (called ubiquitin). This ubiquitination then marks HIFα to be recognized and degraded by the proteasomal complex within the cell. *HIFα* Hypoxia Inducible Factor alpha, *VHL* von Hippel Lindau, *Ub* ubiquitin, *HRE* hypoxia response element.

These HREs are found in the regulator region, called the promoter, of genes important in the cell's response to hypoxia. When a transcriptional regulator, such as the HIFα/β complex, binds to the response element (HRE) in the promoter of a gene, the transcriptional machinery of the cell is turned on and *messenger RNA (mRNA)* specific for that gene is produced in a process called gene *transcription* (see Fig. 12.3). These mRNA molecules then translocate to the cell's cytoplasm where the code embedded in the mRNA is translated into a series of amino acids to generate the specific protein corresponding to that gene (gene *translation*). In the case of HIF and hypoxia, these correspond to a variety of genes that are critical to the cell's response to hypoxia. These include vascular endothelial growth factor (VEGF), platelet derived growth factor (PDGF), transforming growth factor alpha (TGFα), carbonic anhydrase IX (CA-IX), erythropoietin, glucose transporter 1 (GLUT-1), and others. The VHL-HIF axis serves as a good example, then, of a tumor suppressor (VHL) regulating an *oncogene* (HIFα) that in turn transcriptionally regulates a series of other genes that are important to normal cellular function.

In the setting of clear cell RCC, the normal balance in the cell is upset. When the VHL protein either cannot function or is abnormally low/absent in the cell, then no matter the oxygen levels in the cell, HIFα is always at a high level since it cannot be marked for degradation (see Fig. 12.2). Thus, VHL protein is functioning as a tumor suppressor. High levels of HIFα in turn mean the HIFα/β complex will interact with the HREs in the nucleus and the genes normally regulated by HIF will be transcribed and translated at an abnormally high rate (see Fig. 12.3). It is this upregulation of genes such as *VEGF*, *PDGF*, and *TGFα* that is thought to lead to clear cell RCC. Therefore, HIFα is acting as an oncogene.

It is worth pausing for a moment to review a number of general techniques and concepts that are important in the context of molecular biology. These concepts have been part of some of the studies discussed in this chapter and are an integral part of many, as yet unpublished work that is still ongoing in many centers across the world. These involve different ways of interrogating the genetic makeup of tissues (such as tumors) and how these tissues express different proteins that regulate their function.

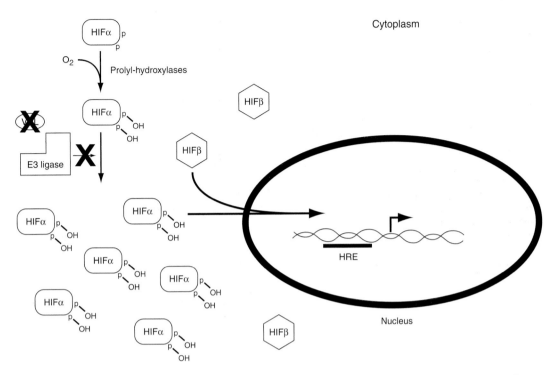

Figure 12.2. Accumulation of HIFα: under conditions of hypoxia, prolyl-hydroxylases cannot hydroxylate HIFα and so it will not bind to the VHL-E3 Ligase complex. Alternatively (as depicted here), if VHL protein is mutated, nonfunctional, or not present the VHL-E3 Ligase cannot bind to HIFα. In either case, HIFα is not ubiquitinated, and so is not degraded by the proteasome. It accumulates within the cell and associates with the constitutively present related molecule, HIFβ. This *heterodimer* now translocates to the nucleus where it binds to specific regions (hypoxia response elements or HRE's) in the promoters of genes upregulated by HIF. The binding of the HIFα-HIFβ heterodimer to this promoter region at the HRE turns on gene transcription. Note that if VHL is absent or not functional, then no matter what the oxygenation level, HIFα cannot be recognized by the E3 Ligase complex and is not degraded. HIFα accumulates in the cell even in the absence of hypoxia. *HIFα* Hypoxia Inducible Factor alpha, *HIFβ* Hypoxia Inducible Factor beta, *VHL* von Hippel Lindau, *HRE* hypoxia response element.

For example, one of the major advances in the study of biology has been the technique of the *polymerase chain reaction (PCR)*. This is essentially a technique to significantly amplify a specific stretch of DNA using a set of DNA primers that the investigator can design to home in on an area of interest. The primers specify exactly what stretch of DNA is amplified. This technique has revolutionized the entire field of gene discovery and cloning. A variation of this can now be done whereby the mRNA in a cell can be reversely transcribed into DNA, and PCR then done on this, so called *RT-PCR*. This technique can now allow biologists to measure the relative expression levels of different genes in cells to see which are up- or downregulated. Further refinements using these basic principles have allowed such studies to be done on a mass scale using "gene chips" that now allow for measurement of thousands of genes at once. This large scale, rapid screen of gene expression across the entirety of the cell's DNA, that is, its genome, is referred to as *genomics*. Other techniques can now screen the entirety of a cell's protein mix using a variety of techniques generally referred to as *proteomics*. Indeed, the number of "-omics" has continued to expand including metabolomics, lipidomics, and others. Mass scale screenings of gene and protein expression is allowing investigators to create a signature for individual patients and tumors (or other diseased tissue). It is these approaches that hold the promise of "individualized" medicine for the future.

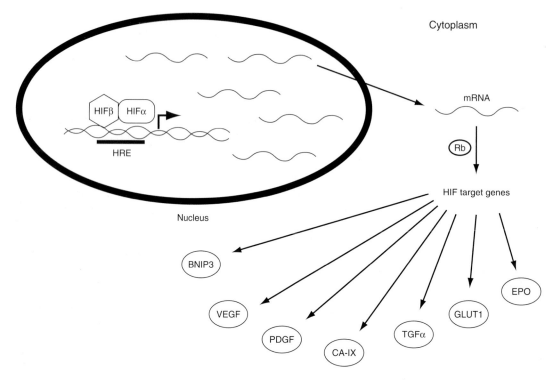

Figure 12.3. Hypoxia responsive genes: binding of the HIFα-HIFβ heterodimer to the HRE in the promoter region at HRE's turns on gene transcription resulting in upregulation of messenger RNA (mRNA) of genes that are responsive to hypoxia and controlled/regulated by HIF. These include vascular endothelial growth factor (VEGF), platelet-derived growth factor (PDGF), transforming growth factor alpha (TGFα), carbonic anhydrase IX (CA-IX), erythropoietin, glucose transporter 1 (GLUT-1), and others. The mRNA translocates from the nucleus to the cytoplasm where it associates with ribosomes, tRNA, and the translational machinery. The code in the mRNA is now translated into the corresponding amino acid sequence forming the relevant proteins. These proteins accumulate and help the cell respond to the hypoxic conditions or, in the case of RCC, may go on to contribute to malignant transformation. *HIFα* Hypoxia Inducible Factor alpha, *HIFβ* Hypoxia Inducible Factor beta, *HRE* hypoxia response element, *Rb* ribosome, *EPO* erythropoietin, *VEGF* vascular endothelial growth factor, *PDGF* platelet derived growth factor, *CA-IX* carbonic anhydrase IX, *TGFα* transforming growth factor alpha, *GLUT1* glucose transporter 1.

VEGR and Cell Signaling

VEGF has stimulated particular interest given its central role in the process of *angiogenesis* (the process of developing new blood vessels), the growing recognition that angiogenesis is a critical component of malignant tumor progression, combined with the clinical observation that clear cell RCCs are often hypervascular tumors.[47-49] The VEGF protein family includes multiple subtypes; VEGF-A, -B, -C, -D, -E, and placenta growth factor-1 (PIGF-1).[50-53] The majority of these are regulated by VHL and HIF using the regulatory system discussed previously. These proteins can in turn bind to

one of three different receptors located at the cell surface, VEGFR-1 (Flt-1), VEGFR-2 (KDR/Flk-1), and VEGFR-3 (Flt-4).[50-53] Of these, VEGFR-1 and -2 are thought to be more important for angiogenesis whereas VEGFR-3 is thought to be more important for lymphangiogenesis.[53] Thus, VEGF is termed a *ligand*, the molecule that is soluble or "mobile," which will bind to its *receptor*, which is less mobile and soluble, in this case positioned in the cell surface membrane. The binding of a ligand to its receptor leads to signaling that affects a cells behavior.

The members of the VEGF receptor family are cell membrane associated *tyrosine kinases.* What this means, is that when VEGF binds to one of these receptors at the cell surface, it induces a change in the receptor that gets passed along to its intracellular (or *cytoplasmic*) portion. In that cytoplasmic portion of the receptor, specific tyrosine amino acid residues in the protein become *phosphorylated*, a reaction that is generally carried out by a class of enzymes termed *kinases*. Therefore, a tyrosine kinase membrane receptor is one that phosphorylates tyrosines (in this case on itself) when it becomes activated by binding to its ligand (in this case VEGF). Once the receptor is activated and its cytoplasmic tyrosine residue(s) is phosphorylated, this then leads to a downstream cascade of signaling events (see Fig. 12.4). There are thought to be at least two main pathways these cascades follow. One is via the Raf-Mek-Erk series of kinases and the other is via the phosphatidylinositol-3 kinase-AKT-mTOR pathway. The activation of these pathways in turn leads to endothelial cell activation, proliferation, migration, and cell survival.[50–54] These effects

on the cell, through a process yet to be fully explained in all its complexity, ultimately lead to carcinogenesis.

A key point for both the Raf-Mek-Erk and PI3K-AKT-mTOR pathways is that they also involve kinases, that is, enzymes that phosphorylate other proteins to regulate their activity. Another important observation relates to the mammalian target of rapamycin (mTOR), which is downstream of VEGF but can also act to increase the cellular levels of HIFα.[55] In principle, the abnormal function of VHL in clear cell RCC can set up a vicious, positive feedback loop in which HIFα levels rise, leading to high levels of VEGF, which binds to its receptor VEGFR resulting in its activation, that in turn signals through the phosphatidylinositol-3 kinase-AKT pathway to activate mTOR (by phosphorylation as with many of these proteins), which can in turn lead to even higher levels of HIFα. This positive feedback loop can accelerate and ramp up signaling via the oncogene HIF.

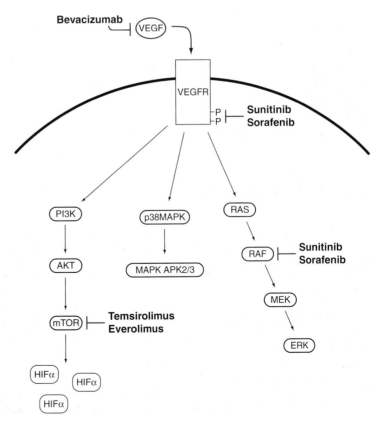

Figure 12.4. Ligand-receptor interaction and downstream signaling: increased expression of proteins such as VEGF (the ligand) allows them to diffuse and bind to their receptor (in this case VEGFR). The VEGF receptor is a tyrosine kinase. When VEGF binds its receptor, a tyrosine is phosphorylated which in turns leads to downstream signaling through a series of other kinases. Note that activation of the PI3K-Akt-mTOR pathway leads to increased HIFα in the cell, which can contribute to a positive feedback loop as HIFα in turn leads to increased signaling along this pathway. Shown within these pathways are some of the known target sites for the monoclonal antibody to VEGF (Bevacizumab), the tyrosine kinase inhibitors (or TKI's, sorafenib and sunitinib), and the mTOR inhibitors (temsirolimus and everolimus).

Moving from Biology to Targeted Therapy

The basic biology of the VHL-HIF cascade described above is an elegant example of how years of work by many talented investigators has shed light on the inner workings of a particular cancer. Had the story ended there, however, one might argue what the relevance is to modern medicine. How does this impact on health care and our patient's well being? The real beauty of this story lies in the movement in the last several years from the "bench top" to the bedside of patients with clear cell RCC. For several decades the management of metastatic RCC was based on the use of immunotherapy including interferon α(IFNα) and interleukin 2 (IL-2).[56] These agents produced response rates on the order of only 10–20%, only a minority of which were durable complete responses. For the remainder the responses were temporary such that the 5 year survival of metastatic RCC was between 0% and 23%.[57,58] Essentially, this meant that 80–90% of patients with advanced RCC did not respond to any appreciable degree to therapy, a situation that cried out for new and innovative agents.

A look again at the VHL-HIF-VEGF pathway we have described so far suggests that if one can interfere with the cascade of events, then in theory one ought to be able to treat clear cell RCC. Stated another way, if one targeted components of the pathway, then the process of carcinogenesis and tumor progression should be reversible. This concept of so called "*Targeted* Therapies," in which specific components of the tumor's biology are attacked and interrupted, forms the basis for many of the therapies that have become the standard of care for advanced clear cell RCC. Given the connection between aberrations in VHL protein function, leading to accumulation of HIF, and subsequent upregulation of VEGF, it was logical to explore the use of an inhibitor of VEGF as one of these novel approaches.

Conceptually the easiest way to block the action of elevated VEGF would be to directly inhibit the molecule itself (see Fig. 12.4). One such approach utilizes a humanized *monoclonal antibody* to bind and sequester VEGF, Bevacizumab (Avastin, Genentech, Inc.).[59] The antibody has been designed so that each antibody molecule is identical (monoclonal or originating from the same cell clone). It has also been

humanized, meaning it has been modified to resemble antibodies normally produced by humans (as opposed to rabbits, mice, or other mammals). This modification is what permits the antibody to be used repeatedly in the same patient without the body automatically recognizing it as foreign and eliminating it from circulation. This novel, targeted agent was first tested in a randomized phase II trial and found to increase the time to progression of advanced RCC when compared to placebo.[59] It has now been tested in a large scale phase III trial in combination with IFNα for men with previously untreated advanced renal cell carcinoma.[60] The combination regimen improved the progression free survival from 5.4 months to 10.2 months when compared to interferon alone. Based on these studies, Bevacizumab in combination with IFNα is now one of the frequently utilized therapies for advanced RCC.

The Tyrosine Kinase Inhibitors (TKIs)

An alternate approach to blocking VEGF is to abrogate the downstream signaling after it binds to its receptor (see Fig. 12.4). As we discussed, the receptor for VEGF (as well as PDGF and TNFα) are tyrosine kinases. When the ligand (VEGF) binds to the receptor (VEGFR) a tyrosine in the receptor is phosphorylated, allowing further downstream signaling to take place via at least one of the two pathways, the Raf-MEK-ERK and the PI3-kinase-AKT-mTOR pathways. Many of the members of these downstream signaling cascades also rely on kinase activity. It would seem logical, then, to look for agents that can block this signaling cascade and thereby interrupt the oncogenic signaling downstream of VHL and HIF. The early attempts developing these *tyrosine kinase inhibitors (TKIs)* were relatively specific for the VEGF receptors' tyrosine kinase activity.[61,62] The results were generally disappointing and these agents have largely been abandoned. In the course of these studies, though, it rapidly became apparent that less specific tyrosine kinase inhibitors, ones that could affect several different signaling molecules simultaneously, were more effective. This is presumably due to the ability to interrupt the signaling cascade at multiple levels simultaneously utilizing one agent. This conceptual framework has resulted in the development, testing, and now approval of several agents in this drug class. There is a rapidly expanding pool of potentially active drugs of this type (eq. AG-013736, GW572016, PTK787/ZK222584, plus others) but for the purpose of this chapter we discuss the two with large scale, published phase three trial data confirming their clinical utility and which are now both approved for use in metastatic RCC (for a more in depth review of the other agents see Lane et al.,[54] Shaheen and Bukowski,[63] and Amato[64]).

Sunitinib is an orally bioavailable multitargeted tyrosine kinase inhibitor. It has been shown to block the downstream signaling from several tyrosine kinase receptors important in RCC, including the receptors for VEGF and PDGF.[65,66] Phase I studies showed promising results in the setting of advanced RCC[67] prompting investigators to initiate two phase II studies in patients who had failed prior systemic cytokine therapy followed by a large, prospective, randomized phase III trial in patients who had not received prior systemic therapy.[68–70] In the phase II trials, both designed to test the efficacy of Sunitinib in the setting of patients with metastatic RCC who had failed prior systemic cytokine therapy (with either interferon or interleukin-2) the partial response rates were 34–40% and the median time to progression was 8.3–8.7 months.[69,70] Based on these promising results, a large scale, international, multicenter, prospective, randomized, phase III trial was completed that enrolled 750 patients with clear cell RCC who had not received prior systemic therapy.[68] Patients were randomized to either Sunitinib or IFNα with the primary endpoint of the trial being progression free survival (PFS). The partial response rate for Sunitinib was 31%, significantly better than the 6% for patients randomized to IFNα. The median progression free survival was significantly better in patients who received Sunitinib (11 months) compared to 5 months for those in the IFNα arm. Toxicity was generally manageable. These results demonstrated the superiority of the oral TKI Sunitinib over IFNα in the front line setting for advanced RCC. The critical point to note is the development and testing of this tyrosine kinase inhibitor flowed directly from an understanding of the molecular biology that underlies the disease it is treating (advanced RCC).

Sorafenib is also an orally bioavailable, multitargeted tyrosine kinase inhibitor, which was originally developed as a specific inhibitor of Raf-1, a member of the Raf/MEK/ERK pathway downstream of receptors important in the VHL/HIF axis (see Fig. 12.4) such as VEGFR and PDGFR and the same (in principle) to the pathways targeted by Sunitinib.[71] Subsequently, studies showed it could also block the downstream signaling of a variety of other tyrosine kinases, including VEGFR, PDGFR, as well as others. As was the case with Sunitinib, the initial phase II studies with Sorafenib showed promise, with substantial improvements in progression free survival.[39,72] These in turn lead to a large-scale, multicenter, international, randomized, prospective trial of 903 patients with clear cell RCC who had failed at least one prior systemic therapy.[73] Patients were randomized to either oral Sorafenib versus placebo. Sorafenib was superior to placebo with respect to progression free survival and it was generally well tolerated, though there were rare cases of significant hypertension and cardiac ischemia. As with Sunitinib, the salient point is that the success of this oral, small molecule agent lies in its development to specifically target a pathway involved in the disease.

Targeting mTOR

As we have discussed, aberrations in VHL underlies the process of carcinogenesis in clear cell RCC, which in turn leads to accumulation and build up of HIFα in RCC cells. Conceptually, another way to block the buildup of HIFα in the cell is to interrupt its initial or starting levels. There are a number of important pathways that impact on the expression of HIFα, but one of the most important is the Akt/mTOR pathway. Signaling from the mTOR pathway leads to increased expression of HIFα mRNA and then to increased starting levels of the protein. In RCC, buildup of HIFα leads to increased signaling along the Akt-mTOR pathway, which leads to upregulation and increased levels of HIFα, which cannot be targeted for degradation by association with VHL since it is abnormal in clear cell RCC. This vicious cycle, or positive feedback loop, as reviewed already, is thought to be important in RCC. Strategies to interrupt this cycle presumably would be effective in treating patients with the advanced form of the disease (see Fig. 12.4). To date, there are a number of compounds that are inhibitors of the mTOR pathway and decrease HIFα, including rapamycin, temsirolimus, and everolimus (see also Cho et al.,[55] Boulay et al.,[74] and Reddy et al.[75]). Of these, the two that have received the greatest attention and have demonstrated efficacy in the setting of advanced RCC are temsirolimus and everolimus. Temsirolimus is a water-soluble ester of sirolimus, which is able to inhibit mTORs kinase activity, leading to *cell cycle* arrest. Phase II trials evaluating its efficacy both in combination with IFNα and as a single agent in cytokine refractory advanced RCC suggested it improved progression free survival when compared to historical controls.[76,77] These prompted a large-scale, prospective, randomized, phase III trial of patients with high risk metastatic RCC (based on the Motzer criteria) randomized to receive Temsirolimus alone, IFNα alone, or the combination of both agents.[78] The results demonstrated that Temsirolimus as monotherapy improved not only progression free survival, but overall survival compared to either IFNα or combination therapy. The toxicity noted in the temsirolimus monotherapy arm was manageable. Based on these results, Temsirolimus has now joined both sunitinib and sorafenib as approved agents for use in advanced RCC. More recently, another mTOR inhibitor, everolimus, was tested in a large-scale, prospective randomized placebo-controlled phase III trial in patients who had failed prior targeted therapies such as those described previously.[79] It demonstrated better progression free survival in those taking everolimus compared to patients in the placebo arm. As with the other targeted therapies, the mTOR inhibitors are a logical extension of attacking the known biology of the disease that has now proven its efficacy beyond the laboratory in the "real world" of patient care.

Conclusion

The development of the targeted therapies for advanced RCC illustrates how biology can speak to medical therapeutics and vice versa. The overarching theme in this chapter is that all the targeted therapies were conceived and derived from an in-depth understanding at the molecular level of renal cell carcinoma biology. That knowledge drove the development and testing of the targeted therapies and their success in many ways can be directly attributed to the work that shed light on that biology. This is an obvious and gratifying example of science moving from bench to bedside and proof that an understanding of the biology of cancer can lead to tangible improvements in patient's lives. As more such therapies are developed across a range of other diseases, it is clear that a fundamental understanding of molecular biology and its basic principles will be increasingly important in order to understand how to manage our patients.

References

1. Knudson AG Jr. Mutation and cancer: statistical study of retinoblastoma. *Proc Natl Acad Sci USA*. 1971;68:820
2. Knudson AG. Antioncogenes and human cancer. *Proc Natl Acad Sci USA*. 1993;90:10914
3. Gessler M, Poustka A, Cavenee W, et al. Homozygous deletion in Wilms tumours of a zinc-finger gene identified by chromosome jumping. *Nature*. 1990;343:774
4. Cavenee WK, Hansen MF, Nordenskjold M, et al. Genetic origin of mutations predisposing to retinoblastoma. *Science*. 1985;228:501
5. Fung YK, Murphree AL, T'Ang A, et al. Structural evidence for the authenticity of the human retinoblastoma gene. *Science*. 1987;236:1657
6. Xu GF, O'Connell P, Viskochil D, et al. The neurofibromatosis type 1 gene encodes a protein related to GAP. *Cell*. 1990;62:599
7. Kinzler KW, Vogelstein B. Cancer. A gene for neurofibromatosis 2. *Nature*. 1993;363:495
8. Cohen AJ, Li FP, Berg S, et al. Hereditary renal-cell carcinoma associated with a chromosomal translocation. *N Engl J Med*. 1979;301:592
9. Kovacs G, Brusa P, De Riese W. Tissue-specific expression of a constitutional 3;6 translocation: development of multiple bilateral renal-cell carcinomas. *Int J Cancer*. 1989;43:422
10. Pathak S, Strong LC, Ferrell RE, et al. Familial renal cell carcinoma with a 3;11 chromosome translocation limited to tumor cells. *Science*. 1982;217:939
11. Yoshida MA, Ohyashiki K, Ochi H, et al. Cytogenetic studies of tumor tissue from patients with nonfamilial renal cell carcinoma. *Cancer Res*. 1986;46:2139
12. de Jong B, Oosterhuis JW, Idenburg VJ, et al. Cytogenetics of 12 cases of renal adenocarcinoma. *Cancer Genet Cytogenet*. 1988;30:53
13. Presti JC Jr, Rao PH, Chen Q, et al. Histopathological, cytogenetic, and molecular characterization of renal cortical tumors. *Cancer Res*. 1991;51:1544
14. Kovacs G, Frisch S. Clonal chromosome abnormalities in tumor cells from patients with sporadic renal cell carcinomas. *Cancer Res*. 1989;49:651

15. Szucs S, Muller-Brechlin R, DeRiese W, et al. Deletion 3p: the only chromosome loss in a primary renal cell carcinoma. *Cancer Genet Cytogenet*. 1987;26:369

16. Zbar B, Brauch H, Talmadge C, et al. Loss of alleles of loci on the short arm of chromosome 3 in renal cell carcinoma. *Nature*. 1987;327:721

17. Anglard P, Tory K, Brauch H, et al. Molecular analysis of genetic changes in the origin and development of renal cell carcinoma. *Cancer Res*. 1991;51:1071

18. Seizinger BR, Rouleau GA, Ozelius LJ, et al. Von Hippel-Lindau disease maps to the region of chromosome 3 associated with renal cell carcinoma. *Nature*. 1988; 332:268

19. Lerman MI, Latif F, Glenn GM, et al. Isolation and regional localization of a large collection (2,000) of single-copy DNA fragments on human chromosome 3 for mapping and cloning tumor suppressor genes. *Hum Genet*. 1991;86:567

20. Hosoe S, Brauch H, Latif F, et al. Localization of the von Hippel-Lindau disease gene to a small region of chromosome 3. *Genomics*. 1990;8:634

21. Latif F, Tory K, Gnarra J, et al. Identification of the von Hippel-Lindau disease tumor suppressor gene. *Science*. 1993;260:1317

22. Gnarra JR, Tory K, Weng Y, et al. Mutations of the VHL tumour suppressor gene in renal carcinoma. *Nat Genet*. 1994;7:85

23. Whaley JM, Naglich J, Gelbert L, et al. Germ-line mutations in the von Hippel-Lindau tumor-suppressor gene are similar to somatic von Hippel-Lindau aberrations in sporadic renal cell carcinoma. *Am J Hum Genet*. 1994; 55:1092

24. Shuin T, Kondo K, Torigoe S, et al. Frequent somatic mutations and loss of heterozygosity of the von Hippel-Lindau tumor suppressor gene in primary human renal cell carcinomas. *Cancer Res*. 1994;54:2852

25. Foster K, Prowse A, van den Berg A, et al. Somatic mutations of the von Hippel-Lindau disease tumour suppressor gene in non-familial clear cell renal carcinoma. *Hum Mol Genet*. 1994;3:2169

26. Crossey PA, Richards FM, Foster K, et al. Identification of intragenic mutations in the von Hippel-Lindau disease tumour suppressor gene and correlation with disease phenotype. *Hum Mol Genet*. 1994;3:1303

27. Herman JG, Latif F, Weng Y, et al. Silencing of the VHL tumor-suppressor gene by DNA methylation in renal carcinoma. *Proc Natl Acad Sci USA*. 1994;91:9700

28. Gnarra JR, Duan DR, Weng Y, et al. Molecular cloning of the von Hippel-Lindau tumor suppressor gene and its role in renal carcinoma. *Biochim Biophys Acta*. 1996; 1242:201

29. Linehan WM, Lerman MI, Zbar B. Identification of the von Hippel-Lindau (VHL) gene. Its role in renal cancer. *JAMA*. 1995;273:564

30. Jones PA, Baylin SB. The epigenomics of cancer. *Cell*. 2007;128:683

31. Ballestar E, Esteller M. Epigenetic gene regulation in cancer. *Adv Genet*. 2008;61:247

32. Dressler GR. Epigenetics, development, and the kidney. *J Am Soc Nephrol*. 2008;19:2060

33. Gnarra JR, Zhou S, Merrill MJ, et al. Post-transcriptional regulation of vascular endothelial growth factor mRNA by the product of the VHL tumor suppressor gene. *Proc Natl Acad Sci USA*. 1996;93:10589

34. Iliopoulos O, Levy AP, Jiang C, et al. Negative regulation of hypoxia-inducible genes by the von Hippel-Lindau protein. *Proc Natl Acad Sci USA*. 1996;93:10595

35. Siemeister G, Weindel K, Mohrs K, et al. Reversion of deregulated expression of vascular endothelial growth factor in human renal carcinoma cells by von Hippel-Lindau tumor suppressor protein. *Cancer Res*. 1996; 56:2299

36. Haase VH. Hypoxia-inducible factors in the kidney. *Am J Physiol Ren Physiol*. 2006;291:F271

37. Linehan WM, Walther MM, Zbar B. The genetic basis of cancer of the kidney. *J Urol*. 2003;170:2163

38. Iliopoulos O. Molecular biology of renal cell cancer and the identification of therapeutic targets. *J Clin Oncol*. 2006;24:5593

39. Stadler W. Chromosomes, hypoxia, angiogenesis, and trial design: a brief history of renal cancer drug development. *Clin Cancer Res*. 2007;13:1630

40. Wang GL, Semenza GL. General involvement of hypoxia-inducible factor 1 in transcriptional response to hypoxia. *Proc Natl Acad Sci USA*. 1993;90:4304

41. Maxwell PH, Wiesener MS, Chang GW, et al. The tumour suppressor protein VHL targets hypoxia-inducible factors for oxygen-dependent proteolysis. *Nature*. 1999;399:271

42. Salceda S, Caro J. Hypoxia-inducible factor 1alpha (HIF-1alpha) protein is rapidly degraded by the ubiquitin-proteasome system under normoxic conditions. Its stabilization by hypoxia depends on redox-induced changes. *J Biol Chem*. 1997;272:22642

43. Cockman ME, Masson N, Mole DR, et al. Hypoxia inducible factor-alpha binding and ubiquitylation by the von Hippel-Lindau tumor suppressor protein. *J Biol Chem*. 2000;275:25733

44. Tanimoto K, Makino Y, Pereira T, et al. Mechanism of regulation of the hypoxia-inducible factor-1 alpha by the von Hippel-Lindau tumor suppressor protein. *EMBO J*. 2000;19:4298

45. Ohh M, Park CW, Ivan M, et al. Ubiquitination of hypoxia-inducible factor requires direct binding to the beta-domain of the von Hippel-Lindau protein. *Nat Cell Biol*. 2000;2:423

46. Kamura T, Sato S, Iwai K, et al. Activation of HIF1alpha ubiquitination by a reconstituted von Hippel-Lindau (VHL) tumor suppressor complex. *Proc Natl Acad Sci USA*. 2000;97:10430

47. Folkman J, Shing Y. Angiogenesis. *J Biol Chem*. 1992; 267:10931

48. Bard RH, Mydlo JH, Freed SZ. Detection of tumor angiogenesis factor in adenocarcinoma of kidney. *Urology*. 1986;27:447

49. Rini BI, Small EJ. Biology and clinical development of vascular endothelial growth factor-targeted therapy in renal cell carcinoma. *J Clin Oncol*. 2005;23:1028

50. Roy H, Bhardwaj S, Yla-Herttuala S. Biology of vascular endothelial growth factors. *FEBS Lett*. 2006;580:2879

51. Hicklin DJ, Ellis LM. Role of the vascular endothelial growth factor pathway in tumor growth and angiogenesis. *J Clin Oncol*. 2005;23:1011

52. Carmeliet P. VEGF as a key mediator of angiogenesis in cancer. *Oncology*. 2005;69(Suppl 3):4

53. Donovan EA, Kummar S. Targeting VEGF in cancer therapy. *Curr Probl Cancer.* 2006;30:7

54. Lane BR, Rini BI, Novick AC, et al. Targeted molecular therapy for renal cell carcinoma. *Urology.* 2007;69:3

55. Cho D, Signoretti S, Regan M, et al. The role of mammalian target of rapamycin inhibitors in the treatment of advanced renal cancer. *Clin Cancer Res.* 2007;13:758s

56. Bukowski RM. Cytokine therapy for metastatic renal cell carcinoma. *Semin Urol Oncol.* 2001;19:148

57. Heinzer H, Huland E, Huland H. Systemic chemotherapy and chemoimmunotherapy for metastatic renal cell cancer. *World J Urol.* 2001;19:111

58. Pantuck AJ, Zisman A, Belldegrun A. Biology of renal cell carcinoma: changing concepts in classification and staging. *Semin Urol Oncol.* 2001;19:72

59. Yang JC, Haworth L, Sherry RM, et al. A randomized trial of bevacizumab, an anti-vascular endothelial growth factor antibody, for metastatic renal cancer. *N Engl J Med.* 2003;349:427

60. Escudier B, Pluzanska A, Koralewski P, et al. Bevacizumab plus interferon alfa-2a for treatment of metastatic renal cell carcinoma: a randomised, double-blind phase III trial. *Lancet.* 2007;370:2103

61. Kuenen BC, Giaccone G, Ruijter R, et al. Dose-finding study of the multitargeted tyrosine kinase inhibitor SU6668 in patients with advanced malignancies. *Clin Cancer Res.* 2005;11:6240

62. Kuenen BC, Tabernero J, Baselga J, et al. Efficacy and toxicity of the angiogenesis inhibitor SU5416 as a single agent in patients with advanced renal cell carcinoma, melanoma, and soft tissue sarcoma. *Clin Cancer Res.* 2003;9:1648

63. Shaheen PE, Bukowski RM. Targeted therapy for renal cell carcinoma: a new therapeutic paradigm. *Cancer Invest.* 2006;24:640

64. Amato RJ. Renal cell carcinoma: review of novel single-agent therapeutics and combination regimens. *Ann Oncol.* 2005;16:7

65. Fabian MA, Biggs WH 3rd, Treiber DK, et al. A small molecule-kinase interaction map for clinical kinase inhibitors. *Nat Biotechnol.* 2005;23:329

66. Mendel DB, Laird AD, Xin X, et al. In vivo antitumor activity of SU11248, a novel tyrosine kinase inhibitor targeting vascular endothelial growth factor and platelet-derived growth factor receptors: determination of a pharmacokinetic/pharmacodynamic relationship. *Clin Cancer Res.* 2003;9:327

67. Faivre S, Delbaldo C, Vera K, et al. Safety, pharmacokinetic, and antitumor activity of SU11248, a novel oral multitarget tyrosine kinase inhibitor, in patients with cancer. *J Clin Oncol.* 2006;24:25

68. Motzer RJ, Hutson TE, Tomczak P, et al. Sunitinib versus interferon alfa in metastatic renal-cell carcinoma. *N Engl J Med.* 2007;356:115

69. Motzer RJ, Michaelson MD, Redman BG, et al. Activity of SU11248, a multitargeted inhibitor of vascular endothelial growth factor receptor and platelet-derived growth factor receptor, in patients with metastatic renal cell carcinoma. *J Clin Oncol.* 2006;24:16

70. Motzer RJ, Rini BI, Bukowski RM, et al. Sunitinib in patients with metastatic renal cell carcinoma. *JAMA.* 2006;295:2516

71. Wilhelm S, Carter C, Lynch M, et al. Discovery and development of sorafenib: a multikinase inhibitor for treating cancer. *Nat Rev Drug Discov.* 2006;5:835

72. Rosner GL, Stadler W, Ratain MJ. Randomized discontinuation design: application to cytostatic antineoplastic agents. *J Clin Oncol.* 2002;20:4478

73. Escudier B, Eisen T, Stadler WM, et al. Sorafenib in advanced clear-cell renal-cell carcinoma. *N Engl J Med.* 2007;356:125

74. Boulay A, Zumstein-Mecker S, Stephan C, et al. Antitumor efficacy of intermittent treatment schedules with the rapamycin derivative RAD001 correlates with prolonged inactivation of ribosomal protein S6 kinase 1 in peripheral blood mononuclear cells. *Cancer Res.* 2004; 64:252

75. Reddy GK, Mughal TI, Rini BI. Current data with mammalian target of rapamycin inhibitors in advanced-stage renal cell carcinoma. *Clin Genitourin Cancer.* 2006; 5:110

76. Atkins MB, Hidalgo M, Stadler WM, et al. Randomized phase II study of multiple dose levels of CCI-779, a novel mammalian target of rapamycin kinase inhibitor, in patients with advanced refractory renal cell carcinoma. *J Clin Oncol.* 2004;22:909

77. Smith JW, Ko Y-J, Dutcher J, et al. Update of a phase I study of intravenous CCI-779 given in combination with interferon-a to patients with advanced renal cell carcinoma. *Proc Am Soc Clin Onc.* 2004;23: 4513A

78. Hudes G, Carducci M, Tomczak P, et al. Temsirolimus, interferon alfa, or both for advanced renal-cell carcinoma. *N Engl J Med.* 2007;356:2271

79. Motzer RJ, Escudier B, Oudard S, et al. Efficacy of everolimus in advanced renal cell carcinoma: a double-blind, randomised, placebo-controlled phase III trial. *Lancet.* 2008;372:449

13

Chemotherapeutic Agents for Urologic Oncology

Hendrik Van Poppel and Filip Ameye

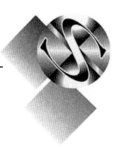

Introduction

The main goal of chemotherapy is to cure cancer by killing the neoplastic cells. To keep the cancer from metastasizing, chemotherapy may be used in combination with other cancer treatments, such as surgery and radiotherapy. In widespread, fast-growing cancers, chemotherapy reduces cellular proliferation, eases symptoms, and improves the quality of life. When it is employed after the primary tumor has been treated by some other modality, it is called adjuvant chemotherapy. Sometimes neoadjuvant chemotherapy is employed, which refers to the initial use of chemotherapy in patients with localized cancer in order to reduce tumor burden, there by rendering local therapy (surgery or radiotherapy) more effective. A common procedure in human cancer therapy is combination chemotherapy that refers to the parallel or sequential use of several different antineoplastic agents in order to enhance their effectiveness. Combining chemotherapy with targeted therapies is an investigational approach under development. This chapter presents a comprehensive overview of the use of chemotherapeutics and targeted agents in the treatment of urologic malignancies.

Bladder Cancer

Bladder cancer is the most common malignancy of the urinary tract and as the incidence of the disease rises, more effective treatment options are urgently needed.

Non-muscle Invasive (TaT1) Bladder Cancer

At initial diagnosis, most bladder tumors are stage Ta or T1 papillary tumors. Non-muscle invasive papillary bladder cancer is managed with transurethral resection (TUR) of the tumor and for most patients with one immediate postoperative intravesical instillation of chemotherapy within 6 h after tumor resection. The choice of drug (mitomycin C, epirubicin or doxorubicin) is optional, and no single drug can be considered superior with regards to efficacy.[1,2] Further treatment depends on the patient's risk of recurrence and progression to muscle-invasive disease. In order to predict this risk, a scoring system and risk tables have been developed based on the European Organisation for Research and Treatment of Cancer (EORTC) database, which provided individual data of 2,596 patients diagnosed with TaT1 tumors and randomized in seven studies.[2,3] Table 13.1 provides a scoring system based on the most significant clinical and pathological characteristics. The European Association of Urology (EAU) working group suggests to use a three-tier system reflecting the EORTC risk tables, which defines low-, intermediate-, and high-risk groups for recurrence and progression (Table 13.2). In patients at low risk of tumor recurrence and

C.R. Chapple and W.D. Steers (eds.), *Practical Urology: Essential Principles and Practice*,
DOI: 10.1007/978-1-84882-034-0_13, © Springer-Verlag London Limited 2011

Table 13.1. Weighting used to calculate the recurrence and progression scores in patients with non-muscle invasive (TaT1) bladder cancer (Reprinted with permission from Babjuk et al.[2])

Factor	Recurrence	Progression
Number of tumors		
Single	0	0
2–7	3	3
≥8	6	3
Tumor diameter		
<3 cm	0	0
≥3 cm	3	3
Prior recurrence rate		
Primary	0	0
≤1 recurrence/year	2	2
<1 recurrence/year	4	2
Category		
Ta	0	0
T1	1	4
Concomitant CIS		
No	0	0
Yes	1	6
Grade (1973 WHO)		
G1	0	0
G2	1	0
G3	2	5
Total score	0–17	0–23

CIS carcinoma in situ.

progression, no further treatment is recommended before recurrence.[1,2] Immediate instillation of chemotherapy is contraindicated in patients with known or suspected bladder perforation following TUR as severe complications related to extravasation of the drug have been reported. In patients at an intermediate or high risk of recurrence and an intermediate risk of progression, one immediate instillation of chemotherapy should be followed by additional adjuvant intravesical chemotherapy or a minimum of 1 year Bacillus Calmette-Guérin (BCG) immunotherapy. A meta-analysis comparing intravesical chemotherapy to TUR alone, showed

that chemotherapy prevents recurrence but not progression.[4] The efficacy of intravesical chemotherapy in reducing the risk of recurrence was confirmed by two other meta-analyses.[5,6] Intravesical chemotherapy decreased tumor recurrence from 30% to 80% depending on the outcome of interest (i.e., recurrence at 1, 2, or 3 years post-TUR). In a more recent meta-analysis of seven randomized studies with median follow-up of 3.4 years intravesical chemotherapy after TUR reduced, the percentage of patients with recurrence by 12% (from 48.4% to 36.7%) and the odds of recurrence by 39%.[1] In patients at high risk of progression, one immediate instillation of chemotherapy should be followed by intravesical BCG for at least 1 year. Radical cystectomy is advocated in T1 patients failing intravesical BCG therapy.[2] No consensus exists regarding the optimal schedule and duration of intravesical chemotherapy instillations.[2,7] Furthermore, it is recommended to use the chemotherapeutic drug at its optimal pH and to maintain the concentration of the drug during instillation by asking the patient not to drink the morning before instillation.[2]

Muscle Invasive Bladder Cancer

For patients with stage T2 or higher muscle invasive cancers, treatment is usually radical cystectomy. However, this standard treatment only provides 5-year survival in about 50% of patients.[8,9] Several randomized phase III studies have demonstrated a 5–7% improvement in survival at 5 years after neoadjuvant cisplatin-containing combination chemotherapy in muscle invasive bladder cancer, irrespective of the type of definite treatment (about 82% chemo combination regimens).[10-12] This strategy is not recommended in patients with performance status≥2 and impaired renal function. It is important to note that chemotherapy alone is not recommended as primary therapy for localized bladder cancer.[9] Chemotherapy can be used as a component of a bladder-preserving strategy that combines TUR and chemotherapy with or without radiation.[9,13] This multimodality bladder-preserving strategy is a reasonable option for carefully selected patients seeking an alternative to radical cystectomy with a comparable long-term survival rate of 50–60% at 5 years' follow-up. Although bladder-preserving

Table 13.2. Probability of recurrence and progression of non-muscle invasive (TaT1) bladder cancer according to total score (Reprinted with permission from Babjuk et al.[2])

Recurrence score	Probability of recurrence at 1 year		Probability of recurrence at 5 years		Recurrence risk group
	%	(95% CI)	%	(95% CI)	
0	15	(10–19)	31	(24–37)	Low risk
1–4	24	(21–26)	46	(42–49)	Intermediate risk
5–9	38	(35–41)	62	(58–65)	
10–17	61	(55–67)	78	(73–84)	High risk
Progression score	Probability of progression at 1 year		Probability of progression at 5 years		Progression risk group
	%	(95% CI)	%	(95% CI)	
0	0.2	(0–0.7)	0.8	(0–1.7)	Low risk
2–6	1	(0.4–1.6)	6	(5–8)	Intermediate risk
7–13	5	(4–7)	17	(14–20)	High risk
14–23	17	(10–24)	45	(35–55)	

Note: Electronic calculators for Tables 13.1 and 13.2 are available at http://www.eortc.be/tools/bladdercalculator.

strategies may be appealing in a small proportion of patients, these protocols should be considered investigational because cystectomy and bladder-sparing strategy have never been directly compared in a randomized trial.[9,13] Even if a patient has shown a complete response, close surveillance for the potential development of recurrences remains necessary. To date, the use of adjuvant chemotherapy after radical cystectomy for patients with pT3/4 and/or lymph node positive disease (N+) without clinically detectable metastases is still debated. So far, it should only be used in the context of clinical trials.[9]

Metastatic Bladder Cancer

Responses with single-agent chemotherapy in patients with metastatic bladder cancer are usually of short duration and complete responses are rare. The median survival in these patients is only about 6–9 months.[9] Cisplatin-containing combination chemotherapy with gemcitabine-cisplatin (GC), methotrexate-vinblastine-adriamycin-cisplatin (M-VAC), preferably with granulocyte-colony stimulating factor (G-CSF), or high-dose intensity M-VAC (HD-MVAC) with G-CSF is the standard first-line chemotherapy for "fit" patients with metastatic bladder cancer. Cisplatin-containing combination chemotherapy (M-VAC and GC) is able to achieve a median survival of up to 14 months,[9,14-16] while before the development of effective chemotherapy patients with metastatic urothelial cancer rarely exceeded the median survival of 3–6 months.[9,17] HD-MVAC with GCSF is less toxic and more efficacious than classic M-VAC in terms of dose density, complete response, and 2-year survival rate. However, there is no significant difference in median survival between the two regimens (15.1 months for HD-MVAC and 14.9 months for M-VAC).[9,18] Several newer regimens have failed to demonstrate superiority in terms of overall survival (OS) when compared to classic M-VAC. The addition of a third agent to doublet combinations is still being studied. Performance status and the presence or absence of visceral metastases are independent prognostic factors for survival and are at least as important as the type of chemotherapy administered. Besides these prognostic factors, treatment decisions should be based on a patient's renal function to decide whether the patient is "fit" enough to receive a cisplatin-containing combination chemotherapy regimen (creatinine clearance ≥ 60 mL/min, PS, comorbidity). To date, there is no generally accepted definition for "fit" or "unfit" patients. Carboplatin-containing combination chemotherapy or single agents are suggested as first-line treatment in patients "unfit" for cisplatin. It should be noted that carboplatin-combination chemotherapy is less effective than cisplatin-based chemotherapy in terms of complete response and survival.[9] At present, there is no standard of care for the treatment of patients with bladder cancer after failure of cisplatin-containing combination chemotherapy in the first-line setting. If the patient has a good performance status, single agents or paclitaxel/gemcitabine can be considered as second-line treatment. Attempts to improve second-line treatment have directed to the assessment of single agents such as vinflunine and pemetrexed[9] and multidrug combinations with cytotoxic and targeted agents, including trastuzumab and bevacizumab.[19] Post-chemotherapy surgical resection after a complete or partial response may contribute to long-term disease control in selected patients.[9]

Conclusion

Further investigations and randomized studies are required to clarify the exact role of chemotherapy in patients with bladder cancer. Progress in the understanding of the molecular biology of bladder cancer and identification of newer drug combinations and targeted agents directed at specific molecular pathways will provide less toxic and perhaps more active regimens. In the meantime, bladder removal continues to be a necessary life-saving operation that must be considered in all high-risk cases that fail to immediately respond to other treatment options.

Prostate Cancer

Traditionally, chemotherapy has not been offered as routine treatment for patients with hormone refractory prostate cancer (HRPC) because of treatment-related toxicity and poor responses. Major adverse events associated with chemotherapeutics are myelosuppression, gastrointestinal toxicity, cardiac toxicity, neuropathy, and alopecia. Therefore, urologists have been using second-line hormonal manipulations such as ketoconazole and aminoglutethimide. Recently abiraterone has been tested with success after first-line hormonal manipulation. Over the past 2 decades, chemotherapy for advanced prostate cancer has evolved from a therapy having a limited role in HRPC to a therapy that may provide a short survival benefit, but more importantly that can provide effective palliation of the symptoms.

Estramustine, Mitoxantrone, and Docetaxel

To date, three drugs (estramustine, mitoxantrone, and docetaxel) have gained approval by the US Food and Drug Administration (FDA) for first-line chemotherapy in HRPC. Estramustine and mitoxantrone could not cause a survival advantage compared to control treated patients with HRPC, although they did reduce pain. More recently, data from two large randomized phase III trials, TAX 327 and SWOG 9916, have demonstrated an acceptable tolerability and a significant improvement in OS for patients with HRPC treated with three-weekly docetaxel, although the increase was small (< 2.5 months).[20-22] In the SWOG 9916 and TAX 327 study, the median survival was 17.5 and 18.9 months in the three-weekly docetaxel group, while 15.6 and 16.5 months in the mitoxantrone group. Weekly docetaxel in the TAX 327 study did not result in a significant survival benefit. Patients treated with three-weekly docetaxel plus prednisone in the TAX 327 study experienced improved pain relief and quality of life compared to mitoxantrone plus prednisone.[21,22] The combination of three-weekly docetaxel with estramustine in the SWOG 9916 study was associated with increased toxicity and did not appear to have improved efficacy compared with the three-weekly docetaxel plus prednisone regimen in the TAX 327 study. These findings supported the approval of docetaxel-based chemotherapy for the treatment of HRPC by the FDA in May 2005. Three-weekly docetaxel (75 mg/m^2) plus low-dose prednisone regimen has widely become the current standard of care as first-line chemotherapy for treating HRPC.[23] An updated survival analysis of TAX 327 showed that the significant improvement in survival associated with three-weekly docetaxel compared with mitoxantrone has persisted after 3 years follow-up with a slightly increased median survival difference of 3 months.[24] Furthermore, in patients with symptomatic osseous metastases due to HRPC, either docetaxel or mitoxantrone with prednisone or hydrocortisone are possible therapeutic options.[20]

Nevertheless, answers to the questions which need to be treated, when to initiate docetaxel-based chemotherapy and on the duration of therapy remains unclear. In the updated survival analysis of TAX 327, patients with PSA level < 114 ng/mL and PSA doubling time (PSADT) ≥ 55 days have a median OS of 24.7 months, while those with PSA level ≥ 114 ng /mL and a PSADT < 55 days have a median OS of only 13.8 months. The investigators suggest that in patients with fast disease progression chemotherapy may be started earlier when metastases are not yet symptomatic.[25] However, the optimal timing of docetaxel-based chemotherapy is still debated. Regarding the duration of treatment, studies investigating interruptions in treatment schedules for patients who experience an initial response to chemotherapy are needed to define the future role of intermittent chemotherapy for the treatment of prostate cancer. This approach with chemotherapy holidays may avoid or delay the development of progressive toxicity.[26]

Other Chemotherapeutic Drugs or Combinations for Treating HRPC

Second-line hormonal manipulation includes antiandrogen withdrawal, the use of glucosteroids, estrogens, ketaconazole, liarozole, and aminoglutethimide. Abiraterone that targets adrenal androgens is currently being evaluated as a potential drug for the treatment of HRPC. Once these drugs have been exhausted, the limited treatment options that are left include radionuclides and cytotoxic chemotherapy. Mitoxantrone plus prednisone has become the second-line regimen with palliative activity for docetaxel-resistant HRPC. Another option is the epitholone B analog ixabepilone currently under evaluation in ongoing clinical trials. Next to taxanes, other drugs are investigated for treating HRPC. Although earlier studies in HRPC suggested a lack of activity, recent studies of platinum drugs such as carboplatin and

cisplatin, using PSA and palliation endpoints, have demonstrated greater evidence of benefit.[27] Treatments under investigation include the first orally available platinum drug satraplatin, combinations of docetaxel with another agent and the tyrosine kinase receptor inhibitors sunitinib and sorafenib. Cyclophosphamide seems to be an interesting agent for the treatment of docetaxel-resistant HRPC.[28] Furthermore, a phase I trial reported that the combination of thalidomide and oral cyclophosphamide is well tolerated and appears to be associated with biochemical response in patients with HRPC.[29]

Conclusion

Chemotherapy should be considered as a treatment option for patients with HRPC. Hopefully one or more combinations with docetaxel or new agents with improved survival benefit and reasonable tolerability will be developed for treating HRPC in the near future. The optimal timing of docetaxel-based chemotherapy is still unknown. Therefore, the benefits of early chemotherapy should be carefully balanced against its potential toxicity risk. In addition, further investigation through randomized clinical trials is warranted to define the precise role of neoadjuvant and adjuvant chemotherapy in high-risk populations with prostate cancer.

Renal Cell Carcinoma

Renal cell carcinoma (RCC) accounts for 2–3% of all adult cancers. About 20–30% of patients develop metastatic disease.[30] The prognosis for patients with advanced metastatic RCC is poor with a 5-year survival rate of less than 10%.[31] Since RCCs arise from the cells of proximal tubules, they have high levels of expression of the multiple drug resistance protein P-glycoprotein. This explains the resistance of RCC to chemotherapeutic agents.[30]

Chemotherapy

Chemotherapy alone is generally considered ineffective in patients with metastatic RCC (mRCC). It seems to be effective only if 5-fluorouracil (5-FU) is combined with immunotherapeutic agents.[30]

Immunotherapy

Until recently, treatment of mRCC has been based on nephrectomy and limited use of toxic and often ineffective immunotherapy with interferon-alpha (IFN-α) and interleukin-2 (IL-2). Both are beneficial only for mRCC patients with a good performance status and clear cell subtype histology. IFN-α (alpha) can be used as comparative control arm for studies investigating the efficacy of new drugs for mRCC patients. High-dose IL-2 may induce durable complete responses in a minority of patients ranging from 7% to 27%; however, it has more side effects than IFN-α (alpha). Combination of cytokines, with or without additional chemotherapy, does not improve OS compared with monotherapy.[30]

Angiogenesis Inhibitor Drugs

Major advances in the understanding of the molecular biology of RCC have led to the development of several new therapies that target ligands at the molecular level, so-called "targeted therapies". Figure 13.1 presents the major targets for these targeted therapies. Small molecule tyrosine kinase inhibitors (sunitinib and sorafenib), mammalian target of rapamycin inhibitors (temsirolimus), and monoclonal antibodies (bevacizumab) appear to be the most promising agents for treatment of mRCC. Table 13.3 presents a summary of phase III randomized controlled trials of targeted therapies in renal cell carcinoma. Sunitinib, sorafenib, temsirolimus, and the combination bevacizumab with interferon-alpha are approved for treatment of mRCC.[33-37] Sunitinib is advised as first-line therapy in low-and intermediate-risk mRCC patients. Bevacizumab and interferon-alpha can be considered as an additional option for first-line therapy in these patients. Temsirolimus should be considered as first-line treatment in poor-risk mRCC patients. Sorafenib has proven efficacy as second-line therapy for mRCC after failure of cytokine therapy. These new agents improve quality of life and seem able to stabilize mRCC for a prolonged period of time.[30] The mTOR inhibitor everolimus also shows promising results in patients with mRCC.[38] Studies are ongoing to compare combination therapies with single agents and to determine the efficacy of single agents as adjuvant therapy after nephrectomy.

Conclusion

Angiogenesis inhibitor drugs have an important role in the management of mRCC. However, for a selected group of patients, high-dose IL-2 remains an option. More research and clinical studies are required to identify the optimal combination therapy for patients with mRCC and to define strategies for non-clear cell cancer. Questions regarding optimal sequence and timing of treatment options still need to be addressed.

Testicular Cancer

Testicular cancer is rare and rapidly progressive, but cure rates are almost 100%, regardless of treatment modality. Treatment of patients with testicular cancer is described in the European Germ Cell Cancer Consensus Group (EGCCG) report (part I and II).[39,40]

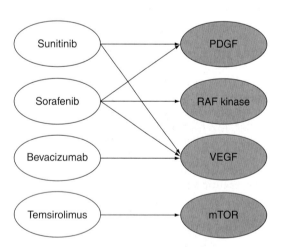

Figure 13.1. Targeted drugs with major inhibited targets for treatment of renal cell carcinoma. mTOR: mammalian target of rapamycin kinase, PDGF: platelet-derived growth factor, VEGF: vascular endothelial growth factor.

Table 13.3. Randomized controlled trials of targeted therapies in renal cell carcinoma (From Vakkalanka et al.[32])

Study	Randomization		No. of patients	Objective response rate (%)	Progression-free survival (months)
Escudier et al.[33]	Bevacizumab (10 mg/kg) i.v. every 2 weeks and IFN-α2a 9 MU s.c. three times per week	vs. placebo and IFN-α2a9 MU s.c. three times per week	649	31 vs. 13	10.2 vs. 5.4 ($p = 0.0001$)
Rini et al.[34]	Bevacizumab (10 mg/kg) i.v. every 2 weeks and IFN-α 9 MU s.c. three times per week	vs. IFN-α9 MU s.c. three times per week	732	25.5 vs. 13.1 ($p < 0.0001$)	8.5 vs. 5.2 ($p < 0.0001$)
Motzer et al.[35]	Sunitinib (50 mg) p.o. daily	vs. IFN-α9 MU s.c. three times per week	750	31 vs. 6 ($p < 0.001$)	11 vs. 5 ($p < 0.001$)
Escudier et al.[36]	Sorafenib (400 mg) p.o. twice daily	vs. placebo	903	10 vs. 2	5.5 vs. 2.8 ($p < 0.01$)
Hudes et al.[37]	Temsirolimus (25 mg) i.v. weekly	vs. IFN-α 3–18 MU s.c. three times per week vs. temsirolimus (15 mg) i.v. weekly and IFN-α 6 MU s.c. three times per week	626	4.8 vs. 8.6 vs. 8.1	3.1 vs. 5.5 vs. 4.7

IFN interferon, *i.v.* intravenous, *MU* million units, *p.o.* orally, *s.c.* subcutaneous.

Stage I Seminoma

The initial treatment is radical inguinal orchidectomy. Acceptable therapeutic options following
orchidectomy comprise surveillance, radiotherapy, or chemotherapy. A phase-III trial between
the Medical Research Council (MRC) and EORTC
suggested that adjuvant chemotherapy with one
cycle of carboplatin area under curve (AUC) 7
can be recommended as alternative to adjuvant
radiotherapy. There were no significant differences in relapse rate, time to relapse and survival
after a median of 4-yr follow-up.[41,42] Two cycles of
carboplatin seem to further reduce the relapse
rate to the order of 1–3%, but longer follow-up is
essential to confirm the data.[42]

Stage I non-seminomatous Germ Cell Tumours (NSGCT)

Patients with stage I NSGCT can be offered
nerve-sparing retroperitoneal lymph node dissection (RPLND), surveillance, or adjuvant
cisplatin-based chemotherapy.[42] Risk-adapted
treatment is currently based on the risk factor
vascular invasion. Standard treatment for low-
risk stage 1A NSGCT tumors without evidence
of vascular invasion consists of close surveillance after orchidectomy. Adjuvant chemotherapy or nerve-sparing retroperitoneal
lymph node dissection (RPLND) remain
options for patients not suitable for surveillance. In the case of positive lymph nodes, chemotherapy with two cycles of bleomycin,
etoposide, and cisplatin (BEP) should be considered.[42] Patients with high-risk stage 1B
NSGCT tumors with evidence of vascular invasion (having about 50% risk of relapse) should
receive chemotherapy with two cycles of BEP.
In several studies involving more than 200
patients, a relapse rate of only 2.7% was
reported with very little long-term toxicity.
The efficacy and toxicity compared well with
the results of surveillance strategies or RPLND
in these patients. Two cycles of BEP do not
seem to adversely affect fertility or sexual
activity. In patients unwilling to undergo chemotherapy, surveillance or nerve-sparing
RPLND remain alternative options. In the case
of positive lymph nodes, further chemotherapy
should be considered.[42]

Metastatic Germ Cell Tumours

In 1997, the International Germ Cell Cancer
Collaborative Group (IGCCCG) defined prognostic factors for metastatic testicular cancer to
categorize patients into "good," "intermediate,"
and "poor" prognosis groups (Table 13.4).[42,43]

Low-Volume Metastatic Disease (Stage II A/B)

Until now, the standard treatment of stage II A/B
seminoma has been radiotherapy. An alternative
for those with stage IIB seminoma unwilling to
undergo radiotherapy is chemotherapy with
three cycles BEP or alternatively four cycles
etoposide – cisplatin (EP).[42] NSGCT stage II A/B
without elevated tumor markers can be treated
either by RPLND or close surveillance. If the
tumor markers are high after orchidectomy,
patients require chemotherapy (three or four
cycles of BEP), according to IGCCCG "good or
intermediate prognosis" NSGCT followed by
surgical resection of residual disease. Patients
unwilling to undergo primary chemotherapy in
the case of metastatic disease may choose for
primary RPLND with adjuvant chemotherapy
(two cycles BEP). In terms of outcome both treatment options are similar but adverse events and
toxicity are different which may influence the
patient in selecting the treatment of choice.[42]

Advanced Metastatic Disease

The treatment for advanced disease is three or
four cycles of BEP chemotherapy based on the
IGCCCG risk stratification (Table 13.4).[42,43] In
metastatic NSGCT (≥ stage IIC) with a "good
prognosis," the primary treatment of choice is
three cycles of BEP or alternatively four cycles of
EP. In those with an "intermediate prognosis",
four cycles of BEP are given. For patients with a
"poor prognosis", the standard treatment is four
cycles of BEP, or alternatively four cycles of PEI
(cisplatin, etoposide, ifosfamide), although this
regimen is more toxic.[42] High-dose chemotherapy as part of first-line therapy may be considered. However, there is no evidence from
randomized trials that it increases survival in
patients with poor prognosis. The exact role of
high-dose chemotherapy still needs to be identified. Surgical resection of all post-chemotherapy residual disease in NSGCT is indicated in

Table 13.4. Prognostic-based staging system for metastatic germ cell cancer (From International Germ Cell Cancer Collaborative Group (IGCCCG).[43] Reprinted with permission.©2008 American Society of Clinical Oncology. All rights reserved)

Prognosis group	Non-seminoma	Seminoma
Good	5-year PFS 89% 5-year survival 92% All of the following criteria: • Testis/retroperitoneal primary • No non-pulmonary visceral metastases • AFP < 1,000 ng/mL • hCG < 5,000 IU/L (1,000 ng/mL) • LDH < 1.5 × ULN	5-year PFS 82% 5-year survival 86% All of the following criteria: • Any primary site • No non-pulmonary visceral metastases • Normal AFP • Any hCG • Any LDH
Intermediate	5-year PFS 75% 5-year survival 80% All of the following criteria: • Testis/retroperitoneal primary • No non-pulmonary visceral metastases • AFP > 1,000 ng/mL and < 10,000 ng/mL or • hCG > 5,000 and < 50,000 IU/L or • LDH > 1.5 and < 10 × ULN	5-year PFS 67% 5-year survival 72% All of the following criteria: • Any primary site • Non-pulmonary visceral metastases • Normal AFP • Any hCG • Any LDH
Poor	5-year PFS 41% 5-year survival 48% All of the following criteria: • Mediastinal primary • Non-pulmonary visceral metastases • AFP > 10,000 ng/mL or • hCG > 50,000 IU/L (10,000 ng/mL) or • LDH > 10 × ULN	No patients classified as poor prognosis

PFS progression-free survival, *AFP* alpha-fetoprotein, *hCG* human chorionic gonadotrophin, *LDH* lactate dehydrogenase.

the case of visible residual masses and tumor marker normalization.[42]

Salvage Chemotherapy for Relapsed or Refractory Disease

For patients with good prognostic factors at first relapse, salvage chemotherapy (four cycles of standard dose) is recommended. The regimens of choice are four cycles of PEI/VIP (cisplatin, etoposide, ifosfamide), four cycles of TIP (paclitaxel, ifosfamide, cisplatin) or four cycles of VeIP (vinblastin, ifosfamide, cisplatin). In patients with poor prognostic features at relapse

and for all patients with second or subsequent relapse, high-dose chemotherapy plus autologous stem cell support is suggested.[42] These patients should be treated at specialized high-volume centers and within prospective randomized studies.

Conclusion

Chemotherapy has a place in selected patients with testicular cancer. Future research will focus on further reduction of chemotherapy's related morbidity without compromising the high rates of cure.

Penile Cancer

Penile carcinoma is an uncommon malignancy. Treatment options include surgery, radiotherapy and chemotherapy. Chemotherapy should preferably be given in the context of clinical trials. Adjuvant chemotherapy consisting of two cycles of cisplatin and 5-fluorouracil may be sufficient. The combination chemotherapy regimen with vincristine, methotrexate, and bleomycin given once a week for 12 weeks on an outpatient basis appears to be a promising option. Neoadjuvant chemotherapy may be administered to patients with fixed inguinal nodes and includes three or four cycles of cisplatin and 5-fluorouracil. Chemotherapy for advanced penile cancer has not been widely used. The most commonly used combinations are cisplatin and 5-fluorouracil and cisplatin, bleomycin, and methotrexate. The response rates of both treatment combinations are similar, but the tolerability is much better with no treatment-related deaths in patients treated with cisplatin and 5-fluorouracil.[44] An emphasis of future research should be to reduce toxicity. New combinations are currently tested in clinical trials, e.g., taxane-based chemotherapy.

Side Effects of Chemotherapy

Chemotherapy can be physically exhausting for the patient. Side effects mainly affect the fast-dividing cells of the body. Table 13.5 presents possible side effects of chemotherapy (dependent on the agent).

Conclusion

Chemotherapy is evolving in the management of urologic malignancies. Urologists and oncologists should work together to optimize patient care. Further investigations and randomized studies are required to clarify the exact role of chemotherapy in urologic oncology. More insight in the molecular biology of the urologic tumors will lead in the future to the development of more effective drugs or combinations with better tolerability profile.

Table 13.5. Possible side effects of chemotherapy

- Pain
- Nausea and vomiting
- Diarrhea or constipation
- Anemia
- Malnutrition
- Hair loss
- Memory loss
- Depression of the immune system, hence (potentially lethal) infections and sepsis
- Weight loss or gain
- Hemorrhage
- Secondary neoplasms
- Cardiotoxicity
- Hepatotoxicity
- Nephrotoxicity
- Ototoxicity

References

1. Sylvester RJ, Oosterlinck W, van der Meijden AP. A single immediate postoperative instillation of chemotherapy decreases the risk of recurrence in patients with stage Ta T1 bladder cancer: a meta-analysis of published results of randomized clinical trials. *J Urol.* 2004;171:2186-2190

2. Babjuk M, Oosterlinck W, Sylvester RJ, Kaasinen E, Böhle A, Palou J. Guidelines on TaT1 non-muscle invasive bladder cancer. European Association of Urology. 2008. http://www.uroweb.org/professional-resources/guidelines. Accessed September 17, 2008

3. Sylvester RJ, van der Meijden AP, Oosterlinck W, et al. Predicting recurrence and progression in individual patients with stage Ta T1 bladder cancer using EORTC risk tables: a combined analysis of 2596 patients from seven EORTC trials. *Eur Urol.* 2006;49:466-477

4. Pawinski A, Sylvester R, Kurth KH, et al. A combined analysis of European Organization for Research and Treatment of Cancer, and Medical Research Council randomized clinical trials for the prophylactic treatment of stage TaT1 bladder cancer. European Organization for Research and Treatment of Cancer Genitourinary Tract Cancer Cooperative Group and the Medical Research Council Working Party on Superficial Bladder Cancer. *J Urol.* 1996;156:1934-1941

5. Huncharek M, Geschwind JF, Witherspoon B, McGarry R, Adcock D. Intravesical chemotherapy prophylaxis in primary superficial bladder cancer: a meta-analysis of 3703 patients from 11 randomized trials. *J Clin Epidemiol.* 2000;53:676-680

6. Huncharek M, McGarry R, Kupelnick B. Impact of intravesical chemotherapy on recurrence rate of recurrent superficial transitional cell carcinoma of the bladder: results of a meta-analysis. *Anticancer Res.* 2001;21: 765-769

7. Sylvester RJ, Oosterlinck W, Witjes JA. The schedule and duration of intravesical chemotherapy in patients with non-muscle-invasive bladder cancer: a systematic review of the published results of randomized clinical trials. *Eur Urol.* 2008;53:709-719

8. Stein JP, Skinner DG. Radical cystectomy for invasive bladder cancer: long-term results of a standard procedure. *World J Urol.* 2006;24:296-304

9. Stenzl A, Cowan NC, De Santis M, et al. Guidelines on bladder cancer; muscle-invasive and metastatic. *Eur AssocUrol.* 2008. http://www.uroweb.org/professional-resources/guidelines. Accessed September 17, 2008

10. Advanced Bladder Cancer Meta-analysis Collaboration. Neoadjuvant chemotherapy in invasive bladder cancer: a systematic review and meta-analysis. *Lancet.* 2003;361: 1927-1934

11. Winquist E, Kirchner TS, Segal R, Chin J, Lukka H. Neoadjuvant chemotherapy for transitional cell carcinoma of the bladder: a systematic review and meta-analysis. *J Urol.* 2004;171:561-569

12. Advanced Bladder Cancer (ABC) Meta-analysis Collaboration. Neoadjuvant chemotherapy in invasive bladder cancer: update of a systematic review and meta-analysis of individual patient data advanced bladder cancer (ABC) meta-analysis collaboration. *Eur Urol.* 2005;48:202-206

13. Rodel C, Grabenbauer GG, Kuhn R, et al. Combined-modality treatment and selective organ preservation in invasive bladder cancer: long-term results. *J Clin Oncol.* 2002;20:3061-3071

14. Sternberg CN, Yagoda A, Scher HI, et al. M-VAC (methotrexate, vinblastine, doxorubicin and cisplatin) for advanced transitional cell carcinoma of the urothelium. *J Urol.* 1988;139:461-469

15. Sternberg CN, Yagoda A, Scher H, et al. Methotrexate, vinblastine, doxorubicin, and cisplatin for advanced transitional cell carcinoma of the urothelium. Efficacy and patterns of response and relapse. *Cancer.* 1989;64: 2448-2458

16. von der Maase H, Hansen SW, Roberts JT, et al. Gemcitabine and cisplatin versus methotrexate, vinblastine, doxorubicin, and cisplatin in advanced or metastatic bladder cancer: results of a large, randomized, multinational, multicenter, phase III study. *J Clin Oncol.* 2000;18:3068-3077

17. Sternberg CN, Vogelzang NJ. Gemcitabine, paclitaxel, pemetrexed and other newer agents in urothelial and kidney cancers. *Crit Rev Oncol Hematol.* 2003;46(suppl): S105-115

18. Sternberg CN, de Mulder P, Schornagel JH, et al. Seven year update of an EORTC phase III trial of high-dose intensity M-VAC chemotherapy and G-CSF versus classic M-VAC in advanced urothelial tract tumours. *Eur J Cancer.* 2006;42:50-54

19. Gallagher DJ, Milowsky MI, Bajorin DF. Advanced bladder cancer: status of first-line chemotherapy and the search for active agents in the second-line setting. *Cancer.* 2008;113:1284-1293

20. Heidenreich A, Aus G, Abbou CC, et al. Guidelines on prostate cancer. *Eur Urol.* 2007. http://www.uroweb.org/professional-resources/guidelines. Accessed September 17, 2008

21. Tannock IF, de Wit R, Berry WR, et al. Docetaxel plus prednisone or mitoxantrone plus prednisone for advanced prostate cancer. *N Engl J Med.* 2004;351:1502-1512

22. Petrylak DP, Tangen CM, Hussain MH, et al. Docetaxel and estramustine compared with mitoxantrone and prednisone for advanced refractory prostate cancer. *N Engl J Med.* 2004;351:1513-1520

23. Calabro F, Sternberg CN. Current indications for chemotherapy in prostate cancer patients. *Eur Urol.* 2007;51: 17-26

24. Berthold DR, Pond G, de Wit R, Eisenberger M, Tannock IF. Docetaxel plus prednisone or mitoxantrone plus prednisone for advanced prostate cancer: updated survival of the TAX 327 study. *J Clin Oncol Suppl.* 2007; 25:5005

25. de Wit R. Chemotherapy in hormone-refractory prostate cancer. *BJU Int.* 2008;101(suppl 2):11-15

26. Lin AM, Ryan CJ, Small EJ. Intermittent chemotherapy for metastatic hormone refractory prostate cancer. *Crit Rev Oncol Hematol.* 2007;61:243-254

27. Oh WK, Tay MH, Huang J. Is there a role for platinum chemotherapy in the treatment of patients with hormone-refractory prostate cancer? *Cancer.* 2007;109: 477-486

28. de Kernion JB, Lee AK, Vogelzang NJ. Treatment of organ-confined, locally advanced and metastatic prostate cancer. American Urological Association (*AUA*) Annual Meeting Highlights; May 19–24, 2007; 7–9. Anaheim, CA. http://www.auanet.org/cme/amhighlights/proscanchemo07.pdf. Accessed September 22, 2008

29. Di Lorenzo G, Autorino R, De Laurentiis M, et al. Thalidomide in combination with oral daily cyclophosphamide in patients with pretreated hormone refractory prostate cancer: a phase I clinical trial. *Cancer Biol Ther.* 2007;6:313-317

30. Ljungberg B, Hanbury DC, Kuczyk MA, et al. Guidelines on renal cell carcinoma. *Eur Assoc Urol.* 2007;51:1502–10 http://www.uroweb.org/professional-resources/guidelines. Accessed September 25, 2008

31. Schrader AJ, Varga Z, Hegele A, Pfoertner S, Olbert P, Hofmann R. Second-line strategies for metastatic renal cell carcinoma: classics and novel approaches. *J Cancer Res Clin Oncol.* 2006;132:137-149

32. Vakkalanka BK et al. Targeted therapy in renal cell carcinoma. *Curr Opin Urol.* 2008;8(5):481-487

33. Escudier B, Pluzanska A, Koralewski P, et al. Bevacizumab plus interferon alfa-2a for treatment of metastatic renal cell carcinoma: a randomised, double-blind phase III trial. *Lancet.* 2007;370:2103-2111

34. Rini BI, Halabi S, Rosenberg JE, et al. CALGB 90206: A phase III trial of bevacizumab plus interferon-alpha monotherapy in metastatic renal cell carcinoma [abstract 350]. In: Genitourinary cancers symposium; February 14–16, 2008; San Francisco: *AM Soc Clinl Oncol,* 2008

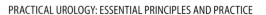

35. Motzer RJ, Hutson TE, Tomczak P, et al. Sunitinib versus interferon alfa in metastatic renal-cell carcinoma. *N Engl J Med*. 2007;356:115-124

36. Escudier B, Eisen T, Stadler WM, et al. Sorafenib in advanced clear-cell renal-cell carcinoma. *N Engl J Med*. 2007;356:125-134

37. Hudes G, Carducci M, Tomczak P, et al. Temsirolimus, interferon alfa, or both for advanced renal-cell carcinoma. *N Engl J Med*. 2007;356:2271-2281

38. Motzer RJ, Escudier B, Oudard S, et al. Efficacy of everolimus in advanced renal cell carcinoma: a double-blind, randomised, placebo-controlled phase III trial. *Lancet*. 2008;372:449-456

39. Krege S, Beyer J, Souchon R, et al. European consensus conference on diagnosis and treatment of germ cell cancer: a report of the second meeting of the European Germ Cell Cancer Consensus Group (EGCCCG): part I. *Eur Urol*. 2008;53:478-496

40. Krege S, Beyer J, Souchon R, et al. European consensus conference on diagnosis and treatment of germ cell cancer: a report of the second meeting of the European Germ Cell Cancer Consensus Group (EGCCCG): part II. *Eur Urol*. 2008;53:497-513

41. Oliver RT, Mason MD, Mead GM, et al. Radiotherapy versus single-dose carboplatin in adjuvant treatment of stage I seminoma: a randomised trial. *Lancet*. 2005;366: 293-300

42. Albers P, Albrecht W, Algaba F, et al. Guidelines on testicular cancer. *EurAssoc Urol*. 2008. http://www.uroweb.org/professional-resources/guidelines. Accessed September 26, 2008

43. International Germ Cell Consensus Classification: a prognostic factor-based staging system for metastatic germ cell cancers. International Germ Cell Cancer Collaborative Group. *J Clin Oncol*. 1997;15: 594–603

44. Solsona E, Algaba F, Horenblas S, Pizzocaro G, Windahl T. Guidelines on penile cancer. *Euro Assoc Urol*. 2008;54: 631–639 http://www.uroweb.org/professional-resources/guidelines. Accessed September 29, 2008

14

Tumor and Transplant Immunology

Sean C. Kumer and Kenneth L. Brayman

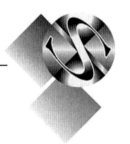

The realm of immunology encompasses basic science and clinical applied medicine. It continues to evolve from its initial studies of innate immunity and resulting physiologic response. Its entirety includes the primary therapy of cancers and the modulation of the immune system in cancer therapy as well as the suppression during transplantation to prevent recognition of non-self.

William Coley first recognized the potential immune system role in cancer therapy. Coley identified patients with sarcoma had spontaneous tumor regression. He found that those patients with concomitant or preceding bacterial infection experienced this regression. As a result, Coley is credited with the earliest attempts of using the immune system to combat cancer.[1] He proceeded to deliberately infect his cancer patients with bacteria. He utilized dead bacterial vaccines to stimulate the immune system to attack the offending malignancy. He actually observed total tumor regression in a small subset of his patients.[2] At this early time in history, however, the molecular aspects of cancer recognition and rejection were not completely understood.

In the mid 1970s, interleukin-2 was identified and cloned. This allowed for experimentation on T-cells in the laboratory setting. Cytokines such as interleukin-2 (IL-2) are now established agents for the treatment of tumors. As we have discovered more players within the immune system, we have explored their potential roles in cancer therapy. These discoveries have led to the underlying basis for immune modulation and immune suppression in transplantation.

The basic premise of cancer immunotherapy is to stimulate the immune system to treat and prevent cancer. We know that the immune system clearly regulates or modulates cancer progression. As a corollary, we have witnessed that immunosuppression is associated with a proclivity toward cancer development and progression. Malignancies have been reported to be up to 100 times more likely in patients who are immunosuppressed such as those patients having undergone previous organ transplantation.[3]

Skin cancers and lymphomas are the most common types of cancer associated with immunosuppression. For instance, patients who have undergone renal transplantation have approximately three to five times higher incidence of malignancy than the general population.[4] Those transplant patients found to have a posttransplant lymphoproliferative disease (PTLD) are often treated with chemotherapy and weaning of their immunosuppression. Furthermore, antitumor activity of the immune system has been implicated in spontaneous cancer regression.[5]

The exact role of the immune system in cancer occurrence and regression as well as immune suppression remains controversial and is an active area of research. The immune system, specifically antibodies and T-cells do not recognize or respond to defective genes, but they do recognize and respond to the abnormal proteins the cancer-causing genes encode. The obvious targets of therapy often revolve around B-and

C.R. Chapple and W.D. Steers (eds.), *Practical Urology: Essential Principles and Practice*,
DOI: 10.1007/978-1-84882-034-0_14, © Springer-Verlag London Limited 2011

T-lymphocytes as mediators in the stimulation or suppression of the immune system to attack cancer or prevent organ rejection.

Antibodies

Antibodies are proteins made by B cells in response to a foreign antigen. Each antibody binds to a specific antigen. The more specific the antibody, the greater the strength of the antibody–antigen bond.[6] All antibodies are composed of light and heavy polypeptide chains. The number of chains may vary, but usually there are two of each type. Every heavy chain is paralleled by a light chain.[6] Fc receptors on the heavy chain regions which allow for antibody function.

Antibodies function in two distinct manners. They either directly attack the antigen or they activate the complement system. Direct attack initiates agglutination, precipitation, neutralization, or lysis. Agglutination involves binding multiple large particles with antigens on their surfaces. The antigen–antibody bonding can also create a molecular complex so large that it is rendered insoluble and precipitates. Neutralization occurs when the antibodies envelope the antigen. Lysis occurs when specific and potent antibodies directly attack the cell membranes and rupture the cell.

The direct attack of antibodies on antigens is not usually completely sufficient. Antibodies compound their effect by activating the cascade of the complement system consisting of approximately 20 different proteins.[6] These proteins are usually inactive enzyme precursors that are activated by the antigen–antibody complex. When an antibody binds with an antigen, a specific reactive site on the antibody is activated. This reactive site initiates a cascade of reactions within the complement system. A single antibody–antigen combination activates many molecules of the complement system and increasing amounts of enzymes. The multiple end products formed help prevent damage by the offending agents.

Importantly, the complement system in turn initiates opsonization and phagocytosis. A product of the complement cascade strongly activates phagocytosis by neutrophils and macrophages. The neutrophils and macrophages dock onto the Fc receptor and literally digest the bound cell. This type of antibody-mediated process is antibody-dependent cell-mediated cytotoxicity (ADCC). ADCC also accelerates T-cell activity. The digested foreign cell proteins are presented on the major histocompatibility complex (MHC) molecules of the antigen-presenting cell (APC) as peptides.

Antibodies have assisted with the detection, prognosis, and treatment of urologic cancers. Oncofetal antigens such as AFP and β-hCG have been identified as important markers in germ cell tumors. Several growth factor receptors have also been associated with tumors and have become important prognostic factors as well as potential therapeutic targets. Prostate cancer has received the most notoriety in the development of antibodies to PSA. Other antibodies being tested for prostate cancer include prostatic acid phosphatase and prostate-specific membrane antigen. B-hCG and CEA are expressed on some transitional cell carcinomas, although this tends to be a minority of these cancers. Germ cell tumors appear to have the largest potential for therapeutic intervention in that β-hCG and AFP are commonly used to detect and prognose outcome with regard to cancer. The relative levels of each of these tumor markers enable classification of the tumors with regard to risk and survival. Monoclonal antibody immunotherapy has met with limited success. In some cases, tumor cell death has been accomplished; however, only with unacceptable side effect risk profiles. Limited or incomplete tumor cell killing therapies have also been utilized with moderate success. Most of these therapies remain investigational at this point.

Cytotoxic and T-helper Cells

T-cells are either cytotoxic (CD8+) or helpers (CD4+). Unlike antibodies, which react to intact proteins only, the cytotoxic T-cells react to peptide antigens expressed on the surface of a cell. Peptide antigens are proteins that have been digested and presented as peptides displayed on the MHC. The peptide and the MHC together attract T-cells. Cytotoxic T-cells are specific for class I MHC molecules, while T helper cells are specific for class II MHC molecules.

After attaching to the MHC-peptide complex expressed on a cell, the cytotoxic T-cell destroys the cell by enzymatically perforating the membrane or by apoptosis. The cytotoxic T-cell will continue to progress to other cells expressing the same MHC-peptide complex and repeat the process. As a result, cytotoxic T-cells neutralize a large number of invasive cells.

The T helper is the major regulator of virtually all immune system activities.[7] These cells form a series of protein mediators or lymphokines that regulate other cells of the immune system. Some of the most important lymphokines secreted by the T helper cells include IL-2, IL-3, IL-4, IL-5, IL-6, granulocyte-monocyte colony stimulating factor (GM-CSF), and interferon-gamma. Without these lymphokines, the remainder of the immune system does not function as effectively as it would with the appropriate cytokine environment.

T helper cells also recognize MHC-peptide complexes, but they are of the class II variety. T helper cells augment the immune response by secreting cytokines that stimulate either a cytotoxic T-cell response (Th1 helper T-cells) or an antibody response (Th2 helper T-cells). These cytokines can initiate B-cells to produce antibodies or enhance the cytotoxic T-cell production. The function of the T helper cell depends upon the type of antigen it recognizes, and the type of immune response required.

Lymphokines produced by T helpers regulate macrophage response. The lymphokines adjust the migration of macrophages and allow macrophages to accumulate at the site. These lymphokines also stimulate more efficient phagocytosis. The T helper amplifies itself by secretion of lymphokines, most importantly IL-2. This action enhances the immune system's response to foreign antigens. (Fig. 14.1)

There appear to be several cell-mediated scenarios in which tumor cells are attacked. Spontaneous regression of RCC metastases following removal of the primary has been observed. This phenomenon occurs in the minority of patients; however, this suggests that elimination of a potential inhibitor of cell-mediated immunity may allow for regression of RCC metastases.

Both active and passive forms of cell-mediated immunity appear to offer a role in prospective immunotherapy. Vaccines are considered forms of active yet experimental therapy. Autologous and allogeneic vaccines have been utilized. Autologous vaccines are tumor- and patient-specific, in that they are extracts from the patient's own tumor. Allogeneic vaccines identify tumor-specific antigens and can be mass-produced; however, the target antigens may not be specific for certain patient's tumors. Active immunotherapy trials have involved prostate cancer cell lines transfected with GM-CSF as well as PSA to treat prostate cancer patients.

Bacillus Calmette-Guérin (BCG) has also proven to be an effective active immunotherapy in the treatment of superficial bladder cancers. It is unclear how BCG is able to elicit local immune responses, although it is hypothesized to activate macrophages and lymphocytes as well as recruit natural killer cells. Furthermore, IL-2 and alpha-interferon are other naturally occurring cytokines which appear to have anti-tumor properties and are in clinical use today in the treatment of RCC.

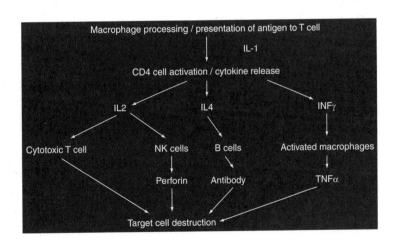

Figure 14.1. Overview of immune reaction.

Immunosuppression

The underlying premise of organ transplantation is to promote acceptance of a foreign organ while attempting to prevent rejection and maintain the immune system's integrity. This is a delicate balance to strike. Complicating the issue is individualizing patients' sensitivities to immunosuppressive medications as well as specific physiologic states that may affect their levels of tolerance or rejection.

The first successful renal transplant with long-term function was performed by Joseph Murray between twin males in 1954. During this time, they realized that foreign organs were rejected at alarming rates. This necessitated matching between twin siblings during this era of transplantation. The progression of immunosuppression began with the institution of total body irradiation, thoracic duct drainage, and splenectomy. During the late 1950s and early 1960s, pharmacologic methods of immune suppression became prevalent. Corticosteroids were employed in 1956 and azathioprine was introduced in 1962. Polyclonal antibodies were developed in the mid-1960s. These advances were brought from the basic science laboratories to the clinical bedside and permitted for the prevention of rejection and long-term maintenance of the functioning allograft.

Major advances in the field of transplantation mirrored such advancements in immunosuppression. With the discoveries of cyclosporine and tacrolimus, the field of transplantation was transformed. It became commonplace to expect and achieve long-term graft survival with more easily treatable and less frequent allograft rejections. The mechanism of action of cyclosporine and tacrolimus is the inhibition of calcineurin. This prevents the transcription of IL-2, and its subsequent actions on T-cells as described above.

The pharmacologic principles of immunosuppression have evolved since their inception. The goal is to titrate the immune response to prevent rejection while attempting not to over-immunosuppress and elicit infection. Immunosuppression is usually initiated before or during surgery. Furthermore, other drugs have been developed such as mycophenolate mofetil, an inosine monophosphate dehydrogenase inhibitor, to assist as antirejection therapies. The concomitant use of all of these therapies has allowed for lower doses of all drugs, which minimizes the potential side effects and toxicities of these powerful antirejection medications. Overall, there are no absolute rules in determining which and how much of each antirejection drug to utilize. There is significant bias from one transplant center to another, and pharmaceutical companies compete actively.

Modern immunosuppressive therapy may be broken down into three distinct types. The initial exposure to immunotherapy is induction therapy. This entails the use of antibody preparations within the first week posttransplant to reduce exposure to calcineurin inhibitor toxicity or to decrease the incidence of rejection within the first 6 months. Maintenance therapy is the lifelong use of immunosuppression to prevent rejection. This therapy is frequently fine-tuned over the lifetime of the allograft. Often, the therapy is weaned to lower levels as some level of tolerance is achieved. Furthermore, the incidence of rejection is highest during the first 6 months of transplantation. Finally, rejection is observed when the innate immune system recognizes the foreign organ and begins to mount a response. This occurs secondary to many causes including drug noncompliance, malabsorption of drug, etc. Most often, use of high-dose steroids or antibody preparations are employed to reverse rejection.

Induction Therapy

The goal of induction therapy is to provide potent immunosuppressive activity during the initial 7–14 days following transplantation. This allows for coverage of the patient while introducing and titrating maintenance immunosuppressive drugs. Induction has been demonstrated to be extremely effective in decreasing rates of rejection. Its use has increased as has its effectiveness. Polyclonal antibody preparations include Atgam and Thymoglobulin, while monoclonal preparations include OKT3, Basiliximab, Alemtuzumab, and Daclizumab. Standard for induction therapy has been the use of high-dose steroids and, in some cases, an antilymphocyte antibody preparation. Unfortunately, it is an expensive endeavor, costing $1,000–$1,500 per day of treatment.

Thymoglobulin induces dose-dependent T-cell depletion in both the blood and peripheral lymphoid tissues. This depletion is thought to involve complement-dependent lysis and activation-associated apoptosis. Thymoglobulin also modulates several functional molecules that mediate the interaction between leukocytes and the endothelium. As a result, there is decreased leukocyte adhesion and translocation into sites of inflammation (Figs. 14.2 and 14.3)[8-11]. The monoclonal antibody preparations have gained some acceptance as well. The original monoclonal antibody, OKT3, is T-cell directed. It binds CD3 and was historically used for induction as well as treatment of rejection. Unfortunately, it may cause a cytokine release syndrome initiating a life-threatening anaphylactoid reaction resulting in hypotension and pulmonary edema. Newer monoclonal preparations include Daclizumab and Basiliximab. They are monoclonal antibodies directed at the IL-2 receptor. They are primarily utilized for induction and have few, if any, side effects.

There are as many derivations of induction therapy as there are transplant centers. There is obviously no clear and correct manner to administer induction therapy. Some centers will administer the entire induction at once during the operative and immediate postoperative period, while other centers administer the doses split over several days. Of course, many centers fall in between these two extremes. Others advocate the use of induction in only select cases. What is clear is that highly sensitized patients benefit from the use of a combined steroid and antilymphocyte regimen as induction. These highly sensitized patients include those with previous exposure to blood transfusions, previous transplantation, and African-Americans.

Induction therapy occasionally prolongs hospitalization. As a result, some centers have begun to alter the administration schedule as outlined above. Antilymphocyte antibody preparations are often given as a single dose initiated perioperatively and continued until the final and goal dose is achieved. Many agree that a full dose constitutes 6 mg/kg. Significant side effects can be observed secondary to induction therapy. Many cytokines are released as a consequence of induction. Potential opportunistic infections occur at an increased rate and pose a significant threat to the patient as well as the allograft viability. Rarely, a patient may also develop antibodies to the antilymphocyte antibody.

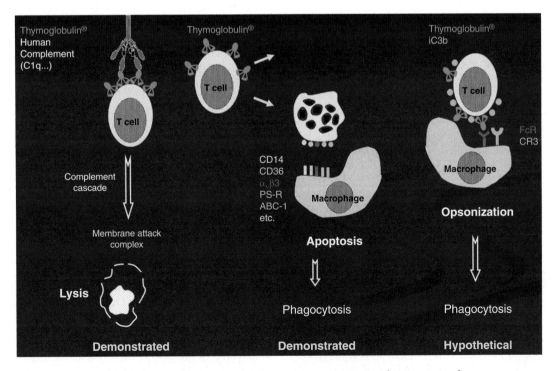

Figure 14.2. Thymoglobulin® T-cell depletion: possible mechanisms (Adapted from Brennan[8] and von Andrian[9]).

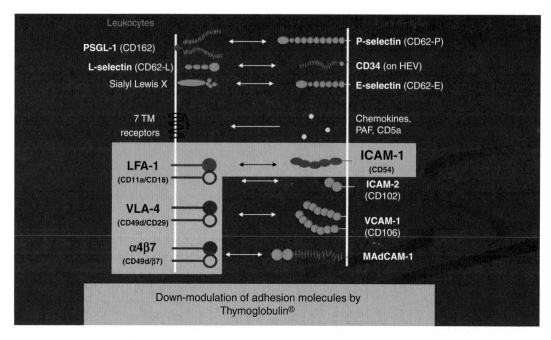

Figure 14.3. Thymoglobulin® down-modulation: interactions between leukocytes and endothelium. (Courtesy of Genzyme Corporation; Adapted from Genestier et al.[10] and Préville et al.[11])

Maintenance Therapy

Allograft tolerance remains the "Holy Grail" for the field of transplantation. Unfortunately, only limited success has been achieved with regard to this goal. Consequently, maintenance therapy is required for the life of the allograft. Commonly accepted practice with regards to posttransplant immunosuppression involves the use of one to three drugs for the life of the allograft. The decision to utilize one drug versus another depends on the type of organ transplanted and is often transplant center dependent. If no rejection is encountered, the general premise is to reduce the dose of immunosuppression or discontinue the use of some of the drugs with time. If the patient experiences rejection, the immunosuppression is most often increased or different drug therapies are employed.

The discussion on which immunosuppressants to utilize usually begins with the calcineurin inhibitors, namely, Cyclosporine and Tacrolimus. The calcineurin inhibitors exert their mechanism of action as inhibition of T-cells by preventing the transcription and subsequent release of IL-2. They have transformed solid organ transplant significantly. The rates of

rejection have plummeted since their inception. Furthermore, allograft survival has greatly increased since their introduction. Unfortunately, they do have common and significant side effect profiles. Cyclosporine has been associated with hirsutism, gingival hyperplasia, hyperlipidemia, hypertension, hypomagnesemia, and nephrotoxicity. Tacrolimus is slightly more potent than cyclosporine. It has similar drug interactions as cyclosporine but has a greater propensity to cause hyperglycemia. Tacrolimus also has better bioavailability than cyclosporine and has enabled steroid reduction protocols. With renal transplantation, there appears to be a less rapid decline in glomerular filtration rates.[12] Furthermore, several studies have suggested that lower rates of rejection are observed with tacrolimus use.[13,14] As a result, tacrolimus has gained wider acceptance nationally. Another immunomodulator, Sirolimus, has gained recent acceptance for having less nephrotoxicity and less likelihood in causing PTLD. Sirolimus binds to immunophilin (FK Binding Protein-12) to generate an immunosuppressive complex. The sirolimus:FKBP-12 complex does not affect calcineurin activity. Rather, this complex binds to and inhibits the activation of the mammalian

Target Of Rapamycin (mTOR), a key regulatory kinase. This inhibition suppresses cytokine-driven T-cell proliferation, inhibiting the progression from the G1 to the S phase of the cell cycle. Its main side effect is the inhibition of the healing process; however, it may also cause hyperlipidemia and bone marrow suppression. Sirolimus use has become more popular because of lower rates of chronic rejection relative to cyclosporine-based therapy.[15]

The second drug added to the immunosuppression regimen is often mycophenolate mofetil (Cellcept, MMF), mycophenolic acid (Myfortic, enteric-coated MMF), or azathioprine (Imuran). Azathioprine was one of the first drugs developed for immunosuppression and has a storied role in the early progression of kidney and liver transplantation. It decreases both T- and B-cell production by antagonizing purine metabolism. As a result, it inhibits synthesis of DNA, RNA, and proteins. Azathioprine may also interfere with cellular metabolism and inhibit mitosis. Azathioprine unfortunately has been associated with bone marrow suppression, pancreatitis, and has significant drug interactions. Mycophenolate mofetil and mycophenolic acid primarily decrease B-cell production, although they exert some effect on T-cells. They are selective but reversible inhibitors of inosine monophosphate dehydrogenase, which is a critical enzyme for the de novo synthesis of guanosine nucleotides. They have been found to decrease the incidence of antibody-mediated rejection and reduce the prevalence of chronic rejection.[13,16] They have some minor bone marrow suppressive effects, but their primary side effect is gastrointestinal disturbance, which may be decreased with the enteric-coated form.

Corticosteroids are the third drug class in the armamentarium of maintenance therapy. They are usually used in the IV or PO forms, methyl-prednisolone or prednisone, respectively. Steroids have a broad set of physiologic effects and subsequent side effects. In the field of solid organ transplantation, they are employed in the prevention as well as the treatment of rejection. With regard to immunosuppression, they inhibit T-cells, IL-2, and antibody formation. Unfortunately, steroids have serious deleterious effects. Centrally, they can often cause mood swings and psychoses as well as cataracts and glaucoma. From a gastrointestinal standpoint, they are associated with increased appetite and weight gain, ulcers, and nausea. They cause hyperglycemia and promote diabetes mellitus. Acne, hirsutism, skin atrophy, and easy bruising are frequent side effects. Muscle weakness and osteoporosis often ensue. Many patients experience edema, hypertension, and hypernatremia. Ultimately, a subset of patients with long-term steroid use may develop Cushing's syndrome.

Transplant physicians and surgeons are constantly adjusting immunosuppression on a personalized patient basis for the life of the allograft and patient. These judgments are made based on each patient's clinical presentation, laboratory values, and other associated or unassociated illnesses. In general, patients require higher levels of immunosuppression early in their postoperative course; however, immunosuppression may be weaned to lower levels within 3–6 months posttransplant in most cases. The balance between excessive and inadequate imunosuppression must be found. A steady-state immunosuppressive regimen may be altered by the patient's pharmacokinetics and dynamics or a concomitant illness. As a result, immunosuppression should be adjusted accordingly. Over-immunosuppression may result in an opportunistic infection, malignancy, or PTLD. Under-immunosuppression will almost inevitably result in organ rejection.

Rejection

Organ rejection manifests as an innate immunologic reaction to donor tissue. There are four main types: hyperacute, accelerated, acute, and chronic. The outcome may result in organ damage with the possible eventual loss of the allograft. Moreover, only acute rejection is completely responsive to therapy. Hyperacute rejection is extremely rare and, in most cases, preventable. These are the so-called pre-formed antibodies that immediately attack the foreign organ. Anti-HLA antibodies within the serum of the recipient react towards the donor organ. The onset is nearly immediate within minutes to hours. Vascular damage begins immediately resulting in inflammation, congestion, thrombosis, and necrosis. Unfortunately, the only recourse is to remove the offending organ.

Accelerated rejection is a more indolent form of hyperacute rejection. There is usually a low level of circulating non-HLA antibody against donor tissue. The onset occurs 3–10 days posttransplant. The allograft vessels are most often involved and not the parenchyma. Therapy is not often helpful secondary to the antibody mechanism and most of the drugs are directed toward T-cells. However, IVIG and plasmapheresis may play a role.

Acute rejection is T-cell-mediated. These types of rejections are more common, and their onset can be weeks to months to years. Lymphocytes and macrophages infiltrate the allograft. Damage ensues to the parenchyma, and scarring damages the structural integrity of the organ. The initial hint that a rejection episode has begun is usually organ dysfunction, fever, malaise, or allograft tenderness. The differential diagnosis must always include rejection; however, the patient's presentation is most often not easily discernible. A biopsy of the organ can confirm or dismiss the diagnosis. Fortunately, therapies are usually successful in reversing this type of rejection if treated promptly. The treatments often include the use of large pulse doses of steroids and/or antilymphocyte antibody preparations as described above. The successful treatment of rejection is often accompanied with the adjustment of the patient's maintenance immunosuppression.

Chronic allograft rejection appears to affect nearly every transplanted organ. Most often it occurs over the lifetime of a transplanted organ at clinically undetectable levels. Its etiology is unknown; however, its incidence is increased in those patients who have experienced previous acute rejection episodes. Its onset is months to years following the transplant. The appearance on organ biopsy presents as persistent perivascular and interstitial inflammation. There is little to no lymphocyte involvement. Tailoring the immunosuppression regimen aims to prevent persistent rejection while attempting to minimize the side effects of the drugs on the allograft. This strategy occasionally will extend graft survival; however, the results are not overly encouraging. Unfortunately, the only definitive remedy for this type of rejection remains re-transplantation.

Posttransplant Lymphoproliferative Disease

Posttransplant lymphoproliferative disease (PTLD) is the other spectrum of chronically immunosuppressed transplant patients. PTLD is a relatively uncommon complication of both solid organ and bone marrow transplantation. Most cases of PTLD are associated with an Epstein-Barr virus (EBV) infection. This occurs as a consequence of reactivation of the recipient's virus after transplantation or from a donor-acquired primary posttransplantation EBV infection. T-cell lymphoproliferative disorders not associated with EBV infection have also been documented, yet the vast majority are B-cell proliferations.[17]

Most cases of PTLD are observed in the first year following transplant. Higher levels of immunosuppressive regimens are associated with a higher incidence of PTLD. Successful treatment of PTLD involves the reduction or withdrawal of immunosuppressive medications. Unfortunately, this approach risks significant allograft rejection and possible allograft loss. Other treatment modalities that have been demonstrated as effective include surgical excision of the lesion, radiation therapy, chemotherapy, monoclonal antibodies, and interferon.

PTLD is an uncommon phenomenon; however, it has been described in all types of solid and bone marrow transplants. Up to 60% of patients with renal allografts who develop PTLD do so within 6 months of their transplant. Cardiac transplant patients had an incidence ranging from 5% to 13% with half developing PTLD within 6 months of transplantation. In liver transplantation, the incidence is 2% with most developing PTLD within 1 year of transplantation.[17] Renal allograft patients had an overall incidence of PTLD of approximately 2%; however, it was slightly higher in the pediatric population (1–10%).[18,19]

Summary

Overall, immunosuppression has transformed the field of transplantation. Unfortunately with great advances, confounding factors are often encountered. Immunosuppression is a powerful tool in combating rejection; however, the underlying auspices of infection must not be allowed to prevail. Initially, induction therapy prevents early rejection and allows for the titration of maintenance therapy. Maintenance therapy is frequently adjusted for the life of the allograft to accommodate physiologic changes in the recipient. The ultimate goal remains the prevention of rejection and avoidance of over-immunosuppression and opportunistic infections. The use of combined therapies allows for lower doses and minimization of potential side effects as well as a multifaceted approach to suppress the innate immune response.

References

1. Old LJ. Immunotherapy for cancer. *Sci Am*. 1996;275: 136-143

2. Coley WB. The treatment of malignant tumors by repeated inoculations of erysipelas. With a report of ten original cases. 1893. *Clin Orthop Relat Res*. 1991;262: 3-11

3. Berkow R, Beers MH. Cancer and the immune system. In: *The Merck Manual of Medical Information*. Whitehouse Station, NJ: Merck Research Laboratories; 1997: 792-794

4. Zeir M, Hartschuh W, Wiesel M, Lehnert T, Ritz E. Malignancy after renal transplantation. *Am J Kidney Dis*. 2002;39:E5

5. Challis GB, Stam HJ. The spontaneous regression of cancer. A review of cases from 1900 to 1987. *Acta Oncol*. 1990;29:545-550

6. Guyton AC, Hall JE, eds. Immunity, allergy, blood groups, and transfusion. In: *Human Physiology and Mechanisms of Disease*. 6th ed. Philadelphia, PA: W.B. Saunders Company;1997:291-293

7. Guyton AC, Hall JE, eds. Resistance of the body to infection: II. Immunity and allergy. In: *Textbook of Medical Physiology*. 10th ed. Philadelphia, PA: W.B. Saunders Company;2000: 408-410

8. Brennan D. Faith supported by reason: mechanistic support for the use of polyclonal antibodies in transplantation. *Transplantation*. 2003;75:577

9. von Andrian UH, Mackay CR. T-cell function and migration: two sides of the same coin. *N Engl J Med*. 2003; 343:1020

10. Genestier L, Fournel S, Flacher M, Assossou O, Revillard JP, Bonnefoy-Berard N. *Blood*. 1998;91:2360

11. Préville X, Flacher M, LeMauff B, et al. Mechanisms involved in antithymocyte globulin immunosuppressive activity in a nonhuman primate model. *Transplantation*. 2001;71:460

12. Gill JS, Tonelli M, Mix CH, et al. The effect of maintenance immunosuppression medication on the change in kidney allograft function. *Kidney Int*. 2004;65(2):692-699

13. Ahsan N, Johnson C, Gonwa T, et al. Randomized trial of tacrolimus plus mycophenolate mofetil or azathioprine versus cyclosporine oral solution (modified) plus mycophenolate mofetil after cadaveric kidney transplantation: results at 2 years. *Transplantation*. 2001;72(2): 245-250

14. Mourad G, Garrigue V, Squifflet JP, et al. Induction versus non induction in renal transplant recipients with tacrolimus-based imunosuppression. *Transplantation*. 2001;72(6):1050-1055

15. Kahan BD, Knight R, Schoenberg L, et al. Ten years of sirolimus therapy for human renal transplantation: the University of Texas at Houston experience. *Transplant Proc*. 2003;35(suppl 3):25S-34S

16. Pescovitz MD, Govani M. Sirolimus and mycophenolate mofetil for calcineurin-free immunosuppression in renal transplant recipients. *Am J Kidney Dis*. 2001;38(4 suppl 2):S16-S21

17. Cohen JI. Epstein-Barr virus infection. *N Engl J Med*. 2000;343(7):481-492

18. Shapiro R, Nalesnik M, McCauley J. Posttransplant lymphoproliferative disorders in adult and pediatric renal transplant patients receiving tacrolimus-based immunosuppression. *Transplantation*. 1999;68(12):1851-1854

19. Srivastava T, Zwick DL, Rothberg PG. Posttransplant lymphoproliferative disorder in pediatric renal transplantation. *Pediatr Nephrol*. 1999;13(9):748-754

15

Pathophysiology of Renal Obstruction

Glenn M. Cannon and Richard S. Lee

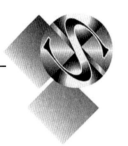

Causes of Renal Obstruction

Renal obstruction can be caused by intrinsic or extrinsic factors that affect the ureters, bladder, or urethra. Most of the literature concerning the pathophysiology of renal obstruction has focused on unilateral ureteral obstruction (UUO) or bilateral ureteral obstruction (BUO). Table 15.1 lists possible causes of renal obstruction.

Effects on Prenatal Development

Prenatal Hydronephrosis

Ultrasound has remained the main diagnostic tool in evaluation of prenatal hydronephrosis since its introduction in 1980.[1] Historically, the degree of anteroposterior renal pelvic diameter has been used as an indicator to predict need for surgery. A renal pelvic diameter of <12 mm without caliectasis poses a minimal risk of eventually requiring surgery, while severe dilatation of >50 mm may inevitably require surgery.[1] Diuretic renal scanning aids the evaluation of infants between these two extremes and has been demonstrated to be reliable over the age of 6 weeks to 2 months.[2] Serial ultrasound examination is frequently utilized and a trend of progressive hydronephrosis on two consecutive examinations serves as an early diagnostic sign of obstruction.[3] Society of Fetal Urology (SFU) Grade of 3–4 of postnatal hydronephrosis and a relative renal function of <40% are both independent risk factors for the eventual need for surgery.

Lee et al. performed a meta-analysis including 1,308 patients with prenatal hydronephrosis and postnatal follow-up that concluded that children with any degree of prenatal hydronephrosis are at greater risk of postnatal pathology compared with the normal population.[4] They found that children with moderate hydronephrosis (defined as AP diameter 7–10 mm for second trimester, 9–15 mm for third trimester) and severe hydronephrosis (AP diameter > 1m for second trimester, >15 mm for third trimester) were at significant risk for postnatal pathology, and postnatal diagnostic studies should be considered. The authors also concluded that even children with mild prenatal hydronephrosis may carry a greater risk as compared to the normal population for postnatal pathology. The optimal postnatal management of patients with mild prenatal hydronephrosis is controversial and further prospective studies are needed.

Spectrum of Renal Abnormalities

Congenital ureteropelvic junction obstruction (UPJO) can cause a spectrum of renal abnormalities.[5,6] In its mildest form, UPJO represents the radiological demonstration of reversible hydronephrosis without permanent renal damage. Its most severe form represents a hypertrophic and fibrotic UPJ with renal parenchymal changes such as glomerulosclerosis, chronic tubulointerstitial injury, and dysplasia that may

C.R. Chapple and W.D. Steers (eds.), *Practical Urology: Essential Principles and Practice*,
DOI: 10.1007/978-1-84882-034-0_15, © Springer-Verlag London Limited 2011

Table 15.1. Possible causes of renal obstruction

Ureter

Intrinsic

    Ureteropelvic junction obstruction

    Ureterovesical junction obstruction

    Ureteral valve

    Ureteritis cystica

    Tuberculosis

    Schistosomiasis

    Ureteral carcinoma

    Papillary necrosis

    Calculus

    Endometriosis

    Blood clot

    Fungal bezoar

Extrinsic

    Crossing lower pole vessel at ureteropelvic junction

    Retroperitoneal fibrosis

    Retroperitoneal tumor

    Abdominal aortic aneurysm

    Cervical cancer

    Prostate cancer

    Retrocaval ureter

    Tubo-ovarian abscess

    Diverticulitis

    Gravid uterus

Bladder

Intrinsic

    Bladder carcinoma

    Calculi

    Neurogenic bladder

Extrinsic

    Pelvic lipomatosis

Urethra

Intrinsic

    Posterior urethral valve

    Urethral stricture

    Urethral carcinoma

    Urethral atresia

Extrinsic

    Prostate carcinoma

    Penile carcinoma

necessitate nephrectomy.[7] Renal biopsies performed in patients after pyeloplasty demonstrate relatively well-maintained parenchyma in which the only overt changes are mainly glomerular.[7]

Signaling Pathways and Tissue Interactions

Recent finding from gene expression studies and embryological mutants have resulted in a better understanding of ureteral development and its effect on the developing renal parenchyma. Glial-derived neurotropic factor (Gdnf) is released from the metanephric blastema and induces ureteral bud growth from the Wolffian duct.[8] Airik et al. have demonstrated that the transcription factor gene *Tbx18* is initially expressed between the Wolffian duct and metanephric mesenchyme in mouse embryos and is later found exclusively at the distal ureteric stalk.[9] This implies that the ureteric mesenchyme is differentiated shortly after ureteral budding, which occurs before the differentiation of ureteric epithelium. Several investigators have identified that the signaling molecule Bmp4 also plays a key role in the specification and differentiation of the ureteric bud.[10-12] Both urothelial and smooth muscle development are significantly impaired after inactivation of the *Bmp4* gene. Deletion of the signaling molecule Bmp4 or the angiotensin type II receptor can result in ectopic Gdnf signaling that results in multiple ureteric buds.[13-15] Multiple other genes have been identified as playing a role in ureteral development and mutations in any of them may result in urinary tract obstruction.[8]

Renal Functional Changes

Renal Growth/Counterbalance

Hinman initially described compensatory growth of the contralateral kidney in rats with UUO.[16] Obstruction at a younger age is associated with a greater degree of ipsilateral growth impairment and contralateral increased growth.[17] It has also been demonstrated in neonatal rats that an increased duration of obstruction results in a greater degree of growth in the contralateral kidney.[18] Compensatory renal growth has also been demonstrated in human fetuses.[19] A greater degree of contralateral compensatory renal growth has been associated with a greater severity of obstruction in infants with ureteropelvic junction obstruction.[20]

Vascular Changes

High renal vascular resistance in the fetus and neonate is the result of activation of the renin-angiotensin system (RAS).[21] Chronic UUO results in increase of RAS activity and renal vascular resistance, which resolves by relief of the obstruction.[22] Chronic UUO also results in vasodilatation of the contralateral kidney.[23,24] The vasodilator nitric oxide plays a role in regulating renal vascular resistance. After UUO, nitric oxide synthase activity is increased as a counterbalance to the increased renal vascular resistance brought about by RAS activation.[25]

Changes to Electrolyte Transport/ Renal Concentrating Ability

Normally, the proximal nephron is responsible for reabsorption of 60–70% of the filtered sodium and water and 90% of the filtered bicarbonate.[26,27] The thick ascending loop of Henle reabsorbs 20–30% of filtered sodium via sodium-chloride -potassium cotransporters. Approximately, 5–10% of filtered sodium is reabsorbed by the distal tubule through sodium chloride cotransport in the luminal membrane. As for water, the collecting duct can reabsorb 10–15% of that filtered. Under normal conditions, urinary excretion of sodium and water can range from 0.1% to 3%, and 0.3 to 15% of the filtered load, respectively.[26]

During acute UUO, electrolyte and renal concentrating ability is altered. Obstruction results in a significant decrease in sodium, potassium, and solute excretion. This results in a decrease in urine sodium concentration and an increase in urine osmolality.[28] However, during chronic UUO the literature is conflicting regarding the effects on electrolyte transport. With chronic UUO, sodium, potassium, and osmotic excretion can either increase or decrease depending upon the overall renal function and physiologic homeostasis.[17,29-33]

Ureteral obstruction also results in decreased renal concentrating ability and urinary acidification. The reduction in concentrating ability is thought to be a result of medullary and inner cortical dysfunction caused by decreased sodium absorption in the distal tubule and medullary nephrons.[28] Under normal conditions, one of the major tasks of the renal proximal tubule is acid secretion. The proximal tubule reabsorbs up to 90% of the filtered bicarbonate and can generate additional bicarbonate in order to regulate blood pH.[34] Ureteral obstruction causes urinary acidification dysfunction that may be secondary to alteration in the reabsorption of bicarbonate in the juxtamedullary nephrons as well as decreased acid secretion in the distal tubules.[28]

Inflammatory Mediators

Interstitial inflammation is an early response to UUO.[35] This inflammation can contribute to tubular apoptosis and interstitial fibrosis.[36] Monocyte chemoattractant protein-1 (MCP-1) is believed to be a mediator of the intrarenal inflammation that occurs after obstruction.[37] MCP-1 is suppressed by heme oxygenase-1 (HO-1) that provides negative feedback to this inflammatory pathway.[38]

After renal obstruction, the upregulated renin-angiotensin system acts to recruit inflammatory cells through activation of AT_1 and AT_2 receptors and the NF-κB pathway.[39] Angiotensin also increases production of TGF-1 and Smad3, which cause apoptosis and interstitial fibrosis.[40]

Glomerular Development Changes

There is irreversible nephron loss that occurs with UUO in the developing kidney. Chronic

UUO impairs nephrogenesis and glomerular development in both animals and humans.[41] Nephron number is decreased in fetal rabbits and pigs that experience chronic UUO.[42,43] Relief of obstruction does not result in subsequent increased nephron development in the obstructed kidney, but rather hyperfiltration in the remaining nephrons.[44] Hyperfiltration can result in injury to the remaining nephrons and future glomerular sclerosis even in the presence of a normal contralateral kidney.[41,45,46]

Mechanical Stretch of Renal Tubules

Mechanical stretching of renal tubules is a significant step in the progression of obstructive nephropathy.[47] Integrins are cell surface receptors that can sense extracellular mechanical signals and transmit them across the cell membrane.[48,49] After mechanical stretch occurs, cation channels are activated with leads to Ca^{2+} influx.[47] Increased calcium levels result in the activation of several pathways that lead to increased TGF-β_1 expression and induction of oxidative stress, which ultimately results in renal inflammation and fibrosis.[47]

Unilateral Versus Bilateral

There are major differences in renal function before and after release of UUO and bilateral ureteral obstruction (BUO).[28] During UUO and BUO, GFR decline occurs secondary to a decrease in intraglomerular capillary pressure. However, with BUO a persistent elevation in intratubular pressure occurs that also contributes to GFR decline.[50] Although kidneys with both forms of obstruction experience an initial increase in intratubular pressure, kidneys with UUO experience a return to baseline intratubular pressure within 24 h. However, BUO kidneys have persistently elevated intratubular pressure even after 24 h.[50] Another difference with BUO is that intravascular increases of atrial natriuretic peptide and prostyacyclin occur that do not occur with UUO.[51]

After the release of obstruction, kidneys with BUO experience a postobstructive diuresis and natriuresis that does not typically occur with UUO. Urinary concentrating ability is decreased and fractional sodium excretion is increased with release of BUO versus release of UUO. In addition, fractional potassium excretion is also increased after release of BUO but significantly decreased after release of UUO.[28]

Figure 15.1 summarizes the differential effects on renal blood flow and glomerular filtration rate in unilateral and bilateral ureteral obstruction.

Limitations of Animal Models

Much of the knowledge on the pathophysiology of renal obstruction is derived from animal models. Although animal models have greatly enhanced the understanding of renal injury, they have limitations.[52] Effective treatment of acute renal failure in animal models has not translated to successful outcomes in human.[53] This may be secondary to the variations in pathophysiology between humans and animals. For instance, in acute tubular necrosis, animals have different locations of necrosis as compared to humans.[52] Overall, animal models of obstruction and / or renal damage that are more translatable to the human condition are needed. To better assess the applicability of a particular animal model of renal injury, applications such as the quantitation of excreted proteins or the assessment of renal oxygenation by radiographic imaging techniques may be utilized to test the efficacy of the animal model.[52]

Future Research

Current and future research efforts continue to focus on understanding the basic pathophysiology of UUO in an attempt to identify potential new therapeutic targets to protect or improve renal function. For example, it was believed that the antioxidant therapies had limited effect on mitochondria, the primary source of intracellular reactive oxygen species, and previous attempts at using antioxidant therapies to mitigate the effects of UUO have had disappointing outcomes. However, recently, Mizuguchi et al. demonstrated that peptides, which protect mitochondria in vitro can provide protection from renal damage in a UUO model.[54] This and other research are encouraging and will hopefully identify new pathways of investigation.

Other research efforts on UUO have focused on identifying new biomarkers of renal obstruction to help guide therapy and potentially

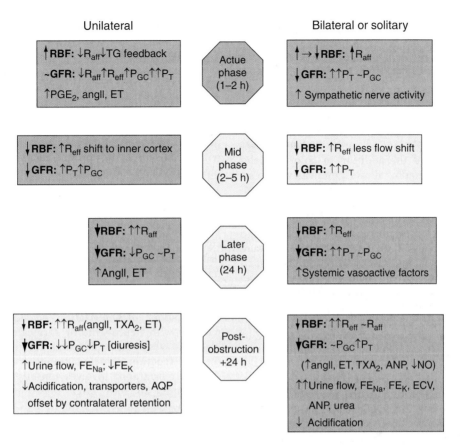

Figure 15.1. Differential effects on RBF and GFR in UUO and BUO (Reprinted with permission from Pais et al.[66] Copyright Elsevier 2006).

identify novel therapeutic targets. Previous efforts to identify markers of obstruction have focused on studying one or a few potential markers in a subjective fashion. Recently, in an effort to identify new biomarkers or panels of disease biomarkers, many researchers are turning toward Proteomics as a rapid unbiased screening tool for identifying new targets of interest. Evaluating proteins using proteomic technologies has the ability to increase the understanding of protein / protein interaction, protein modification, and protein interaction in the context of systems biology. As an example of expanding the use of animal models, a temporal interrogation of the normal postnatal rodent urinary proteome demonstrated dramatic changes in the urinary proteome secondary to physiologic changes related to nephrogenesis and developmental maturation.[55] This work identified a potential set of proteins

that may indicate normal development; may provide the basis for future studies on renal development or renal dysfunction; and allow for future comparative studies in rat renal obstruction models. One significant study on human urinary obstruction using proteomics has been reported. In this study, a portion of the urinary proteome of children with hydronephrosis (e.g., polypeptides < 30 kDa) were analyzed using various proteomic techniques. Using discovery-based proteomic methods, a potential polypeptide pattern was identified that may help determine which children require surgery.[56] Further prospective validation work will determine the potential of these markers. In summary, these and other research efforts will hopefully further the understanding of obstructive nephropathy, and uncover new clinical significant markers and therapies for this disease.

Issues in Patient Management

Diagnostic Imaging

Ultrasound

Ultrasound imaging is frequently utilized in the diagnostic management of suspected renal obstruction. Ultrasound can easily detect hydronephrosis, and the addition of color Doppler duplex sonography allows noninvasive assessment of renal perfusion.[57] Ultrasound is advantageous in that it is noninvasive, portable, relatively inexpensive, and does not require ionizing radiation, or contrast media.[58] Ultrasound has the potential to detect characteristics of renal parenchymal disease that may be associated with obstruction such as increased echogenicity, loss of corticomedullary differentiation, or cystic disease.

Doppler ultrasound can be utilized to calculate the resistive index (RI), which is defined as (peak systolic velocity-lowest diastolic velocity) / peak systolic velocity.[59] A RI above 0.70 has been thought to be associated with renal obstruction.[58] In diagnosing obstruction in adults with renal dilatation, an RI above 0.70 has 92% sensitivity and 88% specificity.[59] In children with hydronephrosis, the sensitivity of RI to diagnose obstruction decreases to 82% and specificity decreases to 63%.[60]

Intravenous Urography

Over the last couple of decades, intravenous urography (IVU) has been replaced by other imaging modalities. IVU provides anatomic information such as degree of hydronephrosis and possible level of obstruction, and also functional information. IVU may be particularly useful in diagnosis of calyceal obstruction (e.g., calyceal diverticulum), or complex duplex or ectopic ureteral anatomy. Since it is dependent upon renal excretion of contrast medium, IVU should not be used in patients with renal insufficiency or patients with contrast allergy.

Antegrade Urography and the Whitaker Test

The Whitaker test was first described in 1973 to diagnosis upper urinary tract obstruction, but is currently not commonly used.[61] A percutaneous renal catheter and bladder catheter are placed.

Saline or contrast material is infused at 10 mL/min into the renal access, while pressures within the kidney and bladder are monitored. Intravesical pressure is subtracted from intrarenal pressure and a difference between these pressures greater than 22 cm H_2O is considered obstructive, 15–22 cm H_2O is considered indeterminate, and less than 15 cm H_2O is considered nonobstructive. The Whitaker test is associated with poor sensitivity and specificity for renal obstruction and is rarely utilized today.[62]

Nuclear Renography

Radionucleotide imaging provides a noninvasive means to assess for renal obstruction and differential renal function. The current radiopharmaceutical of choice is Tc-99m MAG_3.[63] Adequate hydration is essential prior to the study as dehydration can mimic renal obstruction. Bladder catheterization is required in patients with neurogenic or surgically altered bladders, vesicoureteral reflux, lower urinary tract obstruction, or pelvic kidneys.[63] Standard diuretic renography involves administration of furosemide 20 min after injection of the radiotracer. In patients with equivocal results, administering furosemide 15 min before the radiotracer can improve sensitivity and specificity for obstruction.[64,65]

Obstruction is assessed by determining the time it takes for 50% of the radiotracer to clear from the kidney ($t_{1/2}$). In a standard renogram where furosemide is administered 20 min after radiotracer injection: $t_{1/2}$ greater than 20 min is consistent with obstruction, $t_{1/2}$ between 10 and 20 min is equivocal, and $t_{1/2}$ less than 10 min is normal.[66] These values will change if other methodology is used. For example, if furosemide is administered 15 min before the radiotracer: $t_{1/2}$ greater than 10 min is consistent with obstruction, $t_{1/2}$ between 5 and 10 min is equivocal, and $t_{1/2}$ less than 5 min is normal.[66]

Computed Tomography

Unenhanced computed tomography (CT) is the most accurate radiologic study for the diagnosis of renal calculi with a sensitivity of 97% and a specificity of 96%.[67] CT is able to image all types of radiolucent calculi with the exception of protease inhibitor stones.[68] Utilization of intravenous contrast in CT is useful for anatomical assessment of UPJO. CT with arterial and venous phase contrast-enhanced images has 97% sensitivity and 92% specificity in the detection of a lower pole crossing vessel.[69] The symmetry of parenchymal opacification can serve as a surrogate marker of renal function.[70] In the last several years, techniques such as small section multidetector row CT and multiplanar reformation allow for excellent 3D reconstruction of UPJ anatomy.[70]

Magnetic Resonance Urography

Magnetic resonance (MR) urography is an evolving group of technique that allows for optimal visualization of many urinary tract abnormalities without the use of ionizing radiation.[71] It can be performed in two ways: static-fluid MR urography (T2-weighted MR urography) and excretory MR urography (T1-weighted MR urography). Static-fluid MR urography is well suited for patients with dilated collecting systems because it is dependent on the presence of urine in the collecting systems and not on renal function.[71] In excretory MR urography, a gadolinium-based contrast agent is administered and the collecting system is imaged. A low dose of furosemide given 2 min prior to contrast injection is typically administered during excretory MR urography.[72] Utilizing excretory MR urography, Karabacakoglu et al. reported 92.8% accuracy for diagnosing stone disease and 100% accuracy at diagnosing other causes of obstructive uropathy.[72] The technique of MR urography is becoming more widely available, especially because imaging processing software is now available in the public domain.[73]

Hypertension

Hypertension is rarely a consequence of congenital UPJ obstruction. In a literature review, Farnham et al. only identified 15 cases of hypertension attributed to UPJ obstruction from 1960–2005.[74] One series followed 71 adults with UPJO an average of 17 years and found only four patients developed hypertension.[75] Parkhouse et al. reviewed a series of 88 boys with posterior urethral valves (PUV) followed for 11–22 years after diagnosis.[76] During that time, seven patients developed hypertension. However, other possible causes of hypertension were not reported.

Based on current existing literature, it is difficult to draw conclusions regarding the relation of hypertension to UPJO or PUV.[74]

Postobstructive Diuresis

Postobstructive diuresis is a significant loss of water and possibly solute that can occur after relief of urinary obstruction. It is usually arbitrarily defined as a persistent urine output great than 200 mL/h.[77-79] Most commonly, this occurs after relief of BUO (or UUO in a solitary kidney), but it has been reported after relief of UUO with a normal contralateral kidney.[80] Postobstructive diuresis can be severe enough to cause life-threatening dehydration and electrolyte disorders.

Several physiological derangements have been discovered to occur in postobstructive diuresis. Investigators have identified a decreased expression of aquaporin genes and proteins with BUO.[81,82] Having a decreased number of aquaporin channels in the collecting tubules impairs renal reabsorption of water and contributes to ongoing diuresis. Ureteral obstruction has also been demonstrated to decrease the activity of Na^+K^+-ATPase that contributes to postobstructive diuresis and naturalis.[83] Recently, Norregaard et al. have demonstrated that cyclooxygenase-2 activity transiently contributed to increased water and sodium excretion after release of ureteral obstruction.[84] They reported that treatment of rats with COX-2 inhibitor parecoxib decreased the downregulation of aquaporin channels with BUO.

Patients more likely to experience significant postobstructive diuresis have preexisting volume overload, severe renal impairment, or central nervous system manifestations.[77] Management initially includes urethral catheter placement. In the setting of urinary retention, there is no benefit to gradual bladder decompression.[79] Serum electrolytes and urine osmolarity should be monitored at least every 12 h. In a clinically stable patient, oral fluid replacement alone is recommended as excessive intravenous fluids may prolong the period of diuresis.[66] It has also been suggested that fluid replacement be two-thirds of the fluid output.[77] Unstable patients are best monitored in a critical care setting with specific fluid replacement dictated by serum electrolytes.

References

1. Dhillon HK. Prenatally diagnosed hydronephrosis: the Great Ormond Street experience. *Br J Urol*. 1998;81 (suppl 2):39-44

2. Chung S et al. Diuretic renography in the evaluation of neonatal hydronephrosis: is it reliable? *J Urol*. 1993;150 (2 pt 2):765-768

3. Hafez AT et al. Analysis of trends on serial ultrasound for high grade neonatal hydronephrosis. *J Urol*. 2002; 168(4 pt 1):1518-1521

4. Lee RS et al. Antenatal hydronephrosis as a predictor of postnatal outcome: a meta-analysis. *Pediatrics*. 2006; 118(2):586-593

5. Huang WY et al. Renal biopsy in congenital ureteropelvic junction obstruction: evidence for parenchymal maldevelopment. *Kidney Int*. 2006;69(1):137-143

6. Elder JS et al. Renal histological changes secondary to ureteropelvic junction obstruction. *J Urol*. 1995;154(2 pt 2): 719-722

7. Rosen S et al. The kidney in congenital ureteropelvic junction obstruction: a spectrum from normal to nephrectomy. *J Urol*. 2008;179(4):1257-1263

8. Airik R, Kispert A. Down the tube of obstructive nephropathies: the importance of tissue interactions during ureter development. *Kidney Int*. 2007;72(12):1459-1467

9. Airik R et al. Tbx18 regulates the development of the ureteral mesenchyme. *J Clin Invest*. 2006;116(3):663-674

10. Brenner-Anantharam A et al. Tailbud-derived mesenchyme promotes urinary tract segmentation via BMP4 signaling. *Development*. 2007;134(10):1967-1975

11. Miyazaki Y et al. Bone morphogenetic protein 4 regulates the budding site and elongation of the mouse ureter. *J Clin Invest*. 2000;105(7):863-873

12. Miyazaki Y et al. Evidence that bone morphogenetic protein 4 has multiple biological functions during kidney and urinary tract development. *Kidney Int*. 2003; 63(3):835-844

13. Chevalier RL. Perinatal obstructive nephropathy. *Semin Perinatol*. 2004;28(2):124-131

14. Oshima K et al. Angiotensin type II receptor expression and ureteral budding. *J Urol*. 2001;166(5):1848-1852

15. Dunn NR et al. Haploinsufficient phenotypes in Bmp4 heterozygous null mice and modification by mutations in Gli3 and Alx4. *Dev Biol*. 1997;188(2):235-247

16. Hinman F. Renal counterbalance. *Cal West Med*. 1926;24(3):333-335

17. Taki M, Goldsmith DI, Spitzer A. Impact of age on effects of ureteral obstruction on renal function. *Kidney Int*. 1983;24(5):602-609

18. Chevalier RL et al. Unilateral ureteral obstruction in early development alters renal growth: dependence on the duration of obstruction. *J Urol*. 1999;161(1):309-313

19. Mandell J et al. Human fetal compensatory renal growth. *J Urol*. 1993;150(2 pt 2):790-792

20. Koff SA et al. The assessment of obstruction in the newborn with unilateral hydronephrosis by measuring the size of the opposite kidney. *J Urol*. 1994;152(2 pt 2): 596-599

21. Gruskin AB, Edelmann CM Jr, Yuan S. Maturational changes in renal blood flow in piglets. *Pediatr Res*. 1970; 4(1):7-13

22. Chevalier RL, Gomez RA. Response of the renin-angiotensin system to relief of neonatal ureteral obstruction. *Am J Physiol*. 1988;255(6 pt 2):F1070-7

23. Chevalier RL, Thornhill BA. Ureteral obstruction in the neonatal rat: renal nerves modulate hemodynamic effects. *Pediatr Nephrol*. 1995;9(4):447-450

24. Chevalier RL, Kaiser DL. Chronic partial ureteral obstruction in the neonatal guinea pig I. Influence of uninephrectomy on growth and hemodynamics. *Pediatr Res*. 1984;18(12):1266-1271

25. Chevalier RL, Thornhill BA, Gomez RA. EDRF modulates renal hemodynamics during unilateral ureteral obstruction in the rat. *Kidney Int*. 1992;42(2): 400-406

26. Greger R. Physiology of renal sodium transport. *Am J Med Sci*. 2000;319(1):51-62

27. Alexander RT, Grinstein S. Na+/H + exchangers and the regulation of volume. *Acta Physiol (Oxf)*. 2006;187 (1–2):159-167

28. Wen JG et al. Obstructive nephropathy: an update of the experimental research. *Urol Res*. 1999;27(1):29-39

29. Stecker JF Jr, Gillenwater JY. Experimental partial ureteral obstruction. I. Alteration in renal function. *Invest Urol*. 1971;8(4):377-385

30. Wilson DR. Micropuncture study of chronic obstructive nephropathy before and after release of obstruction. *Kidney Int*. 1972;2(3):119-130

31. Tanagho EA. Surgically induced partial urinary obstruction in the fetal lamb. 3. Ureteral obstruction. *Invest Urol*. 1972;10(1):35-52

32. Olsen L. Renal function in experimental chronic hydronephrosis. III. Glomerular and tubular functions in relation to renal pelvic volume. *Scand J Urol Nephrol*. 1976;(suppl 32):5-13

33. Josephson S. Experimental obstructive hydronephrosis in newborn rats III. Long-term effects on renal function. *J Urol*. 1983;129(2):396-400

34. Boron WF. Acid-base transport by the renal proximal tubule. *J Am Soc Nephrol*. 2006;17(9):2368-2382

35. Misseri R et al. Inflammatory mediators and growth factors in obstructive renal injury. *J Surg Res*. 2004;119(2): 149-159

36. Sean Eardley K, Cockwell P. Macrophages and progressive tubulointerstitial disease. *Kidney Int*. 2005;68(2): 437-455

37. Wada T et al. Gene therapy via blockade of monocyte chemoattractant protein-1 for renal fibrosis. *J Am Soc Nephrol*. 2004;15(4):940-948

38. Pittock ST et al. MCP-1 is up-regulated in unstressed and stressed HO-1 knockout mice: pathophysiologic correlates. *Kidney Int*. 2005;68(2):611-622

39. Esteban V et al. Angiotensin II, via AT1 and AT2 receptors and NF-kappaB pathway, regulates the inflammatory response in unilateral ureteral obstruction. *J Am Soc Nephrol*. 2004;15(6):1514-1529

40. Inazaki K et al. Smad3 deficiency attenuates renal fibrosis, inflammation, and apoptosis after unilateral ureteral obstruction. *Kidney Int*. 2004;66(2):597-604

41. Chevalier RL. Molecular and cellular pathophysiology of obstructive nephropathy. *Pediatr Nephrol*. 1999;13(7): 612-619

42. McVary KT, Maizels M. Urinary obstruction reduces glomerulogenesis in the developing kidney: a model in the rabbit. *J Urol*. 1989;142(2 pt 2):646-651. discussion 667-8

43. Peters CA et al. The response of the fetal kidney to obstruction. *J Urol*. 1992;148(2 pt 2):503-509

44. Chevalier RL et al. Recovery following relief of unilateral ureteral obstruction in the neonatal rat. *Kidney Int*. 1999;55(3):793-807

45. Okuda S et al. Influence of age on deterioration of the remnant kidney in uninephrectomized rats. *Clin Sci Lond*. 1987;72(5):571-576

46. O'Donnell MP et al. Age is a determinant of the glomerular morphologic and functional responses to chronic nephron loss. *J Lab Clin Med*. 1985;106(3):308-313

47. Quinlan MR et al. Exploring mechanisms involved in renal tubular sensing of mechanical stretch following ureteric obstruction. *Am J Physiol Ren Physiol*. 2008; 295(1):F1-F11

48. Alenghat FJ, Ingber DE. Mechanotransduction: all signals point to cytoskeleton, matrix, and integrins. *Sci STKE*. 2002;2002(119):PE6

49. Wang N, Butler JP, Ingber DE. Mechanotransduction across the cell surface and through the cytoskeleton. *Science*. 1993;260(5111):1124-1127

50. Klahr S, Ishidoya S, Morrissey J. Role of angiotensin II in the tubulointerstitial fibrosis of obstructive nephropathy. *Am J Kidney Dis*. 1995;26(1):141-146

51. Chertin B et al. Conservative treatment of ureteropelvic junction obstruction in children with antenatal diagnosis of hydronephrosis: lessons learned after 16 years of follow-up. *Eur Urol*. 2006;49(4):734-738

52. Rosen S, Heyman SN. Difficulties in understanding human "acute tubular necrosis": limited data and flawed animal models. *Kidney Int*. 2001;60(4):1220-1224

53. Lieberthal W, Nigam SK. Acute renal failure II. Experimental models of acute renal failure: imperfect but indispensable. *Am J Physiol Ren Physiol*. 2000;278 (1):F1-F12

54. Mizuguchi Y et al. A novel cell-permeable antioxidant peptide decreases renal tubular apoptosis and damage in unilateral ureteral obstruction. *Am J Physiol Ren Physiol*. 2008;295(5):F1545-F1553

55. Lee RS et al. Temporal variations of the postnatal rat urinary proteome as a reflection of systemic maturation. *Proteomics*. 2008;8(5):1097-112

56. Decramer S et al. Predicting the clinical outcome of congenital unilateral ureteropelvic junction obstruction in newborn by urinary proteome analysis. *Nat Med*. 2006;12(4):398-400

57. Mostbeck GH, Zontsich T, Turetschek K. Ultrasound of the kidney: obstruction and medical diseases. *Eur Radiol*. 2001;11(10):1878-1889

58. Shokeir AA. The diagnosis of upper urinary tract obstruction. *BJU Int*. 1999;83(8):893-900. quiz 900–1

59. Platt JF, Rubin JM, Ellis JH. Distinction between obstructive and nonobstructive pyelocaliectasis with duplex Doppler sonography. *Am J Roentgenol*. 1989;153(5):997-1000

60. Shokeir AA et al. Renal doppler ultrasound in children with obstructive uropathy: Effect of intravenous normal saline fluid load and furosemide. *J Urol*. 1996;156(4): 1455-1458

61. Whitaker RH. Diagnosis of obstruction in dilated ureters. *Ann R Coll Surg Engl*. 1973;53(3):153-166

62. Sperling H et al. The Whitaker test, a useful tool in renal grafts? *Urology*. 2000;56(1):49-52

63. Dubovsky EV, Russell CD. Advances in radionuclide evaluation of urinary tract obstruction. *Abdom Imaging*. 1998;23(1):17-26

64. English PJ et al. Modified method of diuresis renography for the assessment of equivocal pelviureteric junction obstruction. *Br J Urol*. 1987;59(1):10-14

65. Upsdell SM, Testa HJ, Lawson RS. The F-15 diuresis renogram in suspected obstruction of the upper urinary tract. *Br J Urol*. 1992;69(2):126-131

66. Pais VM, Strandhoy JW, Assimos DG. Pathophysiology of urinary tract obstruction. In: Wein AJ et al., eds. *Campbell-Walsh Urology*. Philadelphia, PA: Saunders; 2006

67. Smith RC et al. Diagnosis of acute flank pain: value of unenhanced helical CT. *Am J Roentgenol*. 1996;166(1): 97-101

68. Gentle DL et al. Protease inhibitor-induced urolithiasis. *Urology*. 1997;50(4):508-511

69. El-Nahas AR et al. Role of multiphasic helical computed tomography in planning surgical treatment for pelviureteric junction obstruction. *BJU Int*. 2004;94(4): 582-587

70. Lawler LP et al. Adult ureteropelvic junction obstruction: insights with three-dimensional multi-detector row CT. *Radiographics*. 2005;25(1):121-134

71. Leyendecker JR, Barnes CE, Zagoria RJ. MR urography: techniques and clinical applications. *Radiographics*. 2008;28(1):23-46. discussion 46–7

72. Karabacakoglu A et al. Diagnostic value of diuretic-enhanced excretory MR urography in patients with obstructive uropathy. *Eur J Radiol*. 2004;52(3):320-327

73. Lefort C et al. Dynamic MR urography in urinary tract obstruction: implementation and preliminary results. *Abdom Imaging*. 2006;31(2):232-240

74. Farnham SB et al. Pediatric urological causes of hypertension. *J Urol*. 2005;173(3):697-704

75. Kinn AC. Ureteropelvic junction obstruction: long-term followup of adults with and without surgical treatment. *J Urol*. 2000;164(3 pt 1):652-656

76. Parkhouse HF et al. Long-term outcome of boys with posterior urethral valves. *Br J Urol*. 1988;62(1):59-62

77. Vaughan ED Jr, Gillenwater JY. Diagnosis, characterization and management of post-obstructive diuresis. *J Urol*. 1973;109(2):286-292

78. Jones DA, George NJ, O'Reilly PH. Postobstructive renal function. *Semin Urol*. 1987;5(3):176-190

79. Nyman MA, Schwenk NM, Silverstein MD. Management of urinary retention: rapid versus gradual decompression and risk of complications. *Mayo Clin Proc*. 1997;72(10):951-956

80. Schlossberg SM, Vaughan ED Jr. The mechanism of unilateral post-obstructive diuresis. *J Urol.* 1984;131(3): 534-536

81. Kim SW et al. Diminished renal expression of aquaporin water channels in rats with experimental bilateral ureteral obstruction. *J Am Soc Nephrol.* 2001;12(10): 2019-2028

82. Frokiaer J et al. Bilateral ureteral obstruction downregulates expression of vasopressin-sensitive AQP-2 water

channel in rat kidney. *Am J Physiol.* 1996;270(4 pt 2): F657-F668

83. Kim SW et al. Diminished expression of sodium transporters in the ureteral obstructed kidney in rats. *Nephron Exp Nephrol.* 2004;96(3):e67-76

84. Norregaard R et al. COX-2 activity transiently contributes to increased water and NaCl excretion in the polyuric phase after release of ureteral obstruction. *Am J Physiol Ren Physiol.* 2007;292(5):F1322-1333

16

Pathophysiology of Lower Urinary Tract Obstruction

Marcus J. Drake and Ahmed M. Shaban

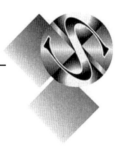

Introduction

Lower urinary tract obstruction signifies imped-ance of urine expulsion. It can give rise to symp-toms, though some people who appear to have outlet obstruction do not complain of any symp-tomatic problem. Classically associated with benign prostate enlargement in men, obstruction is being increasingly recognized in women, and there is ongoing debate on how to diagnose the problem. In particular, symptoms similar to those of obstruction can derive from reduced expulsive ability associated with impaired bladder contrac-tility, and the latter complicates the objective evaluation of outlet function. Mechanisms of obstruction can be either anatomical or func-tional, and the fundamental role of the central nervous system in regulating the phases of the micturition cycle and ensuring the synergic activity of the lower urinary tract means outlet obstruction in neurological disease is an impor-tant consideration.

The Normal Lower Urinary Tract

Anatomy

The lower urinary tract comprises the bladder and the bladder outlet. The bladder serves as the urine reservoir for storage and the expulsive organ for voiding. The muscle of the bladder wall is the detrusor, and the bladder lumen is lined by functionally active urothelium, subja-cent to which is a dense plexus of nerves and interstitial cells.

The bladder outlet comprises the urethra and urethral sphincters; it is anatomically complex and is different for men and women. In men, the urethra is of greater length and is subdivided into membranous, bulbar, and pendulous parts. At the start of the male urethra, the bladder neck serves as a genital sphincter, constricting at the time of seminal emission and ejaculation to ensure semen is propelled without passing ret-rogradely into the bladder. Just distal to the male bladder neck is the prostate, a secretory organ, which houses the ends of the ejaculatory ducts. The urethral sphincters are located just distal to the apex of the prostate, at the level of the pelvic floor. In women, the urethra is comparatively short (2–3 cm), and the bladder neck is anatom-ically poorly defined, probably serving no major functional role for continence. The urethral sphincters lie at the level of the pelvic floor, approximately at the midpoint of the urethra.

For both genders, the urethral sphincter com-prises smooth muscle (leiosphincter), which provides the background continuous contrac-tion, and an external skeletal muscle component (rhabdosphincter), for voluntary and reflex increases in urethral closure. The muscular com-ponent is distributed asymmetrically.[1] In women, supportive anchoring to the pelvic floor and ligaments is a key aspect for normal function,[2] along with a firm "back-plate0065" for urethral compression.[3,4]

C.R. Chapple and W.D. Steers (eds.), *Practical Urology: Essential Principles and Practice*,
DOI: 10.1007/978-1-84882-034-0_16, © Springer-Verlag London Limited 2011

Storage Function

Urinary storage is dependent on relaxation of the bladder to maximize reservoir capacity, combined with simultaneous closure of the outlet. The detrusor has some specific properties that allow it to elongate substantially without generating force during storage[5]; in addition, the muscle is inhibited by the sympathetic nervous system.

The nature of the sphincter activity can be demonstrated by urethral pressure profilometry, in which a catheter is drawn along the urethra, while measuring the pressure needed to keep continuous perfusion of saline through holes in the side of the catheter.[6] This technique provides an indication of tonic background contraction, additional superimposed voluntary contraction and the tone of the non-sphincteric parts of the urethra.

In men, circular constriction by sphincter activity is crucial for continence. In addition, the bladder neck is kept closed by sympathetic innervation, acting through alpha-1 adrenergic receptors.[7] Furthermore, tonic urethral contraction, sustained by intrinsic urethral cellular mechanisms,[8] means that the greater length of the male urethra renders men less prone to urinary incontinence. Finally, the prostate provides both active (contractile) and passive (elastic) contributions to outlet resistance, which are affected by ongoing prostate growth.[9] Nonetheless, while the bladder neck, prostate, and urethra provide some additional outlet closure, their removal by standard prostate surgery does not normally result in incontinence.

In women, sphincteric contraction serves both to elongate the urethra[10] and to "kink" it.[11] Additionally, the closure of the urethra is maintained by coaptation of the lining urothelium. Overall, continence is maintained by numerous factors.[12]

Voiding Function

Voiding represents a reversal of the bladder and outlet roles from that during storage, with global contraction of the detrusor muscle providing expulsive pressure, and synchronous outlet relaxation to permit flow. Detrusor contraction is achieved by widespread release of acetylcholine from the parasympathetic nerves ramifying throughout the muscle, which binds to muscarinic receptors.[13] In addition, intrinsic cellular structures may provide the sustained contraction that maintains voiding until bladder emptying is complete.[14] Synchronously, outlet relaxation permits the easy flow of urine along the urethra, with the peripheral nerves crucial in ensuring active relaxation of the smooth muscle components of the outlet.[15,16]

Voiding can be evaluated urodynamically, by simultaneously recording pressure within the bladder, the abdomen, and the urinary flow rate. Subtraction of abdominal pressure allows estimation of the component of the bladder pressure that is due to active detrusor contraction. In men, this detrusor pressure shows a clear increase at the time of voiding (Fig. 16.1); the pressure rise is less clearly apparent in women, because the overall lower outlet resistance results in pressure dissipation (Fig. 16.2).

Neural Control

The central nervous system (CNS) is responsible for regulating lower urinary tract function, imposing several crucial properties which define normal function;

1. During urine storage, activity in Onuf's nucleus in the ventral horn of the sacral part of the spinal cord maintains outlet closure.
2. During urine storage, the sympathetic neurones in the intermediolateral horn of the thoracolumbar spinal cord inhibit detrusor activity and maintain bladder neck closure.
3. The pontine part of the brainstem ("pontine micturition center") and parts of the midbrain ensure the synergic function of the bladder outlet and detrusor, such that only one element is actively contracting at any given moment. During voiding, the PMC actively relaxes the outlet by inhibition of Onuf's nucleus, while the parasympathetic neurones in the intermediolateral horn of the sacral spinal cord are activated to drive detrusor contraction.
4. The frontal cortex allows volitional control, so an individual has executive control on timing of micturition, which is thereby possible regardless of extent of bladder filling.

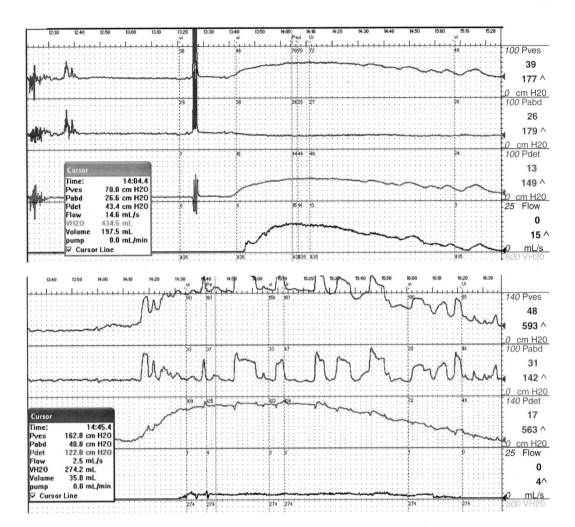

Figure 16.1. Male voiding cystometrogram; simultaneous pressure recordings have been made from a catheter in the rectum (*red line*) as a measure of abdominal pressure, and another catheter in the bladder (*blue line*). Since the bladder is an intra-abdominal organ, abdominal pressure change is visible in the bladder; subtracting the abdominal pressure allows the investigator to see when the bladder itself is contracting, which is plotted as the "subtracted detrusor pressure" (*green line*). Flow rate is shown in black. The top panel shows a normal male; at the time of the maximum flow of 14.6 ml/s, the subtracted detrusor pressure is 43.4. From the equation $P_{det}Q_{max} - 2Q_{max}$, this gives a BOOI of 14.2; anything below 20 is defined as not obstructed. In the *lower panel*, the study is of a man with bladder outlet obstruction. $P_{det}Q_{max}$ is 122, and Q_{max} is 2.5, giving a BOOI of 117; anything above 40 is taken as unequivocally obstructed. This man is also straining in an attempt to improve his flow rate, shown by the simultaneous intermittent increases in both abdominal and bladder pressure during the time of urine flow.

5. Additional CNS functions include sensory awareness of bladder filling, emotional aspects, and coordination with other vegetative functions such as bowel opening and blood pressure

The complexity of CNS control means that lower urinary tract dysfunction is a common consequence of clinical neurological disease.

Diagnosing Bladder Outlet Obstruction

Symptoms

Bladder outlet obstruction (BOO) represents a problem whereby some impedance, whether functional or anatomical, prevents the free flow

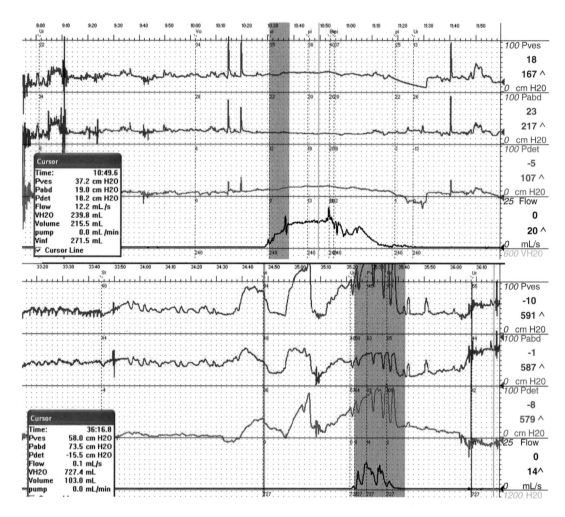

Figure 16.2. Female voiding cystometrogram; both women in this figure have previously had stress incontinence surgery. In the top trace, a lady who previously had had a colposuspension; the urine flow rate is fairly good (Q_{max} 12.2 mL/s), and associated increase in detrusor pressure to achieve this is very small (which is common in women). In the *lower panel*, from a lady with outlet obstruction after TVT, there is a greater increase in detrusor pressure, flow fails to start for some time, flow is intermittent, and the patient is straining. There was a significant post-void residual in the TVT patient, and no residual in the colposuspension patient.

of urine from the bladder. This may be asymptomatic if the detrusor contractility increases the pressure of expulsion. Nonetheless, in many patients there will be lower urinary tract symptoms (LUTS), including "voiding symptoms" experienced during voiding, and post-micturition symptoms immediately afterward (Table 16.1). A combination of BOO and reduced contractility can result in a post-void residual and chronic urinary retention. Ultimately, complete inability to void can arise from severe BOO, culminating as acute urinary retention – a painful bladder distension which presents as an emergency to

relieve the obstruction. Any of the symptoms listed in Table 16.1 suggests the possibility of BOO. However, very similar symptoms arise in people with reduced bladder contractility; thus, symptoms alone are inadequate for diagnosing BOO.[19] A complicating factor is the high prevalence of storage phase symptoms in people with BOO. It is unclear whether BOO gives rise to secondary bladder changes predisposing to storage LUTS. Certainly, BOO in the experimental setting leads to detrusor hypertrophy and abnormal detrusor contractions during bladder filling.[20] However, in the clinical setting, the relationship

Table 16.1. Voiding and post-micturition symptoms as defined by the International Continence Society (ICS) Standardisation Committee in 2002[17,18]

Voiding symptoms	
Slow stream	The patient's perception of reduced urine flow, usually compared to previous performance or in comparison with others
Intermittent stream	The urine flow stops and starts, on one or more occasions, during micturition
Hesitancy	Difficulty initiating micturition, resulting in a delay in the onset of voiding after the individual is ready to pass urine
Straining	Describes the muscular effort used to initiate, maintain, or improve the urinary stream
Terminal dribble	The term used to describe a prolonged final part of micturition, when the flow has slowed to a trickle/dribble
Post-micturition symptoms	
Feeling of incomplete emptying	A self-explanatory term for a feeling experienced by the individual after passing urine
Post micturition dribble	Involuntary loss of urine immediately after he or she has finished passing urine, usually after leaving the toilet in men, or after rising from the toilet in women

is not so clear-cut, since relief of obstruction with prostate resection surgery does not lead to resolution of storage urinary problems.[21]

Flow Rate and Post-void Residual

Flow rate machines measure flow volume over time and evaluate various parameters, of which the maximum flow rate (Q_{max}), flow pattern and post-void residual (PVR) volume are most widely used clinically. Findings have to be interpreted in the light of clinical circumstances; checking the voided volume (VV) falls into a

suitable range, and is comparable to the typical voided volume on the individual's frequency volume chart, is a means by which to ascertain that the flow rate test is representative and informative. Q_{max} is affected by VV, so nomograms have been developed to aid interpretation, exemplified by the Liverpool nomograms for men and women[22] and the Siroky nomogram for men.[23,24] At low VV, the bladder has insufficient volume to expel and Q_{max} may be reduced as a result; nonetheless, informative conclusions can sometimes be drawn regardless of low VV.[25] Above 550 mL, the bladder starts to overfill and efficiency declines,[26] again causing artefactual reduction in Q_{max}. Failure of expulsion of the entire bladder contents, leading to a PVR, signifies inefficient bladder emptying; this suggests either reduced bladder contractility or outlet obstruction, or both.

The normal flow curve should have a rapid upstroke, a clear Q_{max}, and decline quickly to end cleanly. Abnormal patterns include;

1. Prostatic (men): Characterized by a slow upstroke, reduced Q_{max}, and prolonged downstroke.
2. Urethral stricture (men): the pattern has a "plateau" appearance.
3. Intermittent (men or women): several peaks in the flow curve can result if the patient strains during voiding. Likewise, a poorly sustained detrusor contraction causes the stream to fluctuate.

In men of the appropriate age group, a prostatic pattern with a reduced Q_{max} when VV is adequate is suggestive of BOO but accuracy is inadequate by itself.[27] Where Q_{max} is above the expected range, outlet obstruction is unlikely. However, sensitivity of flow rate testing by itself as a diagnostic test for BOO is inadequate.

Voiding Cystometry

BOO is characterized by increased detrusor pressure and reduced urine flow rate.[17] It is usually diagnosed by studying the synchronous values of flow rate and detrusor pressure, and is thus a urodynamic diagnosis.[17]

Consensus on what constitutes BOO in men has been achieved because of the relatively homogeneous nature of male BOO, reflecting high prevalence of benign prostate enlargement in older men, and the availability of transurethral resection surgery to relieve obstruction. This provided suitable circumstances to derive urodynamic nomograms[28]; the nomogram of Abrams and Griffiths was adopted and adapted by the International Continence Society as a standardized criterion for diagnosing male BOO. Thus a plot of Q_{max} against simultaneous detrusor pressure ($P_{det}Q_{max}$) allows derivation of the bladder outlet obstruction index (BOOI), from which a definite diagnosis of BOO, equivocal BOO or unobstructed can be made, as illustrated in Fig. 16.1. The concept superseded the earlier concept of a urethral resistance factor, which originated from rigid tube hydrodynamics. Since the urethra is an irregular and distensible conduit, whose walls and surroundings have active and passive elements which influence the flow, a resistance factor does not reliably provide a valid comparison between patients.[29]

While measurements to derive a BOOI are generally made by invasive urodynamic testing, noninvasive techniques are now emerging[30,31] which may be able to derive an estimate of the detrusor pressure generating maximum flow (i.e., with no catheter within the bladder lumen to measure pressure). Penile cuff intermittent urethral compression[32] is one approach and a nomogram has been developed for the technique.[33] Similar noninvasive pressure measurement can be derived from a modified condom collecting device.[34] Detrusor wall thickness is another parameter which may also indirectly signify the presence of BOO.[35,36]

Diagnosis of BOO in women has not been standardized and remains an area of ongoing discussion.[37] Proposals for urodynamic diagnosis of BOO have been made as follows;

1. Female BOO nomogram[38]; derived a nomogram based on study of several hundred women defined as obstructed on clinical grounds, with quite a heterogeneous group of causative pathologies. The study estimated the prevalence of female BOO at 6.5%. The nomogram employs somewhat different parameters from the male BOOI, using the maximum detrusor pressure ascertained during invasive urodynamics and the maximum flow rate on free flow testing.

2. An alternative nomogram has been proposed by a different group.[39]

3. The BOOI is applicable in men with benign prostate enlargement and no relevant neurological problem. Nonetheless, the parameters of the BOOI have been evaluated in women, such that the BOOI evaluated in conjunction with Q_{max} could be a usable urodynamic parameter of female BOO.[40] A separate study came to similar conclusions, but cut-off values were different.[41]

4. An alternative compared women with anatomical BOO against women with stress urinary incontinence,[42] with revisions using a larger study group in 2000,[43] and a control group without stress incontinence in 2004.[44]

5. A panel of criteria derived during videourodynamic evaluation has been proposed based on study of a group of women clinically felt to have BOO.[45]

6. Area under the curve of detrusor pressure during voiding, adjusted for voided volume, is a proposed parameter for diagnosing female BOO, though more work is needed.[46]

7. Abnormalities of free flow pattern are seen in a greater proportion of women subsequently concluded to be obstructed on urodynamic evaluation.[47]

Causes of Bladder Outlet Obstruction

Male

The additional anatomical structure of the male bladder outlet is the prostate gland, which encompasses the urethra between the genital and urethral sphincters. With aging, the gland undergoes benign prostate enlargement (BPE), which can typically be shown to be a consequence of benign prostate hyperplasia (BPH); BPH can only be diagnosed where pathological specimens by biopsy or resection are available.[48] The prevalence of BPH determined from autopsy studies shows that it does not occur below the age of 30 years and that almost 90% of men have developed BPH by their ninth decade.[49] Likewise,

Figure 16.3. *Left panel;* a urethroscopic view of the intrusion of the lateral lobes and median lobe of a benignly enlarged prostate gland. *Right panel;* urethroscopic view of a dense fibrotic urethral stricture.

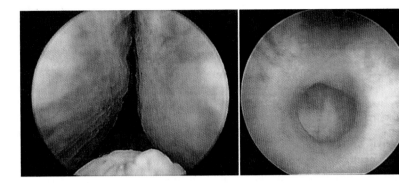

there is a steady increase in both LUTS[50] and BPE,[51] and all three processes are clearly interrelated with ageing in men.[52]

Implicitly, the intrusion of the prostate into the urethral lumen in BPE (Fig. 16.3) can be expected to provide a degree of anatomical impedance to urine flow during voiding by direct flow impedance, and by distortion of the bladder outlet. Thus, flow rate does decline with ageing in a population of men with BPE.[25] The role of anatomical impedance to flow is supported clinically by the response to treatment aimed at reducing male sex hormones, which reduces the trophic factors giving rise to BPH and thereby can partly reverse the enlargement. Within the prostate, the conversion of androgens to dihydrotestosterone by 5-alpha reductase is a means by which this can be achieved.[53] A second contribution to BOO in BPE is the active contraction of smooth muscle in the prostate stroma. The smooth muscle of the prostate expresses alpha-adrenergic receptors, falling into at least two subtypes in the human prostate.[54] Clinically, alpha-adrenergic antagonists relax prostate smooth muscle, indicating a contribution of functional prostate muscle activity in BOO.[55] On this basis, alpha-adrenergic antagonists and hormonal therapy may respectively decrease BOO by relaxing or shrinking the prostate. These clinical observations support the hypothesis that there are both dynamic and static components of BOO associated with BPE.

The Olmstead County Study of Urinary Symptoms and Health Status[56] studied 2,115 men between 40 and 79 years of age and showed that the severity of LUTS, peak flow rate, and extent of prostate enlargement were all age-dependent and interrelated. However, the Veterans Affairs Cooperative Study[57] comparing

placebo, the alpha-blocker terazosin, the 5-alpha reductase inhibitor finasteride and combination therapy, suggested that factors other than BOO alone almost certainly contribute to LUTS in BPH. Recent studies using botulinum injections within the prostate suggest that afferent nerve activity may also be an element of LUTS in BPE.[58] Furthermore, the persistence of LUTS after effective surgical management of BPE[21] strongly suggests that age-related changes in bladder function contribute to male LUTS as a codependent variable alongside BPE.[59] The inherent difficulties of controlling for the range of contributory variables means that the pathophysiology of male LUTS will remain a source of considerable scientific debate for the foreseeable future.

Urethral strictures are another mechanism giving rise to BOO in men. They comprise an inelastic circumferential fibrous constriction (Fig. 16.3), and thereby differ from BPE in that there is not contribution of active muscle contraction to the BOO. They can be present at any point along the urethra; postsurgical bladder neck stenosis is a related situation. Strictures have comparatively little effect on lower urinary tract function until they cause significant constriction of the lumen. Characteristically, the pattern of urine flow differs from that seen in BPE. Strictures usually arise as a consequence of urethral trauma, which can be iatrogenic. Congenital male urethral strictures have been described. Cobb's collar is a congenital narrowing in the male urethral bulb of uncertain etiology.[60]

BPE and urethra stricture are by far the most common causes of BOO in men. Rare causes of obstruction in men include congenital urethral abnormalities,[61,62] foreign bodies,[63] ureterocoele,[64] adult onset voiding dysfunction.[65]

Female

In women, several factors can contribute to BOO (Table 16.2), which consequently represents a more diverse situation pathophysiologically than is the case in men. As discussed above, this renders formal standardized diagnosis problematic.

1. Pelvic Organ Prolapse (POP). Deficiency of ligamentous support of the pelvic floor and weakness of the musculature results in prolapse of pelvic and abdominal organs. Where the anterior vaginal compartment is affected, the altered configuration may distort the urethra, which can impair voiding. Where middle compartment prolapse to the level of the vaginal introitus is present, a direct compression effect on the urethra could also occur. Obstructive voiding, LUTS, in general, and occult stress incontinence can all coexist.[72] Some women with prolapse find that voiding is impeded during the daytime, as a consequence of upright posture, and complain of incontinence overnight, when the supine position reduces the prolapse. The precise effect can be hard to evaluate urodynamically,[73] since effects on voiding are dependent on the patient's position, which will affect the anatomical relationship between the abnormally mobile structures and markedly influence their function.

2. BOO caused by stress incontinence surgery is symptomatic of the conflicting roles of the lower urinary tract in being responsible both for urinary storage and intermittent expulsion of the urine. In women with incontinence, the need to improve urine storage surgically carries an implicit risk that voiding may be impaired. For most women, voiding function is satisfactorily preserved, but a minority do suffer impaired voiding, taking the form of voiding symptoms, an increased post-void residual or acute urinary retention. This is recognized for the main surgical options available, including midurethral slings,[74] other forms of sling[75] and colposuspension,[76] along with techniques no longer in general use such as the Stamey procedure[77] and bone-anchored slings.[78]

3. Functional causes; the lower urinary tract musculature and the range of CNS structures contributing to their regulation requires coordinated activity to achieve normal function. Some women manifest voiding abnormalities, which appear to derive from excessive activity, failure of relaxation, or impaired coordination of some of these complex components. In part, this can derive from failure to acquire normal toileting habits in childhood, or acquired in adulthood,[65] leading to dysfunctional voiding[79] and "pseudo-dyssynergia." Fowler's syndrome is an acute onset condition arising in adult women, characterized by painless retention, and diagnosed by high urethral closure pressures and abnormal urethral sphincter EMG activity [80] (Fig. 16.4).

Neurourology

Impaired voiding function is common in patients with neurological disease, resulting from reduced bladder contractility (Fig. 16.4), BOO, or both. In lower motor neurone neurological lesions, BOO can be a consequence of pelvic floor denervation, leading to pelvic organ prolapse and urethral distortion. For upper motor neurone neurological lesions, the problem is one of failure of the urethral sphincter to relax appropriately at the time of voiding. This can

Table 16.2. Causes of female bladder outlet obstruction

Anatomical	Functional
Gynecological; pelvic organ prolapse, fibroids, lichen sclerosus[66]	Bladder neck obstruction
Postsurgical	Pseudodyssynergia
Urethral abnormalities, such as diverticulum,[67] stenosis[68]	Fowler's syndrome
Mass lesions such as uterine fibroids,[69] other intra-abdominal lesions[70]	
Ureterocoele[71]	

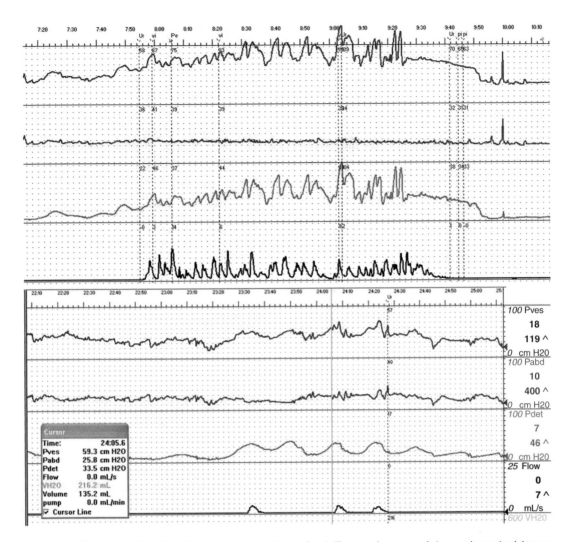

Figure 16.4. Two women with an intermittent urinary stream. In the *top panel*, a neurologically normal woman with dysfunctional voiding and outlet obstruction due to Fowler's syndrome. *Lower panel*; voiding cystometrogram from a female patient with multiple sclerosis. The trace shows a wandering, poorly sustained detrusor contraction, resulting in an intermittent and very poor flow, with incomplete emptying. It would be extremely hard to ascertain whether outlet obstruction is also present in this patient.

occur as a consequence of problems in the sacral part of the spinal cord causing tonic contraction.[81] It is also seen when there is loss of communication between the brainstem and the lower urinary tract, which results in detrusor sphincter dyssynergia (DSD).[82] DSD is common in high spinal cord injury and also occurs in advanced multiple sclerosis. It gives rise to a characteristically intermittent flow rate, and post-void residuals tend to be significant. Because of the high pressures generated during voiding, upper urinary tract function can be impaired, leading to hydronephrosis and renal failure.[83] When examined endoscopically, the bladder neck of these patients is often hypertrophied, and the bladder wall itself is trabeculated and diverticulated.

Conclusions

Both men and women are at risk of BOO, but the more homogenous nature of BOO in men has allowed a standard approach to diagnosis, which is lacking in women. Anatomical constriction or distortion (or direct blockage from a foreign body) result in BOO. In addition, excessive sphincter activity, as a result of neurological disease of the CNS, or idiopathic overactivity of the sphincter muscles themselves, is an unusual but important patient group. Diagnosis cannot rely on symptoms alone, and an overall impression, using symptoms, flow rate testing, cystometrogram, and imaging all have a part to play.

References

1. Yucel S, Baskin LS. An anatomical description of the male and female urethral sphincter complex. *J Urol.* 171:1890-1897

2. Wallner C, Dabhoiwala NF, Deruiter MC, Lamers WH. The anatomical components of urinary continence. *Eur Urol.* 2009;55(4):932-943

3. Ashton-Miller JA, DeLancey JO. Functional anatomy of the female pelvic floor. *Ann NY Acad Sci.* 2007;1101: 266-296

4. DeLancey JO. Structural support of the urethra as it relates to stress urinary incontinence: the hammock hypothesis. *Am J Obstet Gynecol.* 1994;170:1713-1720. discussion 20–3

5. Brading AF. Spontaneous activity of lower urinary tract smooth muscles: correlation between ion channels and tissue function. *J Physiol.* 2006;570:13-22

6. Brown M, Wickham JE. The urethral pressure profile. *Br J Urol.* 1969;41:211-217

7. Bolton JF, Whittlestone TH, Sibley GN. Comparisons of the responses of anterior and posterior human adult male bladder neck smooth muscle to in vitro stimulation. *BJU Int.* 2008;102:1737-1742

8. Sergeant GP, Thornbury KD, McHale NG, Hollywood MA. Interstitial cells of Cajal in the urethra. *J Cell Mol Med.* 2006;10:280-291

9. Ichiyanagi O, Sasagawa I, Suzuki Y, Ishigooka M, Nakada T. Relation between urethral elasticity and bladder outlet obstruction and histologic composition of the prostate in patients with benign prostatic hyperplasia. *Urology.* 1999;53:1149-1153

10. Mitterberger M, Pinggera GM, Neuwirt H, et al. Three-dimensional ultrasonography of the urinary bladder: preliminary experience of assessment in patients with haematuria. *BJU Int.* 2007;99:111-116

11. Sebe P, Fritsch H, Oswald J, et al. Fetal development of the female external urinary sphincter complex: an anatomical and histological study. *J Urol.* 2005;173:1738-1742. discussion 42

12. Petros PE, Woodman PJ. The integral theory of continence. *Int Urogynecol J Pelvic Floor Dysfunct.* 2008;19: 35-40

13. Andersson KE. Detrusor contraction – focus on muscarinic receptors. *Scand J Urol Nephrol Suppl.* 2004; 215:54-57

14. Drake MJ. The integrative physiology of the bladder. *Ann R Coll Surg Engl.* 2007;89:580-585

15. Ho KM, McMurray G, Brading AF, Noble JG, Ny L, Andersson KE. Nitric oxide synthase in the heterogeneous population of intramural striated muscle fibres of the human membranous urethral sphincter. *J Urol.* 1998;159:1091-1096

16. Ho KM, Ny L, McMurray G, Andersson KE, Brading AF, Noble JG. Co-localization of carbon monoxide and nitric oxide synthesizing enzymes in the human urethral sphincter. *J Urol.* 1999;161:1968-1972

17. Abrams P, Cardozo L, Fall M, et al. The standardisation of terminology of lower urinary tract function: report from the Standardisation Sub-committee of the International Continence Society. *Neurourol Urodyn.* 2002; 21:167-178

18. Abrams P, Cardozo L, Fall M, et al. The standardisation of terminology of lower urinary tract function: report from the Standardisation Sub-committee of the International Continence Society. *Am J Obstet Gynecol.* 2002;187:116-126

19. de la Rosette JJ, Witjes WP, Schafer W, et al. Relationships between lower urinary tract symptoms and bladder outlet obstruction: results from the ICS-"BPH" study. *Neurourol Urodyn.* 1998;17:99-108

20. Pandita RK, Fujiwara M, Alm P, Andersson KE. Cystometric evaluation of bladder function in non-anesthetized mice with and without bladder outlet obstruction. *J Urol.* 2000;164:1385-1389

21. Thomas AW, Cannon A, Bartlett E, Ellis-Jones J, Abrams P. The natural history of lower urinary tract dysfunction in men: minimum 10-year urodynamic followup of transurethral resection of prostate for bladder outlet obstruction. *J Urol.* 2005;174:1887-1991

22. Haylen BT, Ashby D, Sutherst JR, Frazer MI, West CR. Maximum and average urine flow rates in normal male and female populations – the Liverpool nomograms. *Br J Urol.* 1989;64:30-38

23. Siroky MB, Olsson CA, Krane RJ. The flow rate nomogram: I. Development. *J Urol.* 1979;122:665-668

24. Siroky MB, Olsson CA, Krane RJ. The flow rate nomogram: II. Clinical correlation. *J Urol.* 1980;123: 208-210

25. Reynard JM, Yang Q, Donovan JL, et al. The ICS-"BPH" study: uroflowmetry, lower urinary tract symptoms and bladder outlet obstruction. *Br J Urol.* 1998;82: 619-623

26. Pernkopf D, Plas E, Lang T, et al. Uroflow nomogram for male adolescents. *J Urol.* 2005;174:1436-1439. discussion 9

27. Idzenga T, Pel JJ, van Mastrigt R. Accuracy of maximum flow rate for diagnosing bladder outlet obstruction can be estimated from the ICS nomogram. *Neurourol Urodyn.* 2008;27:97-98

28. Abrams PH, Griffiths DJ. The assessment of prostatic obstruction from urodynamic measurements and from residual urine. *Br J Urol.* 1979;51:129-134

29. Abrams P, Blaivas JG, Stanton SL, Andersen JT. The standardisation of terminology of lower urinary tract function. The International Continence Society Committee on Standardisation of Terminology. *Scand J Urol Nephrol Suppl.* 1988;114:5-19

30. Belal M, Abrams P. Noninvasive methods of diagnosing bladder outlet obstruction in men. Part 2: noninvasive urodynamics and combination of measures. *J Urol.* 2006;176:29-35

31. Belal M, Abrams P. Noninvasive methods of diagnosing bladder outlet obstruction in men. Part 1: nonurodynamic approach. *J Urol.* 2006;176:22-28

32. Harding CK, Robson W, Drinnan MJ, Griffiths CJ, Ramsden PD, Pickard RS. An automated penile compression release maneuver as a noninvasive test for diagnosis of bladder outlet obstruction. *J Urol.* 2004;172:2312-2315

33. Griffiths CJ, Harding C, Blake C, et al. A nomogram to classify men with lower urinary tract symptoms using urine flow and noninvasive measurement of bladder pressure. *J Urol.* 2005;174:1323-1326. discussion 6; author reply 6

34. Pel JJ, van Mastrigt R. A flow rate cut-off value as a criterion for the accurate non-invasive measurement of bladder pressure using a condom-type catheter. *Urol Res.* 2003;31:177-182

35. Oelke M, Hofner K, Jonas U, de la Rosette JJ, Ubbink DT, Wijkstra H. Diagnostic accuracy of noninvasive tests to evaluate bladder outlet obstruction in men: detrusor wall thickness, uroflowmetry, postvoid residual urine, and prostate volume. *Eur Urol.* 2007;52:827-834

36. Oelke M, Hofner K, Wiese B, Grunewald V, Jonas U. Increase in detrusor wall thickness indicates bladder outlet obstruction (BOO) in men. *World J Urol.* 2002;19:443-452

37. Akikwala TV, Fleischman N, Nitti VW. Comparison of diagnostic criteria for female bladder outlet obstruction. *J Urol.* 2006;176:2093-2097

38. Blaivas JG, Groutz A. Bladder outlet obstruction nomogram for women with lower urinary tract symptomatology. *Neurourol Urodyn.* 2000;19:553-564

39. Di Grazia E, Troyo Sanroman R, Aceves JG. Proposed urodynamic pressure-flow nomogram to diagnose female bladder outlet obstruction. *Arch Ital Urol Androl.* 2004;76:59-65

40. Gravina GL, Costa AM, Ronchi P, Galatioto GP, Luana G, Vicentini C. Bladder outlet obstruction index and maximal flow rate during urodynamic study as powerful predictors for the detection of urodynamic obstruction in women. *Neurourol Urodyn.* 2007;26:247-253

41. Kuo HC. Urodynamic parameters for the diagnosis of bladder outlet obstruction in women. *Urol Int.* 2004;72:46-51

42. Chassagne S, Bernier PA, Haab F, Roehrborn CG, Reisch JS, Zimmern PE. Proposed cutoff values to define bladder outlet obstruction in women. *Urology.* 1998;51:408-411

43. Lemack GE, Zimmern PE. Pressure flow analysis may aid in identifying women with outflow obstruction. *J Urol.* 2000;163:1823-1828

44. Defreitas GA, Zimmern PE, Lemack GE, Shariat SF. Refining diagnosis of anatomic female bladder outlet obstruction: comparison of pressure-flow study parameters in clinically obstructed women with those of normal controls. *Urology.* 2004;64:675-679. discussion 9–81

45. Nitti VW, Tu LM, Gitlin J. Diagnosing bladder outlet obstruction in women. *J Urol.* 1999;161:1535-1540

46. Cormier L, Ferchaud J, Galas JM, Guillemin F, Mangin P. Diagnosis of female bladder outlet obstruction and relevance of the parameter area under the curve of detrusor pressure during voiding: preliminary results. *J Urol.* 2002;167:2083-2087

47. Klijer R, Bar K, Bialek W. Bladder outlet obstruction in women: difficulties in the diagnosis. *Urol Int.* 2004;73:6-10

48. Abrams P. LUTS, BPH, BPE, BPO: a plea for the logical use of correct terms. *Rev Urol.* 1999 Spring;1:65

49. Berry SJ, Coffey DS, Walsh PC, Ewing LL. The development of human benign prostatic hyperplasia with age. *J Urol.* 1984;132:474-479

50. Parsons JK, Bergstrom J, Silberstein J, Barrett-Connor E. Prevalence and characteristics of lower urinary tract symptoms in men aged > or = 80 years. *Urology.* 2008;72:318-321

51. McConnell JD, Roehrborn CG, Bautista OM, et al. The long-term effect of doxazosin, finasteride, and combination therapy on the clinical progression of benign prostatic hyperplasia. *N Engl J Med.* 18, 2003;349:2387-2398

52. Roehrborn CG. BPH progression: concept and key learning from MTOPS, ALTESS, COMBAT, and ALF-ONE. *BJU Int.* 2008;101(Suppl 3):17-21

53. Shirakawa T, Okada H, Acharya B, et al. Messenger RNA levels and enzyme activities of 5 alpha-reductase types 1 and 2 in human benign prostatic hyperplasia (BPH) tissue. *Prostate.* 1, 2004;58:33-40

54. Maruyama K, Fukutomi J, Chiba T, et al. Two district alpha(1)-adrenoceptor subtypes in the human prostate: assessment by radioligand binding assay using 3H-prazosin. *Gen Pharmacol.* 1996;27:1377-1381

55. Garg G, Singh D, Saraf S. Management of benign prostate hyperplasia: an overview of alpha-adrenergic antagonist. *Biol Pharm Bull.* 2006;29:1554-1558

56. Girman CJ, Jacobsen SJ, Guess HA, et al. Natural history of prostatism: relationship among symptoms, prostate volume and peak urinary flow rate. *J Urol.* 1995;153:1510-1515

57. Lepor H, Williford WO, Barry MJ, Haakenson C, Jones K. The impact of medical therapy on bother due to symptoms, quality of life and global outcome, and factors predicting response. Veterans Affairs Cooperative Studies Benign Prostatic Hyperplasia Study Group. *J Urol.* 1998;160:1358-1367

58. Ilie CP, Chancellor MB. Perspective of botox for treatment of male lower urinary tract symptoms. *Curr Opin Urol.* 2009;19:20-25

59. Housami F, Abrams P. Persistent detrusor overactivity after transurethral resection of the prostate. *Curr Urol Rep.* 2008;9:284-290

60. Cranston D, Davies AH, Smith JC. Cobb's collar – a forgotten entity. *Br J Urol.* 1990;66:294-296

61. Kajbafzadeh A. Congenital urethral anomalies in boys. Part I: posterior urethral valves. *Urol J.* Spring 2005;2:59-78

62. Kajbafzadeh A. Congenital urethral anomalies in boys. Part II. *Urol J.* Summer 2005;2:125-131

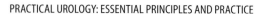
63. Kim ED, Moty A, Wilson DD, Zeagler D. Treatment of a complete lower urinary tract obstruction secondary to an expandable foam sealant. *Urology*. 2002;60:164

64. Shetty BP, John SD, Swischuk LE, Angel CA. Bladder neck obstruction caused by a large simple ureterocele in a young male. *Pediatr Radiol*. 1995;25:460-461

65. Groutz A, Blaivas JG, Pies C, Sassone AM. Learned voiding dysfunction (non-neurogenic, neurogenic bladder) among adults. *Neurourol Urodyn*. 2001;20:259-268

66. Attaran M, Rome E, Gidwani GP. Unusual presentation of lichen sclerosuis in an adolescent. *J Pediatr Adolesc Gynecol*. 2000;13:99

67. Chou CP, Levenson RB, Elsayes KM, et al. Imaging of female urethral diverticulum: an update. *Radiographics*. 2008;28:1917-1930

68. Keegan KA, Nanigian DK, Stone AR. Female urethral stricture disease. *Curr Urol Rep*. 2008;9:419-423

69. Novi JM, Shaunik A, Mulvihill BH, Morgan MA. Acute urinary retention caused by a uterine leiomyoma: a case report. *J Reprod Med*. 2004;49:131-132

70. Advincula AP, Hernandez JC. Acute urinary retention caused by a large peritoneal inclusion cyst: a case report. *J Reprod Med*. 2006;51:202-204

71. Merlini E, Lelli Chiesa P. Obstructive ureterocele – an ongoing challenge. *World J Urol*. 2004;22:107-114

72. Romanzi LJ, Chaikin DC, Blaivas JG. The effect of genital prolapse on voiding. *J Urol*. February 1999;161:581-586

73. Mueller ER, Kenton K, Mahajan S, FitzGerald MP, Brubaker L. Urodynamic prolapse reduction alters urethral pressure but not filling or pressure flow parameters. *J Urol*. 2007;177:600-603

74. Ordorica R, Rodriguez AR, Coste-Delvecchio F, Hoffman M, Lockhart J. Disabling complications with slings for managing female stress urinary incontinence. *BJU Int*. 2008;102:333-336

75. Hilton P. A clinical and urodynamic study comparing the Stamey bladder neck suspension and suburethral sling procedures in the treatment of genuine stress incontinence. *Br J Obstet Gynaecol*. 1989;96:213-220

76. Wang AC, Chen MC. Comparison of tension-free vaginal taping versus modified Burch colposuspension on urethral obstruction: a randomized controlled trial. *Neurourol Urodyn*. 2003;22:185-190

77. Wang AC. Burch colposuspension vs. Stamey bladder neck suspension. A comparison of complications with special emphasis on detrusor instability and voiding dysfunction. *J Reprod Med*. 1996;41:529-533

78. Goldman HB, Zimmern PE. The treatment of female bladder outlet obstruction. *BJU Int*. 2006;98:359-366

79. Bael A, Lax H, de Jong TP, et al. The relevance of urodynamic studies for urge syndrome and dysfunctional voiding: a multicenter controlled trial in children. *J Urol*. 2008;180:1486-1493. discussion 94–5

80. Swinn MJ, Fowler CJ. Isolated urinary retention in young women, or Fowler's syndrome. *Clin Auton Res*. 2001;11:309-311

81. Sakakibara R, Hattori T, Uchiyama T, Yamanishi T, Ito H, Ito K. Neurogenic failures of the external urethral sphincter closure and relaxation; a videourodynamic study. *Auton Neurosci*. 14, 2001;86:208-215

82. Karsenty G, Reitz A, Wefer B, Boy S, Schurch B. Understanding detrusor sphincter dyssynergia – significance of chronology. *Urology*. 2005;66:763-768

83. Ahmed HU, Shergill IS, Arya M, Shah PJ. Management of detrusor-external sphincter dyssynergia. *Nat Clin Pract Urol*. July 2006;3:368-380

17

Urologic Endocrinology

Paolo Verze and Vincenzo Mirone

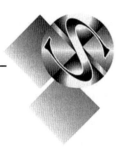

Urology is a specialist discipline having both medical and surgical aspects. In recent years, a growing interest in medical urological diseases of mainly endocrinological origin has emerged. Within this context, age-related male hypogonadism is of paramount importance. Recent preclinical and clinical data has demonstrated the critical consequences of hypogonadism not only on sexual behavior, but also on the entire psychophysical health of men as testosterone regulates the functional properties of multiple body tissues.

The Testis

Normal Androgen Metabolism

Testosterone, mainly secreted by Leydig's cells into the testes, is the major active sex hormone circulating in the blood of males. Its production is regulated by a negative feedback system involving a gonadotropin-releasing hormone (GnRH) and a luteinizing hormone (LH).[1] Testes produce 0.24 μmol/day of testosterone. The adrenal cortex contributes to circulating androgen levels by producing 0.002 μmol/day of androgens, mainly as androstenedione. In males, testosterone secretion begins in fetal life with peak concentrations seen at 12 weeks of gestation. A second testosterone secretion peak is observed at birth. Then, up until puberty, testosterone levels in males are low and similar to those in females. Pulsatile secretion of gonadotropin-releasing hormones and

luteinizing hormones begins at the onset of puberty and results in the maturity of the Leydig cells. Testosterone is metabolized into dihydrotestosterone by 5-alpha reductase and to estradiol by aromatase. In young men, there is a diurnal variation in serum testosterone concentration, with the highest values seen at 8 AM and the lowest in late afternoon.[2] Total testosterone circulates mostly in the blood and is 98% bound to serum proteins, primarily a sex hormone-binding globulin (SHBG) and albumin; only 1–2% of serum testosterone is free of bound protein. The combination of albumin-bound (weakly bound) testosterone and free testosterone is referred to as bioavailable testosterone, which is available to target tissues for androgenic action.[3]

Hypogonadism: Definition and Classification

Hypogonadism represents a state of impaired testosterone secretion, which may occur if the hypothalamic-pituitary-gonadal axis is interrupted at any level. Primary (hypergonadotropic) hypogonadism refers to testicular disorders and is characterized by low serum testosterone levels despite high levels of the follicle-stimulating hormone (FSH) and the luteinizing hormone (LH). Secondary (hypogonadotropic) hypogonadism is characterized by failure of gonadal function

C.R. Chapple and W.D. Steers (eds.), *Practical Urology: Essential Principles and Practice*,
DOI: 10.1007/978-1-84882-034-0_17, © Springer-Verlag London Limited 2011

secondary to deficient gonadotropin secretion, the result of either a pituitary or hypothalamic defect, and is commonly seen in association with structural lesions or functional defects affecting this region. Causes of primary hypogonadism include genetic conditions (e.g., Klinefelter syndrome, gonadal dysgenesis); anatomic defects; infection; tumor; injury; iatrogenic causes (surgery or certain medications); and/or alcohol abuse.[4] Hypogonadotropic hypogonadism may result from failure of the hypothalamic LHRH pulse generator or from the inability of the pituitary to respond with secretions of LH and FSH. It is most commonly observed as one aspect of multiple pituitary hormone deficiencies resulting from malformations (e.g., septo-optic dysplasia or other midline defects) or lesions of the pituitary that are acquired postnatally (such as tumors, infectious diseases, trauma, vascular diseases or radiation.[4] In 1944, Kallmann and colleagues were the first to describe familial isolated

gonadotropin deficiency.[5] Recently, many other genetic causes for hypogonadotropic hypogonadism have been identified such as mutations in the gene coding for the GnRH (LHRH) receptor.[6] According to Australian consensus guidelines, secondary (hypogonadotropic) hypogonadism is indicated by $T < 231$ ng/dL without LH elevations.[7] The clinical picture of testosterone deficiency is dependent on the time at which this deficiency appears and the extent of the deficiency (Table 17.1).[9] Treatment of patients with hypergonadotropic hypogonadism involves replacement of sex steroids. For treatment of patients with hypogonadotropic hypogonadism, the usual approach is the replacement of sex steroids that initiate development and maintain secondary gender characteristics. Sex steroid replacement does not result in increased testicular size in males nor fertility in males or females. Gonadotropin or GnRH replacement is offered to the patient when stimulated fertility is desired.[10]

Table 17.1. Signs of androgen deficiency (Reprinted from Jockenhovel[8]; Table 2.1, p. 31)

Organ	Before end of puberty	After end of puberty
Bones	Excessive eunuchoid growth, osteoporosis	Osteoporosis
Larynx	Voice does not break	No change in voice
Hair	Feminile hair type • Horizontal pubic hair line • Hair at temples straight across • No facial hair • No body hair	Decreasing facial, armpit, pubic and body hair, no androgenic alopecia (at temples)
Skin	Dry skin and no acne in puberty as no sebum produced, pallor	No sebum produced, atrophy, pallor, fine wrinkles
Erythropoiesis	Anemia	Anemia
Musculature	Underdeveloped, no strength	Atrophy, decreasing strength
Fat distribution	Female (pronounced hips)	Increasingly female
Lipid metabolism	Increased HDC-C, decreased LDL-C	Increased HDC-C, decreased LDL-C
Spermatogenesis	Not initiated, infertility	Stops, increasing infertility
Semen	Usually aspermia	Small volume
Libido and potency	Do not develop	Reduced or absent
Penis	Child-like	No change in size
Scrotum	Not very pigmented, slightly wrinkled	No change
Prostate	Small, underdeveloped	Atropy

Aging, Hypogonadism and Sexual Function: New Concepts

Testosterone levels start declining in the fifth decade of life, with the lowest levels seen in men 70 years of age and older.[11,12] The rate of decrease in total testosterone levels is approximately 110 ng/dL per decade (Fig. 17.1). The development of age-related hypogonadism appears to involve deficits at multiple levels of the hypothalamic–pituitary–testicular axis[13-16] (Fig. 17.2). With aging, there is a decrease in the number and volume of the Leydig cells, impaired steroid hormone biosynthesis, impaired blood supply to the gonads and decreased steroid output after administration of human chorionic gonadotropin. In addition, the number, volume and function of Leydig cells decrease with aging and are affected by several medications, including glucocorticoids, spironolactone, opiates, and ketoconazole.[17-20] Alterations in the hypothalamic-pituitary compartment include loss of diurnal variations in gonadotropin levels, blunted luteinizing-hormone response to gonadotropin-releasing hormone stimulation, decreased or absent response of luteinizing-hormone levels to naloxone or tamoxifen, and increased gonadotrophic sensitivity to testosterone feedback.[21,22] Neuroleptic drugs that cause hyperprolactinemia can inhibit the release of gonadotropin-releasing hormones, leading to hypogonadotropic hypogonadism. Longitudinal studies on aging reported an average annual decrease of total serum testosterone of 3.2 ng/dL in men older than 53 years, i.e., about 1% per year based on a low limit of normal 325 ng/dL. According to

recommendations of the International Society of Andrology (ISA), the International Society for the Study of the Aging Male (ISSAM) and the European Association of Urology (EAU), TDS is defined as "a clinical and biochemical syndrome associated with advancing age and characterized by typical symptoms and deficiency in serum testosterone levels." These associations also clarified that TDS may result in a significant decline in the quality of life and adversely affects the functioning of multiple organ systems.[23,24] Testosterone plays a key role in the regulation of erectile function at both the central and peripheral levels. In the brain, low testosterone levels are associated with a reduction in erectile signaling. Studies in hypogonadal patients have shown that testosterone replacement results in a significant increase in brain activity in response to sexual stimulation at levels similar to those seen in men with normal testosterone.[25] At the peripheral level, testosterone promotes biochemical and structural homeostasis of penile tissues. In animal experimental models, hypogonadism has been reported to be associated with cavernous smooth muscle cell apoptosis, abnormal collagen deposition within corpora cavernosa, adypocite accumulation in the subtunical region, penile dorsal nerve atrophy and penile tunica albuginea fibrosis. These structural alterations were partially reverted after testosterone replacement therapy. Another vital role for testosterone is in the regulation of PDE5 expression. The castration of rats has shown a significant reduction in the PDE5 gene and protein expression in the corpus cavernosum as well as an erectile response to electrostimulation. These effects were completely reversed with testosterone substitution. In addition, an ever-increasing number of reports indicate that T deficiency interferes not only with normal function but also with the response to treatments specifically aimed at correcting the inadequate mechanisms of erection.[26] A number of studies have indeed confirmed that testosterone replacement therapy can improve libido and erectile function in a significant proportion of men with testosterone deficiency syndrome.[27]

Epidemiological Aspects

Hypogonadism affects an estimated two to four million men in the United States and its

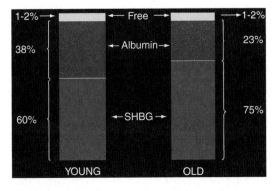

Figure 17.1. Testosterone partition in young and old men.

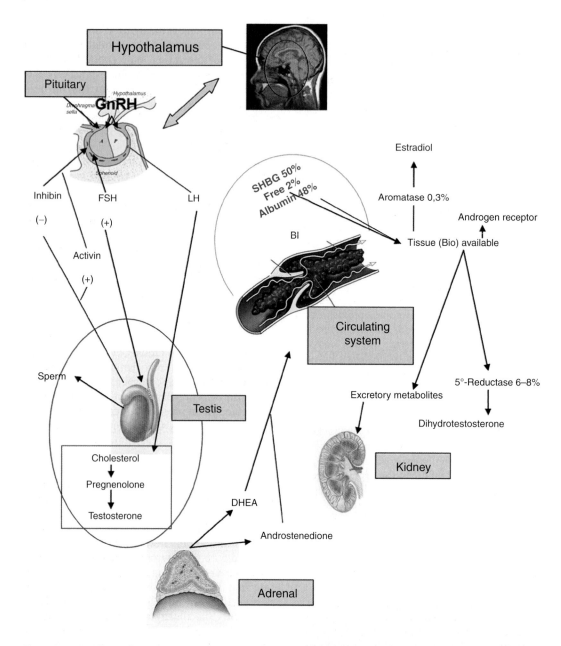

Figure 17.2. Regulation of testosterone in men and age related changes; *SHBG*: sex hormone binding globulin; uncertainty concerning binding; *DHEA* dehydroepiandrosterone, *GnRH* gonadotrophin releasing hormone (Modified from Morley[16]; Fig. 1, p. 369).

prevalence increases with age.[12,28,29] In North America, several cross-sectional and longitudinal studies have confirmed the decline in androgen production associated with age.[12,28,29] It has been estimated that only 5% of affected men currently receive treatment.

Physiological Actions and Tissue Targets of Sexual Hormones

Testosterone regulates morpho-functional homeostasis in multiple organs and body systems.

Prostate

Testosterone is known to be the major growth and functional regulator of the prostate and is essential to the development and maintenance of this organ throughout life. Prostate development, differentiation and maintenance are known to be closely linked to the bioavailability of testosterone and other related sex hormones. Between the ages of 10–20 years when serum testosterone levels rise dramatically in males, there is a pronounced, exponential growth of the prostate controlled by the balanced agonist and antagonist abilities of androgens to stimulate cell proliferation on the one hand, and to inhibit the rate of cell death in prostate tissue on the other. After the age of 20, and under the continuing presence of testosterone, the healthy prostate achieves a steady state of self-renewal and maintenance.[30] Within the prostate, testosterone is enzymatically converted to an active metabolite, 5a-dihydrotestosterone (DHT), by 5a-reductase. Once formed, DHT can bind reversibly to the androgen receptor to regulate prostatic cellular proliferation and survival. It is thought that normally the prostatic level of DHT remains constant even during diurnal and episodic variations in the serum levels of both free and total testosterone. The presence of DHT and its binding to androgen receptors can directly up-regulate the expression of prostate-specific differentiation markers such as PSA and locally active growth factors known as andromedins.[31]

Brain

Androgens have been shown to enhance both memory and spacial skills in rats.[32] Some epidemiological studies have found correlations between serum testosterone levels and general or spatial cognition.[33] Experimental data exists demonstrating that 5 alpha-reduced metabolites of T may have effects in the hippocampus that result in enhanced cognitive performance; however, it remains still unknown whether DHT or T can improve or maintain cognitive function.[34,35] Hypogonadal young and middle-aged men frequently complain of symptoms of depression and a decreased sense of well-being and non-placebo-controlled studies have suggested that mood is improved after testosterone treatment.[36] More detailed studies of the effect of androgen replacement on cognition in older testosterone-deficient men are needed, as are studies on the benefits on cognitive function in dementia associated with aging.[37]

Muscle Mass and Adipose Tissue

Testosterone is known to increase muscle protein synthesis and increase muscle strength.[38] Muscle mass is also correlated with serum testosterone and free testosterone in older men whereas data on muscle strength is not conclusive.[39] Testosterone deficiency results in decreased muscle mass and strength in hypogonadal young and middle-aged men. Multiple non-placebo-controlled studies have demonstrated the positive effects of androgen replacement on these functions in these age groups.[38] In several reported studies that included men with low baseline testosterone levels, testosterone treatment in older men increased muscle mass.[27,40] Testosterone replacement therapy results in decreased abdominal fat and total fat mass in elderly men.[41] Rajan et al hypothesized that testosterone may regulate body composition by preferentially inducing pluripotent mesenchymal cell differentiation toward a myogenic lineage and away from an adipogenic lineage.[42]

Bones

Androgen receptors are present on osteoblasts, and androgens are known to stimulate osteoblast differentiation in utero.[43] The beneficial effects of androgens on bone may be secondary to their aromatization to estrogen or through the anabolic affects of dihydrotestosterone. Dihydrotestosterone enhances mitogenesis in bone cells by inducing the transforming growth factor beta mRNA and by enhancing the binding of the insulin-like growth factor II to osteoblasts. Moreover, androgens inhibit the expression of interleukin-6, also known as osteoclast activating factor.[44] Studies have demonstrated a clear correlation between bioavailable testosterone and bone mineral density.[45,46] A direct link between testosterone deficiency in aging males and hip fracture was demonstrated in a casecontrol study showing that 48% of subjects with hip fractures were hypogonadal, compared with only 12% of a control group; a statistically significant difference.[47] The association between hypogonadism and hip fractures was confirmed in another study on aging men, and it was suggested that early diagnosis and treatment of hypogonadism might prevent hip fractures in an aging population.[48] Additional potential contributing mechanisms are increased mechanical loading via anabolic effects on muscle.

Ematopoiesis

Androgens stimulate erythropoiesis in mammallians by enhancing renal erythropoietin production by means of receptor-mediated transcription and by a direct effect on erythropoietic stem cells in the bone marrow. Androgen receptors are present on cultured erythroblasts and exogenous androgens have direct stimulatory effects on bone marrow stem cells.[49,50] Testosterone also enhances the production of heme and globin. Testosterone deficiency results in a 10–20% decrease in the blood hemoglobin concentration which can bring about anemia. Young hypogonadal men usually have fewer red blood cells and lower hemoglobin levels than age-matched controls, while healthy older men may also have lower hemoglobin levels than normal young men.[51]

Metabolism

Observational studies support the hypothesis that low testosterone is a component of a multidimensional metabolic syndrome characterized by obesity, diabetes mellitus, hypertension, dyslipidemia and a procoagulant/antifibrinolytic state. At physiological doses, testosterone is known to have beneficial effects on glucose regulation. In human studies of obese, diabetic and hypogonadal men, testosterone administration resulted in decreased fasting glucose, increased insulin sensitivity and decreased glycosylated-hemoglobin A1.[52] Laaksonen et al reported that hypogonadism can predict the subsequent development of diabetes and metabolic syndrome in middle aged men. They also hypothesized that, in addition to being an early marker of metabolic syndrome or overt diabetes, hypogonadism may also be involved in the pathogenesis of these disease processes.[53] Hypogonadism was associated with abdominal obesity. Testosterone levels were negatively associated with levels of triglycerides and lipoprotein (a) and positively correlated with HDL levels. Androgen receptors have been identified on adipocytes,

and testosterone administration results in lipolysis. Testosterone replacement in hypogonadal men with abdominal obesity enhances triglyceride turnover in abdominal adipose tissue.[54]

Cardiovascular System

In recent years exciting evidence has proven that androgens favorably influence cardiovascular risk through their influence on arteriosclerosis[55]. Beyond the beneficial effects on cardiovascular risk profile, Testosterone has been reported to exert direct effects on cardiovascular tissues. Both classical genomic (nuclear androgen-receptor mediated) and rapid, non-genomic (mediated by membrane androgen receptor) signaling pathways have been described as mediating the effects of Testosterone on the cardiovascular system.[56] Testosterone exerts acute vasorelaxant effects on peripheral and coronary circulation by modulating membrane ion-channel function. Moreover, physiological testosterone levels are involved in vascular structural homeostasis preservation. Testosterone has been reported to promote endothelial integrity through stimulating endothelial progenitor cells within the bone marrow to proliferate, migrate into the peripheral blood and repair endothelium when injuried.[57] Moreover, physiological testosterone levels inhibit vascular smooth muscle cell proliferation and migration thereby counteracting atherosclerotic-related processes such as neointima formation and media thickening.[58]

Male Hypogonadism: Diagnosis and Treatment

In addition to an adequate history and physical examination, physicians have several options for arriving at a TDS diagnosis including questionnaires and a biochemical assessment from peripheral blood.

Clinical Assessment

TDS may encompass numerous, sometimes vague and non-specific symptoms and signs: a decreased sense of well-being; a decrease in muscle mass, strength, energy; reduced virility, libido, and sexual activity, increased frequency of impotence, increased sweating, mood changes, fat mass, dry skin and anemia.[59] Other symptoms are even less specific and include reduced erectile strength, fatigue, mood disturbances comprising of irritability, frustration, lack of motivation and depression. Medical history should be focused on the presence of pituitary disease, primary testicular disease, exposure to radiation, failure to develop at puberty and osteoporosis. Physical examination may detect signs of hypogonadism such as lack of secondary sexual characteristics and fine wrinkling of facial skin. In middle-aged to older men, the symptoms become even less specific because of the higher frequency of co-morbid conditions. Three questionnaires are most widely recognized as improving diagnostic specificity: the St. Louis University Androgen Deficiency in Aging Males (ADAM) (Table 17.2), the Massachusetts Aging Survey (MMAS), and the Aging Male Survey (AMS) (Table 17.3).

Biochemical Assessment

Clinicians should optimize the determination of serum testosterone levels by drawing the blood sample in the morning (between 7 and 10 a.m). Although circadian rhythms in serum testosterone are less marked as men age, the reference ranges are usually obtained in the morning in younger men. In addition, physicians should check the reference range for serum testosterone in the laboratory they use to help them interpret the results. Normal reference ranges for serum total testosterone in adult men is generally considered to be 300–1,000 ng/dL (10–35 nmol/L). Levels of <250 ng/dL (8.7 nmol/L) suggest that the patient is likely to be hypogonadal, whereas levels of >350 ng/dL (12.7 nmol/L) suggest that the symptoms may not be due to androgen deficiency. Some recent publications suggest using cut-off values of between 200 and 400 ng/dL.[61] When morning serum total testosterone levels are <250 ng/dL, luteinizing hormone (LH) and follicle stimulating hormone (FSH) levels should be checked. LH and FSH levels are elevated in primary hypogonadism but are normal or low in secondary hypogonadism. If testosterone, LH, and FSH levels are low, serum prolactin should be checked to exclude a prolactin-secreting pituitary tumor. The International Society of Andrology (ISA), International Society for the Study of the Aging Male (ISSAM), and European Association of Urology (EAU) guidelines recommend that levels <231 ng/dL (8 nmol/L) are representative of hypogonadism and in such cases testosterone replacement may therefore be appropriate while levels above a threshold of 346 ng/dL (12 nmol/L) are normal.[23] Borderline levels of total testosterone should be followed up by measurement of free or bioavailable testosterone. If these levels are

Table 17.2. The St. Louis University androgen deficiency in aging males (ADAM) questionnaire (Reprinted from Carlo Bettocchi[60]; Table 4, p. 7)

Questionnaire (circle one)			
Yes	No	(1)	Do you have a decrease in libido (sex drive)?
Yes	No	(2)	Do you have a lack of energy?
Yes	No	(3)	Do you have a decrease in strength and/or endurance?
Yes	No	(4)	Have you lost height?
Yes	No	(5)	Have you noticed a decreased enjoyment of life?
Yes	No	(6)	Are you sad and/or grumpy?
Yes	No	(7)	Are your erections less strong?
Yes	No	(8)	Have you noticed a recent deterioration in your ability to play sports
Yes	No	(9)	Are you falling asleep after dinner?
Yes	No	(10)	Has there been a recent deterioration in your work performance?

A positive answer represent yes to (1) or (7) or any other three questions

Table 17.3. The aging males' symptoms (AMS) scale (Reprinted from Carlo Bettocchi[60] Table 3, p. 7)

Symptoms		Score				
		1	2	3	4	5
1.	Decline in your feeling of general well-being (general state of health, subjective feeling)	☐	☐	☐	☐	☐
2.	Joint pain and muscular ache (lower back pain, joint pain, pain in a limb, general back ache)	☐	☐	☐	☐	☐
3.	Excessive sweating (unexpected/sudden episodes of sweating, hot flushes independent of strain)	☐	☐	☐	☐	☐
4.	Sleep problems (difficulty in falling asleep, difficulty in sleeping through, waking up early and feeling tired, poor sleep, sleeplessness)	☐	☐	☐	☐	☐
5.	Increased need for sleep, often feeling tired	☐	☐	☐	☐	☐
6.	Irritability (feeling aggressive, easily upset about little things, moody)	☐	☐	☐	☐	☐
7.	Nervousness (inner tension, restlessness, feeling fidgety)	☐	☐	☐	☐	☐
8.	Anxiety (feeling panicky)	☐	☐	☐	☐	☐
9.	Physical exhaustion / lacking vitality (general decrease in performance, reduced activity, lacking interest in leisure activities feeling of getting less done, of achieving less of having to force oneself to undertake activities)	☐	☐	☐	☐	☐
10.	Decrease in muscular strength (feeling of weakness)	☐	☐	☐	☐	☐
11.	Depressive mood (feeling down, sad, on the verge of tears, lack of drive, mood swings, feeling nothing is of any use)	☐	☐	☐	☐	☐
12.	Feeling that you have passed your peak	☐	☐	☐	☐	☐
13.	Feeling burnt out, having hit rock-bottom	☐	☐	☐	☐	☐
14.	Decrease in beard growth	☐	☐	☐	☐	☐
15.	Decrease in ability/frequency to perform sexually	☐	☐	☐	☐	☐
16.	Decrease in the number of morning erections	☐	☐	☐	☐	☐
17.	Decrease in sexual desire/libido (lacking pleasure in sex, lacking desire for sexual intercourse)	☐	☐	☐	☐	☐
Have you got any other major symptoms?		Yes ☐		No ☐		
If yes please describe:						

low, then the patient is a candidate for testosterone replacement therapy. Values between these limits warrant a repeat morning serum testosterone determination with direct measurement of free testosterone by equilibrium dialysis or calculated by measurements of sex hormone-binding globulin (SHBG) and total testosterone levels.

Treatment Indications and Pre-treatment Evaluations

Testosterone replacement therapy is indicated in patients with morning serum total testosterone levels of <250 ng/dL and signs and symptoms of androgen deficiency (Fig. 17.3).[62] In patients with borderline testosterone levels and symptoms suggestive of androgen deficiency, a short trial of testosterone replacement may be justified.[23] Testosterone administration is absolutely contra-indicated in men suspected of, or having, carcinoma of the prostate or breast. Relative contra-indications include: significant polycythemia (hematocrit ≥ 55%), untreated sleep apnea, severe gestive heart failure, severe symptoms of lower urinary tract obstruction evidenced by high scores on the International Prostate Symptom Score or clinical findings of bladder outflow obstruction (increased postmicturition residual volume, decreased peak urinary flow, pathological pressure flow-studies) due to an enlarged, clinically benign prostate. Moderate obstruction represents a partial contraindication. After successful treatment of the obstruction, the contraindication is lifted.[23] A prerequisite test before initiating testosterone supplementation should include the prostate-specific antigen (PSA) and a digital rectal examination (DRE) in men older than 45 years.

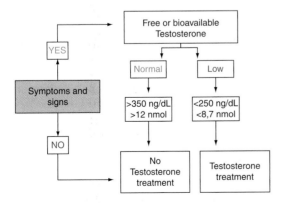

Figure 17.3. Diagnostic flow-chart of patients suitable for testosterone replacement therapy.

Treatment Modalities

Current available testosterone preparations and delivery forms are reported in Table 17.4. Neither injectable preparations nor slow-release pellets can reproduce the circadian pattern of testosterone production of the testes. This is accomplished best by the transdermal preparations. Oral testosterone may also approximate a circadian rhythm by dose adjustments even if the relevance of reproducing a circadian rhythm during testosterone therapy remains unknown. The choice of appropriate testosterone delivery should be based on safety and efficacy while also taking into consideration factors such as cost and convenience. Selection will of course also depend on the patient's preference and that of his physicians.[63]

Oral Preparations

Oral androgen preparations have become popular because of their convenience aspects such as dose flexibility, possibility of immediate discontinuation and self-administration. However, they demand special consideration because they undergo rapid hepatic and intestinal metabolism. An oral preparation that is widely used throughout the world is testosterone undecanoate. This product is designed to deliver testosterone to the systemic circulation via the intestinal lymphatic route, thereby circumventing first-pass inactivation in the liver. Therefore, it is free of liver toxicity and brings serum testosterone levels within the physiological range.[8] One of the newest testosterone replacement therapy modalities is transbuccal testosterone. Since buccal testosterone is transported directly into the superior vena cava from the buccal venous system, it avoids the first-pass effect of hepatic metabolism. Levels peak within 30 min. attain a steady state within 24 h and then drop below normal 2–4 h after the tablet is removed. Transbuccal administration maintains testosterone at levels within the physiological range, comparable to testosterone gel.[64]

Table 17.4. Common testosterone preparations and their recommended doses (Reprinted from Jockenho[63]; Table 1, p. 294)

	Generic name	Trade name	Dose
Injectable	Testosterone cypionate	Depo-testosterone cypionate	200–400 mg every 2–4 weeks
	Testosterone enanthate	Testoviron depot	200–400 mg every 2–4 weeks
	Testosterone undecanoate	Nebido	1,000 mg every 12 weeks
Oral	Testosterone undecanoate	Andriol	120–240 mg daily
Transdermal	Testosterone patch	Androderm	2.5–5 mg daily
	Testosterone gel	Testogel	50–100 mg daily
	Testosterone gel	Testim	50–100 mg daily
Buccal	Buccal testosterone	Striant	30 mg twice a day

Parenteral Preparations

Injectable esters of testosterone have been available for the longest time and their effects are well recognized. They are inexpensive and safe but their use carries several major drawbacks which include: the need for periodic (every 2–3 weeks) deep intramuscular injection, swings in serum levels and initially (within about 72 h) they result in supraphysiological levels of serum testosterone followed by a steady decline over the next 10–14 days. The steady decline frequently results in a very low nadir immediately before the next injection. Parenteral androgens do not evoke the normal circadian patterns of serum testosterone, and the intermittent supraphysiological levels that they produce may result in the development of breast tenderness and gynecomastia. The most widely used parenteral preparations are the 17-b-hydroxyl esters of testosterone, which include the short-acting propionate and the longer acting enanthate and cypionate. Testosterone propionate is rarely used because its short half-life requires administration every other day.[65] A new testosterone preparation for intramuscular injection has recently been developed that consists of a depot formulation of testosterone undecanoate dissolved in castor oil. This new formulation allows for the extension of the injection interval from 10 to 14 weeks (i.e., usually four injections a year in long-term therapy) thus improving both the acceptability and tolerability of testosterone injection therapy.[66]

Transdermal Preparations

Transdermal testosterone therapy permits a close reflection on the variable levels in testosterone production manifested in normal men over the 24 h circadian cycle. Transdermal testosterone therapy is available in both scrotal and non-scrotal patches and in a gel form. The scrotal patches lost their appeal because of inconveniences such as their ability to remain in place and the need for frequent shaving of the scrotal skin. In addition, because of the high concentrations of 5a-reductase in the scrotal skin, they produce abnormally high levels of dihydrotestosterone (DHT).[67] Trans-dermal nonscrotal patches produce normal levels of estradiol but, as opposed to the scrotal ones, result in normal levels of DHT. Most common side effects of the body patches are related to the need to use enhancers to facilitate absorption. This frequently results in various degrees of skin reactions which occasionally result in significant chemical burns.[68] The testosterone gel offers all the advantages of the patches without the frequent skin reactions. Its only drawbacks reside in the potential for contamination of others, drying time and the existence of few long-term studies of its use.

Side Effects and Treatment Monitoring

Follow-up monitoring at 3–6 months for the first year, then yearly thereafter is recommended.[69] Prostate biopsy is warranted in cases where PSA is higher than 4 ng/mL or abnormal DRE. When hematocrit is elevated during the therapy, dosage reduction or cessation of treatment should be considered according to severity. Potential Risks Associated with Testosterone-Replacement Therapy are reported in Table 17.2.

Testosterone Replacement Therapy and Prostate Safety

The prostate is an androgen dependent organ, with a high concentration of testosterone receptors and a high 5-alpha reductase activity. As growing numbers of aging males receive testosterone substitution for management of the signs and symptoms of hypogonadism, there has been a renewed interest in the role of testosterone in prostate health, particularly with regards to the safety profile in terms of BPH and prostate cancer.

Testosterone Replacement Therapy and BPH Progression

Clinical studies have failed to demonstrate exacerbation of voiding symptoms attributable to benign prostatic hyperplasia during testosterone replacement therapy, and complications such as urinary retention have not occurred at higher rates than in controls receiving placebo. Prostate volume, as determined by ultrasonography, increases significantly during testosterone-replacement therapy, mainly during the first 6 months, to a level equivalent to that of men without hypogonadism. However, urine flow rates, postvoiding residual urine volumes, and prostate voiding symptoms do not change significantly in patients receiving testosterone replacement therapy. This apparent paradox is explained by the poor correlation between prostate volume and urinary symptoms.[69,70]

Testosterone Replacement Therapy and Prostate Cancer

The theory that testosterone may stimulate the growth of prostate cancer derives from the original studies conducted by Huggins and Hodges in 1941, where the authors demonstrated that the marked reductions in serum testosterone following castration resulted in a regression of metastatic prostate cancer.[71] Although very clear evidence indicates that a reduction in serum testosterone due to castration concentrations is able to reduce levels of prostate-specific antigen (PSA) and delay the progression of established prostate cancer, it is difficult to prove the converse. Since 1941, a clear relationship between circulating testosterone levels and prostate cancer has not been identified and still remains the subject of intense research study and debate.[71] Clinical studies and basic investigations have shown that the development and growth of prostate cancer are much more complex than simply an excess or lack of androgens. Testosterone regulates prostate growth by modulating the balance between proliferative and apoptotic processes. The direct effect of testosterone on prostate epithelial cells induces differentiation, whereas the indirect effects on proliferation is mediated by the growth factor production by the prostate stroma.[72] Moreover, nonsteroidal hormones (insulin, leptin, glucocorticoids, growth hormone), genetic susceptibility, inflammation and environmental factors appear to be significant contributors to prostate growth. Recent evidence demonstrates the absence of a direct correlation between serum and prostate androgen levels. Marks et al. conducted a randomized, double-blind study on 44 healthy men with serum testosterone levels of <300 ng/dL and related symptoms in order to investigate the effects of testosterone replacement therapy on prostate tissue. Patients were treated with 150 mg testosterone enanthate or placebo intramuscularly every 2 weeks for 6 months. Prostate biopsies were available before and after treatment in 40 men. Testosterone therapy resulted in a significant increase in testosterone and dihydrotestosterone (DHT) levels in the serum, but not in prostate tissue. Total PSA levels were significantly increased by both testosterone (from 1.55 to 2.29 ng/mL) and placebo (from 0.97 to 1.10 ng/mL) but still remained relatively low. Four new cases of prostate cancer were diagnosed in the placebo group and two new cases in the testosterone replacement group. Testosterone replacement therapy also had no effect on prostate histology, tissue biomarkers for cell proliferation, androgen receptors, or angiogenesis nor on the expression of known androgen-regulated genes or those related to cell stress or angiogenesis.[73] Apparently, the internal environment of the prostate is buffered against wide fluctuations in circulating androgen levels within a rather broad range.[67] There is actually no compelling evidence that testosterone has a causative role in prostate cancer. Despite initial reports suggesting a possible role for testosterone replacement therapy in converting an occult cancer into a clinically apparent lesion, more recently Rhoden et al. was unable to demonstrate an increased risk of progression to prostate cancer in hypogonadal men with PIN who were treated with testosterone for 1 year. This suggests that PIN does not appear to be a contraindication to testosterone replacement therapy.[74-76] Overall data from prospective longitudinal epidemiologic studies have not provided evidence of a direct correlation between endogenous total testosterone levels and risk of prostate cancer. In recent years, a saturation model has been proposed by Fowler and Whitmore in order to explain the effects of testosterone on prostate cancer growth. This model postulates that physiologic testosterone concentrations provide an excess of testosterone and its intracellular prostatic metabolite DHT, for optimal prostatic growth requirements. However, reducing T concentration below a critical concentration threshold (the Saturation Point) creates an intracellular milieu in which the availability of androgen becomes the rate-limiting step governing prostate tissue growth.[77] Interestingly, several epidemiological studies have recently demonstrated that low testosterone levels could have adverse effects on men newly diagnosed with prostate cancer.[78] Hoffman and coworkers suggested a higher risk of having a positive biopsy and a higher incidence of high-grade tumor in patients with low free testosterone levels.[79] Yamamoto et al demonstrated that preoperative testosterone levels lower than 300 ng/dL were a significant and independent predictor of PSA failure in patients with clinically localized prostate cancer treated with radical prostatectomy alone.[80] Low testosterone levels were found to be predictive of pathologic stage and positive surgical margins in patients undergoing radical prostatectomy.[81]

Androgen Deprivation Therapy (ADT): Adverse Effects

ADT is the mainstay of treatment for metastatic and recurrent prostate cancer and is increasingly utilized as primary therapy or in combination with other therapies for localized disease. Although the use of ADT has been proven to improve oncological outcome, the resulting hypogonadism leads to a number of adverse consequences i.e., altered body composition and metabolic functions, accelerated bone turnover, cognitive decline and increased cardiovascular morbidity.[82]

Body Composition

ADT is associated with significant decrease in lean body mass and increase in fat mass in men with PCa.[83] Changes in body composition are evident within the first year of therapy. Sarcopenia is associated with frailty and fatigue, resulting in an increased risk of falls and a diminished quality of life.[82]

Insulin Resistance and Metabolic Syndrome

Insulin resistance is the condition whereby normal amounts of glucose are inadequate to produce a normal insulin response from the fat, muscle and liver cells. The metabolic syndrome is a clustering of specific cardiovascular-disease risk factors whose pathophysiology appears to be related to insulin resistance. A cross-sectional study reported a higher prevalence of metabolic syndrome in men receiving ADT compared with age-matched control groups of untreated men with prostate cancer and men without prostate cancer.[84] In a study by Braga-Basaria M. et al, metabolic syndrome was present in more than 50% of the men undergoing long-term ADT, predisposing them to higher cardiovascular risk.[84] However, while classic metabolic syndrome is characterized by low levels of adiponectin and elevated markers of inflammation, ADT significantly increases serum adiponectin levels and does not alter C-reactive protein levels nor other markers of inflammation. As a consequence, some researchers have hypothesized that ADT may cause a pattern of metabolic change that is distinct from the standard metabolic syndrome.[85,86]

Cognitive Decline

ADT's effects on cognitive function are controversial. Green et al. evaluated such effects in men with advanced prostate cancer by demonstrating a statistically significant decline in cognitive tests evaluating verbal memory and executive functions after 6 months.[87] In a further study by Jenkins et al., a significant cognitive decline in spatial memory and spatial ability was demonstrated in men with localized prostate cancer who received ADT.[88] On the contrary, however, other studies demonstrated no detrimental effects on cognitive functions brought on by ADT.[89]

Bone Metabolism

Studies demonstrate that ADT may result in a significant decline in bone mineral density (BMD) at multiple sites due to increased bone turnover resulting in a higher risk of developing osteoporosis.[82,90] During initial ADT, the BMD of the hip and spine decrease by approximately 3% per year. Later, BMD continues to decline steadily during the course of long-term therapy. The risk of developing osteoporosis during ADT depends on individual differences in peak bone mass and the amount of adult bone loss occurring before ADT. Individual variations in bone loss rates during ADT have been reported. The decline of BMD due to both medical or surgical castration leads to a statistically significant and clinically meaningful increase in fracture risk within 5 years of commencing therapy.[89] In large population-based studies, ADT was associated with an approximate 21–45% relative increase in the incidence of clinical fractures.[91-93] Longer treatment duration seems to confer greater fracture risk.

The Kidneys

Endocrine Functions of the Kidney

Beyond excretory function, the kidneys act as complex endocrine organs. The main hormones secreted by the kidneys are: erythropoietin (EPO), the active form of Vitamin D (1,25-dihydroxycholecalciferol) and renin.

Erythropoietin

EPO is a 34-kDa glycoprotein hormone mostly synthesized by interstitial cells of the kidney cortex. At the bone marrow level it acts as a hematopoietic growth factor by regulating the feedback control of red cell production thereby adapting the red cell mass volume to the level of the oxygen tissue required to satisfy tissue oxygen demands.[94,95] EPO production is primarily regulated by hypoxia which acts at the gene transcription level by increasing gene expression. At the bone marrow level, EPO regulates erythroid cell proliferation, differentiation, and survival by binding to an EPO receptor which is expressed primarily on the erythroid cells between the colony forming unit-erythroid (CFU-E) and the pronormoblast stage of erythroid cell development. The number of EPO receptors per cell gradually decreases during erythroid cell differentiation and studies have shown that the reticulocyte and mature erythrocyte do not contain EPO receptors.[96-98] In normal human subjects, serum levels of EPO range between 1 and 27 mu/mL.[99] A variety of mechanisms for EPO down regulation have been reported: hyperoxia, increased catabolism by an expanded erythroid progenitor cell pool, blood hyperviscosity, renal disease and cytokine production during inflammatory, infectious and neoplastic disorders.[100] The mechanism for the anemia of chronic renal failure is probably due to the inability of the kidneys with compromised renal function to produce sufficient amounts of EPO to meet the demands for new red cell production. Nevertheless, the uremic state may also blunt the bone marrow response to EPO.[101,102]

Calcitriol

Calcitriol (Vitamin D3 or 1,25 dihydroxycholecalciferol) is a steroid hormone with a wide range of biological effects. It has long been known for its role in regulating serum levels of calcium and phosphorus, and bone mineralization. More recently, it has been demonstrated that receptors for vitamin D are present in a wide variety of cells, and that calcitriol generates multiple biological responses via both genomic and nongenomic pathways. Immune and cardiovascular systems have been identified as critical targets for calcitriol actions.[103] Calcitriol is synthesized through complex *biosynthetic* pathways involving the skin, the liver and the kidneys in a stepwise manner. The final *biosynthetic* step consists of the hydroxylation of the major circulating metabolite, 25-hydroxyvitamin D3, performed by the mitochondrial cytochrome P450 enzyme 25-hydroxyvitamin D-1alpha-hydroxylase (1alpha-HYD). Although 1alpha-HYD activity has been identified at several sites, circulating levels of calcitriol mainly reflect the expression of this enzyme in the kidney.[104] When kidney disease develops, there is a decreased functional renal mass and a tendency to retain phosphorus which reduces renal 1alpha-hydroxylase activity and subsequently, the synthesis of calcitriol, thus leading to secondary hyperparathyroidism and bone disease.[105]

Renin

Renin is an aspartyl-protease acting as key regulator of the renin-angiotensin-aldosterone system which is critically involved in salt, volume, and blood pressure homeostasis.[106] It is mainly produced and released into circulation by the juxtaglomerular epithelioid cells located in the walls of renal afferent arterioles at the entrance of the glomerular capillary network. Renin secretion is controlled by a number of mechanisms: the baroreceptor mechanism (afferent arteriolar transmural pressure); the macula densa mechanism (solute transport in the macula densa segment of the nephron); the beta-adrenergic mechanism (catecholamines released from the renal nerves and the adrenal medulla); extracellular concentrations of angiotensin II, vasopressin, potassium and magnesium.[107]

Primary Hyperparathyroidism (PHP) and Nephrolithiasis

Renal stone disease is frequently associated with metabolic disorders. About 85% of all kidney stones contain calcium salts (calcium oxalate and/or calcium phosphate) as their main crystalline components. Hypercalciuria is the most common identifiable cause of calcium kidney stone disease. It is defined as urinary excretion of more than 250 mg of calcium per day in women and more than 275–300 mg of calcium per day in men who are on a regular, unrestricted diet. Primary hyperparathyroidism (PHP) is one of the most common causes of hypercalcemia with resulting hypercalciuria. It develops as a consequence of the excessive release of the parathyroid hormone (PTH) by

parathyroid glands and affects nearly 1 in 500 women and 1 in 2,000 men per year, most often in the fifth, sixth, and seventh decades of life. PHP is usually the result of a single benign adenoma. A minority of patients have hyperplasia in all four parathyroid glands. In these cases familial-genetic syndromes should be considered such as type I and type II multiple endocrine neoplasia (MEN). Parathyroid carcinoma accounts for an insignificant minority of cases. Traditionally, the diagnosis is confirmed by the presence of elevated intact parathyroid hormone (iPTH) and serum ionized calcium levels.[108] The most frequent complication of PHP is nephrolithiasis, which occurs in about 20% of patients.[109] Routine imaging of the kidneys is necessary when PHP is documented.[110] Patients with PHP have a greater risk of renal stone disease and this risk persists for 10 years after surgery.[111] In 80% of patients with PHP, hypercalcemia symptoms are mild or not noticeable at the time of diagnosis. Management of these patients is not clear-cut because routine laboratory tests have not proven to assist in predicting the development of overt manifestations of the disease. Conversely, patients with overtly symptomatic PHP (e.g., those with urinary tract stones, bone pain, cognitive abnormalities) and those with marked hypercalcemia (calcium levels >10.2 mg/dL) must be referred for parathyroidectomy.

Paraneoplastic Syndromes

Paraneoplastic syndromes are a group of clinical disorders associated with malignant diseases that are not directly related to the physical effects of primary or metastatic tumors.[112] Paraneoplastic hormonal syndromes ("ectopic" or "inappropriate" hormone production) depend on the secretion of hormonal peptides or their precursors, cytokines, and, more rarely, thyroidal hormones and Vitamin D which act in an endocrine, paracrine or autocrine manner.[113] The molecular mechanisms responsible for the development of these syndromes are poorly understood. Mutational events not only may initiate neoplastic transformation but may also lead to the re-expression of genes responsible for hormone production. Additionally, epigenetic events such as methylation may also be responsible for the development of these syndromes.[114] Paraneoplastic endocrine syndromes are very common in patients with Renal Cell Carcinoma (RCC). However, they have been described in patients with other urological malignances as well.

Paraneoplastic Endocrine Syndromes Associated with RCC

Nearly one third of patients affected by RCC show signs and symptoms of a paraneoplastic syndrome which may be both endocrine or non-endocrine in nature.[115] The presence of a paraneoplastic syndrome in a patient with RCC is neither a marker of metastatic disease nor necessarily indicative of a poor prognosis. However, a paraneoplastic syndrome may be the initial clinical presentation of RCC in a significant number of patients and recognition of these syndromes may facilitate early diagnosis. Most paraneoplastic syndromes are associated with RCC remission after resection of the primary tumor or treatment of metastatic sites. RCC tumor cells may elaborate a number of proteins that serve as mediators of endocrine paraneoplastic syndromes such as parathyroid hormone-related peptide (PTHrP), erythropoietin (EPO), insulin, glucagon, or renin.

Hypercalcemia

Hypercalcemia is the most common paraneoplastic syndrome in patients with RCC affecting from 13% to 20% of RCC patients.[116,117] Neither the presence nor the degree of hypercalcemia, have been shown to have a significant correlation with tumor grade or survival.[118] Hypercalcemia secondary to bony metastatic disease is not a true paraneoplastic syndrome. Non metastatic hypercalcemia in patients with RCC is thought to be mainly the consequence of the secretion of PTHrP by RCC cells.[119] PTHrP binds to the PTH receptor in both the bone and renal tissue leading to increased bone re-absorption and decreased renal clearance of calcium as well as increased phosphorus excretion. Additional factors such as transforming growth factors alpha and beta, the osteoclast activating factor, interleukin 1 and tumor necrosis factor are also believed to exacerbate

the nonmetastatic hypercalcemia seen in RCC patients either by distinct mechanisms or by augmenting the actions of PTHrP.[120] Clinically, hypercalcemia presents a wide range of signs and symptoms affecting numerous organ systems. Patients may complain of lethargy, nausea, fatigue, confusion, weakness and constipation. Physical examination may reveal decreased deep tendon reflexes and an impaired level of consciousness. Signs of dehydration may also be present secondary to loss of renal concentrating ability and subsequent polyuria. Electrocardiogram (ECG) findings include increased PR and QT intervals with eventual bradyarrhythmias and asystole. Nephrectomy is the most effective way of treating the non-metastatic hypercalcemia observed in RCC patients.[121]

Hypertension

Potential mechanisms of hypertension in RCC patients include increased renin secretion, ureteral or parenchymal compression, presence of an arteriovenous fistula and polycythemia. Elevated serum rennin levels have been found in 37% of patients with RCC.[122,123] Renin may be secreted either by neoplastic proximal tubular cells or by local renal parenchymal which may be compressed by a subcapsular hematoma or by a large tumor leading to intrarenal ischemia with subsequent increase of rennin excretion by the juxtaglomerular apparatus. Ureteral obstruction may cause renin secretion by a similar mechanism.[124]

Polycythemia

Polycythemia has been reported in a percentage of patients with RCC ranging from 1% to 8%. Elevated serum red blood cell concentrations are believed to be mediated by ectopic secretion of EPO by tumor cells.[125] Ectopic EPO production is found in 66% of RCC cases making this neoplasm the leading cause of ectopic EPO production. Moreover, perineoplastic cells in RCC may also contribute to total EPO levels secondary to local tumor compression and resultant tissue hypoxia. Although two thirds of RCC patients have elevated EPO levels, only 8% experience erythrocytosis.

Nonmetastatic Hepatic Dysfunction (Stauffer Syndrome)

In 1961, Stauffer described hepatic abnormalities in a patient with RCC with no evidence of hepatic metastases. The abnormalities disappeared after nephrectomy but returned with disease recurrence.[126] The syndrome is characterized by elevations in liver enzymes as well as abnormal levels of hepatic synthetic products. Elevations of aspartate aminotransferase, alanine aminotransferase, alkaline phosphatase, and prothrombine exist in 66% of cases. Additionally, elevated levels of gammaglobulin and bilirubin are seen in 54% and 27% of patients with Stauffer's syndrome, respectively.[127,128] The cause of Stauffer's syndrome is poorly understood. It has been hypothesized that RCC itself can secrete hepatotoxins or lysosomal enzymes that stimulate hepatic cathepsins or phosphatases leading to hepato-cellular injury.[129,130] A second theory suggests that tumor-secreted hepatotoxins lead to hepatocyte injury with subsequent activation of the immune system via the local recruitment of T cells and the production of antibodies against liver antigens.[129] Evidence also suggests that aberrant tumor production of interleukin-6 (IL-6), which is known to stimulate hepatic protein production, may play a direct role in Stauffer's syndrome because it is frequently produced by RCC cells.[131] Liver biopsy reveals generalized hepatitis with lymphocytic infiltration and hepatocellular degeneration without biliary obstruction.[128] Clinically, patients may complain about hepatosplenomegaly, fever, and weight loss. Nephrectomy leads to the resolution of hepatitis in 66% of patients.[132]

Other Endocrine Abnormalities

HCG has been found in elevated levels in up to 6% of patients with RCC.[133,134] Abnormalities in glucose metabolism have also been observed in RCC patients. There are several case reports of hyperglycemia and hypoglycemia that disappeared after nephrectomy for RCC. This finding has led to research into the possible mediators that may be either secreted or stimulated by the tumor. Hormones such as insulin and glucagon have all been isolated from RCC tumor extracts.[135] In 1961, a group from the Mayo clinic first described a possible relationship between RCC and Cushing's syndrome.[136] Subsequently, RCC has been found to account for 2% of all neoplasms responsible for Cushing's syndrome. Galactorrhea and elevated serum prolactin levels have been described in two RCC cases.[137]

Paraneoplastic Endocrine Syndromes Associated with Other Urologic Malignances

Gynecomastia and ectopic production of human chorionic gonadotropin (HCG) have been found to be associated with transitional cell carcinoma of the bladder by a number of authors.[138,139] It has been reported that in patients with prostate carcinoma, small-cell de-differentiation of neoplastic cells are associated with Cushing's syndrome due to the ectopic production of ACTH.[140]

References

1. Jeffcoate SL, Brocks RV, Lin NY, London DR. Androgen production in hypogonadal men. *J Endocrinol*. 1967;37: 401-411
2. Wheeler MJ. Determination of bio-available testosterone. *Ann Clin Biochem*. 1995;32:345-357
3. Dunn JF, Nisula BC, Rodbard D. Transport of steroid hormones: binding of 21 endogenoussteroids to both testosterone-bind in globulin and corticosteroid-binding globulin in human plasma. *J Clin Endocrinol Metab*. 1981;53:58-68
4. American Association of Clinical Endocrinologists. Medical guidelines for clinical practice for the evaluation and treatment of hypogonadism in adult male patients: 2002 update. *Endocr Pract*. 2002;8:440-456
5. Ribeiro RS, Abucham J. Kallmann syndrome: a historical, clinical and molecular review. *Arq Bras Endocrinol Metabol*. 2008;52(1):8-17
6. Bhagavath B, Layman LC. The genetics of hypogonadotropic hypogonadism. *Semin Reprod Med*. 2007;25(4): 272-286
7. Conway AJ, Handelsman DJ, Lording DW, Stuckey B, Zajac JD. Use, misuse and abuse of androgens: the endocrine society of Australia consensus guidelines for androgen prescribing. *Med J Aust*. 2000;172:220-224
8. Jockenhovel F. *Male Hypogonadism – Practical Aspect of Androgen Therapy*. Bremen, Germany: Uni-Med Verlag; 2004
9. Nieschlag E, Jockenhovel F. Hypogonadismus beim mann – Androgenmangel-Sdrom. In: Hesch RD, ed. *Endokrinologie*. Munchen, Germany: Urban & Schwarzenberg; 1989:1216-1220

10. Layman LC. Hypogonadotropic hypogonadism. *Endocrinol Metab Clin North Am*. 2007;36(2):283-296

11. Gray A, Feldman HA, McKinley JB, Longcope C. Age, disease and changing sex hormone levels in middle-aged men: results of the Massachusetts male aging study. *J Clin Endocrinol Metab*. 1991;73:1016-1025

12. Morley JE, Kaiser FE, Perry HMIII, et al. Longitudinal changes in testosterone, luteinizing hormone, and follicle-stimulating hormone in healthy older men. *Metabolism*. 1997;46:410-413

13. Deslypere JP, Vermeulen A. Leydig cell function in normal men: effect of age, life-style, residence, diet, and activity. *J Clin Endocrinol Metab*. 1984;59:955-962

14. Morley JE, Kaiser F, Raum WJ, et al. Potentially predictive and manipulable blood serum correlates of aging in the healthy human male: progressive decreases in bioavailable testosterone, dehydroepiandrosterone sulfate, and the ratio of insulin-like growth factor 1 to growth hormone. *Proc Natl Acad Sci*. 1997;94:7537-7542

15. Kaufman JM, Vermeulen A. The decline of androgen levels in elderly men and its clinical and therapeutic implication. *Endocr Rev*. 2005;26(6):833-876

16. Morley J, Perry HM. Androgen treatment of male hypogonadism in older males. *J Steroid Biochem Mol Biol*. 2003;85:367-373

17. Neaves WB, Johnson L, Porter JC, Parker CR, Petty CS. Leydig cell numbers, daily sperm production and serum gonadotrophin levels in aging men. *J Clin Endocrinol Metab*. 1984;59:756-763

18. Vermeulen A, Desylpere JP. Intratesticular unconjugated steroids in elderly men. *J Steroid Biochem*. 1986; 24:1079-1089

19. Sasano M, Ishyo S. Vascular patterns of the human testes with special reference to its senile changes. *J Exp Med*. 1969;99:269-280

20. Suoranta H. Changes in small blood vessels of the adult human testes in relation to age and some pathological conditions. *Virchows Arch A Pathol Anat*. 1971;352: 765-781

21. Vermeulen A, Desylpere JP, Kaufman JM. Influence of anti-opioids and luteinizing hormone pulsatility in aging men. *J Clin Endocrinol Metab*. 1989;68:68-72

22. Winters SJ, Sherins RJ, Troen P. The gonadotropin suppressive activity of androgens is increased in elderly men. *Metabolism*. 1984;33:1052-1059

23. Morales A, Schulman CC, Tostain JCW, Wu F. Testosterone deficiency syndrome (TDS) needs to be named appropriately – the importance of accurate terminology. *Eur Urol*. 2006;50:407-409

24. Nieschlag E, Swerdloff R, Behre HM, et al. Investigation, treatment, and monitoring of late-onset hypogonadism in males: ISA, ISSAM, and EAU recommendations. *J Androl*. 2006;27:135-137

25. Park K, Seo JJ, Kang HK, Ryu SB, Kim HJ, Jeong GW. A new potential of blood oxygenation level dependent (BOLD) functional MRI for evaluating cerebral centers of penile erection. *Int J Impot Res*. 2001;13:73-81

26. Christian Stief. Testosterone and erection: practical management for the patient with erectile dysfunction. *Eur Urol Suppl*. 2007;6(17):868-873

27. Wang C, Swerdloff RS, Iranmanesh A, et al. Transdermal testosterone gel improves sexual function, mood, muscle strength and body composition parameters in

hypogonadal men. *J Clin Endocrinol Metab*. 2000;85: 2839-2853

28. Harman SM, Metter EJ, Tobin JD, Pearson J, Blackman MR. Longitudinal effects of aging on serum total and free testosterone levels in healthy men: Baltimore longitudinal study of aging. *J Clin Endocrinol Metab*. 2001;86:724-731

29. Feldman Ha, Longcope C, Derby Ca, et al. Age trends in the levels of serum testosterone and other hormone in middle age men: longitudinal results of the Massachusetts ale aging study. *J Clin Endocrinol Metab*. 2002; 87:589

30. Isaacs JT. Testosterone and the prostate. In: Nieschlag E, Behre HM, eds. *Testosterone: Action, Deficiency, Substitution*. 3rd ed. Cambridge, UK: Cambridge University Press; 2004:347-374

31. David Crawford E. Testosterone substitution and the prostate. *Eur Urol Suppl*. 2005;4:16-23

32. Frye CA, Seliga AM. Testosterone increases analgesia, anxiolysis, and cognitive performance of male rats. *Cogn Affect Behav Neurosci*. 2001;1:371-381

33. McKeever WF, Deyo A. Testosterone, dihydrotestosterone and spatial task performance of males. *Bull Psychon Soc*. 1990;28:305-308

34. Wang C, Swerdloff RS. Should the nonaromatizable androgen dihydrotestosterone be considered as an alternative to testosterone in the treatment of the andropause? *J Clin Endocrinol Metab*. 2002;87(4): 1462-1466

35. Edinger KL, Frye CA. Testosterone's analgesic, anxiolytic, and cognitive-enhancing effects may be due in part to actions of its 5alpha-reduced metabolites in the hippocampus. *Behav Neurosci*. 2004;118(6): 1352-1364

36. Wang C, Alexander G, German N, et al. Testosterone replacement therapy improves mood in hypogonadal men – a clinical research center study. *J Clin Endocrinol Metab*. 1996;81:3578-3583

37. Morley JE, Perry HM, Kaiser FE, et al. Effect of testosterone replacement therapy in old hypogonadal males: a preliminary study. *J Am Geriatr Soc*. 1993;41: 149-152

38. Brodsky IG, Balagogal P, Nair KS. Effects of testosterone replacement on muscle mass and muscle protein synthesis in hypogonadal men – a clinical research center study. *J Clin Endocrinol Metab*. 1996;81:3469-3475

39. Baumgartner RN, Waters DL, Gallagher D, Morley JE, Garry PJ. Predictors of skeletal muscle mass in elderly men and women. *Mech Aging Dev*. 1999;107:123-136

40. Snyder PJ, Peachy H, Hannoush P, et al. Effect of testosterone treatment on body composition and muscle strength in men over 65 years of age. *J Clin Endocrinol Metab*. 1999;84:2647-2653

41. Marin P, Holmang S, Gustafson C, et al. Androgen treatment of abdominally obese men. *Obes Res*. 1993;1: 245-248

42. Singh R, Artaza JN, Taylor WE, Gonzalez-Cadavid NF, Bhasin S. Androgens stimulate myogenic differentiation and inhibit adipogenesis in C3H 10T1/2 pluripotent cells through an androgen receptor-mediated pathway. *Endocrinology*. 2003;144:5081

43. Kasperk CH, Wergedal JE, Farley JR, Linkhart TA, Turner RT, Baylink DJ. Androgens directly stimulate

proliferation of bone cells in vitro. *Endocrinology.* 1989;124:1576-1578

44. Bellido T, Jilka RL, Boyce BF, et al. Regulation of interleukin-6, osteoclastogenesis, and bone mass by androgens. The role of the androgen receptor. *J Clin Invest.* 1995;95:2886-2895

45. van den Beld AW, de Jong FH, Grobbee DE, Pols HAP, Lamberts SWJ. Measures of bioavailable serum testosterone and estradiol and their relationships with muscle strength, bone density, and body composition in elderly men. *J Clin Endocrinol Metab.* 2000;85:3276-3282

46. Goldray D, Weisan Y, Jaccard N, et al. Decreased bone density in elderly men treated with the gonadotropin-releasing hormone agonist decapeptyl (D-Tryp6-GnRH). *J Clin Endocrinol Metab.* 1993;76:288-290

47. Stanley HL, Schmitt BP, Poses RM, Deiss WP. Does hypogonadism contribute to the occurrence of minimal trauma hip fracture in elderly men? *J Am Gerontol Soc.* 1991;39:766-771

48. Jackson JA, Riggs MW, Spiekerman AM. Testosterone deficiency as a risk factor for hip fractures in men: a casecontrol study. *Am J Med Sci.* 1992;304:4-8

49. Spivak JL. The blood in systemic disorders. *Lancet.* 2000;355:1707-1712

50. Gardner FH, Besa EC. Physiologic mechanisms and the hematopoietic effects of the androstanes and their derivatives. *Curr Top Hematol.* 1983;4:123-195

51. Shahidi NT. Androgens and erythropoiesis. *N Engl J Med.* 1973;289:72-80

52. Boyanov MA, Boneva Z, Christov VG. Testosterone supplementation in men with type 2 diabetes, visceral obesity and partial androgen deficiency. *Aging Male.* 2003;6:1

53. Laaksonen DE, Niskanen L, Punnonen K, et al. Testosterone and sex hormone-binding globulin predict the metabolic syndrome and diabetes in middle-aged men. *Diab Care.* 2004;27:1036

54. Marin P, Oden B, Bjorntop P. Assimilation and mobilization of triglycerides in subcutaneous abdominal and femoral adipose tissue in vivo in men: effects of androgens. *J Clin Endocrinol Metab.* 1995;80:239-243

55. Hak AE, Witteman JC, de Jong FH, et al. Low levels of endogenous androgens increase the risk of atherosclerosis in elderly men: the Rotterdam study. *J Clin Endocrinol Metab.* 2002;87:3632-3639

56. Rahman F, Christian HC. Non-classical actions of testosterone: an update. *Trends Endocrinol Metab.* 2007; 18:371-378

57. Foresta C, Zuccarello D, De Toni L, Garolla A, Caretta N, Ferlin A. Androgens stimulate endothelial progenitor cells through an androgen receptor-mediated pathway. *Clin Endocrinol Oxf.* 2008;68:284-289

58. Bowles DK, Maddali KK, Dhulipala VC, Korzick DH. PKC delta mediates anti-proliferative, pro-apoptotic effects of testosterone on coronary smooth muscle. *Am J Physiol Cell Physiol.* 2007;293:C805-C813

59. Morales A. Andropause (or symptomatic late-onset hypogonadism): facts, fiction and controversies. *Aging Male.* 2004;7:297-303

60. Bettocchi C. Late-onset hypogonadism (LOH): incidence, diagnosis, and short-term effects. *Eur Urol Suppl.* 2005;4:4-9

61. Araujo AB, O'Donnell AB, Brambilla DJ, et al. Prevalence and incidence of androgen deficiency in middle-aged and older men: estimates from the Massachusetts male aging study. *J Clin Endocrinol Metab.* 2004;89:5920-5926

62. Wang C. Challenges in the diagnosis of the right patient for testosterone replacement therapy. *Eur Urol Suppl.* 2007;6:862-867

63. Jockenho F, Kaufman J, Mickisch G, Morales A, Wang C. The good, the bad, and the unknown of late onset hypogonadism: the urological perspective. *J Men Health Gend.* 2005;2(3):292-301

64. Wang C, Swerdloff R, Kipnes M, et al. New testosterone buccal system (Striant) delivers physiological testosterone levels: pharmacokinetics study in hypogonadal men. *J Clin Endocrinol Metab.* 2004;89(8):3821-3829

65. Sokol RZ, Palacios A, Campfield LA. Comparison of the kinetics of injectable testosterone in eugonadal and hypogonadal men. *Fertil Steril.* 1982;37:425-430

66. Schubert M, Minnemann T, Hubler D, et al. Intramuscular testosterone undecanoate:pharmacokinetic aspects of a novel testosterone formulation during long-term treatment of menwith hypogonadism. *J Clin Endocrinol Metab.* 2004;89(11):5429-5434

67. Bradwin SW, Swerdloff RS, Santen RJ. Androgens: risks and benefits. *J Clin Endocrinol Metab.* 1991;73:4-7

68. Arver S, Meikle AW, Dobbs AS, et al. Permeation enhanced testosterone transdermal systems in the treatment of male hypogonadism: long term effects. *J Endocrinol.* 1996;148:254-259

69. Rhoden EL, Morgentaler A. Risks of testosterone-replacement therapy and recommendations for monitoring. *N Engl J Med.* 29, 2004;350(5):482-492

70. Comhaire FH. Andropause: hormone replacement therapy in the aging male. *Eur Urol.* 2000;38:655-662

71. Huggins C, Hodges CV. Studies on prostatic cancer: I. The effect of castration, of estrogen and of androgen injection on serum phosphatases in metastatic carcinoma of the prostate. *J Urol.* 2002;168:9-12

72. Schalken J. Androgen receptor mediated growth of prostate (cancer). *Eur Urol Suppl.* 2005;4:4-11

73. Marks LS, Mazer NA, Mostaghel E, et al. Effect of testosterone replacement therapy on prostate tissue in men with late-onset hypogonadism: a randomized controlled trial. *JAMA.* 2006;296:2351-2361

74. Curran MJ, Bihrle W III. Dramatic rise in prostate-specific antigen after androgen replacement in a hypogonadal man with occult adenocarcinoma of the prostate. *Urology.* 1999;53:423-424

75. Loughlin KR, Richie JP. Prostate cancer after exogenous testosterone treatment for impotence. *J Urol.* 1997; 157: 1845

76. Rhoden EL, Morgentaler A. Testosterone replacement therapy in hypogonadal men at high risk for prostate cancer: results of 1 year of treatment in men with prostatic intraepithelial neoplasia. *J Urol.* 2003; 170(Issue: 6, Part 1):2348-2351

77. Morgentaler A. Testosterone replacement therapy and prostate cancer. *Urol Clin North Am.* 2007;34:555-563

78. Morgentaler A. Testosterone and prostate cancer: an historical perspective on a modern myth. *Eur Urol.* 2006;50:935-939

79. Hoffman MA, DeWolf WC, Morgentaler A. Is low serum free testosterone a marker for high grade prostate cancer? *J Urol.* 2000;163:824-827

80. Yamamoto S, Yonese J, Kawakami S, et al. Preoperative serum testosterone level as an independent predictor of treatment failure following radical prostatectomy. *Eur Urol.* 2007;52:696-701

81. Teloken C, Da Ros CT, Caraver F, Weber FA, Cavalheiro AP, Graziottin TM. Low serum testosterone levels are associated with positive surgical margins in radical retropubic prostatectomy: hypogonadism represents bad prognosis in prostate cancer. *J Urol.* 2005;174: 2178-2180

82. Isbarn H, Boccon-Gibod L, Carroll PR, et al. Androgen deprivation therapy for the treatment of prostate cancer: consider both benefits and risks. *Eur Urol.* 2009; 55(1):62-75

83. Smith MR, Finkelstein JS, McGovern FJ, et al. Changes in body composition during androgen deprivation therapy for prostate cancer. *J Clin Endocrinol Metab.* 2002;87:599-603

84. Braga-Basaria M, Dobs AS, Muller DC, et al. Metabolic syndrome in men with prostate cancer undergoing longterm androgen-deprivation therapy. *J Clin Oncol.* 2006;24:3979-3983

85. Smith MR, Lee H, Fallon MA, Nathan DM. Adipocytokines, obesity, and insulin resistance during combined androgen blockade for prostate cancer. *Urology.* 2008;71:318-322

86. Smith MR, Lee H, McGovern F, et al. Metabolic changes during gonadotropin-releasing hormone agonist therapy for prostate cancer: differences from the classic metabolic syndrome. *Cancer.* 2008;112: 2188-2194

87. Green HJ, Pakenham KI, Headley BC, et al. Altered cognitive function in men treated for prostate cancer with luteinizing hormone-releasing hormone analogues and cyproterone acetate: a randomized controlled trial. *BJU Int.* 2002;90(4):427-432

88. Jenkins VA, Bloomfield DJ, Shilling VM, Edginton TL. Does neoadjuvant hormone therapy for early prostate cancer affect cognition? Results from a pilot study. *BJU Int.* 2005;96(1):48-53

89. Alibhai SM, Gogov S, Allibhai Z. Long-term side effects of androgen deprivation therapy in men with non-metastatic prostate cancer: a systematic literature review. *Crit Rev Oncol Hematol.* 2006;60(3):201-215

90. Daniell HW, Dunn SR, Ferguson DW, Lomas G, Niazi Z, Stratte PT. Progressive osteoporosis during androgen deprivation therapy for prostate cancer. *J Urol.* 2000; 163:181-186

91. Shahinian VB, Kuo YF, Freeman JL, Goodwin JS. Risk of fracture after androgen deprivation for prostate cancer. *N Engl J Med.* 2005;352:154-164

92. Smith MR, Lee WC, Brandman J, Wang Q, Botteman M, Pashos CL. Gonadotropin-releasing hormone agonists and fracture risk: a claims-based cohort study of men with nonmetastatic prostate cancer. *J Clin Oncol.* 2005;23:7897-7903

93. Smith MR, Boyce SP, Moyneur E, Duh MS, Raut MK, Brandman J. Risk of clinical fractures after gonadotropin- releasing hormone agonist therapy for prostate cancer. *J Urol.* 2006;175:136-139

94. Jacobson LO, Goldwasser E, Fried W, Plzak L. Role of the kidney in erythropoiesis. *Nature.* 1957;179:633-634

95. Koury ST, Bondurant MC, Koury MJ. Localization of erythropoietin synthesizing cells in murine kidneys by in situ hybridization. *Blood.* 1988;71:524-527

96. Sawada K, Krantz SB, Dai C-H, et al. Purification of human blood burst-forming units-erythroid and demonstration of the evolution of erythropoietin receptor. *J Cell Physiol.* 1990;142:219-230

97. Wickrema A, Krantz SB, Winkelmann JC, Bondurant MC. Differentiation and erythropoietin receptor gene expression in human erythroid progenitor cells. *Blood.* 1992;80:1940-1949

98. Sawyer ST, Koury MJ. Erythropoietin requirement during terminal erythroid differentiation: the role of surface receptors for erythropoietin (Abs). *J Cell Biol.* 1987;105:1077

99. Garcia MM, Beckman BS, Brookins JW, et al. Development of a new radioimmunoassay for EPO using recombinant erythropoietin. *Kidney Int.* 1990; 38:969-975

100. Spivak JL. Erythropoietin use and abuse: when physiology and pharmacology collide. *Adv Exp Med Biol.* 2001;502:207-224

101. McGonigle RJS, Boineau FG, Ohene-Frempong K, Lewy JE, Shadduck RK, Fisher JW. Erythropoietin and inhibitors of in vitro erythropoiesis in the development of anemia in children with renal disease. *J Lab Clin Med.* 1985;105:449-481

102. Radtke HW, Rege AB, Lamarche MB, Bartos D, Campbell RA, Fisher JW. Identification of spermine as an inhibitor of erythropoiesis in patients with chronic renal failure. *J Clin Invest.* 1980;67:1623-1629

103. Maalouf NM. The noncalciotropic actions of vitamin D: recent clinical developments. *Curr Opin Nephrol Hypertens.* 2008;17(4):408-415

104. Zehnder D, Hewison M. The renal function of 25-hydroxyvitamin D3-1alpha-hydroxylase. *Mol Cell Endocrinol.* 1999;151(1–2):213-220

105. Gal-Moscovici A, Sprague SM. Role of vitamin D deficiency in chronic kidney disease. *J Bone Miner Res.* December 2007;22(2):V91-V94

106. Schweda F, Friis U, Wagner C, Skott O, Kurtz A. Renin release. *Physiol Bethesda.* 2007;22:310-319

107. Churchill PC. Cellular mechanisms of renin release. *Clin Exp Hypertens A.* 1988;10(6):1189-1202

108. Wang G, Zhang XC, Pan BN, Na YQ. Diagnosis and management of primary hyperparathyrodism with urolithiasis. *Zhonghua Yi Xue Za Zhi.* 2005;85(9):618-620

109. Ruda JM, Hollenbeak CS, Stack BC. A systematic review of the diagnosis and treatment of primary hyperparathyroidism from 1995 to 2003. *Otolaryngol Head Neck Surg.* 2005;132:359-372

110. Suh JM, Cronan JJ, Monchik JM. Primary hyperparathyroidism: is there an increased prevalence of renal stone disease? *Am J Roentgenol.* 2008;191(3): 908-911

111. Sorensen HA. Surgery for primary hyperparathyroidism. *BMJ.* October 12, 2002;325(7368):785-786

112. Tonini G, Vincenzi B, Santini D. Paraneoplastic syndromes: what we know and what we should know. *Clin Ter.* 2006;157(2):93-94

113. Forga L, Anda E, de Esteban JP Martínez. Paraneoplastic hormonal syndromes. *An Sist Sanit Navar.* 2005;28(2): 213-226

114. DeLellis RA, Xia L. Paraneoplastic endocrine syndromes: a review. *Endocr Pathol.* Winter 2003;14(4): 303-317

115. Palapattu Ganesh S, Blaine Kristo, Jacob Rajfer. Paraneoplastic syndromes in urologic malignancy: the many faces of renal cell carcinoma. *Rev Urol.* 2002;4(4): 163-170

116. Muggia FM. Overview of cancer-related hypercalcemia: epidemiology and etiology. *Semin Oncol.* 1990;17:3-9

117. Mundy GR, Ibbotson KJ, D'Souza SM, et al. The hypercalcemia of cancer. *N Engl J Med.* 1984;310:1718-1727

118. Plimpton CH, Gellhorn A. Hypercalcemia in malignant disease without evidence of bone destruction. *Am J Med.* 1956;21:750-759

119. Mangin M, Webb AC, Dreyer BE, et al. Identification of a cDNA encoding a parathyroid hormone-like peptide from a human tumor associated with humoral hypercalcemia of malignancy. *Proc Natl Acad Sci USA.* 1988; 85:597-601

120. Mundy GR. Pathophysiology of cancer-associated hypercalcemia. *Semin Oncol.* 1990;17:10-15

121. Ritch PS. Treatment of cancer-related hypercalcemia. *Semin Oncol.* 1990;17:26-33

122. Lindop GBM, Fleming S. Renin in renal cell carcinoma – an immuno-cytochemical study using an antibody to pure human renin. *J Clin Pathol.* 1984;37:27-31

123. Sufrin G, Mirand EA, Moore RH, et al. Hormones in renal cancer. *J Urol.* 1977;117:433-438

124. Dahl T, Eide I, Fryjordet A. Hypernephroma and hypertension. *Acta Med Scand.* 1981;209:121-124

125. Nielsen OJ, Jespersen FF, Hilden M. Erythropoietin-induced secondary polycythemia in a patient with a renal cell carcinoma. *APMIS.* 1988;96:688-694

126. Stauffer MH. Nephrogenic hepatosplenomegaly. *Gastroenterology.* 1961;40:694

127. Boxer RJ, Weisman J, Leiber MM, et al. Nonmetastatic hepatic dysfunction syndrome associated with renal cell carcinoma. *J Urol.* 1978;119:468-471

128. Hanash KA. The nonmetastatic hepatic dysfunction syndrome associated with renal cell carcinoma (hypernephroma): Stauffer's syndrome. In: Kuss R, Khoury S, Murphy GP, et al., eds. *Renal Tumors: Proceedings of the First International Symposium on Kidney Tumors.* New York, NY: Liss; 1982:301-316

129. Eddleston ALWF. Immunology and the liver. In: Parker CW, ed. *Clinical Immunology.* Philadelphia, PA: Saunders; 1980:1009

130. Coukos WS, Kozlowski JM, Bauer KD, et al. Induction of nonmetastatic hepatic dysfunction (Stauffer's syndrome) by a human sarcomatoid renal cell carcinoma in athymic mice. *J Urol.* 1986;135:322A

131. Tsukamoto T, Kumamoto Y, Miyao N, et al. Interleukin-6 in renal cell carcinoma. *J Urol.* 1992;148:1778-1782

132. Walsh PN, Kissane JM. Non-metastatic hypernephroma with reversible hepatic dysfunction. *Arch Intern Med.* 1968;122:214-222

133. Braunstein GD, Vaitukaitis JL, Carbone PP, et al. Ectopic production of human chorionic gonadotropin by neoplasms. *Intern Med.* 1973;78:39-45

134. Kuida C, Braunstein GD, Shintaku P, et al. Human chorionic gonadotropin expression in lung, breast and renal carcinomas. *Arch Pathol Lab Med.* 1988;112: 282-285

135. Pavelic K, Popovic M. Insulin and glucagon secretion by renal adenocarcinoma. *Cancer.* 1981;48:98

136. Riggs BL, Sprauge RG. Association of Cushing's syndrome and neoplastic disease. *Arch Intern Med.* 1961;108:841-849

137. Turkington RW. Ectopic production of prolactin. *N Engl J Med.* 1971;285:1455-1461

138. Nishiyama T, Washiyama K, Tanikawa T, et al. Gynecomastia and ectopic human chorionic gonadotropin production by transitional cell carcinoma of the bladder. *Urol Int.* 1992;48(4):463-465

139. Caron P, Averous S, Combelles JL, Louvet JP, Sarramon JP. Gynecomastia and cancer of the bladder: an ectopic secretion of chorionic gonadotropin hormone. *Ann Urol Paris.* 1984;18(1):42-44

140. Nimalasena S, Freeman A, Harland S. Paraneoplastic Cushing's syndrome in prostate cancer: a difficult management problem. *BJU Int.* 2008;101(4):424-427

18

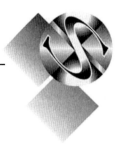

Physiology and Pharmacology of the Prostate

William D. Steers

General Physiology

The physiological properties of the prostate resemble those of other exocrine glands. The precise functions of the prostate remain obscure but some inferences can be made. The prostate is ideally positioned to block the entrance of pathogens into the reproductive tract by secreting potent biological agents that are bacteriostatic. These substances include metal ions, proteases, and highly charged organic molecules such as spermine. The total contribution to seminal fluid (average 3 mL) made by prostate secretions is about 0.5 mL. The pH of these prostate secretions is relatively alkaline and varies from 6 to 8, possibly to counteract the acidic environment of the urethra and vagina. Seminal plasma may increase sperm motility or survival in the male urethra or female genital tract by buffering mechanisms. Constituents of prostatic fluid participate in the clotting (semenogelins I and II) and lysing (prostate specific antigen) of semen. This clotting, then liquefaction may somehow optimize fertility by allowing an initial higher dwell time in the female reproductive tract. A list of components of prostatic fluid is found in Table 18.1.

Access to prostatic fluid by constituents in the blood is limited. Iodine, ethanol, and some antibiotics can directly diffuse into semen. Antibiotics that enter prostatic secretions by virtue of their high lipid solubility include fluoroquinolones, trimethoprim, tetracycline, sulfonamides, erythromycin, clindamycin, and chloramphenicol.[1]

Prostate growth and development from the urogenital sinus is intimately associated with cell–cell communication, most notably stromal–epithelial interactions under endocrine and neural control. An understanding of the tissue matrix in the prostate provides insight into the physiology and growth of the prostate. Laminin surrounds a basement membrane of acinar epithelial cells, capillaries smooth muscle, and nerves. Laminin is important for cellular adhesion, proliferation, differentiation, growth, and migration. Communication via extracellular interactions with the intracellular cytoskeleton regulates prostate cell function.

Cell adhesion molecules determine cellular phenotype and function. Receptors for a number of adhesion molecules span the plasma membrane to bridge cells. Interactions via such receptors are key to the normal growth of the prostate, the pathogenesis of BPH, and the development of prostate cancer.[2] Integrins link extracellular matrix to basement membrane. E-cadherins bind prostate epithelial cells to each other (Fig. 18.1). Selectins link carbohydrates. Immunoglobulins also have a role in cellular adhesion.

Role of Androgens and Other Hormones

The growth, maintenance, and secretory function of the prostate are regulated by androgens, non-androgenic hormones, and growth factors.

C.R. Chapple and W.D. Steers (eds.), *Practical Urology: Essential Principles and Practice*,
DOI: 10.1007/978-1-84882-034-0_18, © Springer-Verlag London Limited 2011

Table 18.1. Components of prostatic secretions

Component	Possible role
Citric acid	Binds metal ions
Polyamines (spermine, putrescene)	Most positively charge organic molecules in nature, involved in cell growth, gate substances through channels
Phosphorylcholine	Reduced in cancer, regulates PSA binding to semenogelins I and II, antibacterial
Prostaglandins (15 types)	
Cholesterol/lipids	
Zinc	
PSA	Inhibits PSA activity, causes semen to clot
Kallikrein 2	
Semenogelins I and II	
Prostase KLK-L1 and 11	Activates alternate pathway
Prostatic acid phosphatase	
Prostate-specific protein	
Prostate-specific membrane antigen	
Prostate stem cell antigen	
Immunoglobulins-IgG	
Transferrin	Binds iron

Androgens affect neural morphology, number, and autonomic receptor function.[3-7] Castration reduces prostate size, the volume of prostatic secretion, muscarinic receptor expression, and noradrenergic innervation of the prostate. The major androgen-regulating prostate physiology and growth is dihydrotestosterone (DHT).[8] The prostate contains five times more DHT than T. DHT is synthesized from testosterone (T) by the action of 5 reductase (5AR) (Fig. 18.2). It exists as two isoforms, Type I and type II. The prostate contains mostly type II. Type I 5AR is found in skin and liver. Expression of 5AR is regulated by androgens. During development, both epithelial and mesenchymal cells contain DHT, which regulates growth. In the adult 5AR is expressed by stromal tissues and basal epithelial cells. DHT is absent in secretory epithelium.

Free T enters cells by diffusion whereupon it is converted to DHT. DHT in epithelial cells exerts its effects on a wide range of cellular functions. After DHT binds to androgen receptors in the cytoplasm the complex is dimerized, then transported to the nucleus where it directs transcription. In the nucleus DHT binds the androgen receptor with much greater potency than T. Dimerized DHT-androgen receptor complex along with coactivators bind to androgen response elements (DNA sequences) on DNA to influence transcription factors and mRNA production (Fig. 18.2). The TATA box DNA sequence determines the RNA polymerase binding start location and the androgen response element dictates how frequently the mRNA is transcribed. These synthetic processes occur over hours to days. However, DHT can also trigger rapid changes in cellular function through separate mechanisms.

Besides DHT, estrogens and adrenal steroids influence prostate function and growth. T can be converted to estradiol and estrone by aromatase in adipose tissues. Another hormone, prolactin, regulates zinc metabolism, citrate and fructose production, as well as androgen uptake and metabolism. Estrogens combined with androgens and possibly prolactin are thought to play a role in the development of BPH.[2]

It is not well understood how signals from neuroendocrine cells in the prostate such as serotonin, paracrine factors (such as basic fibroblast growth factor bFGF), and extracellular matrix regulate the growth and function of the prostate (Fig. 18.1). To a lesser extent DHT also regulates stromal growth factors termed andromedins.

Circulating catecholamines elicit contraction of the prostatic capsule and stroma (norepinephrine, oxytocin).[9,10] Although experiments show that adrenergic mechanisms trigger apoptosis in vitro,[11,12] their long-term administration does not reduce prostate volume, prostate-specific antigen (PSA), or cause histological changes.

Afferent nerves transmit the discomfort of prostatitis and are involved in pathogenesis of male pelvic pain syndrome.[12] Prostate afferents contain neuropeptides that can trigger inflammatory and immune responses. Secretory products, cytokines, and growth factors such as nerve growth factor (NGF), epidermal growth factor (EGF), transforming growth factor beta(TGFβ), insulin growth factor, and basic fibroblast growth factor (bFGF) that are produced in the

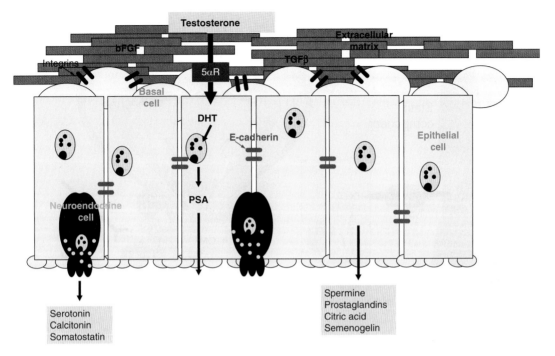

Figure 18.1. Prostate physiology. The prostate is composed of various cell types and extracellular matrix. Integrins link the extracellular matrix to the basement membrane populated by basal epithelial cells. The basal epithelial cells as well as stroma express 5 alpha reductase (5AR). 5AR converts testosterone to dihydrotestosterone (DHT) which diffuses into the secretory epi- thelial cells. Secretory epithelia are attached to each other via cadherins. DHT and other growth factors and hormones regulate synthesis of substances secreted from the epithelium such as the serine protease, prostate-specific antigen (PSA). Interspersed throughout acini close to urethra and lumen are neuroendocrine cells which release a range of compounds.

prostate direct nerve growth and neurotrans- mitter expression in addition to prostate growth and development.[13-16]

Prostate Innervation

Understanding the neurophysiology and auto- nomic pharmacology of the bladder outlet and prostate is of paramount importance for eluci- dating the etiology and designing treatments for lower urinary tract symptoms (LUTS) associated with benign prostatic hyperplasia (BPH). The prostate receives input from parasympathetic and sympathetic nerves.[17-27] Noradrenergic, cho- linergic, peptidergic, and nitrergic nerves have been demonstrated in the prostate.[19-21,28-34] Cell bodies for these neurons reside in the capsule and near the base of the seminal vesicle.[19,27] It is crucial for surgeons to realize that nerves near the lateral aspect of the seminal vesicle

are millimeters from the neurovascular bundle supplying the penis and dissection of these structures must avoid thermal injury. During robotic prostatectomy some nerve fibers within this capsule and fascia can be visualized. Prostatic nerves course within the posterior leaf of Denonvilliers fascia. Often these nerves are mis- taken as branches of the cavernous nerves since those are also NAPHase positive and manufac- ture nitric oxide (NO). Lastly, some branches enter the prostate from the neurovascular bun- dle near the apex. It is tempting to speculate that this abundant innervation implies significant functional importance.

Sympathetic nerves provide most of the effer- ent neural input to the prostate. Nearly 80% of the prostate's innervation is derived from sympa- thetic outflow whereas 21–33% originates from parasympathetic pathways.[25] Nearly two-third of the neurons in the pelvic plexus supplying the prostate are noradrenergic.[35] Noradrenergic nerve fibers are prominent around the prostatic

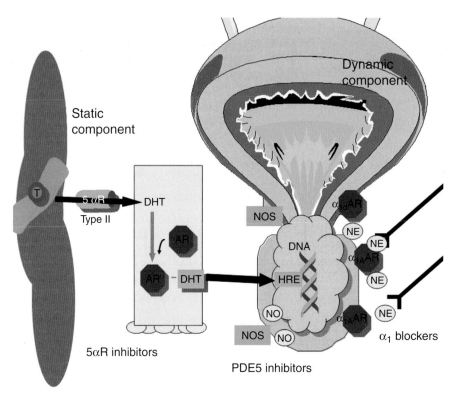

Figure 18.2. Prostate pharmacology. Traditionally, lower urinary symptoms due to benign prostatic hyperplasia (BPH) is attributed to obstruction or increased urethral resistance from prostate growth regulated by dihydrotestosterone (DHT) (STATIC) or increased tone due to norepinephrine (NE) (DYNAMIC) released from noradrenergic postganglionic sympathetic nerves. DHT is synthesized from testosterone by a 5 alpha reductase (5AR) type II in the prostate. After binding to an androgen receptor (AR) the DHT-AR dimmer is transported to the nucleus whereon it binds to a hormone response element (HRE) on DNA to regulate transcription. Nitric oxide (NO) synthesized by nitric oxide synthase (NOS) may also relax the outlet. This action can be enhanced by phosphodiestase type 5 inhibitors (PDE5) which prolong cyclic guanylate cyclase (cGMP) action in smooth muscle.

ducts, especially near their openings into the posterior urethra.

The prostate receives sparse parasympathetic innervation conveyed by the pelvic nerve.[25] Most of the cholinergic fibers are sympathetic in origin. Although less numerous than noradrenergic fibers, cholinergic nerves travel in the dorsal capsule, the fibromuscular stroma, near acini and ducts, and surrounding the vasculature.[29,33,36-38]

Afferent axons whose cell bodies reside in the thoracolumbar and sacral dorsal root ganglia (DRG) travel from the prostate to the CNS in the hypogastric and pelvic nerves, respectively.[25,35] This duality of sensory innervation is most apparent when assessing patterns of referred pain from the prostate. Suprapubic and groin discomfort correspond to referred pain from T12 to L2 levels conveyed from the prostate by

hypogastric nerves,[39] whereas perineal pain signifies input from the pelvic nerve (S2–S4). Prostatic afferents transmit the sensations of pain or contraction, and relay information necessary for reflex phenomena such as emission and ejaculation to the thoracolumbar spinal cord where neurons controlling ejaculation reside.[40] The location of urethral and prostatic nerves, especially sensory fibers, may be relevant for designing therapies for BPH. Thermotherapy for BPH appears to destroy these prostatic nerves or alter neurotransmitter receptor function.[41,42] Relief of symptoms may rely on relative denervation or reduced neurotransmission. Indeed, the ability of prostatic injections of botulinum toxin to relieve symptoms and reduce prostate size suggests an important role for nerves.[43]

In the CNS, pathways receiving input from the prostate participate in an extensive neural network, which interacts with pathways involved in micturition and sexual function.[26] In addition to the expected labeling in autonomic centers, prostate-labeled neurons reside in Barrington's nucleus (micturition center), raphe magnus, reticular formation, A5, A7, periaqueductal gray, red nucleus, and subcoeruleus. The physiological significance of these associations is unclear but they raise the possibility that the function of the prostate or prostatic urethra is somehow linked to that of the bladder/urethra and penis.

CGRP-immunoreactive nerves, considered to represent sensory nerves, are few compared to the other phenotypes characterized. NOS- and CGRP-immunoreactive terminals have similar profiles, but the immunoreactivities are not co-localized.[29] Pituitary adenylate cyclase activating peptide (PACAP), presumably in pelvic afferents, is expressed by nerves supplying the prostate.[29] The proximal central prostate contains more peptidergic fibers (vasoactive intestinal polypeptide [VIP] and opiate-related peptides met- and Leu- enkephalins [ENK],[32,44] neuropeptide Y [NPY], peptide histidine leucine [PHI], somatostatin [SOM], galanin [GAL], bombesin [BOM], substance P [SP], calcitonin gene-related peptide [CGRP], and pituitary adenylate cyclase peptide [PCAP]) than the anterior capsule, which exceeds the distal central zones, which in turn is greater than the peripheral zone.

Neurophysiology and Neuropharmacology

Stimulation of the pelvic nerve produces a slight contraction of the prostate, whereas hypogastric nerve stimulation evokes a profound contraction and secretion.[45] Contraction of the prostatic capsule, due to firing of the hypogastric nerve, increases bladder outlet resistance. Contractile responses are mediated by noradrenergic rather than cholinergic mechanisms. Noradrenaline stimulates contraction-mediating α-adrenoceptors localized to predominately prostatic stroma. Although both α_1 and α_2 receptors can be identified in the human prostate,[46,47] the contractile properties are mediated primarily by α_1-adrenoceptors.[46,48-53] Many clinical investigations have confirmed that α_1-adrenoceptor blockade

relieves storage and voiding components of LUTS in BPH patients.[54-57] The α_{1A}-adrenoceptor is the dominant subtype representing about 60–85% of the α_1-adrenoceptor population. The α_{1A}-adrenoceptor mediates the contractile response of the human prostate in vitro.[58,59] However, there is some variability in expression among men as indicated by differential responses to alpha-subtype drugs that correlate with the α_{1A} and α_{1b} ratio in the specimens.[60]

Noradrenergic nerves are also considered responsible for maintaining prostatic smooth muscle tone,[61] and approximately 50% of the total urethral pressure in BPH patients may be due to α-adrenoceptor-mediated muscle tone.[62,63] Conceivably a global increase in sympathetic tone leads to increased urethral resistance and prostatic tone. Thus α blockers have shown clinical utility for voiding symptoms or painful ejaculation in young anxious men.[64]

In addition to causing contraction of the outlet, hypogastric nerve stimulation (sympathetic) increases secretion.[8,65-68] Yet this secretion is blocked by the muscarinic agonist atropine,[66-68] implying that sympathetic cholinergic nerves control exocrine function (see reviews by Elbadawi and Goodman,[17] Dail,[21] and Smith[69]). Likewise, muscarinic agonists including pilocarpine and urecholine induce prostatic secretion.[8,17,65,66,70] This secretion is mediated by muscarinic receptors expressed by epithelial cells.[46,71,72] Cholinomimetic drugs barely contract prostate capsule accounting for only 10–15% of that of α agonists. Anti-muscarinics such as atropine completely block secretory responses to these agonists as well as hypogastric nerve-evoked secretion. Despite this observation, a decrease in ejaculate volume is rarely a complaint of men on anticholinergics. Of the five molecular muscarinic receptor subtypes the M_1 receptor is expressed by prostatic epithelium, whereas the stroma expresses the M_2 receptor protein.

Many prostatic nerves stain for nitric oxide synthase (NOS) or heme-oxygenase (HO), suggesting that they manufacture nitric oxide and carbon monoxide.[29,33,73-77] NOS is expressed by both sensory and motoneurons. In men with BPH, this finding may explain the efficacy of PDE5 inhibitors to reduce LUTS (Fig. 18.2). NO inhibits secretion and reduces contractile action. NO alone has no consistent effect in the prostate yet relaxes the urethra.[78] Relaxation of NE-contracted prostatic tissue can be prevented by NOS inhibition.[29,42] Similar to its effect on the urethra, exogenous NO relaxes prostatic tissues. NO may play a role in controlling smooth muscle tone in the prostate. Indeed, phosphodiesterase type 5 (PDE5) inhibitors which raise cGMP may increase urine flow rates and lower LUTS in men with BPH.[79-81] Yet, a reduction in symptoms without a corresponding increase in urinary flow suggests actions at other sites than the outlet for PDE5 inhibitors.

Transmitters released from prostatic nerves may alter the composition of prostatic secretions.[68,70,82,83] The concentration of sodium in prostatic secretions is essentially the same as that in plasma. In contrast, sodium and potassium concentrations in neurally evoked prostatic secretions exceed those in plasma. In carbachol-stimulated secretions the protein concentration and prostatic acid phosphatase activity were reduced compared to noradrenaline- or phenylephrine-stimulated secretion.[70]

Nerves maintain the functional integrity of glandular tissue. Several studies have shown that surgical denervation reduces prostatic weight and causes atrophy of acini.[84-86] Similarly, chemical sympathectomy decreases the weight of the prostate and glands appear dilated.[87,88] Botulinum toxin, which prevents neurotransmitter release, causes long-term shrinkage of prostate with a reduction in PSA.[43] Interestingly, men with longstanding spinal cord injury exhibit reduced prostate size, decreased mRNA for the androgen receptor, and lower levels PSA.[89] Whether this is due to changes in neural activity or chronic infections is unclear.

Treatment of LUTS Attributed to BPH

The treatment of LUTS due to BPH has been complicated by the proliferation of clinical trials demonstrating efficacy of agents spanning several drug classes relative to placebo. Traditionally, one is left to believe that LUTS due to BPH results from merely bladder outlet obstruction. Reduction in outlet resistance by relaxation of the urethra and prostatic smooth muscle (dynamic component) or a reduction in prostate size (static component) may be too simplistic a concept and fails to reconcile data that men without urodynamic evidence of reduced obstruction and no change in voiding flow rates can benefit from these drugs (Fig. 18.2). Because LUTS attributed to BPH is multifactorial (increased resistance, changes in the detrusor, urothelium, interstitial cells, or nerves), drugs probably target multiple sites. Indeed, the association of LUTS with metabolic syndrome and erectile dysfunction implies a complex interaction of pathophysiological processes. Moreover, the prevalence of overactive bladder (OAB) increases with age, especially in men. Thus, the multiple sequelae of obstruction combined with underlying OAB suggest that a wide range of therapies may be effective. In fact if one scans the literature for prospective randomized trials for BPH and calculates the potential combinations of approved 5AR inhibitors ($n=2$) α-adrenergic antagonists ($n=7$), PDE 5 inhibitors ($n=4$), and antimuscarinics ($n=6$) used singly, doubly, or in triple drug combinations, greater than 72 regimens can be identified! And this fails to include vasopressin analogs or botulinum toxin.

In general, the rapid onset and relief of most bothersome storage symptoms of urgency, frequency, and nocturia by α-adrenergic antagonist has led to their use as drugs of first choice. The evolution from non-α_1 selective multidose regimens (prazosin, phenoxybenzamine) to once-daily preparations (doxazosin, terazosin, alfuzosin) and then to agents with fewer effects on the vasculature due to α_{1A} selectivity (tamsulosin, silodosin) has occurred. Some agents such as doxazosin GITS with slow release allow initiation at higher doses for non-subtype-selective blockers, thereby avoiding slow dose titration. In a meta-analysis comparing efficacy as indicated by symptom scores and maximal flow rates, all agents are similar.[90] The only exception to this is suggested by a comparative trial between doxazosin and alfuzosin.[91] Although increases in urinary flow rates were similar, symptom improvement was greater for doxazosin. Given similar α-adrenergic antagonist properties, and the major difference being lack of CNS penetration for alfuzosin, implies that central action on α blockers participates in symptom relief especially for storage symptoms. Because the α_{1A} receptor regulates contraction of the seminal vesicles and vas deferens, agents less selective for this receptor (alfuzosin) cause fewer changes in seminal emission and ejaculation than tamsulosin.[92]

For large prostates with increasing likelihood of future urinary retention, hematuria or surgical intervention, especially voiding symptoms (slow stream, hesitancy, dribbling, and double voiding) the 5AR inhibitors (finasteride, dutasteride) are reasonable drugs to treat LUTS in men with large prostates. These agents take 3–6 months to achieve maximal benefit. Additional benefits include reduction in hematuria and a suggested reduction in prostate cancer.[93,94] 5AR inhibition causes a rapid reduction in vascular endothelial growth factor (VEGF) which may explain the reduction in hematuria. The magnitude of clinical benefits of both 5AR inhibitors is similar.[95,96] However, dutasteride has the theoretical advantage in possible greater prophylaxis against prostate cancer and slightly more rapid onset by virtue of blockade of both types I and II AR compared to finasteride, which only acts on type II AR. Ongoing clinical trials are investigating these assertions.

Several large trials (PREDICT, VA CoOP, MTOPS) have shown the benefit of combination therapy with α-adrenergic antagonists and 5AR inhibitors (doxzasosin/finasteride, terazosin/finasteride, alfuzosin/dutasteride).[97-100] Often α blockers can be withdrawn in patients on combination therapy and symptomatic improvement persists.

If men complaining of predominately storage symptoms, especially urge urinary incontinence, have low PSAs (<1.5 ng/mL) and small prostates on digital rectal examination, antimuscarinics may be a good choice alone or in combination with an α-adrenergic antagonist. Because trials excluded men with postvoid residual urines greater than 150 mL, limiting the use of antimuscarinics if the patient has a high residual is prudent. If the patient has cognitive dysfunction antimuscarinics should probably not be initiated.

If a patient has erectile dysfunction plus LUTS, an α-adrenergic antagonist (tamsulosin) combined with daily PDE 5 inhibitor (tadalafil) is reasonable. If ejaculatory dysfunction occurs (up to 20%) then switching to alfuzosin can be considered. The use of 5AR inhibitors, which can cause erectile dysfunction and reductions in ejaculate volume should be limited as well.

Summary

The prostate is an exocrine gland that manufactures an array of substances postulated to play a role in fertility or host defenses. Prostate growth, development of BPH and cancer is attributed to stromal–epithelial interactions mediated by cell–cell interactions via integrins and cadherins as well as a wide range of growth factors and hormones. Growth factors and other substances produced by the prostate are likely to influence neural growth, morphology, and transmitter expression, and function in an autocrine/paracrine-like fashion. The most important of these is DHT. This observation has been exploited to develop drugs that block the production of DHT, namely, 5AR inhibitors, to shrink the prostate and relieve symptoms of BPH. Whether this class of drugs can be used to prevent the development of adenocarcinoma of the prostate is hotly debated.

The prostate receives input from sympathetic and to a lesser extent parasympathetic nerves. In contrast to other genitourinary tissues, postganglionic cholinergic sympathetic nerves are responsible for secretion while postganglionic noradrenergic sympathetic nerves mediate contraction in this organ and the urethra as well as bladder neck via α_{1A} and α_{1D} receptors, respectively. This latter finding forms the principal basis for use of α blockers in men with LUTS due to BPH. Recent data suggesting that PDE5 inhibitors may also be effective for the treatment of LUTS due to BPH could be due to augmentation of NO production and release from nerves in the prostatic stroma and urethra.

Improvement in LUTS following injection of botulinum toxin into the prostate is proof of the principle that abolishing neural input to the prostate reduces LUTS almost to the degree seen with surgery. Exploitation of these findings to further enhance BPH therapy is likely.

References

1. Meares EM. Prostatitis. *Med Clin North Am*. 1991;75: 405-424
2. Veltri R, Rodriguez R, et al. Molecular biology, endocrinology, and physiology of the prostate and seminal vesicles. In: Wein AJ, ed. *Campell-Walsh Urology*. 9th ed. Philadelphia: Saunders; 2007:chap 85

3. Partanen M, Hervonen A. The effect of long-term castration on the histochemically demonstrable catecholamines in the hypogastric ganglion of the rat. *J Autonom Nerv Syst*. 1979;1:139-147

4. Shapiro E, Miller A, Lepor H. Down regulation of the muscarinic cholinergic receptor of the rat prostate following castration. *J Urol*. 1985;134(1):179-182

5. Melvin J, Hamill R. The major pelvic ganglion: androgen control of postnatal development. *J Neurosci*. 1987;7(6): 1607-1612

6. Hamill R, Schroeder B. Hormonal regulation of adult sympathetic neurons: the effects of castration on neuropeptide Y, norepinephrine, and tyrosine hydroxylase activity. *J Neurobiol*. 1990;21(5):731-742

7. Regunathan S, Nassir Y, Sundaram K, et al. Expression of I_2-Imidazoline sites in rat prostate. Effect castration aging. *Biochem Pharmacol*. 1996;51:455-459

8. Farnsworth W, Lawrence M. Regulation of prostate secretion in the rat. *Am J Physiol*. 1965;119:373-376

9. Bodansky M, Sharaf H, Roy J, et al. Contractile activity of vasotocin, oxytocin, and vasopressin on mammalian prostate. *Eur J Pharmacol*. 1992;216:311-313

10. Sharaf H, Foda HD, Said SI, et al. Oxytocin and related peptides elicit contractions of prostate and seminal vesicle. *Ann NY Acad Sci*. 1992;652:474-477

11. Litvak J, Borkowski A, Jacobs S, et al. Induction of apoptosis by doxazosin: targeting alpha-1 blockade in benign prostatic hyperplasia. *J Urol*. 1997;157: 1086A

12. Hellstrom W, Schmidt R, Lue T, et al. Neuromuscular dysfunction in nonbacterial prostatitis. *Urology*. 1987;30(2):183-188

13. Harper G, Barde Y, Burnstock G, et al. Guinea pig prostate is a rich source of nerve growth factor. *Nature*. 1979;279:160-162

14. Collins A, Robinson E, Neal D. Benign prostatic stromal cells are regulated by basic fibroblast growth factor and transforming growth factor beta 1. *J Endocrinol*. 1996;151:315-322

15. Paul A, Grant E, Habib F. The expression and localization of beta nerve growth factor in benign and malignant human prostate tissue: relationship to neuroendocrine differentiation. *Br J Cancer*. 1996;74:1990-1996

16. Story M, Hopp K, Meier D. Regulation of basic fibroblast growth factor expression by transforming growth factor beta in cultured human prostate stromal cells. *Prostate*. 1996;28:219-226

17. Elbadawi A, Goodman D. Autonomic innervation of accessory male genital glands. In: Spring-Mills E, Hafez E, eds. *Male Accessory Sex Glands*. Amsterdam: Elsevier-North-Holland Biomedical Press; 1980

18. Gosling J. Autonomic innervation of the prostate. In: Hinman F, ed. *Benign Prostatic Hypertrophy*. New York: Springer; 1983:349-360:chap 32

19. Higgins J, Gosling J. Studies on the structure and intrinsic innervation of normal human prostate. *Prostate*. 1989;2:5-16

20. Crowe R, Chapple C, Burnstock G. The human prostate gland: a histochemical and immunohistochemical study of neuropeptides, serotonin, dopamine beta-hydroxylase and acetylcholinesterase in autonomic nerves and ganglia. *Br J Urol*. 1991;68(1):53-61

21. Dail WG. Autonomic innervation of male reproductive genitalia. In: Maggi CA, ed. *The Autonomic Nervous System*. Nervous Control of the Urogenital System, vol. 6. London: Harwood Academic Publishers; 1993:69-101:chap 9

22. Benoit G, Merlaud L, Meduri G, et al. Anatomy of the prostatic nerves. *Surg Radiol Anat*. 1994;16(1):23-29

23. Setchell B, Maddocks S, Brooks D. Anatomy, Vasculature Innervation, and Fluids of the Male Reproductive Tract. New York: Raven Press; 1994

24. Vaalasti A. Autonomic innervation of the human male accessory sex glands. In: Riva A, Testa RF, eds. *Ultrastructure of Male Urogenital Glands: Prostate, Seminal Vesicles, Urethral, and Bulbourethral Glands*. New York: Kluwer Academic; 1994:187-196

25. Kepper M, Keast J. Immunohistochemical properties and spinal connections of pelvic autonomic neurons that innervate the rat prostate gland. *Cell Tissue Res*. 1995;281(3):533-542

26. Marson L, Orr R. Identification of rat spinal neurons that innervate the prostate comparison of hypogastric and pelvic inputs using transneuronal tracing with pseudorabies virus. *Soc Neurosci*. 1996;22:1051 (Abstract)

27. Dixon J, Jen P, Gosling J. A double-label immunohistochemical study of intramural ganglia from the human male urinary bladder neck. *J Anat*. 1997;190(1): 125-134

28. Hedlund P, Larsson B, Alm P, et al. Nitric oxide synthase-containing nerves and ganglia in the dog prostate: a comparison with other transmitters. *Histochem J*. 1996;28(9):635-642

29. Hedlund P, Ekstrom P, Larsson B, et al. Heme oxygenase and NO synthase in the human prostate-relation to adrenergic, cholinergic and peptide containing nerves. *J Autonom Nerv Syst*. 1997;63:115-126

30. Gosling J, Thompson S. A neurohistochemical and histological study of peripheral autonomic neurons of the human bladder neck and prostate. *Urol Int*. 1977;32:269

31. Baumgarten H, Falck B, Holstein A, et al. Adrenergic innervation of the human testis, epididymis, ductus deferens and prostate: a fluorescence microscopic and fluorometric study. *Z Fur Zellforsch Und Mikrosk Anat*. 1968;90(1):81-95

32. Alm P, Allumets J, Hakanson R, et al. Peptidergic (vasoactive intestinal peptide) nerves in the genitourinary tract. *Neuroscience*. 1977;2(5):751-754

33. Dunzendorfer U, Jonas D, Weber W. The autonomic innervation of the human prostate. Histochemistry of acetylcholinesterase in the normal and pathologic states. *Urol Res*. 1976;4:29-32

34. Yokoyama R, Inokuchi T, Satoh H, et al. Distribution of tyrosine hydroxylase (TH)-like, neuropeptide Y (NPY)-like immunoreactive and acetylcholinesterase (ACHE)-positive nerve fibers in the prostate gland of the monkey (Macacus fuscatus). *Kurume Med J*. 1990;37(1):1-8

35. Danuser H, Springer J, Katofiasc M, et al. Extrinsic innervation of the cat prostate gland; a combined tracing and immunohistochemical study. *J Urol*. 1997;157(3):1018-1024

36. Dixon J, Jen P, Gosling J. The distribution of vesicular acetylcholine transporter and NPY in and nitric oxide in the human genitourinary organs. *Neurourol Urodynam*. 2000;19:185-194

37. Vaalasti A, Hervonen A. Autonomic innervation of the human prostate. *Invest Urol*. 1980;17(4):293-297

38. Shirai M, Sasaki K, Rikimaru A. A histochemical investigation of the distribution of adrenergic and cholinergic nerves in the human male genital organs. *Tohoku J Exp Med*. 1973;111:281-291

39. Plancarte R, Amescua C, Patt RB, et al. Superior hypogastric plexus block for pelvic cancer pain. *Anesthesiology*. 1990;73(2):236-239.

40. Lique M, Coolen JA, Truitt WA, McKenna KE. Central regulation of ejaculation. *Physiol Behav*. 2004;83(2): 203-215

41. Perichino M, Bozzo W, Puppo P, et al. Does transurethral thermotherapy induce long-term alpha blockade? An immunohistochemical study. *Eur Urol*. 1993;23:299-301

42. Arai Y, Jukuzawa S, Terai A, Yoshida O. Transurethral microwave thermotherapy for benign prostatic hyperplasia – relation between clinical response and prostate histology. *Prostate*. 1996;28(2):84-88

43. Chuang YC, Chiang PH, Yoshimura N, De Miguel F, Chancellor MB. Sustained beneficial effects of intraprostatic botulinum toxin type A on lower urinary tract symptoms and quality of life in men with benign prostatic hyperplasia. *BJU Int*. 2006;98:1033-1037

44. Vaalasti A, Linnoila I, Hervonen A. Immunohistochemical demonstration of VIP, [Met⁵]-and [Leu⁵]-enkephalin immunoreactive nerve fibers in the human prostate and seminal vesicles. *Histochemistry*. 1980;66:89-98

45. Eckhardt C. Untersuchungen uber die Erection des Penis beim Hunde. *Beitr Anat Physiol*. 1863;3:123-166

46. Hedlund H, Andersson K, Larsson B. Alpha-adrenoceptors and muscarinic receptors in the isolated human prostate. *J Urol*. 1985;134:1291-1298

47. Lepor H, Shapiro E. Characterization of alpha₁-adrenergic receptors in human benign prostatic hyperplasia. *J Urol*. 1984;132:1226-1229

48. Hiebel J, Ruffolo R. The use of alpha-adrenoceptor antagonists in the pharmacological management of benign prostatic hypertrophy: an overview. *Pharmacol Res*. 1996;33(3):145-160

49. Shapiro E, Lepor H. Alpha2 adrenergic receptors in hyperplastic human prostate: identification and characterization using 3 H-rauwolscine. *J Urol*. 1986;135: 1038-1043

50. Lepor H, Gup DI, Bauman M, et al. Laboratory assessment of terazosin and a1 blockade in prostatic hyperplasia. *Urology*. 1988;32:21-26

51. Kitada S, Kumazawa J. Pharmacological characteristics of smooth muscle in benign prostatic hyperplasia and normal prostatic tissue. *J Urol*. 1987;138:158-160

52. Chapple CR, Aubrey ML, James S, et al. Characterisation of human prostatic adrenoceptors using pharmacology receptor binding and localization. *Br J Urol*. 1989;63: 487-496

53. Gup D, Shapiro E, Buamann M, et al. Contractile properties of human prostate adenomas and the development of infravesical obstruction. *Prostate*. 1989;15:105-114

54. Eri L, Tveter KJ. a-Blockade in the treatment of symptomatic benign prostatic hyperplasia. *J Urol*. 1995;154: 923-934

55. Andersson KE, Lepor H, Wyllie M. Prostate a1 adrenoceptor and uroselectivity. *Prostate*. 1977;30:202-216

56. Chapple CR. Selective a1-adrenoceptor antagonists in benign prostatic hyperplasia: rationale and clinical experience. *Eur Urol*. 1996;129:144

57. Jardin A, Andersson K-E, Caine M, et al. a-blockers therapy in benign prostatic hyperplasia. In: Cockett ATK, Khoury S, Aso Y, Chatelain C, Denis L, Griffiths K, Murphy C, eds. *The Third International Consultation on Benign Prostatic Hyperplasia (BPH)*. New York: SCI; 1996:527-564

58. Forray C, Bard JA, Wetzel JM, et al. The a1-adrenergic receptor that mediates smooth muscle contraction in human prostate has the pharmacological properties of the cloned human a1c subtype. *Mol Pharmacol*. 1994;45:703-708

59. Marshall I, Burt RP, Chapple CR. Noradrenaline contractions of human prostate mediated by a1a-(a1c-)adrenoceptor subtype. *Br J Pharmacol*. 1995;115:781-786

60. Fabiani ME, Sourial M, Thomas WG, et al. Angiotensin II enhances noradrenaline release from sympathetic nerves of the rat prostate via a novel angiotensin receptor: implications for the pathophysiology of benign prostatic hyperplasia. *J Endocrinol*. 2001;171(1): 97-108

61. Caine M, Raz S, Zeigler M. Adrenergic and cholinergic receptors in the human prostate, prostatic capsule and bladder neck. *Br J Urol*. 1975;47:193-202

62. Appell RA, England HR, Hussell AR, et al. The effect of epidural anesthesia on the urethral closure pressure profile in patients with prostatic enlargement. *J Urol*. 1980;124:410-411

63. Furuya S, Kumamoto Y, Yokoyama E, et al. Alpha-adrenergic activity and urethral pressure in prostatic zone in benign prostatic hypertrophy. *J Urol*. 1982;128:836-839

64. Nickel JC. Alpha-blockers for the treatment of prostatitis-Like syndromes. *Rev Urol*. 2006;8(suppl 4):S26-S34

65. Farrell J, Lyman Y. A study of the secretory nerves and the action of certain drugs on, the prostate gland. *Am J Phys*. 1937;118:64-70

66. Smith E, Lebeaux M. The mediation of the canine prostatic secretion provoked by hypogastric nerve stimulation. *Invest Urol*. 1970;7(4):313-318

67. Smith E, Lebeaux M. The composition of nerve induced canine prostatic secretion. *Invest Urol*. 1971;8(2):100-103

68. Bruschini H, Schmidt R, Tanagho E. Neurologic control of prostatic secretion in the dog. *Invest Urol*. 1978; 15(4):288-290

69. Smith ER. The canine prostate and its secretion. In: Thomas JA, Singhai R, eds. *Molecular Mechanisms of Gonadal Hormone Action*. Baltimore, MD: University Park Press; 1975:167-204

70. Wang J, McKenna KE, Lee C. Determination of prostatic secretion in rats: effect of neurotransmitters and testosterone. *Prostate*. 1991;18:289-301.

71. Lepor H, Khuhar M. Characterization of muscarinic cholinergic receptor binding in the vas deferens, bladder, prostate and penis of the rabbit. *J Urol*. 1984;132: 392-396

72. James S, Chapple C, Phillips M, et al. Autoradiographic analysis of alpha-adrenoceptors and muscarinic cholinergic receptors in the hyperplastic human prostate. *J Urol*. 1989;142(2 Pt 1):438-444

73. Burnett A, Takeda M, Maguire M, et al. Characterization and localization of nitric oxide synthase in the human prostate. *Urology*. 1995;45:435-439

74. Jen P, Dixon J, Gosling J. Co-localisation of tyrosine hydroxylase, nitric oxide synthase and neuropeptides in neurons of the human postnatal male pelvic ganglia. *J Autonom Nerv Syst*. 1996;59(1–2):41-50

75. Jen P, Dixon J, Gerahart J, et al. Nitric oxide synthase and tyrosine hydroxylase are co-localized in nerves supplying the postnatal human male genitourinary organs. *J Urol*. 1996;155(3):1171-1121

76. Jen P, Dixon J. Development of peptide-containing nerves in the human fetal prostate gland. *J Anat*. 1995; 187(Pt. 1):169-179

77. Takeda M, Tang R, Shapiro E, et al. Effects of nitric oxide on human and canine prostates. Urology. 1995;45:440-446

78. Isaacs J, Steinberg G. A guide to the physiology of the prostate. *Cont Urol*. 1990;47:54-66

79. McVary KT, Monnig W, Camps JL Jr, Young JM, Tseng LJ, van den Ende G. Sildenafil citrate improves erectile function and urinary symptoms in men with erectile dysfunction and lower urinary tract symptoms associated with benign prostatic hyperplasia: a randomized, double-blind trial. *J Urol*. 2007;177:1071-1077

80. McVary KT, Roehrborn CG, Kaminetsky JC, et al. Tadalafil relieves lower urinary tract symptoms secondary to benign prostatic hyperplasia. *J Urol*. 2007;177: 1401-1407

81. Stief CG, Porst H, Neuser D, Beneke M, Ulbrich E. A randomised, placebo-controlled study to assess the efficacy of twice-daily vardenafil in the treatment of lower urinary tract symptoms secondary to benign prostatic hyperplasia. *Eur Urol*. 2008;53:1236-1244

82. Smith E, Miller T, Pebler R. Transepithelial voltage changes during prostatic secretion in the dog. *Am Phys Soc*. 1983;245:F470-F477

83. Jacobs SC, Story MT. Autonomic control of acid phosphatase exocrine secretion by the rat prostate. *Urol Res*. 1989;17:311-315

84. Martinez-Pineiro L, Dahiya R, Nunes L, et al. Pelvic plexus denervation in rats causes morphologic and functional changes of the prostate. *J Urol*. 1993;150(1): 215-218

85. Wang J, McKenna K, McVary K, et al. Requirement of innervation for maintenance of structural and functional integrity in the rat prostate. *Biol Reprod*. 1991;44(6):1171-1176

86. McVary KT, Razzaq A, Lee C, et al. Growth of the rat prostate gland is facilitated by the autonomous nervous system. *Biol Reprod*. 1994;51:99-107

87. Vaalast A, Alho AM, Tainio H. The effect of sympathetic denervation with 6-hydroxydopamine on the ventral prostate of the rat. *Acta Histochem*. 1986;79:49-54

88. Lamano-Carvalho TL, Favaretto AL, Petenusci SO, et al. Prepubertal development of rat prostate and seminal vesicle following chemical sympathectomy with guanethidine. *Braz J Med Biol Res*. 1993;26(6): 639-646

89. Huang HFS, Li MT, Linsenmeyer T, et al. The effects of spinal cord injury on the status of messenger ribonucleic acid for TRPM2 and androgen receptor in the prostate of the rat. *J Androl*. 1997;18:250-256

90. Djavan B, Marberger M. A meta-analysis on the efficacy and tolerability of α_1-adrenoceptor antagonists in patients with lower urinary tract symptoms suggestive of benign prostatic obstruction. *Eur Urol*. 1999;36:1-13

91. de Reijke TM, Klarskov P. Comparative efficacy of two α-adrenoreceptor antagonists, doxazosin and alfuzosin, in patients with lower urinary tract symptoms from benign prostatic enlargement. *BJU Int*. 2004;93:757-762

92. Hellstrom WJ, Sikka SC. Effects of acute treatment with tamsulosin versus alfuzosin on ejaculatory function in normal volunteers. *J Urol*. 2006;176:1529-1533

93. Foley SJ, Soloman LZ, Wedderburn AW, et al. A prospective study of the natural history of hematuria associated with benign prostatic hyperplasia and the effect of finasteride. *J Urol*. 2000;163:496-498

94. Thompson IM, Goodman PJ, Tangen CM, et al. The influence of finasteride on the development of prostate cancer. *N Engl J Med*. 2003;349(3):215-224

95. Gormley GJ, Stoner E, Bruskewitz RC, et al. The effect of finasteride in men with benign prostatic hyperplasia. The Finasteride Study Group. *N Engl J Med*. 1992;327:1185-1191

96. Roehrborn CG, Marks LS, Fenter T, et al. Efficacy and safety of dutasteride in the four-year treatment of men with benign prostatic hyperplasia. *Urology*. 2004;63:709-715

97. Roehrborn CG. Alfuzosin 10 mg once daily prevents overall clinical progression of benign prostatic hyperplasia but not acute urinary retention: results of a 2-year placebo-controlled study. *BJU Int*. 2006;97:734-741

98. Kirby RS, Roehrborn C, Boyle P, et al. Efficacy and tolerability of doxazosin and finasteride, alone or in combination, in treatment of symptomatic benign prostatic hyperplasia: the Prospective European Doxazosin and Combination Therapy (PREDICT) trial. *Urology*. 2003;61:119-126

99. Lepor H, Williford WO, Barry MJ, et al. The efficacy of terazosin, finasteride, or both in benign prostatic hyperplasia. Veterans Affairs Cooperative Studies Benign Prostatic Hyperplasia Study Group. *N Engl J Med*. 1996;335:533-539

100. McConnell JD, Roehrborn CG, Bautista OM, et al. The long-term effect of doxazosin, finasteride, and combination therapy on the clinical progression of benign prostatic hyperplasia. *N Engl J Med*. 2003;349:2387-2398

19

Wound Healing and Principles of Plastic Surgery

Timothy O. Davies and Gerald H. Jordan

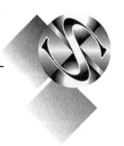

Wound Healing

Wound healing is the natural restorative response to tissue injury. Essential to optimizing surgical procedures and evolving novel techniques, a basic understanding of the basic principles of wound healing is necessary. Types of wound closure are classified as primary, secondary, and tertiary. Primary wound healing refers to those wounds which are immediately closed with direct epithelial/mucosal approximation. Secondary wound healing refers to those wounds that all or a portion are left open to heal, without any attempt at closure. These will heal by granulation, reepithelialization, and wound contraction. Tertiary wound healing refers to wounds closed by delayed primary closure.

The process of wound healing is usually described in three phases: inflammation, proliferation, and remodeling. The inflammatory phase is initiated immediately at the time of injury and consists of hemostasis and debridement of the wound by inflammatory cells. The events of the proliferative phase include epithelialization, fibroplasia, and angiogenesis. The remodeling phase strengthens the wound by reorganizing collagen to increase tensile strength.

Inflammation

Hemostasis and sealing the wound are the first steps to repairing an injury. The release

of epinephrine and norepinephrine, as well as prostaglandins, mediates initial local vasoconstriction. The exposure of collagen (types 4 and 5) and basement membrane proteins from endothelial cells activate platelet aggregation and the coagulation pathway, both intrinsic and extrinsic clotting factors.[1] With the initiation of the clotting cascade, the eventual product – thrombin – catalyzes fibrinogen to fibrin. Fibrin traps red blood cells and clotting ensues to seal the wound. This initial clot is primarily composed of aggregated platelets and fibrin.

Platelets are activated by adherence to exposed collagen and respond with the release of stored factors in alpha granules (storage organelles) and dense bodies. The alpha granules release platelet-derived growth factor (PDGF), transforming growth factor β (TGF-β), fibrinogen, and other vasoactive and chemotatic substances when they degrade. These substances further stimulate platelet aggregation, vasodilation, and increased vascular permeability.[2] The action of phospholipases on disrupted cell membranes causes arachidonic acid release. This results in thromboxane and prostaglandin accumulation in injured tissue promoting further platelet aggregation and vasoconstriction.

The initial vasoconstriction is followed by vasodilation mediated by PDGF, TGF-β, and other vasoactive factors. Vasodilation and increased vascular permeability are also mediated by histamine and endothelial growth factor (EGF). These cytokines are released by injured endothelial cells and local mast cells.[3]

C.R. Chapple and W.D. Steers (eds.), *Practical Urology: Essential Principles and Practice*,
DOI: 10.1007/978-1-84882-034-0_19, © Springer-Verlag London Limited 2011

In addition to furthering the inflammatory process, local vasodilation is responsible for the typical erythema that accompanies acute injury. With the release of these chemotatic substances, leukocytes (neutrophils, monocytes, macrophages, and lymphocytes) are drawn into the wound.

Neutrophils phagocytize necrotic debris, foreign material, and bacteria.[4] They are the dominant white blood cell early in wound healing. After phagocytosis and digestion, neutrophils either die (releasing free oxygen radicals and destructive enzymes) or are engulfed by macrophages.[5] The release of free oxygen radicals and enzymes by the destruction of neutrophils can prolong the inflammatory reaction (oxidizing stress). Areas of encapsulated chronic inflammation, which are termed granulomas, may develop as a result of ongoing release of these enzymes and subsequent continued generation of free oxygen radicals. The recruitment of macrophages to safely remove neutrophils from a wound may help prevent chronic inflammation.

Macrophages are central to wound healing.[6] Following the first 24–48 h, they become the prevailing white blood cells in the wound. As a response to chemotatic agents (like TGF-β), circulating monocytes and tissue macrophages migrate to the wound. They engulf necrotic tissue and bacteria as well as remove the remaining neutrophils preventing ongoing release of inflammatory mediators. Additionally, macrophages release many different growth factors and cytokines. This allows for fibroblast proliferation, angiogenesis, extracellular matrix production, and the recruitment of additional leukocytes. For example, Interleukin-1 (IL-1) is secreted by macrophages, causing lymphocyte activation and is chiefly responsible for the febrile response as a result of circulating IL-1 reaching the hypothalamus.[7] Activated monocytes and macrophages stimulate collagen production and release matrix metalloproteinases (MMPs) – including collagenases – aiding in breaking down and repairing damaged tissue matrix. In order for there to be orderly progress of wound healing, a balance between MMPs and tissue inhibitory metalloproteinases (TIMPs) must exist.[8] If not the effect of MMPs may extend to adjacent uninjured tissues. Repair of the wound begins in the proliferative phase of wound healing.

Proliferation

Wound healing events during this phase of wound healing include mesenchymal cell chemotaxis and proliferation (fibroplasia), angiogenesis, and epithelialization.[9] This phase of wound healing begins with a provisional matrix of fibrin and fibronectin being formed. The matrix consists of a papillary bed, fibroblasts, macrophages, and a loose arrangement of collagen, fibronectin, and bacteria. Macrophages are the principal cell in the initial matrix; however, fibroblasts quickly increase in numbers during this phase of healing. Fibroblasts are normally located in the dermis and are often damaged by the initial insult. Fibroblasts, mediated by cytokines, quickly become the most dominant cell in the proliferative phase. PDGF, fibronectin, and EGF are chemotactic for both fibroblasts and smooth muscle cells.[10]

Fibroblasts divide and produce the components of the extracellular matrix.[8] The extracellular matrix contains collagen, proteoglycans, and attachment proteins such as fibronectin. Over this phase, the amount of collagen increases to become the primary structural element in the wound matrix. Collagen is synthesized primarily by fibroblasts in a complex process that begins 3–5 days after injury.[11] Procollagen, the precursor of collagen is formed within fibroblasts and released. It is composed of long chains which are linked together in a helical configuration and cleaved by proteases to form collagen.[12] TGF-β increases collagen synthesis and glucocorticoids interfere with wound healing during this step by decreasing collagen synthesis. As collagen matures, cross-linking occurs between chains of collagen to form larger collagen fibrils. Vitamin C is a necessary nutrient in hydroxylation, which stabilizes and cross-links collagen. The increased cross-linking increases the tensile strength of the wound. Collagen synthesis is dependent both on local oxygen and vascular supply.

Angiogenesis is stimulated by high lactate levels, an acidic pH, and decreased oxygen tension in the tissue.[9] Fibroblast growth factor (FGF) and vascular endothelial growth factor (VEGF) are important factors in angiogenesis. The epithelial cells secrete VEGF in response to hypoxia signaling to fibroblasts to stimulate angiogenesis. The subsequent release of growth factors from the macrophages stimulates angiogenesis by proliferation and ingrowth of endothelial cells. These new endothelial cells stimulate neovascularization by the formation of capillaries.[13] These new capillaries provide oxygen and nutrients to support ongoing proliferation. Local oxygenation can be impeded by atherosclerosis, local small vessel disease, and preexisting scarring. Edema, which is sequestered extracellular fluid, inhibits wound healing by increasing the diffusion distance of oxygen from its target. Local oxygenation can be augmented with the use of hyperbaric oxygen, although the frequency and duration of such treatment is not fully elucidated.[14]

Regeneration of the epithelium is important to seal the wound and prevent further water loss. The two layers of the skin are the epidermis and the dermis. The epidermis is multilayered. The stratum corneum, the most superficial layer of epidermis, consists primarily of dead cells and keratin. The deeper epidermal layer is composed of a protective layer of the skin which provides protection from water loss. The dermis too is multilayered, consisting of a superficial layer, the periadnexal in areas where adnexal structures are absent, and the deep or reticular layer containing the majority of collagen content and the lymphatics (Fig. 19.1).

The first step in epithelialization is the formation of the clot to seal the wound. This protects against bacterial invasion as well as prevents fluid loss. Initially, the epithelial cells migrate across the wound and can completely cover a surgically coapted wound in 18–24 h.[14] Epithelial cells migrate from epithelium. This can be from the wound edge or in partial thickness wounds – from epithelial appendages (e.g., hair follicles, sweat and sebaceous glands). As epithelial cells cross the wound and contact each other, the speed of migration slows and is stopped by contact inhibition. Epithelial cell migration is decreased by bacteria, large amounts of exudate, and necrotic tissue. Reestablishment of a mature epithelial layer is an important component of scar resolution. In full thickness injuries, epithelialization occurs from the edge of the wound at a rate of 1–2 mm per day.[14] Regenerated epithelium does not retain all the features of normal epithelium. It has fewer basal cells and the interface between dermis and epidermis is abnormal as rete pegs are absent. Without

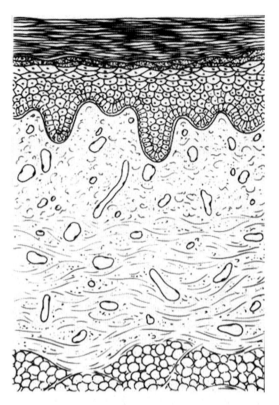

Figure 19.1. Cross-section of the skin (Reprinted with permission from Jordan and McCraw[15].Copyright © American Urological Association Education and Research, Inc).

being anchored to dermis, epithelial cells provide little strength.

The definition of wound contraction is the movement of tissue toward the center of the wound. This should not be confused with wound contracture, which is physically constrained joint motion as a result of wound contraction. Wound contraction typically begins 4–5 days after injury and will continue for 12–15 days.[9] The rate of movement varies by the type of tissue and how much laxity exists at the point of contraction. Contraction is mediated by fibroblasts and myofibroblasts, which act similarly to smooth muscle cells. Pharmaceuticals (e.g., colchicine) that inhibit microtubules (tubulin) minimize wound contraction implicating the important role of microtubules in this phase of wound healing. The process of wound contraction requires cell division and is inhibited by local radiation and systemic chemotherapy drugs.

In those areas with more elastic skin wounds, wound contraction can be augmented greatly by the use of a vacuum-assisted closure (VAC) device. VAC dressings use a sponge with vacuum suction underneath an occlusive dressing to remove exudates from the wound and into the sponge. VAC dressings reduce edema and increase local perfusion as well as decrease bacterial load, facilitating earlier wound closure.[11]

Remodeling

Three to four weeks following the initial injury, collagen synthesis balances collagen destruction resulting in a steady level of collagen within the wound.[14] This collagen equilibrium defines the start of the remodeling phase of wound healing. Collagen makes up 25% of all proteins throughout the body and more than 50% of the protein found in scar tissue. Type III collagen predominates early in the remodeling phase but as collagen matures, type III collagen is replaced by type I. The rate of collagen synthesis increases rapidly and continues at an accelerated rate for 2–4 weeks. Although collagen content is maximal, the strength of the wound can be further increased by polarization of the collagen fibrils from the preliminary random configuration. At 6 weeks after the initial injury, the wound has reached 80–90% of its eventual strength. At this point, the activity of the matrix metalloproteinases (e.g., collagenase) is balanced by the inhibition of tissue inhibitor metalloproteinases (TIMPs) in normal wound healing. The number of capillaries and fibroblasts is decreased thereby reducing the red color of the wound.[16]

Surgical incisions achieve moderate strength by 3 weeks postoperatively. To increase the strength of these wounds, sutures should be placed in high collagen-containing structures (e.g., dermis, muscular fascia, Scarpa's fascia, etc.). Suture for abdominal fascia should be able to hold tension for 6 weeks to gain 50% of its eventual strength. The choice of suture is determined by the strength of the layer and the time needed for suture strength to be replaced by wound strength.[16]

Principles of Plastic Surgery

The principles of plastic surgery, and thereby wound closure, have obvious relevance to surgical practice. The approach to surgical incision and closure of wound defects should be via application of the simplest techniques first termed "the reconstructive ladder". Primary closure and healing by secondary intention are straightforward concepts and this chapter focuses on the principles of tissue transfer. Tissue transfer refers to the movement of tissue for reconstruction, which in the field of urology, chiefly refers to the use of grafts and local flaps. Innovations and improvements in tissue transfer techniques, tissue handling, and tissue engineering have expanded the repertoire of the genitourinary reconstructive surgeon.

The use of tissue transfer for reconstruction requires detailed knowledge of the anatomy of both the donor and the recipient sites as well as of the principles that will allow that tissue to survive once it is transferred. Earlier in the chapter, the two layers of the skin were described (Fig. 19.1). The two layers of the dermis were described, a superficial layer, the adventitial (or periadnexal) dermis, and a deep layer, the reticular dermis. For genitourinary reconstruction, skin without adnexal structures is often used; thus, the papillary dermis is synonymous with the adventitial dermis. Other tissues commonly utilized for genitourinary reconstruction include bladder and buccal mucosa. The bladder epithelium is the superficial layer of the bladder (Fig. 19.2). The deep layer of the bladder, the lamina propria, is composed of superficial and deep layers. The oral mucosa (buccal mucosa) is the superficial layer of much of the oral cavity, which also has a deeper layer termed the lamina propria, again with superficial and deep layers (Fig. 19.3).[18]

Tissue Characteristics

Inherent in the use of tissue is a firm understanding of tissue characteristics. These include extensibility, tissue tension, and the viscoelastic properties. Extensibility is the property of the tissue that allows it to be stretched. This is different from compliance, which is the ability of tissue to be stretched without increasing tissue tension. As mentioned earlier, tissue is mostly a collagen-rich elastin matrix "floating in" mucosal polysaccharide. Extensibility is related to the distance that the collagen fibers can be

Figure 19.2. Cross-section of the bladder wall, with the layers of a bladder epithelial graft demonstrated. Cross-section of anatomy of the vascularity (*bottom*) (Reprinted from Jordan and Schlossberg[17]. Contemporary Urology is a copyrighted publication of Advanstar Communications Inc. All rights reserved).

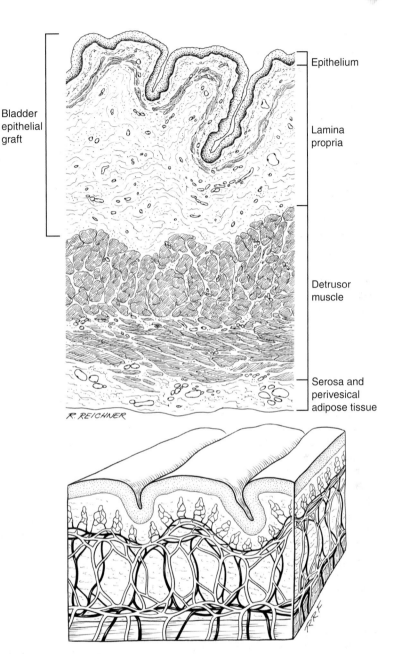

straightened and slide against one another. The amount that these straightened fibers can slide is dependent on the elastin–collagen interaction. The return to normal is related to the structure of collagen and its relation to elastin as well. This concept is what drives the direction of Langer's lines. Langer's lines are drawn to minimize scarring in surgical incisions. These incisions align tissue extensibility with tension, perpendicular to the skin incision thereby minimizing scarring.[19]

The viscoelastic properties relate to the presence of the polysaccharide matrix between the collagen fibers. Two viscoelastic properties have been defined: stress relaxation and creep (Fig. 19.4). Stress relaxation is the property that allows for fixed distension of tissue. The force required to maintain the distension will decrease

Figure 19.3. Cross-sectional anatomy of the oral mucosa. Demonstrated is a buccal mucosa with the layers of the buccal mucosal graft demonstrated. Cross-section of anatomy of the vascularity (*bottom*) (Reprinted from Jordan and Schlossberg[17]. Contemporary Urology is a copyrighted publication of Advanstar Communications Inc. All rights reserved).

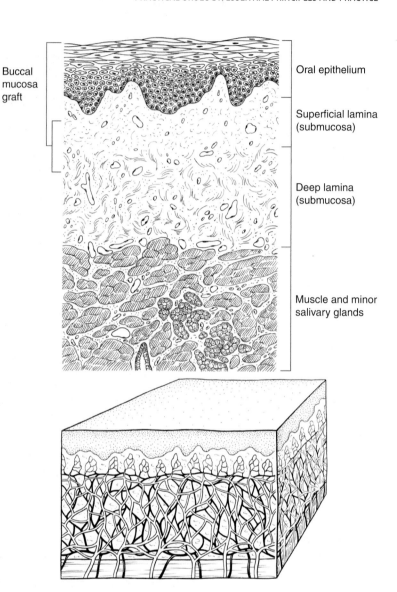

Buccal mucosa graft

Oral epithelium

Superficial lamina (submucosa)

Deep lamina (submucosa)

Muscle and minor salivary glands

over time. However, if the force remains constant, the tissue will continue to distend, and this property is termed creep.[20]

Grafts

Transfer of tissue can be performed via the use of grafts or flaps. A graft is tissue that has been excised and transferred to a graft host bed, where a new blood supply develops by a process termed take. This process is dependent on the bulk of the graft and the number of exposed vessels on the undersurface of the graft as well as the surface of the bed. The initial phase of graft take, imbibition, lasts approximately 48 h. During that phase, the graft survives by "drinking" nutrients from the adjacent graft host bed. The temperature of the graft remains lower than core body temperature. The second phase, inosculation, also requires about 48 h. It is during this phase that true microcirculation is reestablished in the graft and the temperature of the graft rises to core body temperature. The process of take is influenced by both the nature of the grafted tissue and the conditions of the graft

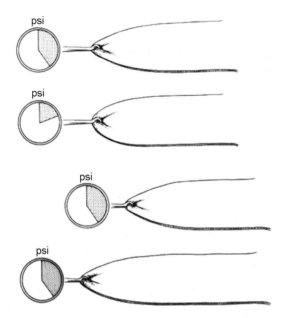

Figure 19.4. Demonstration of the viscoelastic properties: (*Top*) stress relaxation. A force is applied to the tissue, the distension remains constant, the force to maintain that distension decreases; (*Bottom*) Creep. In this model, the force of distension remains constant, over time under that force, the tissue elongates.

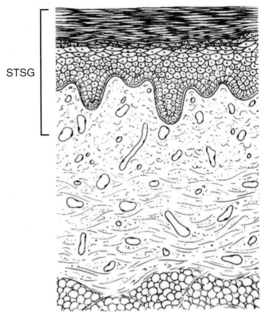

Figure 19.5. Demonstration of the cross-section of anatomy of the skin, with the layers of a split-thickness graft demonstrated (Reprinted with permission from Jordan and Schlossberg[17]. Contemporary Urology is a copyrighted publication of Advanstar Communications Inc. All rights reserved).

host bed. Processes that disrupt or impair the vascularity of the graft host bed thus interfere with graft take.[18]

The epidermal or epithelial layer is a covering, acting as a barrier to the external environment. It lies adjacent to the superficial dermis or superficial lamina. At approximately that interface is the superficial plexus. This plexus is the intradermal plexus in skin. On the undersurface of the deep dermal layer or deep lamina lies the deep plexus. In skin, this is the subdermal plexus. The deep dermis contains most of the lymphatics and greater collagen content than in the superficial dermal layer. The deep or reticular dermis is generally thought to account for the physical characteristics of the tissue.[19]

A *split thickness graft* carries the epidermis, or the covering, and the superficial dermis. This graft exposes the superficial dermal (intradermal or intralaminar) plexus. In most grafts, the superficial plexus is composed of small but numerous vessels allowing for many possible graft-bed connections allowing favorable vascular characteristics. This unit has few lymphatics, and the reticular dermis (and its

physical characteristics) are not carried, which accounts for the tendency of split-thickness units to be brittle and, in some cases, less durable (Fig. 19.5).

A *full-thickness graft* carries the covering, the superficial dermis or lamina and the deep dermis or lamina with all the characteristics attributable to that layer (Fig. 19.6). In skin, the subdermal plexus is exposed. In most cases, that subdermal plexus is composed of larger vessels that are more sparsely distributed (Fig. 19.7). The graft is thus fastidious in its vascular characteristics. A full-thickness unit carries most of the lymphatics, and these physical characteristics are carried with the transferred tissue. If we examine the grafts that are most commonly used in genitourinary reconstructive surgery, the split-thickness skin graft has favorable vascular characteristics but tends to contract. The full-thickness skin graft tends to have more fastidious vascular characteristics, but there is less contraction. There is a difference between genital full-thickness skin (penile and preputial skin grafts) and most areas of extragenital full-thickness skin. This is probably a reflection of the increased mass of the graft

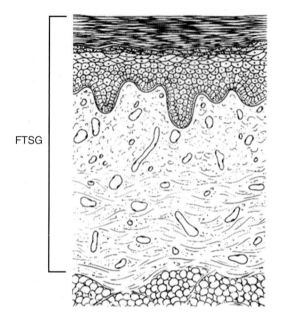

Figure 19.6. Cross-section of anatomy of the skin with the level of a full-thickness skin graft demonstrated (Reprinted with permission from Jordan and Schlossberg[17]. Contemporary Urology is a copyrighted publication of Advanstar Communications Inc. All rights reserved).

FTSG

in extragenital skin grafts. This increased mass makes imbibition more tenuous, and the poor results reported with urethral reconstruction with extragenital full-thickness skin grafts are likely a result of poor take.[18]

The mesh graft is usually an application of the split-thickness graft. After the harvest of a sheet graft, the sheet is placed on a carrier that cuts systematically placed slits in the graft. These slits can expand the graft by various ratios (i.e.,

1.5:1, 2:1, 3:1). For most genital reconstructive surgery, these slits are useful to allow subgraft collections to escape, and the slits allow the graft to conform better to irregular graft host beds (e.g., the testes in split-thickness skin graft scrotal reconstruction).

The *posterior auricular graft, or Wolff graft,* is an exception to the rule concerning extragenital skin. This skin is thin and overlies the temporalis fascia and thought to be carried on numerous perforators. The subdermal plexus of this graft thus mimics the characteristics of the intradermal plexus, and the total mass of the graft is more like that of the split-thickness unit. In the bladder epithelial graft (Fig. 19.2), there is a superficial and a deep plexus; however, the plexuses are connected by many more perforators and the sublaminar lexus is composed of plentiful vessels. Thus, bladder epithelial grafts tend to have more favorable vascular characteristics, and as units are very thin.[18]

There is a panlaminar plexus in oral mucosa, allowing it to be thinned, provided a sufficient amount of deep lamina is carried to preserve the physical characteristics (Fig. 19.3). The oral/buccal mucosal graft is thought to have optimal vascular characteristics. The thinned graft diminishes the total graft mass while preserving the physical characteristics and not adversely affecting the vascular characteristics. The "wet epithelial" surface of buccal mucosa is also thought to be a favorable property for many cases of urethral reconstructive surgery.

The *dermal graft* has been used for years to augment the tunica albuginea of the corpora cavernosa. When it is harvested, the graft exposes both the intradermal plexus and the

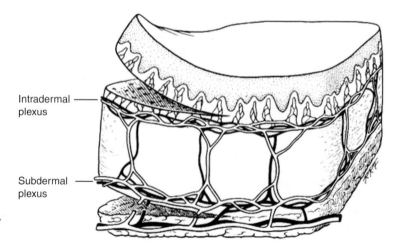

Intradermal plexus

Subdermal plexus

Figure 19.7. Cross-section anatomy of the vascularity of the skin.

deep dermal plexus. The dermal graft thus takes readily and has the physical characteristics of normal skin. Dermal grafts have been used in urethral reconstruction, albeit with poor results. When prepared properly, the *tunica vaginalis graft* is essentially peritoneum. Tunica vaginalis grafts have been shown to be useful for repair of small defects of the tunica albuginea of the corpora cavernosa, but in larger grafts there is a tendency to aneurysmal dilation. Tunica vaginalis grafts have been tried in urethral reconstruction with uniformly poor results.

As an alternative to dermal grafts, the *vein graft* has been used with some success. Initially it was felt that vein grafts did not really take but rather, became directly vascularized. In fact, these grafts seem to take in a similar process as already described. When it is placed under pressure the wall tends to thicken, which has also been called "arterialization." Arterialization is associated with changes in the elastic properties of the vessel wall, and the graft becomes rigid with low compliance. Vein grafts are currently being widely used for replacement of defects of the tunica albuginea of the corpora cavernosa, in some centers. *Rectal mucosal* grafts have been proposed for urethral reconstruction. In general, the vascularity of the bowel mucosa is based on the vascularity of the underlying muscle, with the mucosa carried on perforators. Little is found in the literature regarding the process of take of these grafts; however, it can be presumed to be identical to the processes already described.

The acellular collagen matrices that have been more commonly used with the advances in tissue engineering are incorrectly termed grafts. The precise mechanism by which these collagen matrices are handled by the body and incorporated with living tissues are poorly defined. Any of the "off-the-shelf grafts" used for urologic surgery are essentially an acellular collagen matrix. The future of graft materials seems to lie in the field of tissue engineering. Both urothelium and buccal mucosa have been cultured successfully. However, there is no long-term data to follow the success of these patients, and with many aspects of tissue engineering, the problem is not with the culture of tissues but rather with the correct choice and use of carrier.

Flap

Tissue can also be transferred as a flap. The term flap refers to tissue that is excised and transferred with the blood supply either preserved, or surgically reestablished, at the recipient site. There is some confusion with respect to the terminology of tissue transfer. Many use the term graft to refer to any tissue that is transferred. However, the term graft implies a specific unit of transfer, and using terms such as pedicle graft or free graft are confusing. It is best to avoid these terms in discussing tissue transfer.

Flaps can be classified by a number of criteria. *Flaps* are often classified based on their vascularity and we can thus describe flaps as either random flaps or axial flaps (Fig. 19.8). A *random flap* is a flap without a defined and reproducible cuticular vascular territory. The flap is

Figure 19.8. Demonstration of flaps based on their vascularity. In the case of a random flap, the flap is elevated on the intradermal and subdermal plexuses. There is no defined artery in the base of the flap (Reprinted with permission from Jordan and Schlossberg[17]. Contemporary Urology is a copyrighted publication of Advanstar Communications Inc. All rights reserved).

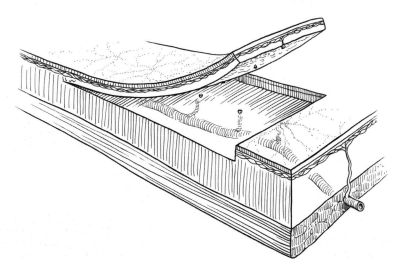

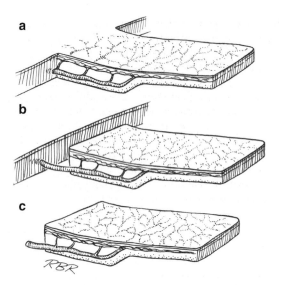

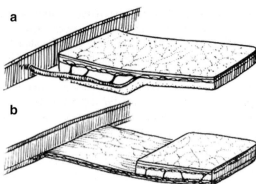

Figure 19.11. Demonstration of the difference between an axial island flap and a skin island or paddle carried on a flap: (**a**) true island flap, (**b**) demonstration of a skin island carried on a fascial flap.

Figure 19.9. Axial flap, there is a defined artery in the base of the flap. Demonstrated are (**a**) axial peninsula flap, (**b**) axial island flap, (**c**) axial microvascular free transfer flap (Reprinted with permission from Jordan and McCraw[15]. Copyright © American Urological Association Education and Research, Inc).

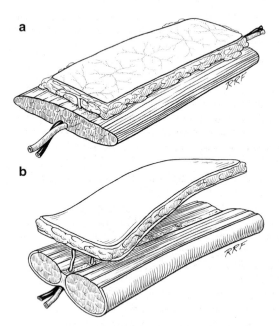

Figure 19.10. (**a**) Demonstration of the musculocutaneous system flap vascularity (Reprinted with permission from Jordan and McCraw[15]. Copyright © American Urological Association Education and Research, Inc) (**b**) Demonstration of the fasciocutaneous system of vascularity (Reprinted with permission from Jordan and Schlossberg[17]. Contemporary Urology is a copyrighted publication of Advanstar Communications Inc. All rights reserved).

carried on the dermal or laminar plexuses; the dimensions of random flaps can vary widely depending on the individual and the flap donor site. The term *axial flap* refers to the presence of a defined vessel in the base of the flap (Fig. 19.9). There are three types of axial flaps. The *direct cuticular axial flap* is a flap based on a vessel superficial to the superficial layer of the deep body wall fascia. The classic example of a direct cuticular flap is the groin flap. A *musculocutaneous flap* (Fig. 19.10), on the other hand, is based on the vascular supply to the muscle. The overlying skin paddle is carried on perforators. If the muscle alone is carried as a flap, the overlying skin survives as a random unit. The *fasciocutaneous flap* has a similar vascular pattern to the musculocutaneous system. However, the deep blood supply is carried on the fascia (both deep and superficial layers), and the overlying skin paddle is based again on perforators. *Familiar to most urologists are the local genital flaps used for hypospadias or other urethral reconstruction.* Thus, one can transfer a fascial flap based on the deep blood supply associated with the flap. It has been argued that fascia is relatively avascular and hence cannot serve as "the blood supply" to the fasciocutaneous unit. In reality, the fascia acts as a trellis and the vessels are carried much like the limbs of a vine.[15]

Flaps can also be classified by elevation technique. A *peninsular flap* is a flap in which the vascular supply and the skin of the flap base are left intact. An *island flap* is a flap in which the skin is divided but the vessels are left intact (or dangling). The microvascular free transfer flap, also referred to as a free flap, has both the vascular supply and skin interrupted. The vascular supply is then reestablished at the recipient site.

Again, there is confusion in terminology. In genitourinary reconstructive surgical procedures, we tend to use the term island flap. As already mentioned, a true island flap is elevated on dangling vessels. The usual case, however, is that a skin island or paddle is elevated either on the muscle, as in the gracilis musculocutaneous flap, or on the fascia, as in local genital skin flaps (Fig. 19.11). The term island flap is not synonymous with the terms skin island and skin paddle. Interest continues in the use of tissue-cultured, or engineered, grafts. The likelihood of being able to successfully use cultured media is right around the corner.

References

1. Meyer FA, Fromjmovic MM, Vi MM. Characteristics of the major platelet membrane site used in binding collagen. *Thromb Res*. 1979;15:755-767
2. Jurk K, Kehrel BE. Platelets: physiology and biochemistry. *Semin Thromb Hemost*. 2005;31(4):381-392
3. Martin P, Leibovich SJ. Inflammatory cells during wound repair: the good, the bad and the ugly. *Trends Cell Biol*. 2005;15(11):599-607
4. Leibovich SJ, Ross R. The role of the macrophage in wound repair: a study with hydrocortisone and anti-macrophage serum. *Am J Pathol*. 1975;78:71-100
5. Clark RAF. Would Repair: overview and general considerations (Chatper1). In *The molecular and Cellular Biology of Wound Repair*, 2nd ed., Springer, 1996
6. Digelmann RF, Cohen IK, Kaplan AM. The role of macrophages in wound repair: a review. *Plast Reconstr Surg*. 1981;68:107-113
7. Rumalla VK, Borah GL. Cytokines, growth factors, and plastic surgery. *Plast Reconstr Surg*. 2001;108:719-733
8. Nwometh BC, Olutoye OO, Diegelmann RF, et al. The basic biology of wound healing. *J Surg Pathol*. 1997;2:143-162
9. Gupta S, Lawrence WT. Wound healing: normal and abnormal mechanisms and closure techniques. In: O'Leary JP, ed. *The Physiologic Basis for Surgery*. 4th ed. Philadelphia, PA: Lippincott Williams & Wilkins; 2008
10. Barrientos S, Stojadinovic O, Golinko MS, et al. Growth factors and cytokines in wound healing. *Wound Repair Regen*. 2008;16(5):585-601
11. Ethridge R, Leong M, Phillips LG. Wound healing. In: Townsend CM, ed. *Sabiston's Textbook of Surgery*. 18th ed. Philadelphia, PA: Saunders; 2007
12. Kavitha O, Thampan RV. Factors influencing collagen biosynthesis. *J Cell Biochem*. 2008;104(4):1150-1160
13. Thackham JA, McElwain DL, Long RJ. The use of hyperbaric oxygen therapy to treat chronic wounds: a review. *Wound Repair Regen*. 2008;16(3):321-330
14. Fine NA, Mustoe TA. Wound healing. In *Greenfield's Surgery: Scientific Principles and Practice*, 4th ed. Lippincott Williams and Wilkins, 2006
15. Jordan GH, McCraw JB. Tissue transfer techniques for genitourinary reconstructive surgery, Part II – Basic flap definitions and techniques/graft techniques. *AUA Update Series*; Lesson 10, Vol VII. 1988
16. Witte MB, Barbul A. General principles of wound healing. *Surg Clin North Am*. 1997;77:509-527
17. Jordan GH, Schlossberg SM. Using tissue transfer for urethral reconstruction. *Contemp Urol*. 1993;5(12):13-23
18. Jordan GH, Schlossberg SM. Surgery of the Penis and Urethra. In: Wein AJ, ed. *Campbell-Walsh Urology*. 9th ed. Philadelphia, PA: Saunders Elsevier; 2007
19. Jordan GH, Schlossberg SM, McCraw JB. Tissue transfer techniques for genitourinary reconstructive surgery, Part I – Principles, definitions, basic techniques and graft techniques. *AUA Update Series*. Lesson 9, Vol VII. 1998
20. Jordan GH, Rourke K. The use of flaps in urethral reconstructive surgery. In *Reconstructive Urethral Surgery* edited by Schreiter and JOrdan; Springer: 2006:16:130-136

20

Overview of the Evaluation of Lower Urinary Tract Dysfunction

Christopher R. Chapple and Altaf Mangera

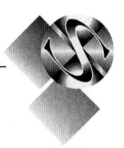

Lower Urinary Tract Symptoms

The idea "the bladder is an unreliable witness" first came into existence with the recognition that lower urinary tract symptoms (LUTS) were not disease or gender specific, could be reported inaccurately by the patient, or could be poorly documented by the investigator.[1] In recent years, attempts have been made to quantify symptoms by the use of disease-specific symptom scores and quality of life measures. Well-known examples include the International Prostate Symptom Score (IPSS) for suspected prostate and the King's Health Questionnaire for incontinence-related problems. Currently, internationally acceptable questionnaires are being evaluated for incontinence.[2]

LUTS are best subdivided into *storage* of urine (also "irritative") or *voiding* (also "obstructive") and post micturition symptom groups (Table 20.1).

Urine storage and voiding are two interrelated yet distinct phases of lower urinary tract function. The bladder and urethra possess intrinsic tone produced by the muscle and connective tissue they contain. At rest, the urethral tone keeps the walls in apposition and aids continence. During filling, the walls of the bladder exhibit receptive relaxation (i.e. the vesical lumen expands without resulting in a concomitant rise in intravesical pressure). Once a threshold level of filling has been achieved (which will depend upon circumstances and vary between individuals), increasing afferent activity will start to impinge on consciousness, resulting in awareness that the bladder is filling up. Except during infancy, there is a complete volitional control over these reflex pathways and voiding will be initiated in appropriate circumstances.

The lower urinary tract function may be divided into two distinct phases:

- The storage phase and
- The voiding phase

Storage Phase

During the storage phase, the bladder is filled with urine from the ureters. For the majority of the time (greater than 99%), the lower urinary tract will be in the storage phase, whilst less than 1% of time is spent voiding. The bladder needs to accommodate to the increase in volume without an appreciable rise in bladder (intra-vesical) pressure. The extent to which a change in volume (δV) occurs in relation to a change in intra-vesical pressure (δP) is known as the bladder compliance ($\delta V/\delta P$).

Factors that contribute to compliance are:

- The passive elastic properties of the tissues of the bladder wall
- The intrinsic ability of smooth muscle to maintain a constant tension over a wide range of stretch or "tonus"
- The neural reflexes which control detrusor tension during bladder filling

C.R. Chapple and W.D. Steers (eds.), *Practical Urology: Essential Principles and Practice*,
DOI: 10.1007/978-1-84882-034-0_20, © Springer-Verlag London Limited 2011

Table 20.1. Lower urinary tract symptoms

Storage symptoms	Voiding symptoms	Post void symptoms
Frequency	Slow/splitting/ intermittent stream	Feeling of incomplete emptying
Urgency	Hesitancy	Post-micturition dribble
Incontinence	Straining	
Increased/reduced/ absent/ painful bladder sensation	Terminal dribble	
Nocturia		

During bladder filling, afferent activity from stretch receptors increases and passes via the posterior roots of the sacral cord and the lateral spinothalamic tracts to the brain, thereby mediating the desire to void. Activity within the striated component of the urethral sphincter is increased and local spinal reflex activity enhances the activity within striated muscles of the pelvic floor and sphincter to tighten up the bladder outlet mechanisms and so augment continence.

Important local factors facilitating bladder filling include both receptive relaxation and the passive viscoelastic properties of the bladder wall. Conditions that contribute to poor bladder compliance and detrusor overactivity include:

- Abnormal bladder morphology resulting from collagenous infiltration, hypertrophy, or altered muscle structure (e.g. obstructed bladder); and
- Abnormal detrusor smooth muscle behavior, either primary or secondary to neural dysfunction.

During the storage phase the urethra and sphincteric mechanisms should be closed, thereby maintaining a high outlet resistance and continence. Storage symptoms (nocturia, frequency, urgency, and urge incontinence – the so-called frequency urgency syndrome/overactive bladder syndrome) may arise from failure of the bladder to store urine. This may be due to a reduced anatomical capacity (shrunken bladder after surgery/radiotherapy/infections such as TB) or a reduced functional capacity resulting from abnormally increased bladder sensation (e.g. interstitial cystitis/painful bladder syndrome – beware the need to exclude carcinoma *in situ* – or bladder overactivity). Nonurological conditions (e.g. diabetes mellitus,

diabetes insipidus, polydypsia) can also present with frequency and nocturia.

Urgency is often considered to be a pivotal symptom in the genesis of overactive bladder syndrome and is defined as a sudden compelling desire to pass urine which is difficult to defer. It may arise as a consequence of disordered peripheral afferent function or central interpretation of afferent symptoms.[3]

Frequency is a very troublesome symptom and is the complaint by the patient who considers that he/she voids too often by day. A frequency of voiding of more than eight times per day is usually taken to be abnormal.

Nocturia (sleep-disturbing voiding) is an interesting symptom since it may result from changes in bladder function, but also as a harbinger of other physiological disorders such as cardiac failure. By the age of 65, a nocturia rate of once a night is taken to be the norm. Indeed, in many elderly patients, a reversal of the normal diurnal voiding pattern is seen, with more than 30% of the 24 h urine volume being produced overnight. In these cases, a frequency–volume chart (measuring and timing fluid intake/ output and incontinence episodes for a minimum of 3 days) is essential in both investigation and treatment.

Incontinence: Urinary incontinence is the involuntary loss of urine. This can be constant or intermittent, and with (urgency) or without (stress) a detrusor contraction.

Enuresis, which represents incontinence occurring at night, can be associated with severe detrusor overactivity, but is also a classical symptom seen in association with chronic retention. Overflow incontinence is the classical cause in elderly men presenting with enuresis. The bladder has become acontractile and overfills, and empties only when the volume exceeds the anatomical capacity, under the influence of the elastic forces in the bladder wall. These patients pass small volumes of urine, frequently without any control. Chronic retention is an important condition to consider in any patient, as many will present with renal impairment.

Voiding Phase

The bladder must cease relaxing and instead contract to expel the urine and the urethra and sphincteric mechanisms must "open" to decrease the outlet resistance and allow passage of urine. Voiding should be efficient and there should be minimal or no urine remaining in the bladder at the end of the voiding phase.

Micturition initiated by the cerebral cortex is likely to involve a complex series of bladder–brain stem reflexes.

During voiding:

- Urethral relaxation precedes detrusor contraction;
- There is simultaneous relaxation of the pelvic floor muscles; and
- There is accompanying funneling of the bladder neck and detrusor contraction occurs to forcefully expel urine

The mechanism of these changes is not clear. It is likely that:

- Increased activity within parasympathetic neurones results in removal of central inhibitory influences acting on the sacral centers; and
- Voiding is initiated under the influence of pontine medullary centers.

There is therefore parasympathetically controlled detrusor contraction associated with a corresponding relaxation of the urethra/prostate/bladder neck complex resulting from reciprocal nerve-mediated inhibition of the sympathetic nerve-mediated outflow.

In addition to these primary actions other important secondary events are:

- Contraction of the diaphragm and anterior abdominal wall muscles;
- Relaxation of the pelvic floor; and
- Specific behavioral changes associated with voiding.

During the voiding phase the reverse activity to the storage phase must occur. Voiding symptoms (poor stream, hesitancy, interruption, and straining) are due to either loss of detrusor power or progressive outflow obstruction which, it is presumed, may progressively lead to detrusor failure and retention.

Return to Storage Phase

At the end of voiding, the proximal urethra is closed in a retrograde fashion, thus milking urine back into the bladder. This "milkback" is seen during contrast studies of the lower urinary tract when the patient is asked to stop voiding. Following this the bladder returns to a state of relaxation. Once these events have been completed, the sacral centers are re-inhibited by the cortex and the next filling cycle starts.

Urodynamic Parameters

Urodynamic Techniques

In any patient presenting with lower urinary tract symptoms, it is essential to carry out a complete evaluation of the patient – both subjectively and objectively. It is imperative that the exact functional derangement is defined and the precise etiological factors identified. Prior to urodynamics a careful history and examination are essential and a balance struck between treatment modalities available and patient expectations.

Urodynamic techniques assume a variety of forms and need to be considered to represent a hierarchical series of increasingly complex tests.

Volume Voided Charts

The urodynamic value of the simple voided volume chart is often overlooked – an important omission since this is a natural volumetric urodynamic record of bladder function. The volume/frequency chart is a simple noninvasive tool used in the evaluation of patients with voiding dysfunction, and in particular, in those with increased urinary frequency and incontinence.[4]

Volume/frequency charts help define severity of symptoms and add objectivity to the history. One can readily diagnose increased urinary frequency secondary to high urinary output and from physiological nocturnal diuresis. A record of fluid intake helps identify an easily treatable cause of urinary frequency. The recommended daily fluid intake of six to eight glasses of fluids (1 glass = 8 oz, 1 oz = 30 mL; so nearly 2 L for all fluids/day) is often misconstrued by the patient as the doctor's recommendation to drink six to eight glasses of water daily in addition to the basic fluid needs. This excessive fluid intake frequently results in frequency, urgency, and may worsen urinary incontinence. It is important to review these simple guidelines with the patient and discover if their craving for fluids is not prompted by a sensation of dry mouth, by the desire to avoid constipation, a fear of another bladder infection, or a special diet to lose weight. The average maximum voided volume represents the patient's functional capacity, knowledge of which is useful to know to prevent overfilling of the bladder during cystometry.

A normal bladder fills to a volume approximating its functional capacity and the chart records a series of sizable (300–500 mL) and fairly consistent volumes.

An overactive bladder contracts at variable degrees of distension before full capacity, erroneously informing the patient that it is full, resulting in urinary frequency and low and varying voided volumes. In addition, frequency/volume charts provide important feedback to the practitioner and patient necessary to objectively evaluate the effectiveness of any therapies used in the treatment of the urinary dysfunction. These charts can be combined with measurements of episodes of urgency, pad usage, or incontinence. They give an indication of the severity of symptoms, add objectivity to the history and allow for temporal relationships to be appreciated. Patients are given a measuring jug and a "diary" and asked to record their urinary activities, keeping to their normal daily routine for up to 1 week. Also recorded are times of sleep and wake (see Table 20.2).

Abnormal findings include:

- Increased frequency and normal volumes – this may be related to a high fluid intake, diabetes mellitus, or insipidus, but is most often habitual
- Reduced volumes with variation in the volume voided – suggestive of detrusor overactivity, due to bladder contraction at different degrees of distension, i.e. abnormal signaling prior to reaching maximum capacity
- Increased nocturnal production (nocturnal polyuria) – where more than one third of the 24 h urine production is produced

Table 20.2. Useful information listed in voiding diaries

24 h frequency	Number of voids in 24 h
Daytime frequency	Number of voids whist awake
Nocturia	Number of voids during sleep
24 h production	Total volume of voids in 24 h
Polyuria	>2.8 L urine production in 24 h
Nocturnal urine volume	Excluding last void before sleep, total volume voided during sleep hours, including first void in morning
Nocturnal polyuria	Nocturnal urine volume/24 h production > 33%
Maximum voided volume	Largest volume voided in a single void
Pad usage	Number of pads used during a specified period
Frequency of incontinence episodes	Number of incontinence episodes in a specified time period
Frequency of urgency episodes	Number of urgency episodes in a specified time period

during the hours of sleep. This is not of urological origin and is commonly due to fluid redistribution whilst lying down such as occurs in congestive cardiac failure

A voiding diary can also be used to evaluate therapeutic responses, and is an excellent tool for providing biofeedback during bladder retraining drills. Bladder retraining programs aim to allow patients to retrain their bladder and work on the principle of holding a voiding desire for progressively longer intervals thus stretching the bladder, to decrease voiding frequency to an acceptable five or six times a day.

Pad Testing

The subjective assessment of incontinence is often difficult to interpret and does not reliably indicate degree of abnormality. Not all patients who complain of urinary incontinence are in fact incontinent during a cystometric examination. Pad testing is a simple, noninvasive objective method for detecting and quantifying urine leakage.[5-7] To obtain a representative result, especially in subjects with variable or intermittent urinary incontinence, the test should occupy as long a period as possible, in circumstances which should approximate those of everyday life; yet be as practical as possible in the available circumstances and be carried out in a standardized fashion.

On the basis of pilot studies performed in various centers, we would recommend a 1 h test period during which a series of standard activities are carried out. This test can be extended by further 1 h periods if the result of the first 1 h test was not considered representative by either the patient or the investigator. Alternatively the test can be repeated having filled the bladder to a defined volume.

The total amount of urine lost during the test period is determined by weighing a collecting device such as a nappy, absorbent pad, or condom appliance. A nappy or pad should be worn inside waterproof underpants or should have a waterproof backing. Care should be taken to use a collecting device of adequate capacity. Immediately before the test begins the collecting device is weighted to the nearest gram.

Typical Test Schedule

a. Test is started without the patient voiding.

b. Pre-weighed collecting device is put on and first 1 h test period begins.

c. Subject drinks 500 mL sodium free liquid within a short period (maximum 15 min), then sits or rests.

d. Half hour period: subject walks, including stair climbing equivalent to one flight up and down.

e. During the remaining period the subject performs the following activities:

   i. Standing up from sitting, ten times

   ii. Coughing vigorously, ten times

   iii. Running on the spot for 1 min

   iv. Bending to pick up small object from floor, five times

   v. Wash hands in running water for 1 min

f. At the end of the 1 h test, the collecting device is removed and weighed.

g. If the test is regarded as representative the subject voids and the volume is recorded.

h. Otherwise the test is repeated preferably without voiding.

If the collecting device becomes saturated or filled during the test it should be removed and weighed, and replaced by a fresh device. The activity programmed may be modified according to the subject's physical ability.

Interpretation: The total weight of urine lost during the test period is taken to be equal to the gain in weight of the collecting device(s). An increase in the weight of the pad of less than 1 g in 1 h is not considered a sign of incontinence since a weight gain of up to 1 g may be due to weighing errors, sweating, or vaginal discharge. Evaporation is not important. The test should not be performed during a menstrual period and be cautious that the patient may influence the test result by voluntarily voiding. A negative result should be interpreted with caution, the test may need to be repeated or supplemented with a longer test. The reproducibility of the 1 h pad test is relatively poor. If substantial variations from the usual test schedule occur, this should be recorded so that the same schedule can be used on subsequent occasions. In principle the subject should not void during the test period. If the patient experiences urgency, then she should be persuaded to postpone voiding and to perform as many of the activities in section (e) as possible in order to detect leakage. Before voiding the collection device is removed for weighing. If inevitable voiding cannot be postponed then the test is terminated. The voided volume and the duration of the test should be recorded. For subjects not completing the full test the results may require separate analysis, or the test may be repeated after rehydration.

Normal values: The hourly pad weight increase in continent women varies from 0.0 to 2.1 g/h, averaging 0.26 g/h. With the 1-h ICS pad test, the upper limit (99% confidence limit) has been found to be 1.4 g/h.

Home pad tests lasting 24–48 h are superior to 1 h test in detecting urinary incontinence. The normal upper limit in a 24 h test is 8 g. Though longer tests are better screening tests for incontinence they are less practical and more cumbersome.

Additional procedures intended to give information of diagnostic value are permissible provided they do not interfere with the basic test. For example, additional changes and weighing of the collecting device can give information about the timing of urine loss. The absorbent nappy may be an electronic recording nappy so that the timing is recorded directly. Coloration of the urine with oral Pyridium before performing pad testing can help differentiate between vaginal discharge and urinary incontinence.

It can be concluded that at this stage, the home and/or office pad-test belongs to the repertoire of pre- and/or postoperative outcome measures in clinical research studies on urinary incontinence. Its role in routine clinical practice remains undetermined.[8]

Uroflowmetry

To assess urinary flow we use uroflowmetry. This measures the volume of urine voided per unit time, expressed as milliliters per second (mL/s). Patients void in to a flow meter (Fig. 20.1), which records the following data as visualized in (Fig. 20.2).

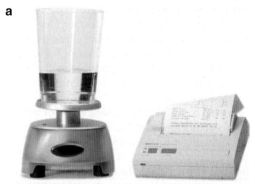

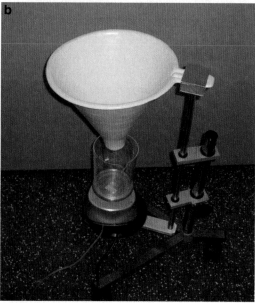

Voided volume	Total volume voided
Maximum flow rate	Maximum flow rate from the entire void
Average flow rate	Volume voided/ total flow time
Flow time	Time over which actual flow occurred
Voiding time	Total duration of micturition, regardless of whether flow was present
Time to maximum flow	Time taken to achieve maximum flow from the onset of flow

Figure 20.1. (a) Photograph of a flowmeter, usually placed under a large funnel (b) into which the patient usually voids in private surroundings. Males stand over the funnel whereas for women it is usually placed under a commode.[22]

The flow rate and pattern give important clues as to the underlying dysfunction. However the major limitation of uroflowmetry is that the flow rate is a composite of both the function of the detrusor and the function of the bladder outlet/urethra, this cannot be resolved easily without pressure/flow urodynamic assessment.

Practical Points: The important factors to consider when interpreting a flow rate are the rate and pattern, in particular whether the flow is continuous or intermittent. A number of characteristic tracings have been reported, but the definition of normal remains debated in women.

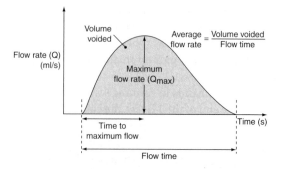

Figure 20.2. A typical flow meter readout demonstrating the International Continence Society nomenclature.[22]

Flow rates are dependent upon bladder volume and age. In carrying out a urinary flow rate, particular attention needs to be paid to certain factors as they can influence the result obtained:

a. Voided volumes of less than 150–200 mL can lead to erroneous results and should be repeated. High voided volumes > 600 mL may lower flow rates by over stretching the bladder resulting in decreased detrusor contractility.
b. If possible the patient should be in favorable surroundings and should not be stressed unduly.
c. Whether the patient is voiding standing, or bending backward, forward, to the side, or half-standing.
d. Whether the flow rate is a so-called free flow rate occurring after natural filling or after mechanical filling at the end of a urodynamic testing or following for example a retrograde bladder filling as part of a stress test or an office cystoscopy

Normal Flow: As discussed normal flow of the human lower urinary tract depends upon integrated coordination of the neural control of the bladder and outflow tract, for which an intact spinal cord is essential (Fig. 20.3a).

Under normal circumstances in adults:

- Bladder capacity is approximately 500 mL and the bladder empties, leaving no residual urine;
- Males void at a pressure of 40–50 cm H_2O and a maximum flow rate of 30–40 mL/s; and
- Females void at a pressure of 30–40 cm H_2O and a maximum flow rate of 40–50 mL/s.

The difference between males and females is a consequence of the higher outflow resistance exerted by the male urethra. Thus women have a lower pressure system as less pressure is required to overcome the urethral outflow resistance. One must also take account of a man's age when interpreting these values, as men over 60 years of age with no urinary obstruction will have flow rates of just over 15 mL/s.

Abnormal Flow: Abnormalities of flow as demonstrated by uroflowmetry involve certain characteristic flow patterns;

- Fast bladder – This is an exaggeration of the normal curve and may be due to a raised end fill bladder pressure associated with detrusor overactivity or due to a significantly low outflow resistance (Fig. 20.3b).
- Prolonged flow – This is a slow flow rate over a prolonged period of time requiring a long time to reach a maximum flow. This is frequently seen with Bladder outlet obstruction (BOO), although a poorly contractile detrusor may give this picture (Fig. 20.3c).
- Intermittent flow – This irregular spiking pattern is frequently due to abdominal straining to augment the pressure required to overcome a bladder outlet obstruction or to add intra-abdominal pressure to a poorly contractile detrusor. Rarely sporadic sphincter contractions may cause this pattern (Fig. 20.3d).
- Flat Plateau – A low maximum flow rate which plateaus throughout the majority of the void, like a "box," is characteristic of a urethral stricture (Fig. 20.3e).

Post Voiding Residual

Ultrasound is combined with a flow rate to provide more detailed information on bladder function. This is a routine investigation for all patients with voiding disorders seen as outpatients; an alternative is to measure the residual by catheterization.

The full bladder is scanned, the patient voids into flow meter in private and a post voiding scan is carried out to assess bladder residual. Interpretation of the flow rate takes into account the factors mentioned above. Any form of ultrasound probe allowing adequate visualization of the bladder is used. The patient should be scanned at the time that they feel "full" thereby providing an idea of the functional bladder capacity. Similarly the patient should be scanned as soon after voiding as possible in order to provide accurate assessment of the true bladder residual.

Figure 20.3. (a) Normal – rapid change before and after peak flow, (b) "Fast Bladder" – exaggeration of normal, (c) Prolonged flow – delayed time to maximum flow and delayed overall void time, (d) intermittent flow – due to abdominal straining, (e) "Box" – showing a long plateau.[22]

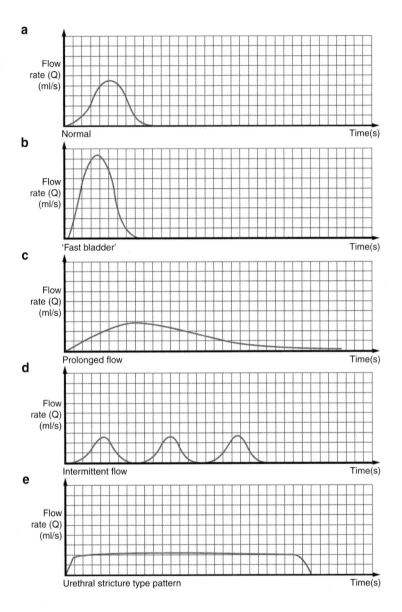

Ensure that the patient has a subjectively full bladder prior to carrying out the study to provide a representative result. Make sure that the study is carried out in circumstances where the patient is relaxed, so as not to introduce error into the results obtained.

This test provides data on bladder capacity, flow rate, and post voiding residual producing a more detailed assessment of the lower urinary tract function than a flow rate alone.[9] It can be carried out easily with little specialized equipment, is noninvasive and does not use ionizing radiation.

It is of particular value in the follow up of patients attending clinics. For instance with a hypocontractile detrusor following surgery for the relief of obstruction or where it is suspected that voiding efficiency may have been compromised e.g. after a repair procedure for stress incontinence.

Patients awaiting an intravenous urogram for imaging of the upper urinary tracts, for another clinical indication, may undergo a complete intravenous urodynamogram, where the addition of uroflowmetry provides a comprehensive assessment of the lower urinary tract, detailing pre and post void residual volumes and also highlighting bladder mucosal abnormalities.

Further Diagnostic Evaluation of Patients

Urodynamic Assessment: When Should Urodynamic Testing Be Performed?

Women with a history of pure stress urinary incontinence associated with urethrovesical hypermobility and no prior history do not necessarily require urodynamic evaluation prior to surgery for stress incontinence.[10,11] However a diagnosis if made on the basis of history alone will not exclude detrusor overactivity in up to 25% of cases. Urodynamic assessment is therefore an important preoperative requisite in women with stress incontinence; particularly those who have other associated abnormalities or risk factors identified from their history and physical examination that may complicate the presentation and thereby influence treatment.[12,13]
These include:

- Women with significant overactive bladder symptoms or mixed stress-urgency incontinence[14]
- Those with recurrent incontinence following previous surgery
- Patients with associated neurological disease, and those whose presentation suggests predominantly intrinsic sphincter deficiency. Women who are dysfunctional voiders with high postvoid residual urine volumes are considered at higher risk of postoperative retention and should be urodynamically evaluated. Pure urgency incontinence not responding to behavioral and pharmacological management is also an indication for study

Male patients can only be clearly defined as being obstructed on the basis of a pressure/flow urodynamic assessment. Whilst the evidence base relating to this is based on observational studies there is a current consensus view that patients are more likely to have a better outcome following surgery for lower urinary tract symptoms if they are obstructed.

Certainly all symptomatic patients with neuropathic bladder dysfunction should undergo urodynamics, and preferably videourodynamics, in order to accurately characterize the detrusor and sphincteric abnormalities, and to help identify patients who are at renal risk from their lower tract abnormality. More sophisticated electrophysiological studies are useful in the diagnosis of neuropathic bladder. The most commonly studied patients are those with multiple sclerosis, stroke, diabetes, Parkinson's disease, and spinal cord injury.

Cystometry with or Without Video

The majority of urodynamic units do not have the benefit of fluoroscopically equipped facilities. In the assessment of the majority of patients presenting with urinary incontinence, frequency and/or urgency simple cystometry provides all of the necessary information. Synchronous cystography and cystometry recordings are most important in the assessment of complex cases, particularly where previous surgery has failed; since this investigation allows a combined anatomical and functional evaluation of lower urinary tract function. Nevertheless it must be remembered that simple cystourethrography can be carried out in all X-ray departments and can provide true, high quality, lateral views of the urethra during voiding.[15,16]

Cystometry

In equivocal or more complex cases, detailed urodynamic investigation is necessary. *Cystometry* is the method by which the pressure/volume relationship of the bladder is measured. The term *cystometry* is usually taken to mean the measurement of detrusor pressure during controlled bladder filling and subsequent voiding with measurement of the synchronous flow rate (filling and voiding cystometry). In *simple cystometry* the intravesical (total bladder) pressure is measured while the bladder is filled. It is not accurate as it assumes that the detrusor pressure approximates the intravesical pressure. However, as the bladder is an intra-abdominal organ, the detrusor pressure is subject to changes in the intra-abdominal pressure which may lead to inaccurate diagnoses. *Subtracted cystometry* involves the measurement of both the intra-vesical and the intra-abdominal pressure simultaneously. Electronic subtraction of the latter from the former enables the detrusor pressure to be determined. Cystometry helps characterize detrusor function by assessing bladder compliance, sensation, stability, and capacity.

Videocystometrography (Cystometry + Cystourethrography)

If appropriate radiological facilities exist, the bladder can be filled with contrast media thus allowing the simultaneous screening of the bladder and outflow tract during filling and voiding to be conducted (cystourethrography). When these two procedures are combined this results in the gold standard investigation, the videocystometrogram or videourodynamic study. Radiological screening provides valuable additional anatomical information on the appearance of the bladder, the presence of vesicoureteric reflux, the degree of support to the bladder base during coughing and by itself is more than adequate for the diagnosis of sphincteric competence, and/or the level of any outflow obstruction in the lower urinary tract on the voiding phase. This information, along with the accompanying pressure flow tracings, can be recorded on a video tape allowing subsequent review and discussion. The majority of patients can be adequately investigated using the simpler urodynamic techniques described including simple cystometry. Videocystometry is however essential for the adequate assessment of complex cases where equivocal results have been obtained from simpler investigations, for the definition of neuropathic disorders, and in situations where there has been an apparent failure of a previous surgical procedure.

Technique for Videocystometrography/Cystometry: The detrusor pressure is estimated by the automatic subtraction of rectal pressure (as an index of intra-abdominal pressure) from the total bladder pressure (intra-vesical pressure), thus removing the influence of artifacts produced by abdominal straining. During this study notice is taken of the initial bladder residual, the bladder volume at the time of the patient's first sensation of filling, the final tolerated bladder volume and the final residual volume after voiding.

Patients, excluding those with indwelling catheters, are asked to void into a flowmeter to allow measurement of a free flow rate. Next, a fluid-filled rectal catheter is introduced into the rectum, the end of the tube being protected with a finger stall to prevent fecal blockage, (a slit is cut in this to prevent tamponade producing artifactual results during the study). With the patient in the supine position, the external urethral meatus is cleaned with antiseptic solution. A 10Ch Nelaton filling catheter with a 1 mm diameter saline-filled plastic pressure catheter inserted into the sub-terminal site hole is gently inserted into the bladder and the two catheters then disengaged. The bladder is filled via the 10 F catheter which is removed prior to the voiding phase leaving the fine catheter in situ. Alternatively a 6, 7, or -8 Fr dual-lumen catheter can be used which avoids the need to use two catheters and then disengage them. The intravesical pressure can also be measured via a suprapubic route. The bladder can be drained of urine and this initial residual volume recorded, alternatively the study can be carried out by filling on top of the initial residual and calculating the residual at the end of the study by subtraction.

The intra-abdominal pressure is measured via a pressure recording rectal catheter, inserted 10–15 cm above the anal verge, but may also be inserted into the vagina or a stoma. The patient is asked to cough to check for dampening of the signal, this is repeated throughout the procedure as a quality control method (a cough should increase both intra-abdominal pressure and intra-vesical pressure but only show as a blip on the detrusor trace). The catheters are then connected to the transducers. The most common transducers are fluid filled and rely on faultless positioning of transducer and meticulous fluid height referencing. Artifacts may be caused by air within the system, dampening waves or kinks within tubing, blocking readings. These must be eliminated. All systems are zeroed at atmospheric pressure. For catheter mounted transducer, the reference point is the transducer itself. For external transducers, the reference point is the level of the superior edge of the symphysis pubis. Newer air charged transducers remove this need and are gaining popularity but still need to be validated. The two pressure measurement lines are then connected to the transducers incorporated in the urodynamic apparatus. The lines are flushed through, great care being taken to exclude all air bubbles from both the tubing and transducer chambers. Contrast medium or saline (in a "non-video" study) at room temperature is then instilled into the bladder at a predetermined rate under the control of a peristaltic pump. Medium and fast fill (50–100 mL/min) is used routinely, although slower filling rates (10–25 mL/min) approaching the physiological range are mandatory in the assessment of the neuropathic bladder.

It is our practice to fill the bladder initially in the supine position and the volume at first sensation of filling is noted. When the subject first experiences discomfort, the radiographic table is tipped toward the standing position and subsequent bladder filling discontinued when at the maximum tolerated capacity. During bladder filling the patient is asked to consciously suppress bladder contraction and may be asked to cough or heel bounce. The patient is then turned to the oblique position relative to the X-ray machine and asked to void into the flowmeter provided.

In units where a tipping table is not available, the study can be carried out in the sitting or standing position initially; but it is important to subsequently stand the patient upright at the end of the study to assess where there is postural detrusor instability and to determine whether there is stress incontinence; in the absence of radiological screening this is assessed with the patient standing with legs slightly apart and squatting.

Throughout the study continuous rectal pressure, total bladder pressure and electronically subtracted detrusor pressure (total bladder pressure minus rectal pressure) measurements are sampled at a predetermined rate (usually 1 Hz) and the results displayed on the video display unit / stored to disc / polygraph chart recorder; depending on the equipment in use. Figure 20.4a and b shows a typical workstation and schematic.

Videodynamics provides an excellent method of evaluating the urethral outlet in female patients with urinary incontinence, males with complex voiding problems and are essential to the optimum management of neurological patients. Standing quietly and partially obliqued, the bladder neck position may be abnormally low, below the level of the upper third of the symphysis pubis, signifying loss of pelvic floor support in female patients with hypermobile urethras/anatomical stress incontinence. Coughing or valsalva maneuvers cause these vesicourethral units to descend and leak. With termination of the increased intra-abdominal pressure the bladder neck quickly "springs back" to its original position terminating leakage. The semi-lateral/oblique position enables to distinguish between the bladder neck from a dependent cystocele and it also helps to evaluate the size and functional significance of the cystocele.

Breaking or funneling of the bladder neck probably represents a normal finding, is common in continent females, but should be distinguished from a rectangular-shaped incompetent bladder neck common in patients with intrinsic sphincter deficiency (ISD). Typically patients with pure ISD as the cause of their incontinence demonstrate severe leakage with minimal intra-abdominal pressure increases and minimal urethrovesical hypermobility. The urethra does not spring back but appears to hold open and continue leaking even after the stress event. Patients often have both bladder neck hypermobility and ISD and experience is necessary in order to interpret their relative functional significance.

Cystourethrography via the adjacent X-ray screening apparatus allows the synchronous display of pressure and flow, and also radiographic data relating to bladder morphology e.g. diverticula, vesicoureteric reflux and the appearances of the bladder outlet and urethra, to be displayed alongside the numerical data on a video display unit.

Cystometric Findings

As filling continues the patient is asked to confirm the following bladder sensations which are recorded on the computer:

- First desire to void
- Strong desire to void
- Desire at which the patient cannot delay micturition (Maximum cystometric capacity)
- Urgency – sudden compelling desire to void
- Bladder pain – should not occur during filling

The computer calculates the pressures and plots them on a temporal graph. The above sensations are recorded at specific times and give an indication of how full the bladder was when these sensations occurred. Figure 20.5 shows a typical readout from the study, showing both storage and voiding phases with regular quality controls (coughing). The detrusor pressure is the result of the intravesical pressure minus the intra-abdominal pressure.

The four graphs in the order produced are:

- Intra-abdominal pressure (P_{abd})
- Intra-vesical pressure (P_{ves})
- Detrusor pressure (P_{det})
- Urinary flow rate (Q)

Figure 20.4. (**a**) A typical workstation comprising: (A) transducers to be placed at height of patients symphysis pubis, (B) Pump for bladder filling, (C) Display, (D) uroflowmeter. (**b**) The bladder is filled at a predetermined rate with a radio-opaque contrast medium, with the simultaneous measurement of intra-vesical pressure and intra-abdominal pressure. The subtracted detrusor pressure is calculated automatically and flow is recorded with the flow meter. This information with accompanying radiographic pictures and a sound track can be recorded allowing subsequent review and analysis.[22]

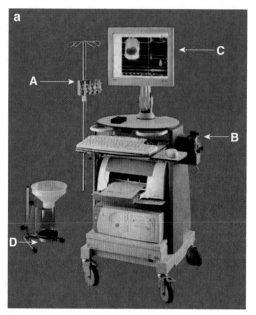

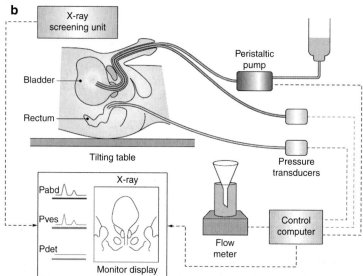

Practical Points: Since a number of variations in technique are currently available, the following points deserve specific consideration.

i. Type of catheter

   a. Fluid-filled catheter – specify number of catheters, single or multiple lumens, type of catheter, size of catheter.

   b. Catheter tip transducer – specifications vary between manufacturers; these catheters tend to be expensive and rather too fragile for routine use.

ii. Measuring equipment.

A number of commercial urodynamic systems are currently available. These vary greatly in terms of sampling rate, associated computer software backup, and price. A major problem with existing computer programs is the ease with which such programs will

Figure 20.5. A typical graphical display of the pressure flow data, showing both storage and voiding phases with regular coughing acting as a quality control (small blips in Pdet). The graph shows good contraction of the detrusor during the voiding phase and no contractions during the storage phase. Not included are the sensations as described by the patient, which will be plotted along the x-axis at the time they occurred, allowing us to calculate volumes at which sensory perceptions occur.[22]

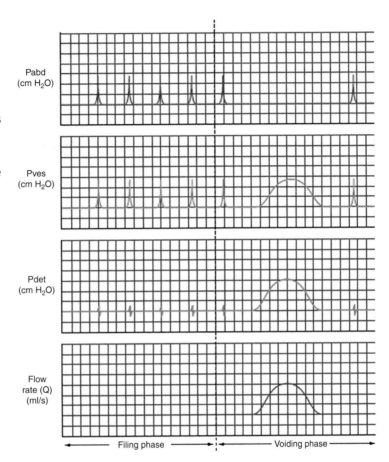

record artifacts which can then bias the results of the subsequent automatic data analysis. The investigator is strongly advised not to rely upon the computer generated data sheets but to use an appropriate standardized reading sheet which allows interpretation of the urodynamic findings by the investigator.

iii. Test medium (liquid or gas)

This is obviously not applicable to catheter tip transducers. The advantage of equipment using gas as a medium is that it can be more compact and is therefore more easily portable. A major drawback with gas cystometry is its susceptibility to artifact being introduced by changes in the temperature of the gaseous medium; a far less important consideration when fluid is used.

iv. Position of patient (e.g. supine, sitting, or standing).

v. Type of filling

This may be by diuresis or catheter. Filling by catheter may be continuous or incremental; the precise filling rate should be stated (vide infra). When the incremental method is used the volume increment should be stated.

vi. Continuous or intermittent pressure measurement

Continuous pressure measurement is of greatest usefulness in clinical practice; in patients for example with a suprapubic catheter and no urethral access, staged measurement of pressures can be carried out through the suprapubic catheter.

vii. Who carries out the study and how? – data quality

It is essential that urodynamic studies are carried out or supervised by experienced investigators:-

a. Always take a clinical history of the patient before carrying out the study and counsel the patient before they attend on the day and at the start of the study as to the nature of the test.

b. Make sure the urodynamic equipment is regularly serviced and calibrate the transducers on a regular basis.

c. Make sure that the lines are zeroed at the start of the study, check subtraction is perfect before starting the study with a detrusor pressure between 0 and 5 cm H_2O, and every minute during the study ask the patient to cough and verify that the rectal and vesical pressure lines track together in their response. If in doubt about artifact, repeat the study.

d. Choose the correct filling rate for the study, e.g. normal filling at 50 mL/min and slower filling at a rate of 10–20 mL/min for neuropaths and patients with a reduced functional capacity.

e. Leak point pressure:

The abdominal pressure or vesical pressure at which leakage occurs is a major problem because there is no standard technique with regard to:

- Catheter caliber
- Presence of prolapse
- Bladder volume at which the leakage is measured
- Valsalva versus cough
- Straining (contraction/relaxation of pelvic floor)
- Absolute measurement or relative measurement compared to baseline
- No defined threshold values for treatment decision

The literature abounds with contradictory reports as to whether there is any correlation between urethral pressure and leak point pressure.[17,18]

Our experience would support the use of graduated coughs as a means of assessing leakage, ideally coupled with cystourethrography or videocystometry. Basically, both tests suffer limitations. Since women leak with stress efforts in their everyday life and not with Valsalva, the Valsalva leak point pressure serves at best as a surrogate marker of sphincter competency. For the urethral pressure profile, the methodology imposed by the test (passive measurement, supine position) negates the real life effect of the stress component over a presumably deficient sphincter.

Comment:

i. Before starting to fill the bladder, the residual urine may be measured. However, the removal of a large volume of residual urine may alter detrusor function especially in neuropathic disorders. Certain cystometric parameters may be significantly altered by the speed of bladder filling.

ii. During cystometry it is taken for granted that the patient is awake, unanasthetized, and neither sedated nor taking drugs that affect bladder function. Any variations from this ideal must be taken into account when interpreting results.

iii. In a small group of women who present with incontinence, urinary leakage cannot be demonstrated either clinically or radiographically. Conventional testing can be repeated or continuous ambulatory urodynamic monitoring considered if available.

Measurements During the Storage Phase:

- Detrusor activity – during the storage phase the detrusor muscle should be inactive. Any activity should be correlated with episodes of urgency and/or incontinence. The volume at which this occurred should be noted. Provocation maneuvers may be employed to stimulate detrusor overactivity.

- Bladder compliance – describes the intrinsic ability of the bladder to change in volume without significantly altering detrusor pressure.

- Bladder capacity – is the volume at the end of the storage phase. It may be reduced in patients with a small contracted bladder and increased due to repeated stretching in patients with chronic outflow obstruction.

- Abdominal leak point pressure – is the intra-vesical pressure at which urine leakage occurs due to increased abdominal pressure in the absence of detrusor contraction. It measures the ability of the bladder neck and the urethral sphincter mechanism to resist increases in intra-abdominal pressure.
- Detrusor leak point pressure – is the lowest detrusor pressure at which urine leakage occurs in the absence of either a detrusor contraction or increased abdominal pressure. It measures the capacity of the bladder neck and urethral sphincter mechanism to resist increased pressure.

Abnormal findings include:

- Detrusor overactivity – activity during storage or associated with episodes of urgency or incontinence
- Poor bladder compliance/capacity – usually noted with small shrunken fibrotic bladders
- Low abdominal leak point pressure – increases in intra-abdominal pressure will precipitate stress urinary incontinence
- Low detrusor leak point pressure – Increases in bladder pressure will precipitate stress urinary incontinence

Measurements During the Voiding Phase:

- Premicturition pressure – pressure recorded prior to the initial isovulometric contraction in the bladder
- Opening pressure – pressure recorded at the onset of urine flow
- Opening time – time from initial rise in detrusor pressure to actual flow
- Maximum pressure – peak amplitude of voiding pressure
- Pressure at maximum flow – lowest pressure recorded at maximum flow rate
- Closing pressure – the pressure as measured at the end of flow
- Minimum voiding pressure – minimum pressure sufficient to produce flow

Abnormal findings include:

- Detrusor underactivity – A detrusor contraction insufficient to achieve complete bladder emptying
- Acontractile detrusor – No detrusor activity
- Bladder outflow obstruction – characterized by increased detrusor pressures and reduced flow rates

Video dynamics during voiding may be able to visualize the bladder outlet and urethra defining the level of obstruction. Also during video urodynamics the stop test maybe performed. The patient is asked to stop their void. During this the urine lying between the bladder neck sphincter and the distal prostatic sphincter is normally pushed back into the bladder, however in patients with bladder neck hypertrophy this urine is unable to return to the bladder and is captured via contrast screening.

Abnormal Function

Disordered lower urinary tract function can result from:

- Disruption of the normal peripheral or central nervous system (CNS) control mechanisms
- Disordered bladder muscle function, either primary (of unknown etiology) or secondary to an identifiable pathology such as prostatic-mediated bladder outflow obstruction.

Patients who have disordered lower urinary tract function in routine clinical practice represent a heterogeneous collection for most of whom there is no identifiable neurological abnormality. Some of these patients will have a primary neural or muscular disorder (e.g. primary idiopathic detrusor overactivity) in contrast to post-obstructive secondary detrusor overactivity where the major etiological factor is likely to be peripheral disruption of local neuromuscular function.

It is essential to use standardized terminology when discussing lower urinary tract symptoms (LUTS) and the results of urodynamic investigations, to allow accurate exchange and comparison of information for clinical and research purposes. The official terminology is as suggested by the International Continence Society (ICS) in 2002.[4]

ICS terminology for LUTS is summarized in Table 20.3: Further information regarding terminology can be found on the ICS Website (www.icsoffice.org).

This terminology refers specifically to symptoms elicited in a history; subtly different definitions are in use in other specific scenarios, for example when using frequency/volume charts. More information on all of the terminology is available in "The Standardisation of Terminology in Lower Urinary Tract Function Report."[19]

Disorders of the Lower Urinary Tract

The vesicourethral unit comprises the bladder and urethra, working in co-operation to store and void urine. Dysfunction occurs when there is breakdown in these fundamental tasks resulting in storage and/or voiding symptoms, urinary retention, or incontinence. Thus disorders of the lower urinary tract can best be subdivided into:

- Disorders of sensation; and
- Disorders of motor function.

Each of these may affect:

- The detrusor muscle; or
- The sphincter-active bladder outflow tract (bladder neck mechanism, distal urethral sphincter mechanism, prostate).

The detrusor muscle and the sphincter-active bladder outflow tract may be normal, overactive, or underactive.

Disorders of Sensation

These disorders represent an important poorly understood group of conditions where investigation is limited by:

- Limited knowledge about the structural and physiological basis for the perception of sensation in the lower urinary tract; and
- The subjective nature of sensation.

Attempts to quantify sensation have included the use of objective or semi-objective tests for sensory function such as evoked potentials and electrical threshold studies.

At present disorders of sensation are usually assessed by asking the patient about voiding pattern and any discomfort felt, based on clinical questioning or cystometry.

Because most sensory disorders are idiopathic, diagnosis of such a disorder can only be considered after other vesical or urethral pathologies (tumor, stone, infection, abnormal detrusor function) have been excluded.

In general terms, sensation can be subdivided as normal, hypersensitive, hyposensitive, and absent. The terminology used to describe disorders of bladder sensation:

- *First Sensation of filling*: Very subjective; a variable and unreliable symptom
- *First desire to void*: can be difficult to interpret; very subjective
- *Strong desire to void*: indicates maximum bladder capacity and signals the end of bladder filling during cystometry
- *Pain*: pain during bladder filling or micturition is abnormal; its site and character should be noted, as well as the volume at which it occurred.

Causes of Hypersensitive Bladder Sensation

The majority of these are idiopathic. However, bladder or urethral inflammation secondary to a number of causes should be excluded such as cystitis due to; bacteria, human papilloma virus, irradiation, cyclophosphamide, chemicals, bladder calculi, and bladder carcinoma. Urethral infections, urethritis, urethral syndrome, and chronic prostatitis are also implicated.

Causes of Hyposensitive Bladder Sensation

Causes of hyposensitivity are idiopathic, neuorgenic, or secondary to bladder stretching as occurs with chronic urinary retention. The neurogenic causes are; Spinal Cord Injury, Pelvic Trauma, Radical Hysterectomy, Abdominoperineal resection of the rectum, Peripheral neuropathy (e.g. diabetes).

Table 20.3. Lower urinary tract symptom terminology

Storage symptoms	
Increased daytime frequency	The complaint by the patient who considers that he/she voids too often by day (term is equivalent to pollakisuria used in many countries).
Nocturia	The complaint that the patient has to wake at night one or more times to void.
Urgency	A sudden compelling desire to pass urine which is difficult to defer.
Urinary incontinence (UI)	Any involuntary leakage of urine
Stress urinary incontinence (SUI)	Involuntary leakage on effort or exertion, or coughing or sneezing
Urge(ncy) urinary incontinence (UUI)	Involuntary leakage accompanied by or immediately preceded by urgency
Mixed urinary incontinence (MUI)	Involuntary leakage associated with urgency and also with exertion, effort, sneezing, or coughing
Enuresis	Any involuntary loss of urine
Nocturnal enuresis	Loss of urine occurring during sleep (involuntary symptom as opposed to nocturia which is a voluntary symptom)
Continuous urinary incontinence	Continuous leakage of urine
Other types of urinary incontinence	May be situational, for example incontinence during sexual intercourse, or giggle incontinence
Bladder sensations during storage phase	
Normal bladder sensation	Aware of bladder filling and increased sensation up to a strong desire to void
Increased bladder sensation	Aware of an early and persistent desire to void
Reduced bladder sensation	Aware of bladder filling but does not feel a definite desire to void
Absent bladder sensation	No awareness of bladder filling or desire to void
Nonspecific bladder sensation	No specific bladder sensation but may perceive bladder filling as abdominal fullness, or spasticity (most frequently seen in neurological patients)
Voiding symptoms	
Slow stream	The perception of reduced urine flow, usually compared to previous performance or in comparison to others
Splitting or spraying	Description of the urine stream
Hesitancy	Difficulty in initiating micturition, resulting in a delay in the onset of voiding after the individual is ready to pass urine
Intermittent stream (intermittency)	Urine flow which stops and starts, on one or more occasions, during micturition
Straining	The muscular effort used to either initiate, maintain, or improve the urinary stream
Terminal dribbling	A prolonged final part of micturition, where the flow has slowed to a trickle/dribble

(*continued*)

Table 20.3. (continued)

Post micturition symptoms	
Felling of incomplete emptying	A feeling experienced by the individual after passing urine
Post micturition dribble	The involuntary loss of urine immediately after an individual has finished passing urine, usually after leaving the toilet in men or after rising from the toilet in women
Other symptoms	
Symptoms associated with sexual intercourse	e.g. dyspareunia, vaginal dryness, and incontinence (should be described as fully as possible – it is helpful to define urine leakage as: during penetration, during intercourse, or at orgasm)
Symptoms associated with pelvic organ prolapse	e.g. "something coming down," low backache, vaginal bulging sensation, and dragging sensation (may need to digitally replace the prolapse in order to defecate or micturate)
Genital and lower urinary tract pain	Pain, discomfort and pressure may be related to bladder filling or voiding or may be felt after micturition, or even be continuous. The terms "strangury," "bladder spasm," and "dysuria" are difficult to define and of uncertain meeting and should not be used, unless a precise meaning is stated. Dysuria literally means "abnormal urination." However, it is often incorrectly used to describe the stinging/ burning sensation characteristic of an urinary infection
Painful bladder syndrome symptoms	
Bladder pain syndrome/ Painful bladder syndrome/ Interstitial cystitis (BPS/PBS/IC)	Suprapubic pain related to bladder filling and associated with other lower urinary tract symptoms, usually increased frequency (but no urgency) (diagnosed only in the absence of UTI or other obvious pathology). This is a specific diagnosis usually confirmed by typical cystoscopic and histological features

Disorders of Detrusor Motor Function

Cystometry is needed to assess detrusor function and not only may detrusor function differ during filling and voiding, but the classification may change between these two phases.

Detrusor function should be considered in the context of coexisting urethral function, but is often the primary cause of marked functional disruption.

Detrusor function may be:

- Normal (stable);
- Overactive;
- Underactive (hypocontractile); or
- Acontractile.

The terminology used to describe the disorders of detrusor motor function:

- *Stable detrusor function*: during filling bladder capacity increases in volume without a marked corresponding rise in pressure
- *Normal detrusor contractility*: normal voiding occurs as a result of a sustained detrusor contraction, which can be initiated and suppressed voluntarily and results in complete bladder emptying over a normal timespan; the magnitude of the recorded detrusor pressure rise depends upon outlet resistance

- *Overactive bladder*: a descriptive term that is applied to the combination in part or together of the lower urinary tract symptoms of urgency plus frequency, nocturia, or urge incontinence

- *Overactive detrusor function*: involuntary detrusor contractions during bladder filling, either spontaneous or provoked by rapid filling (provocation cystometry), provocative tests (hand washing, heel bouncing, alteration in posture, exercise, or coughing)

- *Overactive detrusor*: detrusor that is objectively shown to contract either spontaneously or on provocation during the filling phase during an attempt to inhibit micturition; it may be asymptomatic and it occurs in the absence of a documented neurological disorder

- *Neurogenic detrusor overactivity*: detrusor hyperactivity in the presence of a documented neurological disorder
- *Detrusor overactivity*: detrusor hyperactivity in the absence of a documented neurological disorder
- *Normal compliance*: little or no rise in detrusor pressure during normal bladder filling; at present there are insufficient data to adequately define normal, high, and low compliance
- *Low compliance*: gradual rise in detrusor pressure during bladder filling; usually describes a poorly distensible bladder (e.g. a shrunken fibrotic bladder complicating interstitial cystitis or after radiotherapy); detrusor instability and hyperreflexia also may be associated with low compliance
- *Underactive (hypocontractile) detrusor function*: detrusor contraction during micturition is inadequate to empty the bladder
- *Acontractile detrusor*: no contractile activity on urodynamic investigation
- *Areflexic detrusor*: acontractility resulting from a neurological abnormality
- *Decentralized detrusor*: a specific type of areflexic detrusor that occurs with lesions of the conus medullaris or sacral nerve outflow, where the peripheral ganglia in the wall of the bladder are preserved and the peripheral nerves are therefore intact but "decentralized"; characterized by involuntary intravesical pressure fluctuations of low amplitude, sometimes called "autonomous waves"
- *Urodynamic stress incontinence (Previously Genuine stress incontinence)*: is said to occur when there is demonstrable incontinence associated with a rise in intra-abdominal pressure in the absence of detrusor overactivity. It is due to intrinsic urethral sphincter weakness or hypermobility of the bladder neck/urethra
- *Mixed incontinence*: is a situation where there is a combination of detrusor overactivity and urethral sphincteric weakness
- *Overflow incontinence*: This is the involuntary loss of urine associated with overdistension of the bladder secondary to inefficient bladder emptying
- *Continuous urinary incontinence*: is the complaint of continuous leakage of urine.

This may be due to a vesical fistula for example a vesicovaginal fistula, a congenital abnormality for example an ectopic ureter or possibly due to gross intrinsic sphincter deficiency

Bladder Outflow Tract Dysfunction

The urethral closure mechanisms, including intrinsic urethral muscle and the sphincteric mechanisms (bladder neck and distal urethral) are best considered separately according to the phase of bladder function (either storage or voiding).

Urethral function during storage may be:

- Normal – there is a positive urethral closure pressure that is sufficient to maintain continence in the presence of increased intra-abdominal pressure;
- Incompetent – there is leakage, even in the absence of detrusor contraction; it may result from damage to the urethra or the associated sphincteric mechanisms;
- Underactive; or
- Absent

Urethral function during micturition may be:

- Normal – the urethra opens to allow the bladder to be emptied;
- Obstructive due to overactivity – the urethral closure mechanisms contract against a detrusor contraction or fail to open on attempted micturition – when this occurs in the absence of documented neurological disease it is known as "dysfunctional voiding";
- Obstructive due to nonrelaxation – A nonrelaxing, obstructing urethra may result in reduced urine flow and tends to occur in patients with a sacral or infra-sacral neurological lesion i.e. meningomyelocoele or radical pelvic surgery
- Obstructive due to a mechanical problem – this is uncommon in women, but is the most common cause of bladder outflow tract dysfunction in the male population, usually due to urethral stricture or prostatic enlargement; mechanical obstruction can arise as a consequence of anatomical factors (e.g. prostatic enlargement due to adenomatous hyperplasia) or neural control mechanisms (e.g. providing a functional basis for the relief of obstruction by α_1-adrenoceptor

blockade of the prostate). In this context it is notable that in recent years it has been increasingly recognized that an important component of prostatic obstruction results from smooth muscle contraction within the pathologically enlarged prostate.

Detrusor–Urethral Dyssynergia

In detrusor–urethral dyssynergia there is synchronous contraction of the detrusor and urethra. It can be subdivided depending upon the structures involved into detrusor–bladder neck dyssynergia and detrusor–sphincter dyssynergia.

Detrusor–Bladder Neck Dyssynergia

This refers to a detrusor contraction in the presence of incomplete bladder neck opening on micturition. It is not uncommon in the general population, and is a common cause of voiding dysfunction in younger males. It is thought to be a congenital abnormality, and commonly presents in the third and fourth decades of life.

Detrusor–Sphincter Dyssynergia

Detrusor–sphincter dyssynergia (DSD) describes a detrusor contraction occurring at the same time as an involuntary contraction of the urethral or periurethral striated smooth muscle.

Obstructive overactivity of the striated urethral sphincter muscle may occur in the absence of detrusor contraction, but is not DSD. This condition is uncommon in the general population, it affects women in particular and is most commonly seen in association with polycystic ovary disease.

Detrusor–sphincter dyssynergia is usually associated with neurological disorders, commonly supraspinal lesions, and the diagnosis needs to be treated with caution in the absence of a documented neurological deficit.

Complex Urodynamic Investigation

The current techniques available for the investigation of urethral sphincteric dysfunction are far from satisfactory. Urethral pressure profilometry although useful in the assessment of sympatholytic agents in drug trials is not appropriate as a diagnostic technique. The dynamic evaluation of urethral sphincter function by the use of anal or skin mounted electrodes is inaccurate. Accurate electromyographic evaluation of the urethral sphincter is possible with a concentric needle electrode but it is a painful investigation and cannot be carried out during voiding.

Urethral Pressure Measurement

At rest the urethra is closed and this must be recognized when interpreting the results of urethral pressure studies. The urethral pressure and the urethral closure pressure are therefore idealized concepts which represent the ability of the urethra to prevent leakage. In current urodynamic practice, the urethral pressure is measured by a number of different techniques, which do not always yield consistent values. Not only do the values differ with the method of measurement but there is often lack of consistency for a single method. For example the effect of catheter rotation when urethral pressure is measured by a catheter mounted transducer and the considerable artifacts which automatically result from the introduction of any catheter into the urethra.

Technique

Measurements may be made at one point in the urethra over a period of time, or at several points along the urethra consecutively forming a *urethral pressure profile* (UPP).

At rest the *urethral pressure profile* denotes the intra-luminal pressure along the length of the urethra. All systems are zeroed at atmospheric pressure. For external transducers the reference point is the superior edge of the symphysis pubis. For catheter mounted transducers the reference point is the transducer itself. Intravesical pressure should be measured to exclude a simultaneous detrusor contraction. The subtraction of intravesical pressure from urethral pressure produces the *urethral closure pressure profile*.

Intra-luminal urethral pressure may be measured:

i. At rest(the *storage phase*), with the bladder at any given volume – *Resting urethral pressure profile (UPP)*.
ii. During coughing or straining – *Stress urethral pressure profile*.

Ambulatory Urodynamics: This form of cystometry overcomes some of the problems associated with conventional urodynamics. The equipment is portable, allowing the subject to move freely and void in private. In addition the patient fills her bladder spontaneously after drinking a fluid load. As the technique is not adequately standardized with no internationally accepted diagnostic criteria it is best regarded as a research tool at present, particularly since some studies have reported involuntary detrusor contractions in up to 70% of apparently normal subjects.

Urethral Pressure Profilometry: Although UPP has the potential to be highly informative, the test has multiple problems, the most significant being the large overlap in values obtained from normal and symptomatic patients. UPP does not discriminate SUI from other urinary disorders, provide a measurement of the severity of the condition or predict a return to normal following successful intervention.

Abdominal Leak Point Pressures: Abdominal leak point pressure (ALPP) is defined as the vesical pressure at leakage during abdominal stress in the absence of detrusor contraction. The abdominal stress may be induced by a cough (CLPP) or a Valsalva maneuver (VLPP), with the two stressors differing physiologically in particular with regard to the rate and nature of pressure rise which is seen. Whilst higher abdominal pressures can be achieved with CLPP, the VLPP is better controlled and less variable.[20] Generally, CLPP is used for patients who do not leak during VLPP measurement. The pressure at which the urine is expelled can be measured visually, fluoroscopically, by flowmetry or by electrical conductance.

Although the concept of ALPP as a method of investigating incontinence is empirically sound, its value is limited by a lack of standardized methodology. Variations occur in the type of catheter (transurethral, rectal, vagina), catheter caliber, bladder volume, and patient position. The exact baseline used during the test also varies (e.g. zero level or the level at which the pressure just starts to rise), which can make a dramatic difference to the ALPP value. For ALPP to be a valid test, it is assumed that: the transurethral catheter used does not obstruct the urethra or alter coaptation; straining or coughing does not distort the urethra; and no pelvic relaxation or contraction occurs. However, it is difficult to know whether these are actually occurring during the test, which is a major drawback.

Few data are available on the magnitude of the change in ALPP post-SUI treatment, and how this correlates with cure, improvement, or failure. One general finding is that VLPP does not change significantly if the treatment fails. For example, following suburethral sling operations in 30 women, VLPP increased significantly after a successful operation (mean change: 61.1 cm H_2O; $p < 0.001$) but not after failure (mean change: 9.7 cm H_2O, $p = 0.226$).[21]

Neurophysiological Evaluation

The electrical activity of action potentials of depolarizing striated muscle fibers in the urethra can be studied with electromyography using surface or needle electrodes. Results must be interpreted in the light of symptoms and other investigations. This remains a research tool but has provided valuable insight into the pathophysiology and the effect of treatment on various conditions.

Neurophysiological investigations, like urethral pressure profilometry have not entered widespread usage. Four different neurophysiological methods have been described:

- Electromyography – Needle electrodes are placed in to a muscle mass or surface electrodes are used to record electrical action potentials generated by depolarization of muscle. Potential sampling sites include; the intrinsic striated muscle of the urethra, the periurethral striated muscle, bulbocavernosus muscle, external anal sphincter, and pubococcygeus muscle. These have a characteristic waveform and in disease this may be altered or the impulse may be recorded at an inappropriate time, such as in detrusor sphincter dyssynergia, where the urethral striated muscle contracts during voiding.

- Nerve conduction latency studies – determine time taken (latency) for a response to occur in a muscle following peripheral nerve stimulation
- Reflex latency studies – assess the latency of a reflex arc, assessing the nerve conduction velocity in both the afferent and efferent limbs of the reflex.
- Sensory testing – a standard electrical stimulus is applied to the bladder/urethra to give the least current required for the patient to perceive a stimulus. This is known as the vesical/ urethral sensory threshold.

Conclusion

We can say urodynamics is not an esoteric subject of limited applicability requiring complex equipment. In most cases the basic principles are simple and may be applied to a series of questions formulated from the undertaking of a thorough history and clinical examination. It is useful to view the urinary tract as a sequence of conduits within which urine movement is dictated by chamber pressures and resistance to flow, with intervening sphincters controlling flow. It is advisable to avoid jargon terms and use the nomenclature of the International Continence Society as presented earlier in this chapter.

This chapter outlines the principles and practice of urodynamics used in routine clinical practice. Although we find that the "bladder is an unreliable witness," urodynamic techniques have allowed for objective clarification of these subjective symptoms.

References

1. Chapple CR, Roehrborn CG. A shifted paradigm for the further understanding, evaluation, and treatment of lower urinary tract symptoms in men: focus on the bladder. *Eur Urol.* 2006;49(4):651-659
2. www.iciq.net/. 2009
3. Griffiths D, Tadic SD. Bladder control, urgency, and urge incontinence: evidence from functional brain imaging. *Neurourol Urodyn.* 2008;27(6):466-474
4. Addla S, Adeyouju A, Neilson D. Assessment of reliability of 1-day, 3-day and 7-day frequency volume charts. *Eur Urol Suppl.* 2004;2:30

5. Lose G, Rosenkilde P, Gammelgaard J, Schroeder T. Pad-weighing test performed with standardized bladder volume. *Urology.* 1988;32:78-80
6. Kromann-Andersen B, Jakobsen H, Andersen JT. Pad-weighing tests: a literature survey on test accuracy and reproducibility. *Neurourol Urodyn.* 1989;8:237-242
7. Jorgensen L, Lose G, Thunedborg P. Diagnosis of mild stress incontinence in females: 24-hour pad weighing test versus the one-hour test. *Neurourol Urodyn.* 1987; 6:165-166
8. Gilleran JP, Zimmern P. An evidence-based approach to the evaluation and management of stress incontinence in women. *Curr Opin Urol.* 2005;15:236-243
9. Goode PS, Locher JL, Bryant RL, Roth DL, Burgio KL. Measurement of postvoid residual urine with portable transabdominal bladder ultrasound scanner and urethral catheterization. *Int Urogynecol J Pelvic Floor Dysfunct.* 2000;11:296-300
10. Weber AM, Taylor RJ, Wei JT, Lemack G, Piedmonte MR, Walters MD. The cost-effectiveness of preoperative testing (basic office assessment vs. urodynamics) for stress urinary incontinence in women. *BJU Int.* 2002;89: 356-363
11. Weidner AC, Myers ER, Visco AG, Cundiff GW, Bump RC. Which women with stress incontinence require urodynamic evaluation? *Am J Obstet Gynecol.* 2001;184:20-27
12. Abrams P. *Urodynamics.* London: Springer-Verlag; 1997
13. Agency for Health Care Policy and Research. Clinical practice guideline: urinary incontinence in adults. Rockville MDOHAHSUAFHCPAR, editor. AHCPR Pub. No. 96-0682. 1996
14. Digesu GA, Khullar V, Cardozo L, Salvatore S. Overactive bladder symptoms: do we need urodynamics? *Neurourol Urodyn.* 2003;22:105-108
15. Showalter PR, Zimmern PE, Roehrborn CG, Lemack GE. Standing cystourethrogram: an outcome measure after anti-incontinence procedures and cystocele repair in women. *Urology.* 2001;58:33-37
16. Zimmern P, Lemack G. Voiding cystourethrography and magnetic resonance imaging of the lower urinary tract. In: Corcos I, Schick E, eds. *The Urinary Sphincter.* Marcel Dekker, Inc.: New York; 2001:407-421
17. Hilton P, Stanton SL. Urethral pressure measurement by microtransducer: the results in symptom-free women and in those with genuine stress incontinence. *Br J Obstet Gynaecol.* 1983;90:919-933
18. Bump RC, Norton PA, Zinner NR, Yalcin I. Mixed urinary incontinence symptoms: urodynamic findings, incontinence severity, and treatment response. *Obstet Gynecol.* 2003;102:76-83
19. Abrams P, Cardozo L, Fall M, et al. The standardisation of terminology of lower urinary tract function: report from the Standardisation Sub-committee of the International Continence Society. *Neurourol Urodyn.* 2002;21:167-178
20. Homma Y. The clinical significance of the urodynamic investigation in incontinence. *BJU Int.* 2002;90:489-497
21. Petrou SP, Broderick GA. Valsalva leak-point pressure changes after successful and failed suburethral sling. *Int Urogynecol J Pelvic Floor Dysfunct.* 2002;13:299-302
22. Chapple CR, MacDiarmid SA, Patel A. *Urodynamics Made Easy.* 3rd ed. Edinburgh, UK: Elsevier Churchill Livingstone; 2009

21

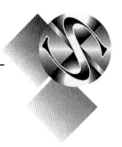

Urologic Instrumentation: Endoscopes and Lasers

Erica H. Lambert, Nicole L. Miller, and S. Duke Herrell

Endoscopy

Cystourethroscopy

Cystourethroscopic examination of the bladder and urethra is the gold standard for the diagnosis of lower urinary tract disorders. It offers direct visualization of the bladder urothelium and provides initial access to the ureteral orifices for assessment and treatment of the upper tracts. It is a cornerstone in the workup for gross and microscopic hematuria and useful in the investigation of lower urinary tract symptoms stemming from anatomic obstruction or neurologic, inflammatory, neoplastic, or congenital disorders. Beyond this, instruments passed through the cystoscope or specially designed resectoscopes allow minimally invasive treatment of identified pathology.

Cystourethroscopy is performed using rigid or flexible endoscopes. Rigid cystoscopes consist of a sheath, an obturator, a bridge, and a telescope (Fig. 21.1). Endoscopes are measured in French scale, which is commonly used to measure the circumference of cylindrical medical instruments including endoscopes, catheters and stents. The diameter in millimeters can be calculated by dividing the number in the French gauge by 3. Endoscopes come in sizes to accommodate both pediatric patients (8–12 Fr) and adult patients (16–25 Fr). For rigid scopes, the sheath provides a connection to the irrigation system. An optional obturator can be placed through the sheath to bluntly enter the urethra or the scope can be passed under visual guidance. Once inside the bladder, the bridge allows the passage of treatment implements (i.e. wires, stents, laser fibers). Various types of bridges exist allowing the passage of multiple catheters, fibers, and wires and even a specialized bridge that allows for deflection of a laser fiber (Alberrans bridge). The light cord connects directly to the telescope, which provides better optics and a rod-lens imaging system that transmits the light and image to the eyepiece. The lens angle enables the endoscopist to adequately evaluate the entire urethra and bladder. The 0° lens allows the best view of the urethra providing a straight image. A 30° lens provides visualization of the base and anterolateral aspect of the bladder. A 70° lens allows improved visual assessmentes of the dome and anterior bladder neck. Rigid cystoscopes provide superior optics and a large working port to accommodate a variety of accessory instruments. The major disadvantage of the rigid endoscope is that it is not well tolerated in nonanesthetized male patients and requires dorsal lithotomy positioning, making it difficult to perform the procedure outside the facilities of the operating room.[1]

Spring-loaded resectoscopes are larger diameter rigid endoscopes (24–27-French) used for the resection of bladder lesions and prostatic hyperplasia. The bladder is typically distended by irrigation, and a multiple channel sheath system is available which allows for continuous flow to maintain a constant bladder volume and

C.R. Chapple and W.D. Steers (eds.), *Practical Urology*: *Essential Principles and Practice*, DOI: 10.1007/978-1-84882-034-0_21, © Springer-Verlag London Limited 2011

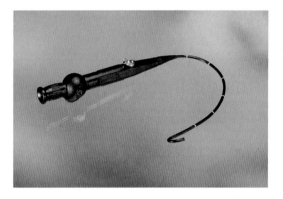

Figure 21.2. Flexible cystoscope.

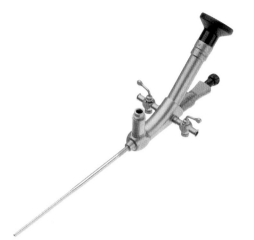

Figure 21.1. Rigid cystoscope.

level of distension. Continuous flow prevents the bladder from collapsing or overdistending. Overdistension results in thinning the overlying bladder musculature, which can predispose to bladder perforation in the area of resection. Continuous flow allows a bladder lesion to remain at a fixed level of distension to facilitate resection. Additionally, some authors feel that it improves visualization in settings of heavy bleeding, particularly during a transurethral resection of the prostate (TURP).

The main advantages of the flexible cystoscope are greater patient tolerability, the ability to perform the procedure supine in the office, the ease of passing the scope over an elevated bladder neck, and the deflection at the end of scope allowing visualization of the entire bladder and retroflexion to visualize the bladder neck. The flexible scope utilizes fiber optic bundles within a flexible shaft to provide illumination and visualization (Fig. 21.2). The tip of the scope can be deflected 180–220°. The irrigation connection and working port are on the instrument's shaft and typically connect to a single common rubber-lined working channel within the scope which can be damaged if instrumentation is passed with the scope in the deflected position.

The newest technology for flexible endoscopy is the distal-sensor digital chip system, which eliminates the need for fiber bundles and the resultant "honeycomb" honeycomb pattern of the image. In a study from University of California at Irvine, three flexible systems, including a new distal-sensor digital cystoscope

with >165,000 effective pixels, were compared to two brand-new standard fiber optic cystoscopes for resolution, contrast, and color discrimination *in vitro*. The group found no difference between the standard fiber optic flexible cystoscopes; however, the distal-sensor all-digital cystoscope was superior to the fiber optic scopes in terms of resolution, contrast discrimination, and red color differentiation.[2]

Video-cystourethroscopy, -ureteroscopy, and -ureteropyeloscopy (discussed below) allow the image in both the rigid and flexible endoscopes to be projected onto a monitor and are currently available in high definition. This obviates the need to look through the eyepiece on the lens. Benefits of the video include avoiding contact with body fluids, improvement in ability to maintain a sterile field, ease in documentation of the procedure, providing patient education during the procedure, aiding in teaching, and improved surgeon ergonomics with potential prevention of cervical injuries, which were common in previous generations of urologists.

Ureteroscopy and Ureteropyeloscopy

Retrograde endoscopic evaluation of the upper urinary tract typically has a much lower morbidity profile than a percutaneous or open renal procedure. Ureteroscopy with laser lithotripsy is the gold standard for the treatment of distal ureteral stones and is commonly utilized for stones throughout the collecting system. AUA guidelines state that the majority of renal calculi can be effectively treated by laser lithotripsy using a flexible ureterscope.[3] Technologic advances in ureteroscopy, ureteropyeloscopy, and laser technology have improved the options for the diagnosis, treatment, and surveillance of select upper tract transitional cell carcinomas. Retrograde technique allows for a closed system, which may potentially lower the risk of tumor seeding and hemorrhage associated with percutaneous procedures.

The first attempt at ureteroscopy was in 1912, when Hugh Hampton Young passed a rigid cystoscope into a massively dilated pediatric ureter. It was not until almost 40 years later that flexible ureteroscopy was performed with a 9 F scope.[4] Currently, with improvements in optics and technology, ureteroscopes range in length (54–70 cm), sizes (6.7–12 F), and degree of deflection in flexible scopes (130–270°). Similar to the cystoscope, the ureteroscope can be either semirigid or flexible. The semirigid ureteroscope contains flexible fiber optic bundles, which allow for some bend in the scope. The scope typically has a single common working and irrigation channel, which is typically larger than that of a flexible scope and allows passage of 3-French instrumentation allowing irrigation serving to distend the ureter and aid in visibility (Fig. 21.1). The semirigid scope is primarily used for the evaluation and treatment of either stones or tumors in the distal to mid portions of the ureter, although in many women and prestented ureters, it can be passed all the way to the renal pelvis. The length and rigidity of the scope as well as the tortuosity of the ureter makes it difficult to reach the renal pelvis with the semirigid scope in some patients.

Modern flexible ureteroscopes haves active deflection at the tip, which has expanded its utilization enabling visualization of the entire collecting system including the lower pole calyces. The newest flexible ureteroscopes have two mechanisms of active deflection; the primary site provides 170–180° of up and down movement; the secondary site proximal to the primary site allows another 130° of downward deflection. This added deflection enables the modern urologist to navigate easily into the lower pole system, which was no small technical feat in some patients prior to the development of the "double deflection" scopes. Contemporary scopes can achieve 270° of deflection. The scopes typically have a common working and irrigation port. The introduction of smaller diameter scopes has allowed increased ease of insertion leading to improved ability to navigate the ureter with less morbidity and without the need for preemptive ureteral dilation by stent placement, which was common in the past. Simultaneously, advances in intracorporeal lithotriptors, including laser lithotrites, have been made facilitating stone fragmentation through a flexible scope. Smaller diameter stone retrieval devices with increased flexibility, such as the nitinol wire basket, have been developed to pass through the working port to aid in stone removal.[5] Disadvantages of the flexible scope include a small working port, which limits irrigation and visualization when instruments, such as baskets and lasers, are being used, and continued difficulty accessing certain calyces despite improvements in flexion.[6]

Nephroscopy

Nephroscopy, which consists of antegrade endoscopic visualization of the renal pelvis and calyces, is generally performed in the setting of percutaneous procedures via a dilated tract. Applications include percutaneous management of renal calculi, tumors, ureteropelvic junction obstruction, and calyceal diverticuli. The nephroscope consists of an inner and outer sheath with a working port, a lens, and an apparatus for continuous flow through irrigation ports (Fig. 21.3). The large bore of the rigid nephroscope provides optimal visualization and a generously sized working channel for graspers or a variety of lithotrite. The rigidity and size,

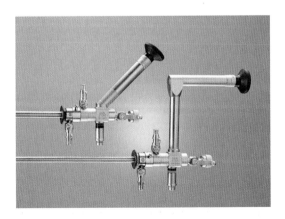

Figure 21.3. Percutaneous nephroscope.

however, may limit the degree of scope movement, resulting in suboptimal access to calyces not favorably aligned to the percutaneous tract. For this reason, a flexible cystoscope (described above) serving as a flexible nephroscope may be utilized, allowing the endoscopist to inspect the entire collecting system without resulting in the same physical torque to the kidney.[7] The use of flexible nephroscopy during the primary PCNL procedure increases the stone-free rate and decreases the need for additional access tracts.[8]

Virtual Reality Simulators

In the modern health care environment a variety of factors including the potential for improved teaching and patient safety combined with decreasing declining reimbursement, decreased available operative time, decreased resident hours and case numbers may increase the use of simulators in resident training. Some authors advocate that simulation systems should be a mandatory part of residency training, to include aptitude skill testing before being able to perform surgical procedures on humans.[9] A potential benefit to the virtual reality simulator is that the trainee can acquire adequate skills in a low-risk environment. "High fidelity" virtual reality trainers consists of a monitor, workstation with an integrated mechatronic unit providing force feedback, and a personalized computer. Endourologic procedures are well replicated in simulator training because of the ability to provide realistic sensations of pressure and force feedback.[10] The software contains procedures including resection of bladder tumors, laser lithotripsy, percutaneous access placement, and ureteroscopy.

Although the use of such simulators is relatively new, several small studies have evaluated the efficacy of the simulator training and found potential benefit.[11,12] One study found that it was possible to tell the difference between "expert" and "novice" endoscopists by evaluating each cystoscopic task and time to complete the task. In another study at University of California, Irvine, medical students were taught ureteroscopic skills on either an ureteroscopy training model (TMU) (Limbs & Things) or the URO Mentor (Simbionix, Israel).[13] After completing the training course, their newly acquired skills were assessed in an animal model of ureteroscopy. Both systems provided for development of an adequate skill set for the medical students to perform basic ureteroscopy. The author concluded that initial training on the simulators might improve a novice's or resident's early clinical experience. The improved familiarity with the instrumentation allowed reduced procedure time and improved competence. Virtual reality simulators, both low and high fidelity, have the potential to play an important role in urologic training, perhaps enhance the historical teacher–apprentice model, and may eventually be incorporated into assessment of procedural competence similar to their use in the aviation industry.

Lasers

Lasers have occupied an increasing role in the treatment of urologic disease. The term "LASER" (Light Amplification by the Stimulated Emission of Radiation) was initially proposed by Albert Einstein in 1917. Forty-three years after Einstein's first theories, Maiman introduced the first visible light laser with synthetic ruby crystals and silver-coated ends surrounded by a flash tube to produce light energy.[14] This marked the beginning of laser use and a bridge between quantum physics and clinical medicine. The earliest use of laser technology in clinical urology started in 1966 with Parsons studies with a ruby laser in a pulsed mode on canine bladders.[14] In 1968, Mulvany fragmented urinary calculi using a similar laser.[14] Currently, lasers are widely used and often the primary tool for the treatment of urolithiasis, endoscopic organ-preserving tumor ablation, ureteral and urethral strictures, and benign prostatic hyperplasia.

Briefly, Einstein's concept of stimulated emission is based on two principles of physics. The first is that light travels as photons or packets of energy. The second is that atoms and molecules exist in a low energy state. Laser energy is produced when an atom becomes excited by an external energy source, such as by electricity, heat, or light energy, causing excited electrons to release excess energy in the form of photons or light energy. The typical energy source in a laser is electric or flashlamp driven, and produces excited atoms as the basis for the laser medium. The photons emitted spontaneously from the excited molecules cause light to travel in all directions within the laser cavity. Different laser source mediums emit photons in different distinct wavelengths. Laser light differs from natural light in that it must have photons in phase, known as coherence, they must travel in parallel, known as collimation, and all must have the same wavelength or color in the visible light spectrum, known as monochromaticity. These properties allow the laser light to be targeted accurately and with very high intensity.[15]

The performance of a laser is based on the power output and the mode of emission. Three types of lasers are important in clinical urologic surgery. Continuous wave lasers emit a steady-state beam. Pulsed lasers produce higher peak power than continuous as power output is built up between pulses. This allows for more precise control and less lateral heat conduction, and pulsed lasers are commonly used for tissue coagulation. The third type is termed Q-switched, a pulsing technique that produces high-peak power output for short duration.[15]

There are 4 physical properties of a laser, which impacts the type of laser used for different procedures. Energy is the amount of work produced (Joules). Rate is described as cycles/s (Hertz). Power is the rate of energy expenditure (measured in Watts = Joules/s). Fluence is the amount of energy delivered per unit area (J/cm^2), which determines the magnitude of the lasers interaction on the tissue. Thus, the smaller the area, the more energy delivered to the tissue. Irradiance or power density is the intensity of the laser beam (W/cm^2) and plays a critical role in determining tissue interaction.

Tissue interaction can be classified as either electromechanical, photoablative, photochemical, or photothermal. Electromechanical causes dielectric breakdown in tissue by shock wave plasma expansion resulting in localized mechanical rupture. Urologists employ the electromechanical property of laser energy for stone fragmentation by spallation and cavitation.[15] Photoablative causes photodissociation or breaking of molecular bonds in tissue. Photochemical causes light-induced chemical reactions to destroy tissue. Finally, photothermal converts light energy into heat energy causing tissue heating and vaporizing. Surgeons commonly use the thermal effect of laser energy to incise, coagulate or ablate tissues and fragment calculi.

The wavelength of the laser of the tissue and characteristics impact the laser effect. Hemoglobin and water absorb light at different wavelengths. These interactions result in different degrees of depth of penetration, absorption, reflection, and scattering of laser energy. In addition, the denser the tissue is or becomes during treatment, the greater the degree of absorption of light energy and the transformation to heat, resulting in decreasing penetration into tissue. Blood flow also acts as a sink to absorb thermal energy, thus reducing the power of the laser at the site of action.[15]

There are many different types of lasers that are used by urologists. Lasers are named after the laser medium generating a specific wavelength. The section below focuses on the different lasers and their applications to treat urologic diseases: condylomata acuminata, urolithiasis, benign prostatic hyperplasia, and ureteral and urethral strictures. Table 21.1 describes a guide to lasers and their applications.

Clinical Application of Lasers

Condylomata Acuminata

The CO_2 laser is often used to treat condylomata acuminata on the skin or urethral meatus. This laser emits light in the far infrared portion (10,600 nm) and has a very short extinction length. Absorption of energy at the surgical site causes thermal coagulation to a depth of approximately 0.5 mm. Infected epithelium from the papillomavirus (HPV) should be ablated precisely to a shallow depth, so that the virus is killed and rapid healing can occur.[16] Most patients can be effectively treated with low morbidity.

Urolithiasis

Endoscopic laser lithotripsy is the most common intracorporeal procedures performed by urologists to treat urolithiasis. Pulsed lasers are effective in stone fragmentation by producing high power density at the stone surface with minimized heat dissipation. The pulsed laser causes the release of electrons and the formation of "plasma" bubbles, which then collapse generating a shockwave.[17] The first pulsed laser for lithotripsy was the coumarin green dye

Table 21.1. Lasers

	Carbon dioxide	KTP Nd:YAG	Nd:YAG	Holmium:YAG
Wavelength (nm)	10,600	532	1,064	2,140
Depth of tissue penetration (mm)	0.5	1–3	10	0.5
Absorption	Water	Hemoglobin	Neither hemoglobin/ water	Water
Irrigant	Water	Saline/water	Saline/water	Saline
Mode of delivery	Continuous/pulsed	Continuous	Continuous/pulsed	Pulsed
Stone disease	NA	NA	NA	A
Prostate coagulation and incision	NA	A	A	A
Stricture disease	NA	A	A	A
Condyloma accuminata	A	NA	A	A

NA not applicable, *A* applicable

medium. Coumarin's wavelength is 504 nm and was absorbed by many stone materials, but not absorbed by the surrounding tissues.[18] Thus, high energies could be used without causing injury to urothelial tissue. Stone composition affected absorption and the efficacy of the coumarin laser. For example, calcium oxalate monohydrate (COM) stones were difficult to fragment. The 200-micron fiber, which allowed for the greatest deflection, could generate only 80 J of coumarin laser energy, which was insufficient to fragment these dense stones. In addition, the coumarin dye laser was ineffective in fragmenting cystine stones. The coumarin laser took approximately 20 min to function and required eye protection with amber glass making visibility difficult.[19]

Today, the most common and most effective laser in the treatment of stones is the Holmium:YAG laser. It is delivered in a pulsatile manner at a wavelength of 2140 nm, which is highly absorbed by water. The holmium laser vaporizes water inside and on the surface of the stone, creating a vaporization or cavitation bubble. The cavitation bubble generates a shock wave, which destabilizes and fragments the stone, by a photothermal mechanism.[20,21] The long pulse duration of 250–350 μs and pulse power of 0.25–2.5 KW produce an elongated cavitation bubble, which generates a weaker shockwave. This reduces the likelihood of retropulsion of the stones, while adequately fragmenting the stone.[22]

Several characteristics of the holmium laser make it both effective and versatile for intracorporeal lithotripsy and tissue treatment. The wavelength can be transmitted through quartz optical fibers making it useful for endoscopic surgery. The pulse duration and power of the holmium laser causes excellent stone fragmentation of all types of stones regardless of composition and can incise tissue at higher energy settings. Multiple fibers are available for endoscopic use, including the 200, 365, 500, and 1,000 μm laser fiber. A 200 or 365 μm laser fiber can be passed via a flexible ureteroscope facilitating intracorporeal lithotripsy throughout the entire collecting system. A side-firing fiber is also available for use in the bladder and for prostatic treatments (discussed below). The Holmium laser treatment of stones typically produces very small fragments and dust particles, which are less likely to obstruct the ureter traveling out of the collecting system and there is often less need to basket the fragments. Furthermore, the Holmium laser is extremely safe and causes less injury than other lithotrites (like EHL) to the ureter, unless directly applied to the tissue.

The zone of thermal injury is approximately 0.5–1.0 mm. Thus, the holmium laser is safely activated at a distance of 0.5–1 mm away from the ureteral wall.[23] Unlike the coumarin pulsed-dye laser, eye protection does not compromise visibility because at levels typically used, the effect on the cornea at a distance from the laser of greater than 10 cm is minimal.[24]

Benign Prostatic Hyperplasia

The use of lasers for the treatment of benign prostatic hyperplasia (BPH) has cycled dramatically over the past decade. The two mechanisms by which lasers function to relieve the obstruction caused by the adenoma are coagulation and vaporization. Coagulative necrosis is caused by focused laser energy heating the tissue to temperatures between 70°C and 100°C. Coagulation may put tissues not being treated, like the sphincter, at risk due to its imprecise mechanism. Vaporization occurs at temperatures of up to several 100°C. The power density is high, but it is delivered through a narrow beam, limiting injury to surrounding tissues.

Initially, the Nd:YAG laser was used for coagulation of the prostate. The combination of neodymium and yttrium aluminum garnet crystal has high efficiency, increased rate of repetition, thermal conductivity, and good optical quality. It emits light at 1,064 nm (poorly absorbed by both hemoglobin and water), which has a tissue penetration of 10 mm and causes deep coagulation and coagulative necrosis of the adenoma.[15] It can be used to coagulate up to 5 mm blood vessels with hemostasis. Treatment of BPH with the Nd:YAG laser typically resulted in extended periods of tissue sloughing and unacceptable rates of irritative voiding symptoms and prolonged catheter time.[25] The deep tissue penetration of the Nd:YAG laser made it effective for BPH, but caused a high rate of tissue injury when applied for lithotripsy.

An alternative technology is the potassium-titanyl phosphate (KTP) "green light" laser, which utilizes the 1,064 nm Nd:YAG laser light that is emitted or passed through a KTP crystal resulting in a green light.[26] This laser technology causes photoselective vaporization of the prostate. The KTP crystal doubles the frequency and halves the wavelength to 532 nm, which is highly absorbed by hemoglobin. This results in less depth of penetration (3 mm) as compared to the Nd:YAG laser (10 mm), which is much safer to use in the prostatic cavity. In addition, it can be delivered at a higher power, either 80 W or 120 W (new HPS system) maximizing the vaporization effect. The technique has decreased bleeding, making photoselective vaporization feasible in patients on anticoagulation.[27] Vaporization is achieved through a side-firing laser in a near contact sweeping technique through a 24 F continuous flow resectoscope. Eye protection is necessary to filter the harmful radiation emitted from the KTP laser.

Gilling et al. are one of the first groups to describe the technique of using the holmium laser to treat BPH.[28] The Ho:YAG laser is highly absorbed by water and causes tissue vaporization. The laser can be used to either vaporize or enucleate the prostate. Advantages of the holmium laser include its pulsed nature and minimal tissue penetration, which provides rapid tissue vaporization, less tissue coagulation, and less injury to surrounding tissues.[29] The laser has excellent hemostatic properties. Holmium laser ablation of the prostate (HoLAP) is performed with a 550-μm side-firing laser fiber at 80–100 W power in a near-contact mode, creating a channel within the prostatic fossa.[30] Contact with the tissue can cause overheating, which degrades the fiber tip and reduces the energy output. The procedure is easily learned, as it does not require resection and retrieval of the tissue. Length of procedure is generally dictated by prostatic size. Thus, HoLAP is best reserved for glands less than 50 g.

Holmium laser enucleation of the prostate (HoLEP) is a minimally invasive alternative to TURP and simulates the open simple prostatectomy. The prostate is divided into 3 anatomic lobes, the two lateral lobes and the median lobe. The high-powered 100 W Holmium laser and a 550-μm end-firing holmium laser fiber are used to delineate the natural tissue plane between the prostate adenoma and the prostatic capsule. Once the three lobes are enucleated in a retrograde fashion, morcellation is carried out to remove the tissue from the bladder.[31] The main advantage of the procedure is that the same amount of tissue is removed as with the open simple prostatectomy but in a minimally invasive technique. Multiple randomized controlled clinical trials comparing HoLEP to TURP and open simple prostatectomy have demonstrated HoLEP to have equal efficacy, improved AUA SS, flow rates with shorter hospital stay, catheterization time, and less blood loss.[32,33] A disadvantage of the procedure has been the perception of a challenging learning curve and translation of the technique to practicing community urologists, although Shah et al. have demonstrated that an endourologist inexperienced in HoLEP can perform the procedure with reasonable efficacy after about 50 cases with comparable outcomes to that of experienced physician.[34]

Ureteral and Urethral Strictures

Ureteropelvic junction obstruction, ureteral strictures, uretero-enteric structures, urethral strictures, and bladder neck contractures have all been treated using laser technology. Minimally invasive techniques for ureteral strictures have come to be the first-line therapy. Specifically, the holmium:YAG laser is often used to treat ureteral strictures due to its good safety profile, precision, incision capability, and minimal collateral injury. In addition, it is compatible with multiple flexible endoscopes providing excellent multifunctionality. A ureterotomy incision should be made from the ureteral lumen to the periureteral fat in a full thickness fashion. The holmium laser pulse energy and frequency are commonly placed at 1 J and 10–15 Hz to make an adequate incision.[35,36] Ho:YAG laser endoureterotomy has been shown to have adequate durability for benign ureteral strictures, ureteropelvic junction, and uretero-enteric strictures than previously accepted minimally invasive modalities, such as balloon dilation.[37-39]

Nd:YAG, KTP, and holmium have treated urethral strictures. Ideally, the type of laser used should vaporize the tissue and exhibit negligible peripheral tissue damage. Nd:YAG laser core-through urethrotomy has been shown to be effective for post-traumatic urethral strictures.[40] However, the drawbacks to using the Nd:YAG laser is that it causes thermal necrosis, which can lead to significant peripheral tissue injury. The KTP laser has less penetration than Nd:YAG, but at the same time is less effective for dense strictures. The holmium:YAG laser has been shown to be the laser of choice for urethral strictures.[41] It provides both direct contact cutting and vaporization with minimal forward scatter. To date, the results of laser urethrotomy have varied durability and the technology may be best for small isolated strictures.

Conclusion

Laser-based therapies are firmly entrenched in the armamentarium of modern urologic surgery and, in some cases, have revolutionized the treatment of urologic disorders including urolithiasis, BPH, stricture disease, and transitional cell carcinoma of the ureter and bladder. With new technological advances and continued understanding of the underlying disease

pathophysiologies, the indications for laser therapy in minimally invasive urologic surgery will continue to expand.

References

1. Wein AJ, Kavoussi LR, Novick AC, Partin AW, Peters CA. Chapter 6 Basic instrumentation and cystoscopy. In: Wein AJ, Kavoussi LR, Novick AC, Partin AW, Peters CA, eds. Campbell-Walsh Urology. 9th ed. Philadelphia, PA: Saunders Elsevier; 2007:168-70

2. Borin JF, Abdelshehid CS, Clayman RV. Comparison of resolution, contrast, and color differentiation among fiberoptic and digital flexible cystoscopes. J Endourol. 2006;20(1):54-58

3. Preminger GM, Tiselius HG, Assimos DG, et al. 2007 guideline for management of ureteral calculi. J Urol. 2007;178:2418-34

4. Wein AJ, Kavoussi LR, Novick AC, Partin AW, Peters CA. Chapter 45 Ureteroscopy and retrograde ureteral access. In: Wein AJ, Kavoussi LR, Novick AC, Partin AW, Peters CA, eds. Campbell-Walsh Urology. 9th ed. Philadelphia, PA: Saunders Elsevier; 2007: 1508

5. Wein AJ, Kavoussi LR, Novick AC, Partin AW, Peters CA. Chapter 43 Evaluation and medical management of urinary lithiasis. In: Wein AJ, Kavoussi LR, Novick AC, Partin AW, Peters CA, eds. Campbell-Walsh Urology. 9th ed. Philadelphia, PA: Saunders Elsevier; 2007:1433

6. Wein AJ, Kavoussi LR, Novick AC, Partin AW, Peters CA. Chapter 49 Management of urothelial tumors of the renal pelvis and ureter. In: Wein AJ, Kavoussi LR, Novick AC, Partin AW, Peters CA, eds. Campbell-Walsh Urology. 9th ed. Philadelphia, PA: Saunders Elsevier; 2007:1674

7. Wein AJ, Kavoussi LR, Novick AC, Partin AW, Peters CA. Chapter 44 Surgical management of upper urinary tract calculi. In: Wein AJ, Kavoussi LR, Novick AC, Partin AW, Peters CA, eds. Campbell-Walsh Urology. 9th ed. Philadelphia, PA: Saunders Elsevier; 2007:1489

8. Beaghler MA, Poon MW, Dushinski JW, Lingeman JE. Expanding role of flexible nephroscopy in the upper urinary tract. J Endourol. 1999;13(2):93-7

9. Nedas T, Challacombe B, Dasgupta P. Virtual reality in urology. BJU Int. 2004;93:255-7

10. Kuo RL, Delvecchio FC, Preminger GM. Virtual reality: current urologic applications and future developments. J Endourol. 2001;15:117-22

11. Reich O, Noll M, Gratze C, et al. High-level virtual reality simulator for endourologic procedures of lower urinary tract. Urology. 2006;67:1144-8

12. Shah J, Darzi A. Virtual reality flexible cystoscopy: a validation study. BJU Int. 2002;90:828-32

13. Chou DS, Abdelshehid C, Clayman RV, McDougall EM. Comparison of results of Virtual-reality simulators

and training model for basic urertoscopy training. J Endourol. 2006;20:266-71

14. Gross AJ, Herrmann TR. History of lasers. World J Urol. 2007;25(3):217-20

15. Grasso M, Green D. Lasers in urology. E Medicine. 2008 http://emedicine.medscape.com

16. Schaeffer AJ. Use of the CO_2 laser in urology. Urol Clin North Am. 1986;3:393-404

17. Floratos DL, de la Rosette JJ. Lasers in urology. BJU Int. 1999;84(2):204-11

18. Grocela JA, Dretler SP. Intracorporeal lithotripsy. Instrumentation and development. Urol Clin North Am. 1997;24(1):13-23

19. Wein AJ, Kavoussi LR, Novick AC, Partin AW, Peters CA. Chapter 45 Ureteroscopy and retrograde ureteral access. In: Wein AJ, Kavoussi LR, Novick AC, Partin AW, Peters CA, eds. Campbell-Walsh Urology. Philadelphia, PA: Saunders Elsevier; 2007:1460

20. Dushinski JW, Lingeman JE. High-speed photographic evaluation of the holumium laser. J Endourol. 1998;12(2):177-81

21. Vassar GJ, Chan KF, Teichman JM, et al. Holmium:YAG lithotripsy: photothermal mechanism. J Endourol. 1999;13(3):181-190

22. Wollin TA, Denstedt JD. The holmium laser in urology. J Clin Laser Med Surg. 1998;16:13-20

23. Santa-Cruz RW, Leveillee RJ, Kronrad A. Ex vivo comparison of four lithotripters commonly used in the ureter: what does it take to perforate? J Endourol. 1998;12(5):417-22

24. Scarpa RM, De Lisa A, Porru D, et al. Holmium:YAG laser ureterolithotripsy. Eur Urol. 1999;35:233-8

25. Gomella LG, Lofti MA, Rivas DA, et al. Contact laser vaporization techniques for benign prostatic hyperplasia. J Endourol. 1995;9:117-23

26. Wang X, Chen J, Jiao D et al. The beam characteristic of Nd:YAG frequency doubling in a KTP crystal by the resonant external ring cavity. Nonlinear Optical Phenomena and Applications. Proc SPIE. 2005;5646: 636-642

27. Reich O, Bachmann A, Siebels M, et al. High power (80 W) potassium-titanyl-phosphate laser vaporization of the prostate in 66 high risk patients. J Urol. 2005;173:158-60

28. Gilling PJ, Cass CB, Malcolm AR, et al. Combination holmium and Nd:YAG laser ablation of the prostate: initial clinical experience. J Endourol. 1995;9:151

29. Johnson DE, Cromeens DM, Price RE. Use of holmium:YAG laser in urology. Lasers Surg Med. 1992;12:353

30. Gilling PJ, Cass CB, Cresswell MD. Holmium laser resection of the prostate: preliminary results of a new method for the treatment of benign prostatic hyperplasia. Urology. 1996;47(1):48-51

31. Gilling PJ. Holmium laser enucleation of the prostate. BJU Int. 2008;101:131-42

32. Tan AHH, Gilling PJ, Kennett KM, et al. A randomized trial comparing holmium laser enucleation of the prostate with transurethral resection of the prostate for the treatment of bladder outlet obstruction secondary to benign prostatic hyperplasia in large glands (40–200 g). J Urol. 2003;170:1270-4

33. Kuntz RM, Lehrich K, Ahyai SA. Holmium laser enucleation of the prostate versus open prostatectomy for prostates greater than 100 g: 5 years follow-up results of a randomised clinical trial. Eur Urol. 2008;53(1):160-6

34. Shah HN, Mahajan AP, Sodha HS, et al. Prospective evaluation of the learning curve for holmium laser enucleation of the prostate. J Urol. 2007;177:1468-74

35. Knudsen BE, Cook AJ, Watterson JD, et al. Percutaneous antegrade endopyelotomy: long-term results from one institution. Urology. 2004;63(2):230-4

36. Springhart WP, Preminger GM. Chapter 11 Retrograde endopyelotomy. In: Nakada SY, Pearle MS, eds. Advanced Endourology: The Complete Clinical Guide. Totowa, NJ: Humana Press; 2006:183-95

37. Watterson JD, Sofer M, Wollin TA, et al. Holmium:YAG laser endoureterotomy for ureterointestinal strictures. J Urol. 2002;167:1692-5

38. Hibi H, Ohori T, Taki T, et al. Long-term results of endoureterotomy using a holmium laser. Int J Urol. 2007;14:872-4

39. Lane BR, Desai MM, Hegarty NJ, Streem SB. Long-term efficacy of holmium laser endoureterotomy for benign ureteral strictures. Urology. 2006;67:894-7

40. Dogra PN, Nabi G. Core-through urethrotomy using the neodymium:YAG laser for obliterative urethral strictures after traumatic urethral disruption and/or distraction defects: long-term outcome. J Urol. 2002;167:543-6

41. Kamp S, Knoll T, Osman MM, et al. Low-power holmium:YAG laser urethrotomy for treatment of urethral strictures: functional outcome and quality of life. J Endourol. 2006;20:38-41

Part II

Clinical Urologic Practice

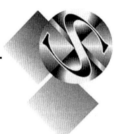

22

Prostatitis and Male Chronic Pelvic Pain Syndrome

J. Curtis Nickel

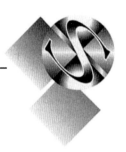

Introduction

Our management of the clinical prostatitis syndromes has evolved significantly from the days of organ centric therapy for prostate infection and inflammation. It was only a decade or so ago when prostatitis seemed easy to understand and for the most part simple to manage. Traditionally, prostatitis involved acute or chronic inflammation of the prostate gland, either bacterial or nonspecific. Our treatment lay then, in eradicating offending organisms and reducing inflammation. Despite new and improved antimicrobials and anti-inflammatories, we realize that the prevalence and burden of prostatitis is as bad today as it was before these pharmacological agents were even discovered.[1] Physicians have become discouraged and patients frustrated by our lack of clinical success. The good news is that our improved understanding of the etiology, pathogenesis, and epidemiology of the prostatitis syndromes has given us the tools to help the majority of patients who have failed our traditional approach of antibiotics and anti-inflammatories.[2,3] This chapter will present important epidemiological data, explain our new understanding of the etiological processes involved, help classify and diagnose patients, outline the new evidence from clinical treatment trials and finally give the reader a blueprint for a therapeutic algorithm that works in clinical practice.

The Prostatitis Syndromes

In the past, most discussion of the prostatitis syndromes centered on acute and chronic bacterial prostatitis, well-defined diseases that could be objectively evaluated with laboratory cultures of urine and prostatic secretions and treated with antibiotics. Very little was discussed, written, or researched about abacterial prostatitis or prostatodynia, nebulous clinical entities that were referred to by many as the "waste basket of urological diagnoses." These traditional diagnostic terms should now be abandoned in favor of the more accepted contemporary diagnostic terminology. The NIH classification of the prostatitis syndromes has been available now for over a decade and is the foundation of our clinical evaluation and treatment.[4] Table 22.1 describes the details of this classification system. In summary, Category I refers to patients with an acute bacterial infection of the prostate, Category II to patients with a chronic infection of the prostate while Category III refers to the vast majority of prostatitis patients in whom a bacterial infection cannot be documented. Category III has been further subdivided into an inflammatory subcategory (IIIA) and a non-inflammatory subcategory (IIIB). Category IV, or asymptomatic inflammatory prostatitis, is not a symptomatic clinical syndrome (diagnosis based on the finding of asymptomatic inflammation localized to the prostate) and will not be addressed in this

C.R. Chapple and W.D. Steers (eds.), *Practical Urology: Essential Principles and Practice*,
DOI: 10.1007/978-1-84882-034-0_22, © Springer-Verlag London Limited 2011

Table 22.1. National Institutes of Health classification system for the prostatitis syndromes

Category	Description	Presentation
Category I Acute bacterial prostatitis	Acute infection of the prostate gland	Acute febrile illness associated with perineal and suprapubic pain, dysuria and obstructive voiding symptoms
Category II Chronic bacterial prostatitis	Chronic infection of the prostate	Recurrent urinary tract infections (usually with the same organism) associated frequently with voiding disturbances[a]
Category III Chronic prostatitis/ chronic pelvic pain syndrome (CP/CPPS)	Chronic genital urinary pain in the absence of uropathogenic bacteria localized to the prostate gland employing standard methodology[a]	Chronic perineal, suprapubic, groin, testicular, penile, ejaculatory pain associated with variable dysuria and obstructive and irritative voiding symptoms
Category IIIA Inflammatory CP/CPPS	Significant[b] number of white blood cells in expressed prostatic secretions, post prostatic massage urine sediment (VB3) or semen	
Category IIIB Non-inflammatory CP/CPPS	Insignificant[b] number of white blood cells in expressed prostatic secretions, post prostatic massage urine sediment (VB3) or semen	

[a]There is still discussion and controversy on how to classify men with chronic symptoms, no history of UTI, but uropathogenic bacterial localization to prostate specific specimens.
[b]There is no consensus on what constitutes significant (or conversely insignificant) number of white blood cells.

chapter (although Category IV is an extremely interesting condition).

The Scope of the Problem

No matter how you look at the epidemiology of prostatitis, there is no getting away from the fact that it is very prevalent and results in a significant impact on patients' quality of life and costs to society as a whole. The prevalence and incidence issue can be examined from a number of view points: we can look at the number of patients diagnosed with prostatitis based on outpatient visit diagnoses or billing data, surveys based on patient's recollections of a diagnosis of prostatitis or determine the prevalence of patients suffering from symptoms that sound like prostatitis (but not necessarily diagnosed). Amongst North American adult males, 4–16% have either a physician or patient self-reported diagnoses of prostatitis, being one of the most common outpatient diagnoses in urology.[5-7] In fact it is the most common outpatient diagnosis in men under 50 years of age in urologic practice.[8] The prevalence for men in the community experiencing chronic-prostatitis-like symptoms ranges from 6.5% to 12%, with moderate symptoms ranging from 2% to 6%.[7,9-12] The impact of these diagnoses and/or these prostatitis symptoms is usually underestimated. In fact, the quality of life of a patient with a chronic prostatitis syndrome rivals that of a patient with active Crohn's disease, severe diabetes and/or congestive heart failure.[13,14] Biopsychosocial parameters such as depression, stress, anxiety, social maladjustment and poor coping behaviors not only exacerbate symptoms but are also associated with poorer quality of life.[15-17] The direct costs to society, in terms of medical care, is also enormous, more than that required for patients with rheumatoid arthritis, amounting to millions of dollars a year in North America alone.[18] The indirect costs (in terms of work and productivity loss) may be incalculable.

The Etiology of the Prostatitis Syndromes

Category I and II: These categories are associated with acute (Category I) infection and chronic infection (Category II) of the prostate with uropathogenic organisms, usally *Enterobacteriaceae* sp. (particularly *E. coli* but also *Klebsiella* sp., *Pseudomonas* sp. and other *Enterobacteriaceae* sp.) and occasionally gram positive *Enterococci* sp.[19] Category II is associated with similar organisms but there is some evidence that other organisms such as *Chlamydia* sp., *Mycoplasma* sp. and perhaps even anaerobic bacteria, *Corynebacterium* sp. and in some specific cases (such as immunocompromised patients) fungi, viruses, etc. may also be involved.[20] In both categories, lower urinary tract infection is associated with the acute exacerbation of symptoms (and in the case of Category I, perhaps even urosepsis). Effective treatment usually eradicates the offending organism in Category I, but in Category II, the patient may continue to have a prostate nidus of infection resulting in the typical clinical picture of recurrent lower urinary tract infections with the same organism. Some patients suffering from these recurrent episodes of infection may develop symptoms between acute episodes or may progress to Category III with chronic symptoms, negative cultures and no improvement with antibiotics.

Category III: By definition, these patients do not have urinary tract infections. There is still disagreement among experts on how to classify patients who do not have infection (or recurrent urinary tract infections), but uropathogenic bacteria are localized to the prostate during evaluation.[2,20] The reason for this controversy is the fact that normal asymptomatic control men localize such bacteria to the prostate gland in similar prevalence as patients clinically categorized as Category III CP/CPPS.[21] Similarly, CP/CPPS does not necessarily imply inflammation in the prostate (histological prostatitis). In fact, there is little correlation between prostate inflammation and symptoms in this condition and it is now recognized that patients without symptoms may have prostate inflammation (Category IV).[21] It is becoming quite evident that the symptom complex associated with Category III CP/CPPS is not secondary to a single defined etiologic agent but is rather a syndrome consisting of a continuous spectrum, initiated and propagated by multiple, and likely inter-related factors.[22,23] The initiators could be infection, high pressure dysfunctional voiding, trauma or some unknown toxin in a genetically or anatomically susceptible man. This initiating event results in either injury and/or inflammation. The initial neuropathy, muscu-

lar dysfunction or immunologic reaction can progress because of persisting initiating factors (persistence of bacteria, dysfunctional voiding, anatomic variance of prostate ducts or perineal trauma) or the pathology could persist even with eradication or amelioration of these factors through self perpetuating stimulatory loops (inflammation by autoimmune mechanism while peripheral neuropathy can progress because of up regulation of the local pelvic neuroloop and "wind up" of the spinal cord). The patients who suffer from chronic prostatitis for many months or many years eventually develop a typical neuropathic pain pattern, associated with local muscular dysfunction. This process is further influenced by supratentorial CNS mechanisms such as depression and maladaptive coping behaviors.[23]

The Diagnosis of the Prostatitis Syndrome

Category I: Acute bacterial prostatitis patients present with lower urinary tract infection symptoms (dysuria, urgency, frequency, suprapubic pain/discomfort, hematuria), varying degrees of urinary obstructive voiding symptoms (including acute urinary retention) and generalized symptoms such as fever.[19] On physical examination the patient is usually uncomfortable, may be feverish, a tender bladder may be palpable, the prostate is usually soft (often referred to as "boggy") and usually exquisitely tender. The white count may be elevated and white cells will be present in the urine (or evidence of infection on dipstick examination). Urine culture and in cases where the patient is clinically septic, blood culture are procured, but therapy is initiated immediately. An ultrasound or bladder scan may be indicated to determine if the patient is in acute urinary retention.[23]

Category II: Chronic Bacterial Prostatitis is traditionally associated with recurring or relapsing lower urinary tract infection, usually with the same organism and usually without clinical sepsis.[2,20,23] The patient may or may not be symptomatic between episodes of treated infection. If symptomatic, the symptoms may be indistinguishable from those of patients with Category III. This category is suspected in men with relapsing symptoms associated with bacteriuria who experience improvement in symptoms with antibiotic therapy. The optimal time to make the diagnosis is between episodes of acute exacerbations employing some form of lower urinary tract localization study. The traditional technique to localize infection to the prostate gland was the Meares-Stamey 4-glass test[24] which included culture of the first initial voided urine (voided bladder 1 or VB1), the midstream urine (voided bladder 2 or VB2), expressed prostatic secretion (EPS) obtained following prostate examination and the initial stream urine specimen collected after prostate massage (voided bladder 3 or VB3). If the colony count of uropathogenic bacteria were significantly higher in EPS and/or VB3 compared to VB1 and VB2, then a diagnosis of chronic prostate infection can be made and patient classified as Category II. However the 4-glass test is cumbersome, expensive, and most physicians, including urologists have abandoned it.[25] A simpler 2-glass test compares the bacterial culture results of the pre-massage urine (Pre-M or VB2) to the post-massage urine specimen (post-M or VB3).[26] A higher bacterial count in the Post-M specimen compared to the Pre-M specimen is indicative of chronic prostate infection. This Pre and Post Massage test (PPMT) provides almost as accurate localization data as the more difficult 4-glass test and can be easily employed in any clinical practice situation.[27]

Category III: By definition chronic prostatitis/chronic pelvic pain syndrome (CP/CPPS) is associated with genitourinary and/or pelvic pain with no evidence of infection.[2,4] Patients have one or more of perineal, ejaculatory, penile, testicular, suprapubic and penile pain/discomfort with variable irritative and/or obstructive voiding symptoms and perhaps some degree of associated sexual dysfunction. Patients experience waxing and waning symptoms that are extremely bothersome and impact on activities. Since this category is a syndrome defined by a symptom complex it is imperative that a comprehensive symptom inventory documenting the location, severity, frequency of the pain, any urinary symptoms and impact on activities and quality of life is undertaken. This can now be accomplished by administering the NIH Chronic Prostatitis Symptom Index (CPSI), a validated and sensitive symptom assessment tool developed for clinical trials in CP/CPPS.[28] Nine separate items that could be answered by most patients in about 5 min addressed all these important issues. The 6 major locations or type of pain or discomfort, the frequency of pain or discomfort and the severity of pain or discomfort are rated on a scale of 0–21. The irritative and obstructive voiding symptoms are rated on a score of 0–10 while the impact on quality of life is rated on a score of 0–12. Each of these domains can be assessed independently or the 3 can be added together for a total NIH-CPSI score of 0–43. The CPSI is a valuable tool for the practicing physician to evaluate a patient at initial presentation and to follow him over time to assess treatment outcomes.[29,30] The NIH-CPSI is presented in Fig. 22.1.

A rather comprehensive evaluation routine should be followed when assessing CP/CPPS patients, particularly during the initial visit.[31] Physical examination may detect suprapubic, perineal, prostate, pelvic floor or external genitalia discomfort or pain or it may be completely noncontributory. The lower abdominal, genital, perineal, rectal and focused neurogenic examinations are primarily necessary to rule out other causes for the patients' symptoms. Urinalysis and urine cytology (particularly important if the patient has hematuria or irritative obstructive voiding symptoms) are collected along with the pre-M urine specimen. Following pelvic and prostate examination, prostate massage is undertaken to produce either EPs or more easily a post-M specimen of urine for culture. Microscopy of the EPS and/or Post-M (VB3) specimen can determine if the patient should be classified as Category IIIA or IIIB, but at the present there is no clinical indication to actually do this step since no clinical trial to date has determined a differential treatment effect between these two categories.[21,32] That may change in the future. If the patient is at an age that prostate cancer is a possibility, a serum prostate specific antigen (PSA) can be collected. Other urologic tests such as cystoscopy, urodynamics and imaging (transrectal ultrasound, CAT scan, etc.) are optional and indications are based on specific findings from history, urinalysis, cytology and physical examination. Table 22.2 represents a suggested diagnostic plan for the prostatitis syndromes.

NIH-Chronic Prostatitis Symptom Index (NIH-CPSI)

Pain or Discomfort

1. In the last week, have you experienced any pain or discomfort in the following areas?

	Yes	No
a. Area between rectum and testicles (perineum)	❑ 1	❑ 0
b. Testicles	❑ 1	❑ 0
c. Tip of the penis (not related to urination)	❑ 1	❑ 0
d. Below your waist, in your pubic or bladder area	❑ 1	❑ 0

2. In the last week, have you experienced:

	Yes	No
a. Pain or burning during urination?	❑ 1	❑ 0
b. Pain or discomfort during or after sexual climax (ejaculation)?	❑ 1	❑ 0

3. How often have you had pain or discomfort in any of these areas over the last week?

- ❑ 0 Never
- ❑ 1 Rarely
- ❑ 2 Sometimes
- ❑ 3 Often
- ❑ 4 Usually
- ❑ 5 Always

4. Which number best describes your AVERAGE pain or discomfort on the days that you had it, over the last week?

❑	❑	❑	❑	❑	❑	❑	❑	❑	❑	❑
0	1	2	3	4	5	6	7	8	9	10

NO PAIN   PAIN AS BAD AS YOU CAN IMAGINE

Urination

5. How often have you had a sensation of not emptying your bladder completely after you finished urinating, over the last week?

- ❑ 0 Not at all
- ❑ 1 Less than 1 time in 5
- ❑ 2 Less than half the time
- ❑ 3 About half the time
- ❑ 4 More than half the time
- ❑ 5 Almost always

6. How often have you had to urinate again less than two hours after you finished urinating, over the last week?

- ❑ 0 Not at all
- ❑ 1 Less than 1 time in 5
- ❑ 2 Less than half the time
- ❑ 3 About half the time
- ❑ 4 More than half the time
- ❑ 5 Almost always

Impact of Symptoms

7. How much have your symptoms kept you from doing the kinds of things you would usually do, over the last week?

- ❑ 0 None
- ❑ 1 Only a little
- ❑ 2 Some
- ❑ 3 A lot

8. How much did you think about your symptoms, over the last week?

- ❑ 0 None
- ❑ 1 Only a little
- ❑ 2 Some
- ❑ 3 A lot

Quality of Life

9. If you were to spend the rest of your life with your symptoms just the way they have been during the last week, how would you feel about that?

- ❑ 0 Delighted
- ❑ 1 Pleased
- ❑ 2 Mostly satisfied
- ❑ 3 Mixed (about equally satisfied and dissatisfied)
- ❑ 4 Mostly dissatisfied
- ❑ 5 Unhappy
- ❑ 6 Terrible

Scoring the NIH-Chronic Prostatitis Symptom Index Domains

Pain: Total of items 1a, 1b, 1c, 1d, 2a, 2b, 3, and 4 = _____

Urinary Symptoms: Total of items 5 and 6   = _____

Quality of Life Impact: Total of items 7, 8, and 9   = _____

Figure 22.1. The National Institutes of Health Chronic Prostatitis Symptom Index (NIH-CPSI) captures the three most important domains of the prostatitis experience: pain (location, frequency and severity), voiding (irritative and obstructive symptoms) and quality of life (including impact). This index is useful in research studies and clinical practice[28] (Reprinted with permission).

Table 22.2. Evaluation of a man presenting with a Prostatitis or CPPS syndrome

Recommendation	Evaluation	Cat I	Cat II	Cat III
Mandatory (all patients)	History	+	+	+
	Physical[a]	+	+	+
	Urinalysis	+	+	+
	Urine culture	+	+	+
	Blood culture	+/−[b]	−	−
Recommended (most patients)	Localization culture [c]	−	+	+
	CPSI	−	+/−[c]	+
	Flow rate	−	+/−[c]	+
	Residual urine	+	+/−[c]	+
	Urine cytology	−	−	+
Optional (selected patients)	Pressure/flow	−	−/+ [c]	+
	Videourodynamics	−	−	−/+
	Urethral culture	−	−	+
	Semen culture	−	+	+
	Cystoscsopy	−	+/−[c]	+
	Imaging[d]	+	+	+
	PSA	−	−	+

[a]Includes Digital Rectal Examination.
[b]If patient has urosepsis.
[c]Should be considered in patients with chronic symptoms between UTIs, exacerbations or failure to respond to antibiotic therapy.
[d]Transrectal ultrasound, abdominal and/or pelvic ultrasound, CAT scan, MRI.

Treatment of the Prostatitis Syndromes

The Bacterial Prostatitis Categories (Categories I and II)

The treatment of the two bacterial categories (I and II) are easier to formulate and results more predictable and therefore these two syndromes will be discussed separately from the much more difficult to manage Category III CP/CPPS. Both categories I and II are associated with bacterial infection in the prostate with uropathogenic bacteria. The role of therapy is to eradicate the bacteria, ameliorate the symptoms and prevent recurrence (not always possible for Category II).

For *Category I acute bacterial prostatitis*, wide spectrum antibiotics (if septic, parenteral is the preferred route) are indicated. The best drugs are either a combination of penicillin (e.g. ampicillin) and an aminoglycoside (e.g. gentamicin), second or third generation cephalosporins or one of the fluoroquinolones.[19,23,33] If the patient is in urinary retention, then insertion of a small caliber foley catheter will be required and depending on the situation can be left indwelling until the acute infection has resolved. If the foley catheter is too uncomfortable and the patient requires continued bladder drainage, then a small suprapubic catheter can be inserted. Once the patient's condition improves, treatment can be switched to oral antibiotics (preferably based on culture and sensitivity results). The most effective are the fluoroquinolones (with ciprofloxacin and levofloxacin being more effective than ofloxacin and all being more effective than norfloxacin) with second line being trimethoprim (with or without sulfamethoxazole). Treatment should be continued for 2–4 weeks. Patients that do not initially respond to this course of therapy should be investigated for the possibility of development of a prostate abscess (CAT scan or transrectal ultrasound) which should be dealt with as an emergency. Transurethral drainage is believed to be the optimal therapy, however transrectal guided needle aspiration may be effective in small localized abscesses.

The definitive therapy for *Category II chronic bacterial prostatitis* is appropriate long term antibiotic therapy.[20,33] Optimal antibiotic therapy includes trimethroprim (or trimethoprim-sulfamethoxazole) and the fluoroquinolones. Although trimethroprim-sulfamethoxazole is the most studied antibiotic in prostatitis, the penetration of the fluoroquinolones into the prostate gland and the increased bacterial susceptibility to this class of drug makes them superior to trimethoprim or trimethoprim-sulfamethoxazole. Clinical studies have confirmed the improved efficacy of fluoroquinolones over trimethroprim or trimethoprim-sulfamethoxazole.[26] Levofloxacin and ciprofloxacin appear to be superior to ofloxacin which is more effective than norfloxacin[34,35] The duration of therapy is controversial and suggestions have ranged from 4 to 12 weeks.[36] Because of the very real possibility of persistence, the physician should err on the side of too much antibiotic rather than too little. Failure of antibiotic therapy is a real possibility (likely secondary to small foci of bacteria forming biofilms in the prostate ducts and acini or associated with prostatic calculi) which becomes a management problem. Switching to a more potent fluoroquinolone (if trimethoprim, norfloxacin or ofloxacin was used as first line therapy) or adding tetracycline (doxycycline) or a macrolide (azithromycin or clarithromycin) may be of benefit. In patients who continue to have recurrent UTIs or in whom symptoms recur when the antibiotics are discontinued, low dose, long term suppressive therapy may have to be considered. Repetitive prostate massage[37,38] and the concomitant use of alpha blockers[39] have been advocated based on low level evidence and prostate massage might be considered for patients who experience symptomatic relief during their diagnostic prostate massage or alpha blockers for those with obstructive voiding symptoms. Surgery is the very last resort[40]

and should be avoided, although there are some case reports of cure after radical TURP and anecdotal reports of improvement after total or radical open prostatectomy in patients with persistently confirmed foci of infection in the prostate.

Category III CP/CPPS

The Goal of Treatment

The treatment options for patients diagnosed with Category III CP/CPPS are more varied, but unfortunately less successful. The most successful therapeutic approach in this syndrome is for both the physician and patient to have realistic expectations or goals in relation to treatment. The patient must realize that the condition is not caused by infection (particularly if a trial of antibiotics have failed), that the symptom complex is not related to cancer or risk of developing prostate cancer and that symptoms will likely wax and wane but may burn themselves out over time. Everyone dealing with this condition (that includes the physician, patient and the patient's partner) must understand that cure may not be possible, but amelioration of symptoms, decrease in impact on daily activities and improvement of quality of life is achievable. Treatment consists of conservative or supportive management, drug therapy, and less frequently surgical intervention.

Conservative Management

Some patient experience exacerbations with selected food (spicy?) or drink (alcohol or acidic?) and while this is not universal, if it can be identified in an individual patient, then avoidance can potentially benefit that individual. Depression, stress and anxiety have been shown to be associated with increased symptoms and poorer quality of life[15-17] and any maneuver that can reduce these issues in a patients' life should be utilized. Some activities, such as high impact sports, bicycle or horseback riding may also exacerbate or be associated with persistence of symptoms and these should be discontinued. Hot sitz baths, the use of a donut cushion and other such options do help patients improve or at least control their symptoms. Other potentially effective therapies include physiotherapy (trigger point massage, repetitive prostate massage, focused pelvic floor massage), exercises (including yoga), biofeedback, acupuncture, and cognitive behavioral therapy.

Drug Therapy

Patients come to the physician hoping that a simple prescription of a medication will resolve their condition. Unfortunately, for most patients, this is usually not the case. However, drug therapy, either monotherapy or in difficult cases, multimodal therapy, do help ameliorate symptoms in the majority of patients.

Antibiotics

Probably the most controversial drug therapy for CP/CPPS is antibiotics. While the benefits of antibiotics are indisputable in Cat I and Cat II Prostatitis, the effect is less evident when employed in patients with no history of bacterial infection. When fluoroquinolones are used in early diagnosed (less chronic), less heavily pretreated patients, it has been shown that antibiotics can result in significant improvement in 50–75%[41,42] of patients. However, when used in more chronic and heavily pretreated (including previous therapy with antibiotics), the benefits of levofloxacin and ciprofloxacin appear to be no more evident than that achieved with placebo.[43,44]

Anti-inflammatories

It is intuitive to consider anti-inflammatory medications for a condition that includes inflammation and pain and while a number of small studies suggest efficacy, the only randomized placebo controlled trial has demonstrated that the COX-2 inhibitor, rofecoxib, may not be beneficial as a monotherapy except as a long-term high dose therapy.[45] Rofecoxib is not available anymore, but it is reasonable that the results can be extrapolated to the class and therefore anti-inflammatories should be considered as an ancillary treatment only. Pentosan-polysulfate sodium, a drug indicated for interstitial cystitis, has demonstrated very modest benefits in some patients when compared to placebo,[46] and may be helpful in men with suprapubic pain associated with voiding symptoms.

Alpha blockers

Five small randomized placebo controlled studies have indicated that the alpha blockers terazosin,[47] doxazosin,[48] tamsulosin[44,49] and alfuzosin,[50] may have a potential role as a primary therapy for CP/CPPS but the results were not conclusive. Analyses trying to explain the discrepancies in these trial results, have concluded that these agents provide the most benefit when used for longer than 6 weeks in alpha blocker naïve men with symptoms of short duration.[51,52] A recently completed NIH trial enrolling newly diagnosed, alpha blocker CP/CPPS men showed that 12 weeks of alfuzosin was not significantly better than placebo therapy.[53] Alpha blockers may not be considered as primary therapy, but may play a role in a multimodal strategy, particularly in men with obstructive voiding symptoms.

Hormone Therapies

A number of small trials including a poorly designed randomized placebo controlled trial suggested that finasteride may provide amelioration of symptoms, however a better designed trial, which showed a numerical improvement in symptom score over placebo, failed to reach statistical significance.[54] However, in older men with concurrent benign prostatic hyperplasia, a 5-alpha reductase inhibitor can be considered.

Phytotherapies

The bioflavonoid, quercetin, was one of the first agents to be evaluated in a randomized placebo controlled trial using the CPSI as the primary outcome. This trial showed a moderate benefit over placebo with quercetin.[55] There is also evidence for the use of pollen extract and saw palmetto, although the main evidence for pollen extract and saw palmetto has published in a peer reviewed journal.

Analgesics, muscle relaxants and neuromodulators

Analgesics can alleviate some of the pain, but narcotics should be avoided except for short term control of serious pain exacerbations. Skeletal muscle relaxants such as diazepam, baclofen and cyclobenzaprine are utilized in men with spastic or dysfunctional pelvic floors with some anecdotal success. Amitriptyline is an important adjunct to neuropathic pain management, has proven efficacious in interstitial cystitis, and should be considered for the neuropathic type pain experienced by many men with CP/CPPS. Similarly, the gabapentinoids are indicated for neuropathic pain control and the results from a recently completed NIH sponsored randomized placebo controlled trial is available soon. Based on the results from other similar pain syndromes, we would expect this drug to prove efficacious in some patients.

Surgery

A number of minimally invasive surgical approaches (transurethral microwave thermotherapy, transurethral radiofrequency needle ablation etc.) have been advocated for CP/CPPS, however no real concrete evidence is available to support any suggestion of efficacy.[23] Radical transurethral and open prostatectomy has similarly been suggested as a last resort and it is evident from anecdotal experience that this may create more harm than benefit for patients with CP/CPPS. Surgery should be restricted to discrete indications, usually those causing lower urinary tract obstruction (urethral meatal stenosis, urethral stricture, bladder neck stenosis).[40]

A Practical Management Plan

Table 22.3 describes the various medical therapies that we employ to treat the prostatitis syndromes and the evidence (or lack of it) to support therapeutic recommendations and suggestions. One can quickly determine, that except for the bacterial prostatitis syndromes (Cat I and II), therapy for the much more prevalent CP/CPPS is poor. Clinical researchers have become frustrated by the lack of efficacy seen in well designed randomized placebo controlled trials in CP/CPPS despite solid theoretical considerations, strong anecdotal evidence from clinical practice, and evidence from numerous small usually single center clinical trials. We have come to the realization that it is the very restrictive nature of these randomized trials, in which we routinely exclude over 90% of the patients we see in our clinics on a daily basis, in order to enroll very homogenous and comparative populations. The patients in our clinical trials may not truly represent patients we see in our clinical practice. In fact, each patient diagnosed with CP/CPPS has a unique clinical phenotype based on etiology, age, duration since diagnosis, concurrent disease, associated conditions, symptom trajectory, and coping behaviors. Based on this new understanding, a clinical phenotyping classification system was developed to describe the characteristics of individual patients. The UPOINT system[56] describes the following phenotypes; Urinary, Psychosocial, Organ specific, Neurogenic/systemic and Tenderness (of muscles). UPOINT is outlined in more detail in Table 22.4. The number of UPOINT domains a patient is classified in is associated with severity of both general CP/CPPS symptoms and CP/CPPS related pain.[57] The domains are not correlated with age, but with duration since diagnosis. Each domain is associated with a slightly different impact on symptoms and pain. By employing this clinical phenotyping system, UPOINT, the physician can categorize patients into one or more domains using standardized workup (perhaps asking a few questions about depression and/or coping) and then use this information to direct specific and usually multi-modal therapies. Table 22.4 describes how therapies can be tailored for individual UPOINT domains experienced by the patient. As we learn more about the etiology and pathogenesis of CP/CPPS (which has so far eluded us), discoveries, including important biomarkers, can be incorporated into the UPOINT system, allowing for stratification of the six domains. The future for patients diagnosed with a prostatitis syndrome is looking brighter as we can now rationalize our clinical approach for this difficult medical condition.

Table 22.3. Medical therapy for the prostatitis syndromes

Class	Medication	Indication	Evidence
Antibiotics	Ciprofloxacin	Category I	Strong
	Levofloxacin	Category II	Strong
	Ofloxacin	Category III	Contradictory
	Norfloxacin	Cat III uropath	Moderate
	Doxycline	Cat III no uropath	Weak
	Azithromycin	Early naïve Cat III no uropath	Moderate
	Clarithromycin	Late Cat III no uropath	Not recommended
Anti-inflammatories	Ibuprofen	Cat III monotherapy	Weak/not recommended
	Diclofenac		
	Indomethocin	Cat III adjuvant therapy	Weak/moderate
	Celecoxib		
Alpha-blockers	Terazosin	Cat III	Contradictory
	Doxazosin	Late Cat III	Not recommended
	Tamsulosin	Early naïve Cat III	Contradictory
	Alfuzosin	Early naïve Cat III voiding symptoms	Suggestive
Glycosaminoglycan	Pentosan	Cat III	Weak
	polysulfate	Cat III suprapubic pain voiding symptoms	Weak/suggestive
5-Alpha reductase inhibitors	Finasteride	Cat III	Not recommended
	Dutasteride	Cat III large prostate over 40 years old	Suggestive
Tricyclic antidepressants	Amitriptyline	Cat III	Suggestive[a]
	Nortriptyline		
Gabapentinoids	Gabapentin	Cat III	Suggestive
	Pregabalin		
Muscle relaxants	Diazepam	Cat III	Suggestive
	Baclofen		
	Cyclobenzaprine		
Phytotherapies	Quercetin	Cat III	Weak/moderate
	Pollen extract		
	Saw palmetto		
Narcotics	Demerol	Cat I	Recommended
	Morphine	Cat II	Recommended
		Cat III	Not recommended
Minimally invasive surgery	TUNA	Cat I, II and III	Not recommended
	TUMT		
	Laser Therapy		

Table 22.3. (continued)

Class	Medication	Indication	Evidence
Invasive surgery	TURP	Cat I, II and III	Not recommended (unless clear surgical indication – see text)
	Radical prostatectomy		
Conservative therapy	Diet modification	Cat III	Suggestive (Anecdotal evidence)
	Lifestyle change		
	Physiotherapy		
	Prostate massage		
	Acupuncture		
	Other alternative therapies		

[a]Publication of recently completed NIH trial evaluating pregabalin in CPPS may change this recommendation.

Table 22.4. The UPOINT clinical phenotyping classification system

Upoint domain	Phenotype presentation	Directed therapies
Urinary	Obstructive voiding symptoms	Alpha blockers
		Anticholinergics
	Irritative voiding symptoms	5-alpha reductase inhibitors
		Pyridium
Psychosocial	Depression	Antidepressants
	Poor coping behaviors	Psychologist intervention
	Poor social support	Counseling
Organ specific	Inflammation	Anti-inflammatories
	Pain localized to prostate	Phytotherapies
Infection	Bacteria localized to prostate specific specimens	Antibiotics
	History of Cat I or II	
Neurogenic/associated conditions	Neuropathic pain	Tricyclic antidepressants
	Neurogenic abnormalities	Gabapentinoids
	Associated Systemic	Specific therapy directed to associated condition
	Syndromes	
Tenderness	Pelvic/perineal muscle spasm	Muscle relaxants
	Pelvic floor or side wall pain or trigger points	Physiotherapy
	Suprapubic/abdominal muscle pain	

References

1. Nickel JC. The three A's of chronic prostatitis therapy; antibiotics, alpha-blockers, and anti-inflammatories: what is the evidence? *BJU Int.* 2004;94:1230-1233

2. Schaeffer AJ. Chronic prostatitis and the chronic pelvic pain syndrome. *N Engl J Med.* 2006;355: 1690-1698

3. Nickel JC. Chronic prostatitis/chronic pelvic pain syndrome: a decade of change. *AUA.* 2006;25: 309-316

4. Krieger JN, Nyberg LJ, Nickel JC. NIH consensus definition and classification of prostatitis. *JAMA.* 1999;282:236-237

5. Roberts RO, Lieber MM, Rhodes T, et al. Prevalence of a physician-assigned diagnosis of prostatitis: the Olmsted County Study of urinary symptoms and health status among men. *Urology.* 1998;51:578-584

6. McNaughton-Collins M, Meigs JB, Barry MJ, et al. Prevalence and correlates of prostatitis in the health professionals follow-up study cohort. *J Urol.* 2002; 167: 1363-1366

7. Nickel JC, Downey J, Hunter D, Clark J. Prevalence of prostatitis-like symptoms in a population based study employing the NIH-chronic prostatitis symptom index (NIH-CPSI). *J Urol.* 2001;165:842–845

8. McNaughton-Collins M, Stafford RS, O'Leary MP, Barry MJ. How common is prostatitis? A national survey of physician visits. *J Urol.* 1998;159: 1224-1228

9. Moon TD, Hagen L, Heisey DM. Urinary symptomatology in younger men. *Urology.* 1997;50:700-703

10. Roberts RO, Jacobson DJ, Girman CJ, et al. Prevalence of prostatitis-like symptoms in a community based cohort of older men. *J Urol.* 2002;168:2467-2471

11. Clemens JQ, Meenan RT, O'Keeffe Rosetti MC, et al. Incidence and clinical characteristics of National Institutes of Health type III prostatitis in the community. *J Urol.* 2005;174:2319

12. McNaughton-Collins M, Joyce GF, Wise M, et al. US Department of Health and Human Services, Public Health Service, National Institutes of Health, National Institute of Diabetes and Digestive and Kidney Diseases. In: Litwin MS, Saigal CS, et al., eds. *Urologic Diseases in America.* Washington, DC: U.S. Government Publishing Office; 2007:9-41

13. Wenninger K, Heiman JR, Rothman I, et al. Sickness impact of chronic nonbacterial prostatitis and its correlates. *J Urol.* 1996;155:965-968

14. McNaughton-Collins M, Pontari MA, et al. Quality of life is impaired in men with chronic prostatitis: the Chronic Prostatitis Collaborative Research Network. *J Gen Int Med.* 2001;16:656-662

15. Tripp DA, Nickel JC, Landis JR, et al. Predictors of quality of life and pain in chronic prostatitis/chronic pelvic pain syndrome: findings from the National Institutes of Health Chronic Prostatitis Cohort Study. *BJU Int.* 2004;94:1279-1282

16. Tripp DA, Nickel JC, Wang Y, et al. Catastrophizing and Pain-Contingent Rest Predict Patient Adjustment in Men with Chronic Prostatitis/Chronic Pelvic Pain Syndrome. *J Pain.* 2006;7:697-708

17. Nickel JC, Tripp DA, Chuai S, et al. Psychosocial parameters impact quality of life in men diagnosed with chronic prostatitis/chronic pelvic pain syndrome (CP/CPPS). *BJU Int.* 2007;101:59-64

18. Calhoun EA, McNaughton Collins M, Pontari MA, et al. Chronic Prostatitis Collaborative Research Network. The economic impact of chronic prostatitis. *Arch Intern Med.* 2004;164:1231-1236

19. Neal DE Jr. Treatment of acute prostatitis. In: Nickel JC, ed. *Textbook of Prostatitis.* Oxford: ISIS Medical Media Ltd.; 1999:279-284

20. Nickel JC, Moon T. Chronic bacterial prostatitis: an evolving clinical enigma. *Urology.* 2005;66:2-8

21. Nickel JC, Alexander RB, Schaeffer AJ, et al. Leukocytes and bacteria in men with chronic prostatitis/chronic pelvic pain syndrome compared to asymptomatic controls. *J Urol.* 2003;170:818-822

22. Pontari MA, Ruggieri MR. Mechanisms in prostatitis/chronic pelvic pain syndrome. *J Urol.* 2004;172:839-845

23. Nickel JC. Inflammatory conditions of the male genitourinary tract: prostatitis and related conditions, orchitis, and epididymitis. In: Walsh P et al., eds. *Campbell-Walsh Urology.* 9th ed. Philadelphia, PA: W. B. Saunders Company; 2006:330-370

24. Meares EM Jr, Stamey TA. Bacteriologic localization patterns in bacterial prostatitis and urethritis. *Invest Urol.* 1968;5:492-518

25. McNaughton-Collins M, Fowler EH, Elliott DB, et al. Diagnosing and treating chronic prostatitis: do urologists use the 4-glass test? *Urology.* 2000;55:403-407

26. Nickel JC. The Pre and Post Massage Test (PPMT): a simple screen for prostatitis. *Tech Urol.* 1997;3:38-43

27. Nickel JC, Shoskes D, Wang Y, et al. How does the pre- and post- massage test (PPMT) 2-glass test compare to the Meares-Stamey 4-glass test in men with chronic prostatitis/chronic pelvic pain syndrome? *J Urol.* 2006;176:119-124

28. Litwin MS, McNaughton-Collins M, Fowler FJ, et al. The National Institutes of Health chronic prostatitis symptom index: development and validation of a new outcome measure. *J Urol.* 1999;162:369-375

29. Nickel JC, McNaughton-Collins M, Litwin SM. Development and use of a validated outcome measure for prostatitis. *J Clin Outcomes Manag.* 2001;8:30-37

30. Propert KJ, Litwin MS, Wang Y, et al. Responsiveness of the National Institutes of Health Chronic Prostatitis Symptom Index (NIH-CPSI). *Qual Life Res.* 2006; 15: 299-305

31. Nickel JC. Clinical evaluation of the man with chronic prostatitis/chronic pelvic pain syndrome. *Urology.* 2000;60:20-23. Suppl 6A

32. Schaeffer AJ, Knauss JS, Landis JR, et al. Leukocyte and bacterial counts do not correlate with severity of symptoms in men with chronic prostatitis: the NIH Chronic Prostatitis Cohort (CPC) study. *J Urol.* 2002;168:1048-1053

33. Shoskes DA. Use of antibiotics in chronic prostatitis syndromes. *Can J Urol.* 2001;8:24-28

34. Naber KJ. Antibiotic treatment of chronic bacterial prostatitis. In: Nickel JC, ed. *Textbook of Prostatitis.* Oxford: ISIS Medical Media Ltd.; 1999:283-292

35. Nickel JC, Weidner W. Chronic prostatitis: current concepts in antimicrobial therapy. *Infect Urol*. 2000;13:S22-S29

36. Bjerklund Johansen T, Gruneberg RN, Guibert J, et al. The role of antibiotics in the treatment of chronic prostatitis: a consensus statement. *Eur Urol*. 1998;34: 457-466

37. Shoskes DA, Zeitlin SI. Use of prostatic massage in combination with antibiotics in the treatment of chronic prostatitis. *Prostate Cancer Prostatic Dis*. 1999;2:159-162

38. Nickel JC, Alexander R, Anderson R, et al. Prostatitis unplugged: prostate massage revisited. *Tech Urol*. 1999;5:1-7

39. Barbalias GA, Nikiforidis G, Liatsikos EN. Alpha-blockers for the treatment of chronic prostatitis in combination with antibiotics. *J Urol*. 1999;159:883-887

40. Kirby RS. Surgical considerations in the management of prostatitis. In: Nickel JC, ed. *Textbook of Prostatitis*. Oxford: ISIS Medical Media Ltd.; 1999:346-364

41. Nickel JC, Downey J, Johnston B, et al. Predictors of patient response to antibiotic therapy for chronic prostatitis/chronic pelvic pain syndrome: a prospective multicenter clinical trial. *J Urol*. 2001;165:1539-1544

42. Nickel JC, Xiang J. Clinical significance of non-traditional uropathogens in the management of chronic prostatitis. *J Urol*. 2008;179:1391-1395

43. Nickel JC, Downey J, Clark J, et al. Levofloxacin for chronic prostatitis/chronic pelvic pain syndrome in men: a randomized placebo-controlled multicenter trial. *Urology*. 2003;62:614-617

44. Alexander RB, Propert KJ, Schaeffer AJ, et al. Ciprofloxacin or tamsulosin in men with chronic prostatitis/chronic pelvic pain syndrome. *Ann Int Med*. 2004;141:581-589

45. Nickel JC, Pontari M, Moon T, et al. A randomized, placebo-controlled, multicenter study to evaluate the safety and efficacy of rofecoxib in the treatment of chronic nonbacterial prostatitis. *J Urol*. 2003;169:1401-1405

46. Nickel JC, Forrest JB, Tomera K, et al. Pentosan polysulfate sodium therapy for men with chronic pelvic pain syndrome: a multicenter, randomized, placebo-controlled study. *J Urol*. 2005;173:1252-1255

47. Cheah PY, Liong ML, Yuen KH, et al. Terazosin therapy for chronic prostatitis/ chronic pelvic pain syndrome: a randomized, placebo controlled trial. *J Urol*. 2003;169: 592-596

48. Tugcu V, Tasci AI, Fazlioglu A, et al. A placebo-controlled comparison of the efficiency of triple- and monotherapy in category III B chronic pelvic pain syndrome (CPPS). *Eur Urol*. 2007;51:1113-1118

49. Nickel JC, Narayan P, McKay J, Doyle C. Treatment of chronic prostatitis/chronic pelvic pain syndrome with tamsulosin: a randomized double-blind trial. *J Urol*. 2004;171:1594-1597

50. Mehik A, Alas P, Nickel JC, et al. Alfuzosin treatment for chronic prostatitis/chronic pelvic pain syndrome: a prospective, randomized, double-blind, placebo-controlled, pilot study. *Urology*. 2003;62:425-429

51. Yang G, Wei Q, Li H, et al. The effect of alpha-adrenergic antagonists in chronic prostatitis/chronic pelvic pain syndrome: a meta-analysis of randomized controlled trials. *J Androl*. 2006;27(6): 847-852

52. Mishra VC, Browne J, Emberton M. Role of alpha-blockers in type III prostatitis: a systemic review of the literature. *J Urol*. 2007;177(1):25-30

53. Nickel JC, Krieger J, McNaughton-Collins M, et al. Effect of Alfuzosin on Symptoms in Men with Chronic Prostatitis / Chronic Pelvic Pain Syndrome. *NEJM* 2008; 359(25):2663-2673, 2008

54. Nickel JC, Downey J, Pontari MA, et al. Randomized placebo-controlled, multi-center study to evaluate the safety and efficacy of finasteride in the treatment of male chronic pelvic pain syndrome: category IIIA CPPS (chronic nonbacterial prostatitis). *BJU Int*. 2004;93: 991-995

55. Shoskes DA, Zeitlin SI, Shahed A, et al. Quercetin in men with category III chronic prostatitis: a preliminary prospective, double-blind, placebo control trial. *Urology*. 1999;54:960-963

56. Shoskes DA, Nickel JC, Rackley RR, Pontari MA. Clinical Phenotyping in Chronic Prostatitis/Chronic Pelvic Pain Syndrome and Interstitial Cystitis: A Management Strategy for Urologic Chronic Pelvic Pain Syndromes. *Prostate Cancer and Prostatic Diseases* 2009;12:177-83

57. Shoskes DA, Nickel JC, Dolinga R, Prots D. Clinical Phenotyping of Chronic Prostatitis/Chronic Pelvic Pain Patients and Correlation with Symptom Severity, Urol 2009;73:538-543

23

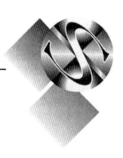

Disorders of Scrotal Contents: Orchitis, Epididymitis, Testicular Torsion, Torsion of the Appendages, and Fournier's Gangrene

Parviz K. Kavoussi and Raymond A. Costabile

Orchitis

Definition and Etiology

Orchitis is defined as inflammation of the testicle.[1] The most common etiology of acute orchitis, and epididymitis, is infection with the sexually transmitted pathogens *C. trachomatis* and *N. gonorrhea* in young men below the age of 35.[2] Epididymorchitis is also the most common cause of the "acute scrotum" in this age-group.[3] The most common organisms to cause orchitis and epididymitis in men over the age of 35 and in prepubertal boys are *E. coli* and *P. mirabilis*.[4]

Less common causes of infectious orchitis and epididymitis include brucellosis (*B. melitensis*), tuberculosis (*M. tuberculosis*), cryptococcus (*C. neoformans*), and the mumps virus. In these cases of epididymorchitis, orchitis develops from the infection spreading contiguously from the epididymis in 20–40%.[5] Mumps is the most common cause of orchitis not associated with epididymitis, with both testicles involved in 14–35% of cases.[6] Mumps orchitis can result in oligospermia and male factor infertility. Childhood vaccination is the best way to prevent mumps orchitis and its sequellae.[7] The incidence of mumps orchitis has diminished with advent of the vaccine, although there have been reports that the measles, mumps, and rubella (MMR) vaccine can induce orchitis in a small number of patients.[8]

Viral orchitis is typically disseminated by hematogenous route.[1] Genitourinary tract tuberculosis can be a source of orchitis. Epididymorchitis has also been reported in men treated with intravesical instillations of bacillus Calmette-Guerin (BCG) therapy for the treatment of bladder cancer.[9]

In the pediatric population, anomalies of the male excurrent duct system can predispose children to epididymorchitis, which is a rare source of the acute scrotum in this population. Epididymorchitis in children is thought to be due to urinary tract infections associated with these anatomic anomalies.[10]

Clinical Signs and Symptoms

The typical symptoms of orchitis include scrotal pain, swelling, tenderness, and skin fixation over the testicle. Prehn's sign has been described in orchitis and epididymitis, when there is relief of pain with elevation of the testicle over the symphysis pubis.[11] Prehn's sign is nonspecific and nondiagnostic and does not necessarily distinguish epididymorchitis from spermatic cord torsion.

Orchitis can cause an irreversible affect on spermatogenesis, impacting the quality and number of spermatozoa. Lymphocytic infiltration and seminiferous tubule damage is seen on testicular biopsies of subfertile men with a history of chronic orchitis.[12]

C.R. Chapple and W.D. Steers (eds.), *Practical Urology: Essential Principles and Practice*,
DOI: 10.1007/978-1-84882-034-0_23, © Springer-Verlag London Limited 2011

Diagnostic Evaluation

A thorough history and physical examination are the most valuable aspects of the diagnostic evaluation of men with acute scrotal pain and swelling. In patients with clinical orchitis, scrotal ultrasound should be obtained as testicular malignancy has been reported to masquerade as orchitis.[13] At least 10% of men with testicular malignancy will initially be incorrectly diagnosed as an acute inflammatory processes or spermatic cord torsion.[14] High-frequency transducer sonography (7.5–10 MHz) is considered the best modality for evaluation of scrotal pathology including orchitis.[5] Heterogeneous echotexture and enlargement of the testicle are typical ultrasound findings in orchitis.[15] Color Doppler ultrasound will show increased blood flow to the epididymis in epididymorchitis[16] (Fig. 23.1). Scrotal wall thickening, hydrocele, or pyocele may also be seen in association with this inflammatory process on sonographic exams.[17]

Treatment of Infectious Orchitis

Doxycycline is effective in treating orchitis due to *C. trachomatis* or *N. gonorrhea*. Third-generation cephalosporins, such as ceftriaxone, are also effective antimicrobial agents for epididymorchitis. *C. trachomatis* is also effectively treated with quinolones and macrolides, and treatment is usually maintained for 3 weeks. Evaluation and treatment of sexual partners is recommended as well. Patients with

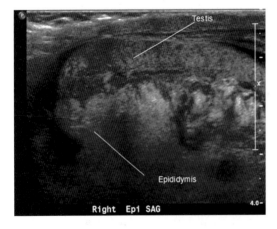

Figure 23.1. Ultrasound image of acute epididymorchitis.

severe bacterial orchitis should be admitted and treated with intravenous antibiotics (aminoglycosides, cephalosporins, or combinations of both) until culture results are available and sensitivity-specific adjustments can be made.[1]

Treatment of Noninfectious Epididymorchitis

Nonspecific therapy for patients with noninfectious epididymorchitis includes nerve blocks, analgesics, scrotal elevation, bed rest, and nonsteroidal anti-inflammatory drugs.[18]

Epididymitis

Definition and Etiology

Epididymitis is defined as inflammation of the epididymis.[1] Epididymitis is the fifth most common urologic diagnosis made in men between the ages of 18 and 59.[19] In the US military, epididymitis is responsible for more man hours lost to illness than any other urologic diagnosis.[20]

There are a number of causes of this inflammatory process including bacterial, viral, and fungal infections; autoimmune disease; trauma; vasculitis; and idiopathic inflammatory causes. Although it is known that a great number of patients with epididymitis do not have an infectious source, there is a paucity of evidence explaining the mechanism of this disease process.[18,21]

Although the pathophysiology of acute epididymitis is not well understood, it is theorized to be secondary to retrograde flow of infected urine into the ejaculatory duct. This theory is supported by the fact that 56% of men diagnosed with acute bacterial epididymitis have concomitant benign prostatic hyperplasia with bladder outlet obstruction, urethral stricture disease, or prostate cancer. Other mechanisms must also be responsible for acute epididymitis as men who have undergone vasectomy develop symptoms of clinical epididymitis.[18,21]

E. coli is the most common infectious pathogen in men older than 35 years of age with infectious epididymitis. Other bacterial pathogens less commonly seen include *U. urealyticum*,

Corynebacteria species, Mycoplasma species, and *M. polymorpha*.[22] *C. trachomatis* is thought to be the primary source of infectious epididymitis in men 35 years of age or younger. Men infected with *C. trachomatis* have a 4.28% incidence of developing acute epididymitis.[23]

Chronic epididymitis has become the terminology of choice for urologists defining a clinical picture of chronic epididymal pain which may or may not be associated with clinical signs. The discomfort may vary in degree and is associated with scrotal, epididymal, or testicular pain lasting for at least 3 months.[24] Chronic epididymitis is thought to account for up to 80% of visits to the urologist for scrotal pain.[25]

Other less common causes of infectious orchitis and epididymitis include *B. melitensis*, *M. tuberculosis*, *C. neoformans*, and the mumps virus.[5] Chronic infectious epididymitis is most commonly due to *M. tuberculosis*, which is thought to be secondary to hematogenous spread.[26] Ten percent of patients with Brucellosis develop epididymitis due to this gram negative coccobacillus.[27]

Other noninfectious sources of chronic epididymitis include sarcoidosis and Behcet's disease. Sarcoidosis is more commonly seen in black patients, and this chronic granulomatous process can affect the genitourinary tract in up to 5% of patients.[28,29] Behcet's disease is a multiorgan vasculitic disease of an idiopathic nature.[30]

Clinicians must also be aware of iatrogenic sources of epididymitis. Clinical noninfectious epididymitis can be a complication of the use of the drug amiodarone for arrhythmias.[14] This is due to anti-amiodarone HCL antibodies which attack the epididymal lining. Clinical epididymitis is seen in 11% of patients on high-dose amiodarone.[31] Prostate biopsy is another iatrogenic source of epididymitis. There is a 0.2% rate of epididymitis after transrectal ultrasound and biopsy of the prostate.[32]

Epididymitis in children is often secondary to systemic viral infection, most commonly secondary to *M. pneumoniae*, enteroviruses, and adenoviruses. Mumps epididymitis is rarely seen in the USA since an effective vaccine was introduced in 1985.[33,34] A vasculitic epididymitis may also develop in children with Henoch-Schonlein Purpura due to immunoglobulin A complex deposition, causing small vessel vasculitis.[35]

Clinical Signs and Symptoms

The mean age of patients presenting with epididymitis is 41. 43% of patients with epididymitis are between the ages of 20 and 39 years. Another 29% are between the ages of 40 and 59 years.[36]

Acute epididymitis typically develops over a course of several days and may present with pain and swelling, often unilateral. Fevers, erythema of the scrotum, hydrocele formation, urethritis, involvement of the testis, leukocytosis, and positive urine cultures may also be seen in the presentation of acute epididymitis.[18] Patients who undergo urinary tract instrumentation or even clean intermittent catheterization are at higher risk of developing infectious epididymitis, especially if they have infected urine during the time of instrumentation.[36-38]

Patients with chronic epididymitis can have painful point tenderness in the epididymis with or without a palpable abnormality on physical examination. Scrotal ultrasound may demonstrate an epididymal abnormality in these men. It is also common that the clinical and ultrasound evaluation in men with chronic epididymitis is completely normal.[39] The majority of patients with chronic epididymitis have had these symptoms for 5 years, and the average age at the time of presentation is 49 years.[24] These men may complain of erectile dysfunction, neurological diseases, and musculoskeletal complaints.[18] When compared to controls, men with chronic epididymitis have a greater number of sexual partners, a more frequent history of sexually transmitted disease, and have used sexually transmitted disease protection less often.[24]

Patients with male factor infertility may reveal a history of chronic epididymitis which has been associated with oligoasthenospermia and alterations in spermatozoa DNA integrity.[40]

Patients with sarcoid epididymitis have progressive enlargement of the epididymis, which can be bilateral in up to 30% of these men. Extragonadal sarcoidosis frequently precedes the diagnosis of sarcoid epididymitis.[29] Patients with epididymitis associated with Behcet's disease may have tender genital ulcers, aphthous ulcers, and uveitis.[30]

Children with epididymitis present with an acute scrotum, sonographic hyperemia on Doppler, and any two of the following: leukocytosis, fever with a temperature greater than

38.5°C, positive urine culture, or pyuria greater than ten leukocytes per high-power field.[41] Henoch-Schonlein Purpura epididymitis occurs in children between the ages of 22 and 11 years. It has been reported that between 22% and 38% of these boys will present with scrotal swelling along with palpable purpura, hematuria, abdominal pain, and joint pain.[35]

Diagnostic Evaluation of Epididymitis

Diagnostic evaluation should begin with a thorough history and physical examination.[22] Patients younger than 35 should undergo gram stain of urethral exudates and if they have greater than five white blood cells per high-power field, a positive leukocyte esterase test, or microscopic examination of first voided urine sediment revealing ten or more white blood cells per high-power field, they should be treated empirically for *N. gonorrhea* and *C. trachomatis*. They should also undergo a culture of nucleic acid amplification test of a urethral swab or urine PCRs for *N. gonorrhea* and *C. trachomatis*. In patients older than 35 years of age, leukocyte esterase test or microscopic examination of first voided urine sediment revealing ten or more white blood cells per high-power field should be treated empirically for a bacterial source. They should also have cultures and gram stains of voided urine obtained.[42](see Table 23.1).

Children, adolescents who are not sexually active, and patients older than 35 years of age should have midstream urine collected. Those with positive dipsticks or microscopic examinations should have urine sent for culture. Patients with indwelling ureteral stents, recent anal intercourse, or recent urinary tract instrumentation should undergo urine culture. Patients with positive results on testing for *C. trachomatis* or *N. gonorrhea* should undergo testing for other sexual transmitted diseases, including HIV.[18] Up to 90% of men in this age group with epididymitis have no evidence of *C. trachomatis* on urethral swab polymerase chain reaction.[43-46]

Ultrasound is utilized primarily to evaluate the acute scrotum with the intent to rule out testicular torsion and is not needed to make the diagnosis of epididymitis or to direct therapy. Only 69% of cases of epididymitis have the classic sonographic features associated with epididymitis. Ultrasound should be reserved for patients without a clear diagnosis of epididymitis.[47] In men with epididymitis, the epididymis may appear hypoechoic, or can appear hyperechoic in the presence of epididymal hemorrhage. Scrotal wall thickening, hydrocele, or pyocele may also be seen in association with inflammatory epididymitis. Color Doppler may show increased blood flow to the epididymis in epididymitis.[17]

In sarcoid epididymitis, scrotal ultrasound may reveal an enlarged, heterogeneous epididymis, which may have distinct nodules.[48,49] Sarcoid epididymitis can lead to azoospermia secondary to extrinsic compression of the epididymal ducts. Patients with the diagnosis of sarcomatoid epididymitis interested in fertility should have a semen analysis performed.[50] Testicular torsion should be ruled out in patients with Henoch-Schonlein Purpura epididymitis as they present with painful scrotal swelling.[35]

Table 23.1. Centers for Disease Control's 2006 guidelines for the diagnosis and management of epididymitis

Age	Younger than 35	Older than 35
Lab tests	Gram stain of urethral exudate for urethritis (> 5 white blood cells/high-power field) or leukocyte esterase test or microscopic examination of first-void urine sediment demonstrating at or above 10 WBC/hpf Culture or nucleic acid amplification test of urethral swab (or urine)	Leukocyte esterase test or microscopic examination of first-void urine sediment demonstrating at or above 10 WBC/hpf Culture and gram stain of voided urine
Treatment	Empiric antibiotics to cover *N gonorrhea* and *C. trachomatis* [a]Ceftriaxone 250 mg intramuscularly x1 and doxycycline 100 mg po bid x10 days	Empiric antibiotics to cover coliform bacteria Levofloxacin 500 mg qd x10 days or ofloxacin 300 mg bid x10 days

[a]Patients younger than 35 with allergies to penicillins or tetracyclines should be treated with levofloxacin or ofloxacin. If *N. gonorrhea* is suspected, patients may need to be desensitized to penicillin on account of the high rate of fluoroquinolone resistance evolving in *N gonorrhea*.[42]

Children with acute epididymitis and a positive urine culture should undergo renal ultrasound and VCUG. Ultrasound examination of the kidneys and urinary bladder without VCUG is adequate for children with acute epididymitis and a negative urine culture.[41]

Treatment of Acute Epididymitis

The evaluation and treatment of epididymitis traditionally includes use of empiric antibiotics when infection is suspected and supportive management such as bed rest, scrotal elevation, analgesics, and nonsteroidal anti-inflammatory drugs. In patients at risk for a sexually transmitted disease, treatment should consist of one dose of Ceftriaxone 250 mg intramuscularly and Doxycycline 100 mg by mouth twice a day for 10 days. Patients older than 35 years of age with a suspected bacterial pathogen should be treated empirically with Levofloxacin 500 mg by mouth daily for 10 days or Ofloxacin 300 mg by mouth twice a day for 10 days.[42]

In patients diagnosed with *C. trachomatis*, sexual partners should be treated as well to prevent pelvic inflammatory disease, infertility, and chronic pelvic pain in the female partner. Without treatment of the partner, the couple will be at risk of transmitting the pathogen back and forth to one another and causing recurrent infections.[51]

If the patient appears toxic, has systemic symptoms (fevers or leukocytosis, necrotizing fasciitis or testicular infarction), or has significant comorbidities (e.g. immunosuppression or uncontrolled diabetes mellitus), then hospitalization is warranted where close observation, supportive care, parenteral antibiotics, and fluid resuscitation should be administered as needed.[18]

Treatment of Chronic Epididymitis

Although there is no level-one evidence for the optimal treatment of chronic epididymitis, local supportive therapy including heat, nerve blocks, analgesics, tricyclic antidepressants, anticonvulsants such as gabapentin, and anti-inflammatory drugs are common practice and may offer some relief.[52] Other treatment options implemented for chronic epididymitis include phytotherapy, anxiolytics, narcotics, acupuncture, and steroid injection therapy.[24] Despite evidence that up to 75% of patients do not have an identifiable bacterial urinary tract infection concomitantly with their clinical epididymitis, antibiotics are routinely given. Empirical antibiotic administration in the absence of positive urine cultures has been steadily increasing, from 75% to 95% between the years of 1965 and 2005. Antibiotic administration does not decrease the length of symptoms or the return to full activity in men without an identifiable bacterial pathogen.[36,53]

Surgical Treatment of Chronic Epididymitis

Surgical treatment for chronic epididymitis is poorly studied in clinical trials with no level-one evidence to support the use of a specific surgical procedure. Fewer than 250 patients with chronic scrotal pain have been treated with differing surgical therapies in the available literature despite the common nature of chronic scrotal pain. The authors do not advocate orchiectomy for chronic orchitis/epididymitis, but if orchiectomy is recommended, the patient should previously have failed conservative therapy and must be apprised of the risks, benefits, and options of orchiectomy. As many patients will continue to have pain or have pain recur after orchiectomy, the surgeon should be aware of the medical legal aspects of this action.

In one study, 10 patients with chronic epididymitis (defined as epididymal pain lasting greater than 3 months), underwent epididymectomy for intractable symptoms. Only one of these patients had significant improvement in pain.[54] Other authors have reported much higher success rates, such as six out of seven patients (86%) having significant improvement in pain after epididymectomy.[55] Chronic or recurrent epididymitis and persistent epididymalgia with point tenderness to the epididymis may be reasonable indications for epididymectomy.[56] Surgical treatment for chronic epididymitis should be considered only after failure of extensive conservative therapy and after appropriate counseling, with the understanding that the symptoms may not improve after surgery, or may indeed worsen. A retrospective review of 32 men who underwent epididymectomy for chronic epididymitis showed that outcomes were best when the patient had a palpable epididymal abnormality on physical examination. Men in this study without a palpable abnormality, but with sonographic changes had slightly worse outcomes, and those without either a palpable abnormality or a demonstrable ultrasound abnormality did not improve with epididymectomy.[39]

Some surgeons have attempted microsurgical denervation of the spermatic cord for symptomatic relief of chronic scrotal pain. Microsurgical denervation of the spermatic cord was performed in 79 men on 95 testicular units for chronic orchalgia over a mean duration of 62 months. There was complete relief of pain in 71% of the patients, partial relief in 17%, and there was no change from the preoperative status in 12%, with no patients experiencing worsened postoperative pain. The mean follow-up was 20.3 months.[57]

Treatment of Purulent and Atypical Epididymitis

The diagnosis of purulent epididymitis is made with the combination of physical examination, ultrasound evaluation, and occasionally needle aspiration of the epididymis. Epididymectomy is performed when possible and orchiectomy is performed when an abscess or necrosis of testicular tissue is present. Common causative organisms include *N. gonorrhea*, *C. trachomatis*, and *E. coli*.[58]

Corticosteroids should be utilized as first-line treatment for pain and swelling in sarcoid epididymitis. In the rare case where surgical exploration is undertaken, a frozen section should be obtained to prevent an unnecessary epididymectomy or orchiectomy.[29] If a patient with sarcoid epididymitis is found to be oligospermic, he should consider sperm storage.[59]

Treatment of Behcet's disease is targeted at symptomatic relief, mainly with corticosteroids.[30]

Treatment of epididymal tuberculosis should consist of a 6 month course using a three drug regimen including isoniazid, rifampin, and pyrazinamide. Ethambutol should be added to the regimen if the patient is from a highly drug-resistant region, until sensitivities are available.[60,61] Men with Bacille Calmette-Guerin epididymitis are treated with isoniazid and rifampin.

Patients with epididymitis due to Brucellosis, (infection with *B. melitensis*), should be treated with doxycycline 100 mg by mouth twice a day for 6 weeks and either streptomycin 1 g intramuscularly daily for 14 days or rifampin 600–900 mg daily by mouth for 6 weeks.[62]

Epididymitis in children is often secondary to viral infections and should be treated conservatively with ice packs and analgesics.[34] Epididymitis associated with Henoch-Schonlein Purpura is a self-limited disease and may improve with the administration of corticosteroids.[35]

Testicular Torsion and Torsion of the Testicular and Epididymal Appendages

Clinical Signs, Symptoms, and Differential Diagnosis of the Acute Scrotum

The acute scrotum includes the diagnoses of testicular torsion, acute epididymorchitis, and torsion of a testicular appendage. A thorough history and physical examination is the key to making an accurate diagnosis. Leukocytosis is frequently not found to be a distinguishing parameter for these diagnoses. Pyuria was found in 26% of patients with epididymorchitis. Color Doppler ultrasound has the highest sensitivity (87.9%) and specificity (93.3%) of differentiating testicular torsion from the other diagnoses of the acute scrotum.[63]

Testicular torsion can be seen in patients of any age, but most commonly occurs in males between the ages of 12 and 18. Testicular torsion occurs in one out of every 4,000 men below the age of 25.[64] The risk of having spermatic cord torsion or torsion of an appendage of the testicle or epididymis is one in 160 by the age of 25.[65] The incidence of bilateral testicular torsion (synchronous or metachronous) is 2%.[66]

The most consistent presentation of testicular torsion is the acute onset of severe testicular pain. Pain may be followed by nausea, vomiting, and even a low-grade fever. The hemiscrotum of the affected side is typically swollen, tender, and inflamed on physical examination. Another typical physical sign is the absence of the cremasteric reflex.[67] Pain is not relieved by elevation of the scrotum.[11] Patients may present with a "bell clapper" deformity, when the tunica vaginalis

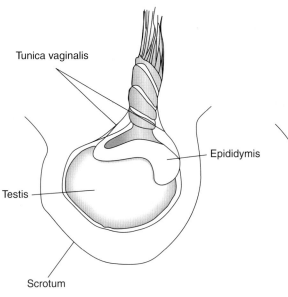

Figure 23.2. Bell clapper deformity.

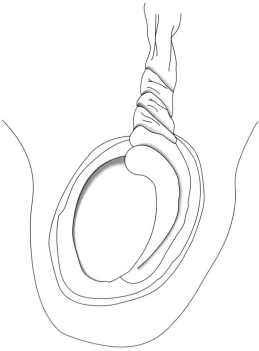

Figure 23.3. Extravaginal torsion.

completely encircles the distal spermatic cord, epididymis, and the testis; instead of attaching to the posterolateral aspect of the testis (Fig. 23.2). This resembles the clapper of a bell, as the testicle is free to rotate and swing freely within the tunica vaginalis. Bell clapper deformities occur bilaterally in 80% of patients who present with testicular torsion.[6,68] On physical examination, the torqued testicle is tender and high riding with a horizontal lie. Irreversible ischemia begins at 6 hours after torsion, or from the onset of symptoms depending on the variability in testicular blood flow following torsion.[69] Torsion of the spermatic cord results in testicular ischemia by causing venous engorgement, edema, and hemorrhage which result in arterial compromise.[70]

Intermittent testicular torsion is episodic twisting of the spermatic cord with spontaneous resolution.[71] Patients in the appropriate age-group with acute scrotal pain and rapid resolution should be suspected of having intermittent testicular torsion, and should be treated with scheduled bilateral orchiopexy.[72]

Clinicians must also be aware of the possibility of testicular torsion in patients who have had prior orchiopexy, as such cases have rarely been reported.[73]

Extravaginal testicular torsion (occurring outside of the tunica vaginalis), when the testis and gubernaculum can rotate freely, occurs exclusively in newborns[74] (Fig. 23.3). Neonates with extravaginal testicular torsion present clinically with scrotal swelling, discoloration, and a firm, painless mass in the scrotum.[75] In these neonates, the testis is usually necrotic from infarction at the time of birth. The sonographic appearance demonstrates an enlarged heterogeneous testicle without color Doppler flow to the testis or spermatic cord, skin thickening, and an ipsilateral hydrocele.[76] Neonatal testicular torsion is estimated to occur in one in 7,500 newborns.[77] Complicated pregnancies and vaginal deliveries are associated with a higher risk for testicular torsion.[78]

Testicular torsion is also more common in a cryptorchid testis. 73% of cases of torsion in cryptorchid testes were reported on the left side. These patients presented with an empty hemiscrotum; a tender, firm mass in the groin; and inguinal swelling and erythema. Doppler ultrasound is useful to confirm the diagnosis. The rates of surgical testicular salvage in these patients are very poor due to delay in presentation, diagnosis, or referral to a urologist.[79]

The primary imaging modality of choice for assistance in evaluation of the acute scrotum is high-frequency transducer sonography including pulsed and color Doppler vascular imaging.[3] A 50% false-positive rate has been reported for the diagnosis of testicular torsion when the diagnosis is made solely on the basis of clinical findings, without the use of imaging.[80] Color Doppler ultrasound is very useful to quantitate intratesticular blood flow.[81] Color Doppler was 86% sensitive, 100% specific, and 97% accurate in diagnosing testicular torsion in patients with a painful scrotum when detection of intratesticular flow was the only criterion utilized.[82]

Subtraction dynamic-contrast enhanced MRI has been utilized to evaluate patients for testicular torsion. Decreased testicular perfusion and hemorrhagic necrosis can be determined with MRI.[83] Scrotal MRI however is presently not a time or cost-effective adjunct to the diagnosis of the acute scrotum.

Torsion of the testicular appendix is the most common cause of the acute scrotum in children.[84] Of all appendiceal torsions, 91–95% involve the appendix testis, and most commonly are seen in boys between 7 and 14 years of age.[3]

The clinical appearance of torsion of the testicular or epididymal appendages is similar to that of testicular torsion, but often with a gradual onset of pain. On physical examination, there is typically a palpable small, firm nodule on the superior portion of the testis. The classic "blue dot sign" refers to bluish discoloration of the appendix, which is visible through the overlying skin.[85] Unlike in testicular torsion, the cremasteric reflex is still present with torsions of the scrotal appendices.

Ultrasound is only useful in cases of appendiceal torsion without a clear diagnosis based on clinical findings. The typical sonographic findings in torsion of the appendix include a circular mass adjacent to the testis or epididymis, with variable echogenicity.[85] There may be peripheral flow by color Doppler around the torqued testicular appendage, and a reactive hydrocele with skin thickening is not uncommon.[81] Ultrasound findings may also include larger testicular appendages than controls, measuring 5 mm or greater, which are spherical in shape, and with increased periappendiceal blood flow. Ultrasound cannot demonstrate blood flow in the torsed or in the normal appendix testis and there is no difference in echogenicity between the normal and the torsed appendix testis.[86]

Torsed testicular appendages should be managed conservatively with analgesics. The pain resolves in 2–3 days with atrophy and sometimes calcification of the appendage.

Treatment of Spermatic Cord Torsion

The ability to salvage a torsed testicle depends on the duration and degree of torsion. If the diagnosis is made and intervention occurs within the first 6 hours after the onset of symptoms, there is a nearly 100% testicular salvage rate. Testicular salvage drops to 70% in the 6–12 hours time frame, and is diminished to 20% between 12 and 24 hours.[87] Age is a significant predictable risk factor for orchiectomy in patients between the ages of one and 25 with testicular torsion, due to the delay in seeking medical attention in older males.[88] Immediate surgical exploration and bilateral orchiopexy is the treatment of choice in acute testicular torsion, although orchiectomy is required with delayed treatment with subsequently infarcted or necrotic testicles.[89] Emergency exploration should be undertaken, and ideally, bilateral orchiopexy should be performed if the torqued testis is found to be viable. Orchiectomy and contralateral orchiopexy should be performed if the testis is not viable. Manual detorsion should be performed if surgical exploration is to be delayed.[69] Manual detorsion is performed by external rotation of the torqued testis with confirmation of intraparenchymal blood flow following detorsion.[64] Manual detorsion is often accompanied by significant and instantaneous relief of symptoms. Orchiopexy is also recommended in these patients.

Patients with intermittent testicular torsion should undergo elective bilateral orchiopexy. If untreated, these patients are at risk for developing an episode of complete testicular torsion with subsequent infarction and testicular loss.[71] Ninety-seven percent of patients treated with prophylactic bilateral orchiopexy have complete resolution of their symptoms with a high likelihood of preventing future infarction.[72]

Some authors feel that urgent surgical exploration and concomitant contralateral orchiopexy is indicated in the case of acute neonatal testicular torsion.[90] The risk of testicular loss must be balanced with the risk of anesthesia in neonates with testicular torsion. Testicles noted to have extravaginal torsion at the time of delivery are never salvageable. It may therefore be argued that emergency exploration is not indicated. There is occasionally a chance for salvage of the testicle in neonatal torsions which are first noted after birth and before 1 month of age, with emergent exploration.[78] Other authors advocate emergent exploration and contralateral orchiopexy in all newborns with intrauterine testicular torsion to decrease their risk of anorchia following contralateral torsion.[91]

Fertility can be adversely affected in men who have had testicular torsion. The development of antisperm antibody levels does not correlate with the patient's age at the time of torsion, ischemia time, seminal parameters, or the type of treatment for torsion. Patients who underwent orchiopexy at the time of surgical exploration for torsion with attempted testicular salvage had poorer sperm motility and morphology when compared to the group which underwent orchiectomy for torsion.[92]

Fournier's Gangrene

Definition and Etiology

Fournier's gangrene is a polymicrobial necrotizing fasciitis involving the scrotum, genitalia, perineum, perirectal area, and can extend to the lower abdominal wall.[93] Fournier's gangrene is a urologic emergency with a rapidly progressive and possibly fatal course if left untreated.[94]

Fournier's gangrene was first described in 1764 by Baurienne, and was thought to only affect men and to have an idiopathic etiology. Necrotizing genital fasciitis is now known to be secondary to infection, and can also occur in women.[95,96] It was named after Jean-Alfred Fournier, a Parisian dermatologist and venereologist, who presented a case in 1883.[96]

Obliterative endarteritis characterizes Fournier's gangrene resulting in cutaneous and subcutaneous necrosis.[95] The hypoperfusion necrosis can result in severe endotoxicosis and subsequent multiorgan failure and death.[97]

The mean age of patients developing Fournier's gangrene is 50 years.[98] Common etiological factors include urinary tract infection, perianal infection, and genital trauma.[99,100] Fournier's has been reported to have a mortality rate as high as 75%.[95,98]

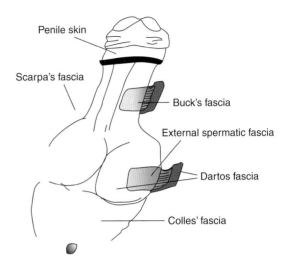

Figure 23.4. Anatomic fascial layers.

Risk Factors

Predisposing risk factors include diabetes mellitus, alcoholism, immunodeficiency, chronic hepatic disease, cardiac disorders, renal failure, advanced age, malignancy, and chemotherapy.[93,100] The most common predisposing risk factor in men and women developing Fournier's gangrene is diabetes mellitus.[98] Liver cirrhosis has been shown to have a high correlation with mortality in patients with Fournier's gangrene.[101] Men are affected more commonly by a ratio of 10:1.[102]

Anatomic Barriers to the Spread of Infection in the Genitalia and Perineum

Anatomic barriers to the spread of necrotizing fasciitis include the dartos fascia of the penis and scrotum, Colles' fascia of the perineum, and Scarpa's fascia of the anterior abdominal wall. The testes and epididymes tend to be spared by this disease process[103] (Figs. 23.4 and 23.5).

Infectious Organisms Associated with Fournier's Gangrene

The most common pathogens in patients with this polymicrobial necrotizing process include *E. Coli*, *Klebsiella*, *Proteus*, *Streptococcus*,

Figure 23.5. Anatomic fascial layers (sagittal view).

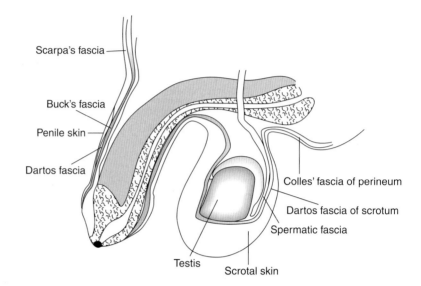

Scarpa's fascia

Buck's fascia

Penile skin

Dartos fascia

Colles' fascia of perineum

Dartos fascia of scrotum

Spermatic fascia

Testis

Scrotal skin

Staphylococcus, Peptostreptococcus, B. fragilis, Enterococcus, and *C. perfringens.*[101,104] *E. coli* is the most commonly isolated bacteria in Fournier's patients, although the infectious process tends to be polymicrobial.[99,100] Candidal infections have been reported to cause Fournier's gangrene in immunocompromised patients.[105]

Clinical Signs and Symptoms

Typical symptoms of Fournier's gangrene include scrotal swelling, pain, and fever. The average duration of symptoms prior to seeking medical care is 3–5 days. 84% of patients with Fournier's gangrene have bilateral scrotal involvement.[99] There is typically erythema and crepitus in the area of necrosis. There may be visible areas of gangrene or skin blistering as well. Nearly 10% of patients are unconscious on presentation. Sepsis can be seen in 43% of patients with Fournier's gangrene, and there is a 50% mortality rate among patients with sepsis. More commonly, necrotizing fasciitis has a rapid onset with a fulminant course, although less commonly it can have an insidious onset and slower progression.[100] Secondary complications of Fournier's that portend a higher risk for mortality are respiratory failure, renal failure, septic shock, hepatic failure, and disseminated intravascular coagulopathy.[101]

Diagnostic Evaluation

Diagnostic evaluation should begin with a thorough history and physical examination. The diagnosis of Fournier's gangrene is made by careful clinical evaluation. Diagnostic imaging can be helpful when the diagnosis is not clear from the clinical evaluation.[6] Plain film radiography, scrotal ultrasound, and computed tomography (CT) may be helpful in uncertain cases if gas is identified in the tissues (18–62% of cases). Subcutaneous gas in the scrotum is the most useful radiological finding to aid in the diagnosis.[106] Other helpful findings on imaging include scrotal wall edema with normal testicular and epididymal echotexture. This must be differentiated from an inguinal scrotal hernia with gas in the bowel lumen protruding into the scrotum.[6] CT may be helpful by demonstrating asymmetric fascial thickening, subcutaneous emphysema, and fluid or abscess formation.[107]

A Fournier's severity index to determine prognostic factors influencing survival has been constructed and validated. If the overall severity score is less than 9, the patient has a 96% chance of survival; whereas if the score is 9 or greater, the mortality rate increases to 46%.[108] Prognostic factors included in the Fournier's severity index include temperature, heart rate, serum sodium, serum potassium, serum creatinine, hematocrit, white blood cell count, and serum bicarbonate. The severity index may be useful in the

Treatment

Treatment should include emergent radical surgical debridement and intravenous broad-spectrum antibiotics. When culture results are available, the antibiotics can be tailored to the organisms based on sensitivities. Treatment should be performed expeditiously and aggressively, as Fournier's gangrene is a life-threatening process. All nonviable and necrotic tissue must be aggressively excised (Fig. 23.6).

An empirical broad-spectrum antibiotic regimen for the initial treatment of Fournier's gangrene includes a third-generation cephalosporin, an aminoglycoside (if the creatinine clearance is acceptable), and metronidazole. Aggressive fluid resuscitation is required including the use of blood and blood products. After debridement, adequate nutrition with early enteral feeding when possible is crucial for wound healing. Repeat debridement should be performed 2 days after the initial exploration to excise any remaining nonviable tissue. Multiple resections may be necessary. If the source of the infection is anorectal or the wound is contaminated, a colostomy should be performed to divert fecal flow.[100] In a likewise fashion, patients may require cystostomies for urinary diversion, especially when there is a urinary source exacerbating the necrotizing fasciitis.

Once the patient has been initially treated and resuscitated and all necrotic tissue has been excised, most wounds can be closed secondarily. Large wounds will often require skin grafts for coverage. Fasciocutaneous rotational thigh flaps may be utilized for coverage with good cosmetic results.[99] Wound closure is performed as soon as there is no evidence of infection of remaining necrotic tissue, and there is a viable bed that will allow reapproximation or grafting.[100] Patients with less than 50% scrotal skin loss can almost always be closed primarily without major difficulty. The testes may be placed in thigh pouches until the time of definitive reconstruction in cases with major scrotal skin loss.[110] Vacuum-assisted closure devices have been utilized to help these complex wounds heal after wide excision and debridement. This technique has been shown to be as effective as conventional wound care in healing wounds. These patients also require fewer dressing changes, have less pain, fewer skipped meals, and greater mobility.[111] The use of a small intestinal submucosa graft and fibrin sealant is an option for closure of scrotal defects after excision for Fournier's gangrene when standard grafting is not possible.[112]

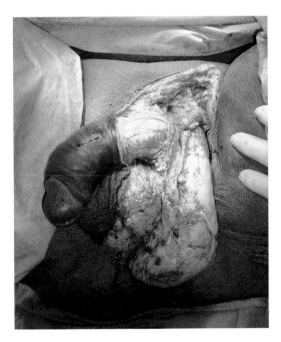

Figure 23.6. Aggressive debridement of Fournier's gangrene.

References

1. Delavierre D. Orchi-epididymitis. *Ann Urol (Paris)*. 2003;37(6):322-338
2. Gift TL, Owens CJ. The direct medical cost of epididymitis and orchitis: evidence from a study of insurance claims. *Sex Transm Dis*. 2006;33(10 Suppl):S84-S88
3. Dogra V, Bhatt S. Acute painful scrotum. *Radiol Clin North Am*. 2004;42(2):349-363
4. Luker GD, Siegel MJ. Color Doppler sonography of the scrotum in children. *AJR Am J Roentgenol*. 1994;163:649-655
5. Lee JC, Bhatt S, Dogra VS. Imaging of the epididymis. *Ultrasound Q*. 2008;24(1):3-16
6. Dogra VS, Gottlieb RH, Oka M, Rubens DJ. Sonography of the scrotum. *Radiology*. 2003;227:18-36
7. Masarani M, Wazait H, Dinneen M. Mumps orchitis. *J R Soc Med*. 2006;99(11):573-575

8. Abdelbaky AM, Channappa DB, Islam S. Unilateral epididymo-orchitis: a rare complication of MMR vaccine. *Ann R Coll Surg Engl*. 2008;90(4):336-337

9. Wise GJ, Shteynshlyuger A. An update on lower urinary tract tuberculosis. *Curr Urol Rep*. 2008;9(4):305-313

10. Oğuzkurt P, Tanyel FC, Büyükpamukçu N. Acute scrotum due to edidymo-orchitis associated with vasal anomalies in children with anorectal malformations. *J Pediatr Surg*. 1998;33(12):1834-1836

11. Noske HD, Kraus SW, Altinkilic BM, Weidner W. Historical milestones regarding torsion of the scrotal organs. *J Urol*. 1998;159:13-16

12. Schuppe HC, Meinhardt A, Allam JP, Bergmann M, Weidner W, Haidl G. Chronic orchitis: a neglected cause of male infertility? *Andrologia*. 2008;40(2):84-91

13. Vaidyanathan S, Hughes PL, Mansour P, Soni BM. Seminoma of testis masquerading as orchitis in an adult with paraplegia: proposed measures to avoid delay in diagnosing testicular tumours in spinal cord injury patients. *Sci World J*. 2008;8:149-156

14. Cook JL, Dewbury K. The changes seen on high-resolution ultrasound in orchitis. *Clin Radiol*. 2000;55: 13-18

15. Farriol VG, Comella XP, Agromayor EG, Creixams XS, Martinez De La Torre IB. Gray-scale and power Doppler sonographic appearances of acute inflammatory diseases of the scrotum. *J Clin Ultrasound*. 2000; 28:67-72

16. Horstman WG, Middleton WD, Melson GL. Scrotal inflammatory disease: color Doppler US findings. *Radiology*. 1991;179:55-59

17. Siegel MJ. The acute scrotum. *Radiol Clin North Am*. 1997;35:959-976

18. Tracy CR, Steers WD, Costabile R. Diagnosis and management of epididymitis. *Urol Clin North Am*. 2008;35(1):101-108

19. Collins MM, Stafford RS, O'Leary MP, et al. How common is prostatitis? A national survey of physician visits. *J Urol*. 1998;159:1224-1228

20. Moore CA, Lockett BL, Lennox KW, et al. Prednisone in the treatment of acute epididymitis: a cooperative study. *J Urol*. 1971;106:578-580

21. Tracy CR, Costabile RA. The evaluation and treatment of acute epididymitis in a large university based population: are CDC guidelines being followed? *World J Urol*. 2009;27(2):259-63

22. Tracy CR, Steers WD. Anatomy, physiology and diseases of the epididymis. *AUA Update Series* 2007; XXVI: lesson 12

23. Trei JS, Canas LC, Gould PL. Reproductive tract complications associated with *Chlamydia trachomatis* infection in US air force males within 4 years of testing. *Sex Transm Dis*. 2008;35(9):827-833

24. Nickel JC, Siemens DR, Nickel KR, Downey J. The patient with chronic epididymitis: characterization of an enigmatic syndrome. *J Urol*. 2002;167(4):1701-1704

25. Nickel JC, Teichman JM, Gregoire M, et al. Prevalence, diagnosis, characterization, and treatment of prostatitis, interstitial cystitis, and epididymitis in out patient urologic practice: the Canadian PIE study. *Urology*. 2005; 66:935-940

26. Heaton ND, Hogan B, Mitchell M, et al. Tuberculous epididymo-orchitis: clinical and ultrasound observations. *Br J Urol*. 1989;64:305-309

27. Pappas G, Akritidis N, Bostilkovski M, et al. Brucellosis. *N Engl J Med*. 2005;352:2325-2336

28. Ulbright TM, Amin MB, Young RH. Miscellaneous primary tumors of the testis, adnexa, and spermatic cord. In: Rosai J, Sobin LH, eds. *Atlas of Tumor Pathology, fasc 25, ser 3*. Washington, DC: Armed Forces Institute of Pathology; 1999:235-266

29. Ryan DM, Lesser BA, Crumley LA, et al. Epididymal sarcoidosis. *J Urol*. 1993;149(1):134-136

30. Cho YH, Lee KH, Band D, et al. Clinical features of patients with Behcet's disease and epididymitis. *J Urol*. 2003;170(4):1231-1233

31. Gasparich JP, Mason JT, Greene HL, et al. Amiodarone-associated epididymitis: drug-related epididymitis in the absence of infection. *J Urol*. 1985;133(6):971-972

32. Chiang IN, Chang SJ, Pu YS, Huang KH, Yu HJ, Huang CY. Major complications and associated risk factors of transrectal ultrasound guided prostate needle biopsy: a retrospective study of 1875 cases in Taiwan. *J Formos Med Assoc*. 2007;106(11):929-934

33. Somekh E, Gorenstein A, Serour F. Acute epididymitis in boys: evidence of a post-infectious etiology. *J Urol*. 2004;171(1):391-394

34. Lau P, Anderson PA, Giacomantonio JM, et al. Acute epididymitis in boys: are antibiotics indicated? *Br J Urol*. 1997;79:797-800

35. Huang LH, Yeung CY, Shyur SD, et al. Diagnosis of Henoch-Schonlein purpura by sonography and nuclear scanning in a child presenting with bilateral acute scrotum. *J Microbiol Immunol Infect*. 2004;37:192-195

36. Tracy CR, Costabile RA. The changing face of epididymitis from 1965 to 2005 [Abstract presentation, 53rd James C. Kimbrough Urological Seminar]

37. Hoppner W, Strohmeyer T, Hartmann M, Lopez-Gamarra D, et al. Surgical treatment of acute epididymitis and its underlying diseases. *Eur Urol*. 1992;22: 218-221

38. Jantos C, Baumgartner W, Durchfield B, et al. Experimental epididymitis due to *Chlamydia trachomatis* in rats. *Infect Immun*. 1992;60(6):2324-2328

39. Calleary JG, Masood J, Hill JT. Chronic epididymitis: is epididymectomy a valid surgical treatment? *Int J Androl*. 2009;32(5):468-72

40. Haidl G, Allam JP, Schuppe HC. Chronic epididymitis: impact on semen parameters and therapeutic options. *Andrologia*. 2008;40(2):92-96

41. Al-Taheini KM, Pike J, Leonard M. Acute epididymitis in children: the role of radiologic studies. *Urology*. 2008;71(5):826-829

42. Korkowski KA, Berman SM. Sexually transmitted diseases treatment guidelines, 2006. *MMWR Recomm Rep*. 2006;5(RR11):1-94. doi:www.cdc.gov/std/treatment

43. Berger RE, Alexander ER, Harnisch JP, et al. Etiology, manifestations, and therapy of acute epididymitis: prospective study of 50 cases. *J Urol*. 1979;121:750-754

44. Pearson RC, Baumber CD, McGhie D, et al. The relevance of *Chlamydia trachomatis* in acute epididymitis in young men. *Br J Urol*. 1988;62:72-75

45. Grant JF, Costello CB, Sequeira PJ, et al. The role of *Chlamydia trachomatis* in epididymitis. *Br J Urol.* 1987;60:355-359

46. Melekos M, Asbach H. Epididymitis: aspects concerning etiology and treatment. *J Urol.* 1987;138:83-86

47. Tracy R, Witmer MT, Costabile RA. The use of ultrasound in patients with clinical epididymitis in a university-based health care system. Poster presentation, 65th Annual Mid-Atlantic Section of AUA; October 18–21, 2008; Southampton, Bermuda

48. Burke BJ, Parker SH, Hopper KD, et al. The ultrasonographic appearance of coexistent epididymal and testicular sarcoidosis. *J Clin Ultrasound.* 1990;18:522-526

49. Suzuki Y, Koike H, Tamura G, et al. Ultrasonographic findings of epididymal sarcoidosis. *Urol Int.* 1994;52:228-230

50. Rudin L, Megalli M, Mesa-Tejada R. Genital sarcoidosis. *Urology.* 1974;3(6):750-754

51. Packel LJ, Guerry S, Bauer HM, et al. Patient-delivered partner therapy for chlamydial infections: attitudes and practices of California physicians and nurse practitioners. *Sex Transm Dis.* 2006;33(7):458-463

52. Davis BE, Noble MJ. Analysis and management of chronic orchalgia. *AUA Update Series 1992*; XI: lesson 2

53. Mittemeyer BT, Lennox KW, Borski AA. Epididymitis: a review of 610 cases. *J Urol.* 1966;95:390-392

54. Davis BE, Noble KJ, Weigel JW. Analysis and management of chronic testicular pain. *J Urol.* 1990;143:936

55. Chen TF, Ball RY. Epididymectomy for post-vasectomy pain: histological review. *BJU Int.* 1991;68:407

56. Padmore DE, Norman RW, Millard OH. Analyses of indications for and outcomes of epididymectomy. *J Urol.* 1996;156:95

57. Strom KH, Levine LA. Microsurgical denervation of the spermatic cord for chronic orchialgia: long-term results from a single center. *J Urol.* 2008;180(3):949-953

58. Arbuliev MG, Arbuliev KM, Gadzhiev DP, Abunimekh BKh. [Diagnosis and treatment of acute epididymoorchitis]. *Urologiia.* 2008;(3):49-52

59. Svetec DA, Waguespack RL, Sabanegh ES Jr. Intermittent azoospermia associated with epididymal sarcoidosis. *Fertil Steril.* 1998;70(4):777-779

60. Al-Ghazo MA, Bani-Hani KE, Amarin ZO. Tuberculous epididymitis and fertility in North Jordan. *Saudi Med J.* 2005;26(8):1212-1215

61. Hinzes JD, Winn RE. Tuberculosis of theurogenital tract. *Infectious diseases.* 2nd edition. Mosby: An Imprint of Elsevier; 2004:773-7

62. Solera J, Geijo P, Largo J, et al. Grupo de Estudio de Castilla-la Mancha de Enfermedades Infecciosas. A randomized, double-blind study to assess the optimal duration of doxycycline treatment for human brucellosis. *Clin Infect Dis.* 2004;39(12):1776-1782

63. Liu CC, Huang SP, Chou YH, et al. Clinical presentation of acute scrotum in young males. *Kaohsiung J Med Sci.* 2007;23(6):281-286

64. Ringdahl E, Teague L. Testicular torsion. *Am Fam Physician.* 2006;74(10):1739-1743

65. Williamson RC. Torsion of the testis and allied conditions. *Br J Surg.* 1976;63:465-476

66. Washowich L. Synchronous bilateral testicular torsion in an adult. *J Ultrasound Med.* 2001;20:933-935

67. Rabinowitz R. The importance of the cremasteric reflex in acute scrotal swelling in children. *J Urol.* 1984;132:89-90

68. Dogra V, Ledwidge ME, Winter TC III, Lee FT Jr. Bell-clapper deformity. *Am J Roentgenol.* 2003;180:1176-1177

69. Kapoor S. Testicular torsion: a race against time. *Int J Clin Pract.* 2008;62(5):821-827

70. Herbener TE. Ultrasound in the assessment of the acute scrotum. *J Clin Ultrasound.* 1996;24:405-421

71. Hayn MH, Herz DB, Bellinger MF, Schneck FX. Intermittent torsion of the spermatic cord portends an increased risk of acute testicular infarction. *J Urol.* 2008;180(4 Suppl):1729-1732

72. Eaton SH, Cendron MA, Estrada CR, et al. Intermittent testicular torsion: diagnostic features and management outcomes. *J Urol.* 2005;174(4 Pt2):1532-1535. discussion1535

73. Mor Y, Pinthus JH, Nadu A, et al. Testicular fixation following torsion of the spermatic cord-does it guarantee prevention of recurrent torsion events? *J Urol.* 2006;175(1):171-173; discussion 173-174

74. Backhouse K. Embryology of testicular descent and maldescent. *Urol Clin North Am.* 1982;9:315-325

75. Hawtrey CE. Assessment of acute scrotal symptoms and findings: a clinician's dilemma. *Urol Clin North Am.* 1998;25:715-723

76. Brown SM, Casillas VJ, Montalvo BM, Albores-Saavedra J. Intrauterine spermatic cord torsion in the newborn: sonographic and pathologic correlation. *Radiology.* 1990;177:755-757

77. Ahmed SJ, Kaplan GW, DeCambre ME. Perinatal testicular torsion: preoperative radiological findings and the argument for urgent surgical exploration. *J Pediatr Surg.* 2008;43(8):1563-1565

78. Kaye JD, Levitt SB, Friedman SC, Franco I, Gitlin J, Palmer LS. Neonatal torsion: a 14-years experience and proposed algorithm for management. *J Urol.* 2008;179(6): 2377-2383

79. Zilberman D, Inbar Y, Heyman Z, et al. Torsion of the cryptorchid testis–can it be salvaged? *J Urol.* 2006;175(6): 2287-2289

80. Dubinsky TJ, Chen P, Maklad N. Color-flow and power Doppler imaging of the testes. *World J Urol.* 1998;16:35-40

81. Lerner RM, Mevorach RA, Hulbert WC, Rabinowitz R. Color Doppler US in the evaluation of acute scrotal disease. *Radiology.* 1990;176:355-358

82. Luker GD, Siegel MJ. Scrotal US in pediatric patients: comparison of power and standard color Doppler US. *Radiology.* 1996;198:381-385

83. Watanabe Y, Nagayama M, Okumura A, et al. MR imaging of testicular torsion: features of testicular hemorrhagic necrosis and clinical outcomes. *J Magn Reson Imaging.* 2007;26(1):100-108

84. Rakha E, Puls F, Saidul I, Furness P. Torsion of the testicular appendix: importance of associated acute inflammation. *J Clin Pathol.* 2006;59(8):831-834

85. Skoglund RW, McRoberts JW, Ragde H. Torsion of testicular appendages: presentation of 43 new cases and a collective review. *J Urol.* 1970;104:598-600

86. Yang DM, Lim JW, Kim JE, Kim JH, Cho H. Torsed appendix testis: gray scale and color Doppler sonographic findings compared with normal appendix testis. *J Ultrasound Med.* 2005;24(1):87-91

87. Patriquin HB, Yazbeck S, Trinh B, et al. Testicular torsion in infants and children: diagnosis with Doppler sonography. *Radiology.* 1993;188:781-785

88. Mansbach JM, Forbes P, Peters C. Testicular torsion and risk factors for orchiectomy. *Arch Pediatr Adolesc Med.* 2005;159(12):1167-1171

89. Taskinen S, Taskinen M, Rintala R. Testicular torsion: orchiectomy or orchiopexy? *J Pediatr Urol.* 2008;4(3):210-213

90. Guerra LA, Wiesenthal J, Pike J, Leonard MP. Management of neonatal testicular torsion: which way to turn? *Can Urol Assoc J.* 2008;2(4):376-379

91. Al-Salem AH. Intrauterine testicular torsion: a surgical emergency. *J Pediatr Surg.* 2007;42(11):1887-1891

92. Arap MA, Vicentini FC, Cocuzza M, et al. Late hormonal levels, semen parameters, and presence of antisperm antibodies in patients treated for testicular torsion. *J Androl.* 2007;28(4):528-532

93. Elem B, Ranjan P. Impact of immunodeficiency virus (HIV) on Fournier's gangrene: observations in Zambia. *Ann R Coll Surg Engl.* 1995;77:283-286

94. Kabay S, Yucel M, Yaylak F, et al. The clinical features of Fournier's gangrene and the predictivity of the Fournier's gangrene severity index on the outcomes. *Int Urol Nephrol.* 2008;40(4):997-1004

95. Vick R, Carson CC III. Fournier's disease. *Urol Clin North Am.* 1999;26:841-849

96. Vaz I. Fournier gangrene. *Trop Doct.* 2006;36(4):203-204

97. Grinev MV, Soroka IV, Grinev KM. [Fournier's gangrene – a model of necrotizing fasciitis (clinical and pathogenetic aspects)]. *Urologiia.* November-December 2007;(6):69-73

98. Cakmak A, Genç V, Akyol C, Ayhan Kayaoğlu H, Hazinedaroğlu SM. Fournier's gangrene: is it scrotal gangrene? *Adv Ther.* 2008;25(10):1065-1074

99. Bhatnagar AM, Mohite PN, Suthar M. Fournier's Gangrene: a review of 110 cases for aetiology, predisposing conditions, microorganisms, and modalities for coverage of necrosed scrotum with bare testes. *NZ Med J.* 2008;121(1275):46-56

100. Ghnnam WM. Fournier's gangrene in Mansoura Egypt: a review of 74 cases. *J Postgrad Med.* 2008;54(2):106-109

101. Kuo CF, Wang WS, Lee CM, Liu CP, Tseng HK. Fournier's gangrene: 10-years experience in a medical center in northern Taiwan. *J Microbiol Immunol Infect.* 2007;40(6):500-506

102. Urdaneta Carruyo E, Méndez Parra A, Urdaneta Contreras AV. Fournier's gangrene current perspectives. *An Med Interna.* 2007;24(4):190-194

103. Gupta A, Dalela D, Sankhwar SN, et al. Bilateral testicular gangrene: does it occur in Fournier's gangrene? *Int Urol Nephrol.* 2007;39(3):913-915

104. Benizri E, Fabiani P, Migliori G, et al. Gangrene of the perineum. *Urology.* 1996;47:935-939

105. Loulergue P, Mahe V, Bougnoux ME, Poiree S, Hot A, Lortholary O. Fournier's gangrene due to *Candida glabrata. Med Mycol.* 2008;46(2):171-173

106. Dogra VS, Smeltzer JS, Poblette J. Sonographic diagnosis of Fournier's gangrene. *J Clin Ultrasound.* 1994;22:571-572

107. Levenson RB, Singh AK, Novelline RA. Fournier gangrene: role of imaging. *RadioGraphics.* 2008;28(2):519-528

108. Corcoran AT, Smaldone MC, Gibbons EP, Walsh TJ, Davies BJ. Validation of the Fournier's gangrene severity index in a large contemporary series. *J Urol.* 2008;180(3):944-948

109. Laor E, Palmer LS, Tolia BM, Reid RE, Winter HI. Outcome prediction in patients with Fournier's gangrene. *J Urol.* 1995;154(1):89-92

110. Gudaviciene D, Milonas D. Scrotal reconstruction using thigh pedicle flaps after scrotal skin avulsion. *Urol Int.* 2008;81(1):122-124

111. Ozturk E, Ozguc H, Yilmazlar T. The use of vacuum assisted closure therapy in the management of Fournier's gangrene. *Am J Surg.* 2009;197(5):660-5; discussion 665

112. Kavoussi PK, Bird ET. Repair of a scrotal wound defect after Fournier's gangrene: a novel approach. *Issues Urol.* 2007;19(2):75-77

24

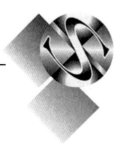

Nonbacterial Infections of the Genitourinary Tract

Ryan N. Fogg and Jack H. Mydlo

Fungal Infections

The presence of fungal infections in genitourinary organs has become a common occurrence with the continuing increase in immunocompromised populations, and improved critical care of the elderly. A variety of fungi, either opportunistic or pathogens endemic to a specific region, cause human disease. Thus, a working knowledge of the common fungal infections, their clinical manifestations, and an awareness of at-risk populations is essential to early diagnosis and aggressive treatment.

Several types of patients are particularly vulnerable to fungal infections. Patients in immunocompromised states such as transplant patients, AIDS, diabetes, malignancies, chemotherapy, and premature infants are more susceptible to opportunistic infections and are vulnerable to endemic fungal dissemination and invasion. Malnutrition such as with chronic alcoholics makes the patients less able to fight systemic infection. Prolonged antibiotic use creates an environment ideal for opportunistic fungal overgrowth. Finally, patients with indwelling invasive catheters including intravenous catheters, particular in patients receiving total parental nutrition (TPN), as well as with indwelling urinary catheters are at increased risk of colonization, infection, and potential dissemination of fungal organisms.[1] In the critical care setting, it is common for all three states to be present, accounting for their increased prevalence in this setting (Table 24.1).

Candidiasis

Candidiasis in the critical care setting comprises 10% of infections[2] increasing with prolonged ICU stay. Candiduria is often seen in patients with prolonged indwelling catheters and antibiotic use exceeding 12–14 days,[3] but its presence in the urine may represent colonization or active infection. The persistence of candiduria in populations at risk can disseminate into systemic invasive infections with mortality of 15–25%.[4] Most patients with candiduria will be asymptomatic[1], but some may present with frequency, urgency, dysuria, or hematuria. Active infections in the bladder typically cause mucosal edema, erythema, and white patches visible on cystoscopy, but may invade the bladder wall resulting in emphysematous cystitis and fungal balls or bezoars with resultant bladder obstruction or rupture.[5] Infection can spread by local extension, perforation, or hematogenously. Invasion into the prostate results in prostatic abscesses and emphysematous prostatitis.[6] In addition, epididymitis, while rare, has been reported.[7] Candidemia in the ICU setting is most commonly caused by hematogenous dissemination of candiduria.[8] Urologic manipulation of patients with candiduria has been demonstrated to cause candidemia. This is a serious sequela and must be aggressively treated as overall mortality approaches 40%.[9] Dissemination can progress to renal involvement by hematogenous spread or as an ascending infection with

Table 24.1. Risk factors for fungal infections

Prolonged urinary catheters

Central venous catheters

Total parental nutrition

Malignancy

HIV

Solid organ transplantation

Broad spectrum antibiotics

Diabetes mellitus

Chemotherapy

Corticosteroids

Neutropenia

Acute renal insufficiency

Hemodialysis

Prematurity

Severe pancreatitis

Gastrointestinal surgery

Ileal conduits

Alcohol abuse

Malnutrition

Cirrhosis

Intravenous drug abuse

resultant pyelonephritis, abscesses, papillary necrosis, renal failure, and obstructive uropathy by fungal bezoars. Patients may present with fevers, colicky flank pain, and pyuria.[5,10]

The diagnosis of candidiasis can be demonstrated in a number of ways. First, the patient population should be considered. In patients with immunocompromise and significant risk factors (See Table 24.1), especially in the ICU setting, a low threshold must be maintained to culture for *Candida sp.* Urine cultures are a mainstay of candiduria diagnosis, with colony counts greater than 10,000 generally considered positive for an active infection.[5] Blood cultures are an insensitive but specific measure of candidemia.[9] In addition to standard culture techniques, a number of immunoassays are available and in development for diagnosis including the latex agglutination assay, beta-glucan assay, Enzyme-Linked ImmunoSorbent Assay (ELISA),

and fluorescence in situ hybridization (FISH). Local availability will determine the most appropriate diagnostic method.

While *Candida albicans* has been the major organism of candidiasis, the emergence of non-albicans infections is becoming more prevalent. *Candida glabrata* has emerged as a common cause of candidiasis in elderly patients with underlying malignancies, *Candida tropicalis* is found in leukemia patients with neutropenia, and *Candida parapsilosis* is the most common cause of candidiasis among neonates.[9] This distinction is important as culture sensitivities are rarely performed in the hospital setting, and each species has unique spectrum of antifungal sensitivities.

Aspergillosis

Aspergilla is a ubiquitous fungus present in soil, vegetation, decaying vegetation, dust, spices, and potted plants. In humans, *Aspergillus fumigatus*, *A. flavus*, and *A. niger* are opportunists causing disease in immunocompromised host.[5,11] Infection typically begins in the respiratory tree, but may disseminate to extra pulmonary sites. The most common genitourinary manifestation is renal aspergillosis, occurring in 12% of disseminated infections. Less common are prostatic, testicular, and adrenal involvement.[12] Renal infection may occur by hematogenous spread or ascending infection. Patients may present with hematuria, fevers, or flank pain due to obstructive uropathy.[11] The sequelae of renal aspergillosis include pyelonephritis, renal abscesses, papillary necrosis, and obstruction by fungus balls or necrotic renal material (Fig. 24.1). Diagnosis is by urine or tissue demonstration of microscopic birfurcate hyphae.[13,14] Mortality is 40–90% necessitating prompt diagnosis and systemic treatment. Prostatic aspergillosis presents with lower urinary tract symptoms and outlet obstruction and is typically diagnosed on histologic analysis of prostatic resection. Aspergillosis epididymo-orchitis has been reported requiring orchiectomy.[5]

Cryptococcosis

Cryptococcus neoformans is an opportunistic fungus found in bird excreta, soil, and decaying matter. Cryptococcosis occurs in many

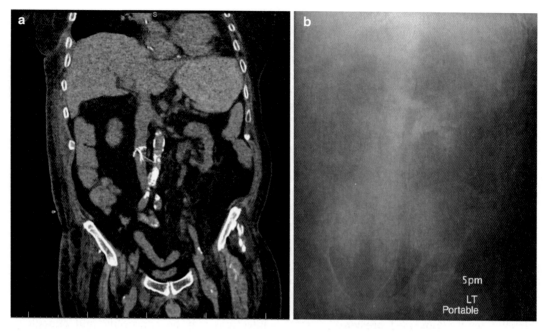

Figure 24.1. Renal aspergillosis. (**a**) Coronal non-contrast CT images of left hydronephrosis and pyelonephritis in 64-year-old male with renal aspergillosis after lung transplant. (**b**) Intraoperative retrograde pyelogram of same patient during stent placement with multiple filling defects.

immunocompromised states but particularly in the AIDS population. Beginning as a pulmonary infection, it can disseminate typically to the nervous system and beyond. Caseating adrenal necrosis with resulting insufficiency has been reported.[15] Renal involvement may be as high as 50% in disseminated cryptococcosis, causing a granulomatous pyelonephritis or renal abscesses with flank pain, fevers, hematuria, or pyuria on presentation. Prostatic involvement may be present in as many as one quarter of disseminated infections. Patients may be asymptomatic, present with prostatism or outlet obstruction and examination may mimic prostatitis or neoplasm.[11,16] Particularly in the AIDS era, the prostate has become a reservoir of infection even after the disseminated infection has been cleared, thus becoming a source of future systemic infections.[17] Penile lesions may occur in cryptococcosis, presenting as ulcers, pseudotumors, or necrotizing infections. Cryptococcal infections can be diagnosed by India ink stain, methenamine silver stain, as well as by serum antigen titers and latex agglutination tests.[11]

Blastomycosis

Blastostomyces dermatitidis is a fungus endemic to the Mississippi, Missouri and Ohio river basins, as well as moist soil near Lake Michigan. It begins as a self-limited pulmonary infection, but in immunocompromised populations it can disseminate into a systemic infections with genitourinary involvement reported in approximately 20% of patients. Most commonly, the prostate, epididymis, and testes are involved.[18] Clinical manifestations range from asymptomatic infection to epididymo-orchitis, irritative voiding symptoms, urinary retention, and prostatic abscesses.[19] Conjugal transmission from infected prostatic and spermatic secretions has been reported.[20] Diagnosis can be made by demonstration of the fungi in tissue, semen or urine by culture, serum blastomyces A antigen, and ELISA.[5]

Coccidioidomycosis

Coccidioides immitis is indigenous to the arid desert regions of western USA and Mexico, preferring hot, dry soil with high saline content.

The primary infection is pulmonary and mild, but rarely disseminated infections occur. Patients at risk for systemic infections include those with immunocompromised states, children younger than 5 years, and adults greater than 50 years old. Postmortem analysis of patients with disseminating infections revealed renal involvement in 35–60% of patients, 17–22% with adrenal infections, 4.6–6% with prostatic infections, 6% with retroperitoneal involvement, and 1–5% with scrotal infections.[21] Additionally, systemic allergic reactions can occur due to the high antigenicity, causing cutaneous manifestations similar to erythema nodosum.[11] Renal coccidioidomycosis presents as graunlomas or microabscesses and may radiographically resemble tuberculosis with renal calcifications, infundibular stenosis or "moth-eaten" calices.[22] Prostatic infections can present with hematuria, pyuria, and bladder outlet obstruction, and examination demonstrates a tender indurated prostate.[23] Scrotal manifestations can include abscesses, sinus tracts, and epididymal graunlomas.[21] Diagnosis can be made by culture of secretions, urine or tissue, as well as by coccidioidal compliment fixation antibody titers, and latex agglutination studies.[5,24,25]

Histoplasmosis

Histoplasma capsulatum has worldwide distribution with a predilection for the Mississippi and Ohio river valleys in soil infused with bird and bat excrement. Infection begins as a mild respiratory infection that can disseminate in the face of immunosuppression with spread to the liver, spleen, bone marrow, reticuloendothelial system, and genitourinary tract. Patients with disseminated infections may present with fever, cough, chest pain, weight loss, hepatosplenomegaly, and lymphadenopathy.[26] Genitourinary manifestations occur most commonly in the adrenal glands, with additional sites including the kidneys, testes, and prostate.[27] Adrenal involvement may result in insufficiency.[28] Patients may also present with renal abscesses, penile ulcers, prostatitis with prostatic abscess, or epididymitis. Diagnosis is made by demonstration of the organism in culture or tissue, Wright-Giemsa-stained blood smears, as well as by serum antigen levels, complement fixation, or immunodiffusion.[11]

Radiographic Findings

The radiographic findings associated with fungal infections of the genitourinary tract differ based on the organ of involvement, but overall have broad similarities that will be present despite the specific organism. Adrenal necrosis will appear heterogeneous and may present with enlargement, or calcification on CT scan. Renal abscesses may be present in the cortex or in the perinephric space seen best by contrast CT, MRI, or ultrasound. Fungus balls or sloughed papilla may be present at any point along the course of the upper tracts and bladder and typically appear as filling defects with or without hydronephrosis on intravenous pyelogram (IVP), CT, and ultrasound. Prostatic abscesses will be well visualized by CT or by transrectal ultrasound. Scrotal abscesses and epididymo-orchitis are well demonstrated by scrotal ultrasound. Overall, the radiographic findings associated with fungal infections may be nonspecific and difficult to distinguish from bacterial infections or malignancy, but must be combined with a low threshold of suspicion in those populations at risk, and with the variety of laboratory tests available diagnose the specific causative organisms.[5,10]

Treatment

Treatment of fungal infections of the genitourinary tract depends upon the specific organism in question as well as the site of infection (Table 24.2). Thus, treatment must be considered on an individual basis and typically with the assistance of the infectious disease specialists. Despite this, several important principles exist. Three classes of antifungal agents are available and include: Amphotericin B, generally considered the gold standard for disseminated fungal infections and may be administered parentally or by bladder irrigation; Fluconazole which may be given intravenously or orally though its effectiveness varies among organisms; and Caspofungin, an effective broad spectrum antifungal. Medication regimens may require different lengths and routes of administration. For example, disseminated infection generally requires systemic intravenous administration, and prostatic infection often requires extended periods of antifungal treatment spanning weeks to months. Antifungal infections often need to be combined with surgical

NONBACTERIAL INFECTIONS OF THE GENITOURINARY TRACT

Table 24.2. Treatment agents (Adapted from Bartlett[29])

Pathogen	Infection	Agent	Dose	Duration
Antifungals				
Candida[a]	Urinary[b]	Fluconazole	200 mg IV or PO	7–14 days
		Amphotericin B[c]	0.3–0.5 mg/kg/day IV	
			50 mg in IL sterile water at 42 cc/h bladder irrigation	5 days
	Systemic infections	Fluconazole	400–800 mg IV × 1 then PO	2 weeks[d]
		Amphotericin B	0.7–1 mg/kg/day IV	
		Caspofungin	70 mg IV daily then 50 mg IV daily	
Aspergillosis[e]		Amphotericin B	1–1.5 mg/kg/day IV	At least 10 weeks
		Voriconazole	6 mg/kg q 12 h × 1 day then 4 mg/kg IV q 12 h then 200 mg PO BID	
Cryptococcus		Amphotericin B + flucytosine then	0.7 mg/kg/day IV 100 mg/kg/day	2 weeks then
		Fluconazole	400 mg PO daily	For 8 more weeks
Blastomycosis		Itraconazole	200 mg PO BID	6–12 months
		Amphotericin B	0.7–1 mg/kg/day	6–12 weeks
Coccidioidomycosis		Itraconazole	200 mg PO BID	At least 1 year
		Fluconazole	400–800 mg daily	
		Amphotericin B	0.5–0.7 mg/kg/day IV	
Histoplasmosis		Itraconazole	200 mg PO BID	6–8 months
		Amphotericin B	0.7–1 mg/kg/day IV	10–12 weeks
Tuberculosis		Isoniazid	5 mg/kg PO daily	6–9 months
		+ Pyrazinamide	15–30 mg/kg PO daily	
		+ Rifampin	10 mg/kg PO daily	
		+ Ethambutol[f]	15–25 mg/kg PO daily	
		+ Vitamin B6	50 mg PO daily	
Schistosomiasis		Praziquantel	20 mg/kg PO BID	1 day
Filariasis		Albendazole	400 mg PO x 1	
		+ Ivermectin	150 μg/kg x1	
		Diethylcarbamazine[g]	2 mg/kg PO TID	2 weeks
Onchocerciasis		Ivermectin	150 μg/kg × 1	Semiannual × 2 years, then yearly

[a]Agents and doses listed are for *Candida albicans*. Other candida species will require consultation with infectious disease specialists for local sensitivities.
[b]Isolated asymptomatic candiduria does not generally require treatment.
[c]Dosages are for amphotericin B deoxycholate. Alternative formulations will require alternative dosage regimens.
[d]Treatment is for 2 weeks after the patient is afebrile and blood cultures are negative.
[e]Itraconazole or caspofungin can be used as alternative agents.
[f]Can discontinue ethambutol after 2 months if sensitivities permit.
[g]Patients with high microfilarial counts may have significant side effects and causes the mazzotti reaction in onchocerciasis.

intervention to promote complete clearance of all infection. Open or percutaneous drainage of abscesses, nephrectomy, adrenalectomy, transurethral resection of the prostate (TURP), orchiectomy and biopsies for tissue diagnosis are a few of the surgical interventions that might adjunct pharmacotherapy. In addition, patients with disseminated infections are often immunocompromised and critically ill with a multitude of comorbid conditions, this can further complicate management.[5,10]

Tuberculosis

The incidence of Tuberculosis (TB) has been on the rise since the introduction of HIV in the 1980s and persistence of other immunocompromised conditions, combined with increased immigration and the upsurge of drug resistant strains of TB.[30]

Tuberculosis typically manifests as pulmonary conditions, but can present in a multitude of ways at a variety of sites, giving it the title "The Great Mimic." Genitourinary TB makes up nearly 30% of all the extrapulmonary sites of manifestation.[31] The great variety of clinical symptoms, combined with the prevalence of immunocompromised states requires a thorough knowledge of the possible presentations of TB, as well as the presence of a high degree of suspicion, and a low threshold to culture.

Tuberculosis is caused by the aerobic organism *Mycobacterium tuberculosis*. This slow growing organism can exist within the host phagocyte, lying indolent for many years before reactivating during a time of host immunocompromise. TB is spread by human droplet exposure and Primary TB may present simply as a self-limited pneumonia-like illness. As the inflammatory process subsides and healing begins, fibrosis and calcification may result in scar formation or strictures.[10]

Populations at increased risk of manifesting genitourinary TB include patients with any condition that creates an immunosuppressed state. This includes patients with chronic renal failure, diabetics, HIV+ patients, particularly those with low CD4 counts, organ transplantation recipients receiving immunosuppressive therapies and IV drug abusers.[32] Recent immigrants and health care workers are also at risk.

Clinical Manifestations

The clinical manifestations of genitourinary TB are a vast and vague collection of symptoms that depend on the organ of involvement. TB can involve nearly all urologic organs as they course from the mid-abdomen to the pelvis and perineum (Table 24.3). Though it is often asymptomatic, it can present with constitutional symptoms (37%), hematuria (51%), irritative voiding symptoms (76%), and recurrent urinary tract infections (22%). Pulmonary manifestations may be absent in as many as 20–30% of patients.[33]

Genitourinary TB can spread hematogenously to the adrenal glands with abscess and necrosis of the adrenals results in the clinical manifestations of Addison's disease. Corticotrophin stimulation testing will confirm the diagnosis with a low response. In addition, bilateral adrenal calcifications may be present by radiographic analysis.[30]

Renal tuberculosis has also been shown to result from direct metastatic hematologic seeding of *M. tuberculosis* to the glomeruli. An acute, then chronic inflammatory reaction occurs resulting in granuloma formation and caseaous necrosis. This inflammation will spread to the renal medulla and papilla with resultant necrosis. Papillary sloughing can result in intermittent renal colic. As extension continues in the renal pelvis, ulceration and calcification with stone formation occur. Calyceal infundibular stenosis can occur in multiple calyces with resultant obstruction.[34] Renal and calyceal abscess can develop (Fig. 24.2).[35] Overall, renal function can be compromised by a combination of destruction of renal parenchyma and obstructive uropathy, resulting in elevated creatinine and renal failure in over 40% of patients.[30] Classic CT finding reveal renal punctuate or curvilinear calcifications, with concurrent deformation and blunting of calyces.[36]

Manifestations of TB in the ureters include inflammation and fibrosis with resultant stricture disease. Continuous or segmental strictures may be seen anywhere along the course of the ureter. Chronic inflammation at the ureteral orifices can result in a "golf hole" appearance, and resultant ureterocoele.[10]

Bladder involvement is typically a sequela of renal tuberculosis. It can be asymptomatic, but more commonly presents with irritative voiding

Table 24.3. Manifestations and treatment of Genitourinary TB

Organ	Clinical manifestation	Radiologic findings	Treatment
Kidney and renal pelvis	− Chronic hematuria/pyuria − Renal failure − Renal colic	− Renal calcifications − Caliectasia − Early calyceal blunting − Late "moth- eaten" appearance − Calyceal infundibular stenosis	− Chemotherapy − Abscess drainage − Partial nephrectomy − Calico/pyelo reconstruction, diversion or excision
Adrenal	− Adrenal insufficiency and no or dampened response to corticotrophin	− Bilateral adrenal calcifications	Cortisol replacement and chemotherapy
Ureter	− Renal colic − Chronic sterile pyuria − Chronic hematuria − Hydronephrosis − Strictures − Renal Failure	− Ureteral narrowing +/− renal calcifications or abscess − Ureterocoele	− Chemotherapy − Removal of obstruction by stenting or PCN − Treatment of renal manifestations
Bladder	− Chronic cystitis − LUTS − Concurrent *Escherichia.coli* UTI's − Pyuria/microhematuria w/ acidic urine − Erythema/bullous edema − Mucosal ulcers/erosions − Mucosal fibrosis	− Contracted bladder − Irregular bladder shape − "Thimble bladder"	− Chemotherapy − Treatment of upper tract abscesses or obstruction
Prostate	− Prostatits − Nodular, fixed, or firm prostate − Elevate PSA	− Calcifications in prostate − Cavitary lesion on MRI	− Chemotherapy − Drainage of absesses
Urethra	− Ulcerative urethritis − Strictures − "Beefy red" mucosa − "Golf hole" prostatic ducts	− "Cyst-like" lesions in prostatic urethra	− Chemotherapy − Endoscopic excision or urethroplasty
Penis	− Indurated tuberculids − Ulcers	− Cavernosal abscess	− Chemotherapy − Biopsy to rule out cancer

(continued)

Table 24.3. (continued)

Organ	Clinical manifestation	Radiologic findings	Treatment
Scrotum	– Granulomatous epididymitis	– Enlarged, heterogeneous epididymis	– Long term (2 years)
			– Chemotherapy
			– Abscess drainage
	– Painful scrotal mass	– Epididymal mass with possible cord extension	– Orchiectomy
Reproductive organs	– Infertility	– Calcifications and thickening of epididymis, seminal vesicles, or vas deferens	– Chemotherapy
	– Epididymal or ejaculatory duct stenosis/ obstruction		– ICSI
			– Microsurgical repair/ excision of obstructed ducts

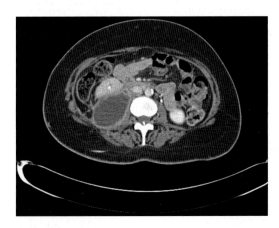

Figure 24.2. Renal tuberculosis. CT scan demonstrating right perinephric abscess in 40-year-old female with multiple sclerosis and renal tuberculosis.

symptoms of urgency, frequency, and microhematuria. A low threshold of suspicion should be applied to patients with chronic cystitis, microhematuria, and sterile pyuria with acidic urine.[30] TB can coexist with a concurrent *Escherichia coli* UTI,[34] but will be resistant to typical antimicrobials. Cystoscopic evaluation will often reveal inflammation with erythema bullous edema surrounding the ureteral orifice resulting in meatal stenosis and hydroureter or ureterocoele. Mucosal ulcerations may develop, and long-term fibrosis results in a contracted, irregularly shaped bladder often termed a "thimble bladder."[35] Bladder capacities will be severely diminished and may be as low as 100–200cc's, Biopsy will reveal caseating granulomas that will help clinch the diagnosis.[30]

Penile tuberculosis, though rare, has been associated with transmission though direct or sexual contact. Patients typically present with tuberculids, or small areas of induration with possible ulceration on the glans of the penis. These lesions are indistinguishable from cancer or syphilis, but histologic analysis may reveal caseating graunlomas.[37] Infection of the cavernosa can occur with penile thickening or abscess formation that may result in peyronie's curvature, loss of erectile function due to fibrosis, and decreased elasticity of the tunica albuginea.[38]

Chronic granulomatous prostatitis is theorized to be spread by hematogenous route. Patients often present with a nodular fixed prostate on rectal examination and elevated prostate specific antigen (PSA). Both parameters will improve after treatment by antituberculin medications. Clinically indistinguishable from, and can coexist with, cancer of the prostate, it can be diagnosed by prostate biopsy or TURP. Tuberculin prostatitis is usually asymptomatic, and can be found in nearly 15% of prostatic specimens of tuberculosis patients. In addition, "golf hole" dilation of the prostatic ducts can be seen on urethroscopy.[33]

Scrotal transmission of TB is thought to spread by hematologic, lymphatic, retrourethral, or by direct contact or extension.[39] Clinical manifestations typically include a painful scrotal mass, with involvement of the epididymis. Epididymal infections occur by hematogenous transmission, beginning at the richest source of epididymal blood supply, the globus minor. Epididymal infection can spread by direct extension to the testicles. Biopsies reveal acid-fast bacteria and caseating granulomas of the tunica vaginalis and testes.[30,33]

Genitourinary tuberculosis can present as male infertility with obstructive azoospermia from fibrosis and scarring of the epididymal and ejaculatory ducts, or leukocytospermia. Physical examination will reveal hardened prostatic nodules, epididymal dilation, and thickened seminal vesicles.

The intravesical administration of the inactive bacilli Calmette-Guerin tuberculosis strain for superficial bladder cancer is most commonly associated with local, mild side effects. Systemic sepsis is a rare complication of this common treatment, characterized by fevers, rigors, hypotension, mental status changes, coagulopathy, and acute lung injury. This serious side effect has significant morbidity and mortality and requires aggressive antituberculin therapy.[40]

Diagnosis

While TB's manifestations are often vague and nonspecific, the clinical genitourinary clinical manifestations will be resistant to standard methods of treatment and antimicrobial therapies.

Diagnosis often starts with a cutaneous purified protein derivative (PPD) skin test, with the injection of purified protein derivative. Results must be interpreted cautiously, as a false-positive is seen in patients previously vaccinated against TB, and false-negatives can be seen with severely blunted immune responses.[30]

The diagnosis of TB can often be made from urine analysis and culture. Initially, pyuria with acidic urine and the absence of typical pathogens with urine culture should prompt special cultures for tuberculosis. These take as long as 8 weeks in a specific culture medium.[32] In addition, drained abscess or tissue cultures may reveal tuberculosis.

Histologic specimens may retrospectively cinch the diagnosis with the presence of acid-fast bacilli as well as caseating granulomas or Langhans giant cells.[30]

Radiographic findings, while generally nonspecific, can suggest the diagnosis of genitourinary TB. CT remains the most accurate method of delineating gross abnormalities commonly seen with tuberculosis.[36] Classically, CT will reveal the presence of renal or caliceal abscesses, blunted calyces, infundibular stenosis, renal curvilinear or punctate calcifications, ureteral stricture, and calcifications or abscesses of the vas deferens, prostate, or seminal vesicles.[41]

Ultrasound can be helpful when elucidating abnormalities in the prostate, seminal vesicles, or scrotum. Findings of calcifications, hypoechoic irregular testicular masses, irregular epididymal-testicular margins, hyperechogenicity of epididymis, and atrophy or swelling of the seminal vesicles are suggestive of TB.[42]

Recently, molecular techniques have been making advances in rapid, specific diagnosis of tuberculosis. Polymerase chain reaction has a demonstrated 94% sensitivity in known TB positive patients.[32]

Treatment

Antituberculosis chemotherapy is the mainstay of all genitourinary tuberculosis (Table 24.2). Recently, an increase in resistant strains of TB, as well as the long duration of chemotherapeutic regimens necessitate aggressive treatment and active follow-up with patient reinforcement and counseling and often directly observed administration. Initially, the patient is treated for 2 months with a four drug combination of isoniazid, pyrazinamide, rifampin, and ethambutol. At the confirmation of culture sensitive lack of resistance, ethambutol may be discontinued. Liver enzymes must be closely monitored during therapy. Patients must be advised to refrain from unprotected sexual activity for 4–6 weeks during initial treatment, due to the risks of sexual transmission of tuberculosis. Completion therapy must be continued for a total of 6–9 months.[33]

In addition to chemotherapeutic regimens, aggressive drainage of all abscesses, debridement of infected tissue, and diversion in the presence of urinary obstruction, many of the long-term sequelae of genitourinary TB require definitive surgical management. Ureteral stricture might require reimplantation, boari flap, or ileal interposition to relieve obstruction. Bladder contractures can be augmented. Urethral strictures may be treated by endoscopic incision or urethroplasty. Seminal vesicle tuberculosis may require abscess drainage, while scrotal tuberculosis can necessitate epididymectomy or orchiectomy.[33] Infertility due to obstruction might be relieved by microsurgical vasovasostomy or vasoepididymostomy. In advanced cases, testicular biopsy with sperm extraction and intracytoplasmic sperm injection (ICSI) can restore fertile potential.[43]

Schistosomiasis

Urinary schistosomiasis is caused by the blood trematode *Schistosoma haematobium*. It is endemic to areas of the Middle East and most of Africa with 90 million infected worldwide, and has become more prevalent in the USA with the increased international travel.[10]

The life cycle of *S. haematobium* in the human host begins with the deposition of ciliated larvae into fresh water from eggs excreted through urine and feces of infected human hosts. The larvae use an intermediate host, *Bulinus* snails, to produce cercariae in freshwater which, using vibratory locomotion, penetrate the unbroken skin of human hosts to become a schistosomulum. Following maturation of 80–110 days, the schistosomulum microembolize to the liver and lung before settling into the pelvic and perivesical venous plexus where paired male and female worms now their adult size of 1.5 cm adhere to the endothelial lining of veins and begin to release eggs into the blood stream. These eggs are ovoid, distinctly terminally spined, and 80–150 μm in length. Twenty percent of these eggs will cross directly into the bladder or rectum where they will be excreted to continue the cycle of infection. The presence of terminally spined eggs in the urine or feces is the gold standard for the diagnosis of schistosomiasis. Adult worms have a typical life span of 3–6 years, but have been demonstrated to live up to 3 decades, and may release as many as 100 eggs per pair daily. During active infection, eggs of all stages are excreted, but in active or cured infections, only degenerated eggs will be excreted.[10,44]

Clinical Manifestations

The clinical sequelae of schistosomiasis come from the eggs which cause significant cellular and humoral host responses that result in the granulomatous encasement of eggs.[45] This inflammatory reaction results in the presence of hyperemic, large, bulky polyps surrounding localized areas of large egg burden within host tissue.[46] As the eggs are destroyed and urinary excretion of eggs ceases, calcification and fibrosis occurs resulting in tan colored flat mucosal lesions, known as the "sandy patches" that characterize chronic schistosomiasis.[10] Patients may be asymptomatic, or present dysuria, hematuria, frequency, colic, incontinence, retention, and stones (Lehman 1973).

Obstructive uropathy is also a long-term sequelae of urinary schistosomiasis. Hydroureter usually precedes hydronephrosis and is typically bilaterally asymmetrical (Lehman 1973). As the obstructive uropathy progresses and ascends to hydronephrosis, long-term dilation leads to atrophy and finally renal failure (Lehman 1973).

Chronic urinary schistosomiasis also produces bladder hyperplasia, metaplasia, dysplasia, and eventually cancer. Metaplasia and dysplasia are usually associated with bladder cancer caused by the chronic inflammatory state. Squamous cell carcinomas make up 50–90% of bladder cancer lesions, with adenocarcinoma accounting for 5–15%. Most are exophytic, but 25% can be endophytic and ulcerative. They tend to occur most frequently on the posterior and lateral walls, typically sparing the trigone.[47] Unlike other squamous cell carcinomas, those associated with schistosomiasis tend to be well differentiated, have a good prognosis, and have low metastatic potential.[45]

In addition to malignant sequelae, the bladder can develop painful ulcers with the sloughing of necrotic papules. More common with chronic schistosomiasis, patients may present with suprapubic or pelvic pain and dysuria.[47] During the very late stages of the disease process, the detrusor can become indurated and thicken, markedly reducing bladder capacity causing the patient abdominal pain and voiding dysfunction. As with bladder cancers, the trigonal region is typically spared.[10]

S. haematobium eggs can invade epididymal structures and ejaculatory ducts, and blood and eggs may be present in the ejaculate even before the urine. A painful scrotal mass may be mistaken for cancer and only discovered after orchiectomy. Women with schistosomiasis may manifest eggs on routine Papanicolaou smear due to asymptomatic cervicitis or vaginitis.[45]

Patients with urinary schistosomiasis may also have concurrent superinfections with a variety of pathogens. In endemic regions, chronic infections with *Salmonella* commonly recur and are resistant to antimicrobial therapy alone (Lehman 1973).

Diagnosis

The diagnosis of schistosomiasis requires a high index of suspicion. Information elicited during the history may increase suspicion for schistosomiasis, such as time spent in or near those regions where the trematode is endemic. Typically, patients require chronic exposure to water, but recent travelers may be more likely to present with acute symptoms.

The gold standard to diagnose schistosomiasis is the demonstration of terminally spined eggs in urine sediment. Egg excretion is highest midday, and the proportion of eggs excreted in the urine is an indication of overall egg burden. Eggs may also be demonstrated on pathologic specimens from bladder biopsy (Fig. 24.3b), which may be necessary in latent infections where active eggs are no longer being excreted in the urine. The schistosomiasis eggs also invade rectal tissue, thus when negative urinalysis necessitates the need for pathologic diagnosis, rectal biopsies might be preferential and less invasive.[10,47] Western blot assays are available, and have a high sensitivity and specificity, but do not differentiate between acute and chronic infections, but this method can make the diagnosis in cases with low egg excretion.[48]

The long-term sequelae of schistosomiasis may be very apparent on x-ray of the kidneys, ureter, bladder (KUB). The presence of rim of calcified bladder resembling a fetal head is pathognomonic for urinary schistosomiasis (Fig. 24.3). In addition, calcifications may also be seen in the wall of the distal ureters, prostate and seminal vesicles, posterior urethra, and even the colon. CT will demonstrate these calcifications with or without concurrent obstructive uropathy.[49] Ultrasound reveals a thick walled, calcified bladder, while voiding cystourethrogram (VCUG) may show vesicoureteral reflux, which can be present in as many as 25% of ureteral infections.[10]

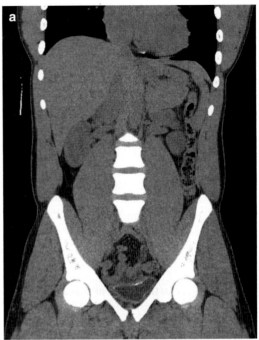

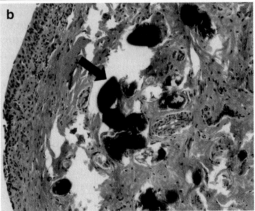

Figure 24.3. Schistosomiasis. (a) Coronal non-contrast CT images demonstrating bladder calcifications in 20-year-old African student with hematuria and schistosomiasis. (b) Histologic demonstration of fibrosis and terminally spined eggs in bladder biopsy.

Treatment

The mainstay of treatment of urinary schistosomiasis is medical treatment with Praziquantel (Table 24.2). Generally well tolerated, it produces cure rates approaching 100%. Many of the clinical manifestations respond to medical therapy alone including obstructive uropathy caused by polypoid lesions, with marked improvement in obstruction and resulting renal impairment in about 2 weeks. For this reason, surgical intervention should be withheld until after the initiation of medical therapy and applied only to those sequelae resistant to medication, or those requiring acute intervention such as severe hematuria.[10,44]

Thus, surgical intervention must be applied on a case by case basis with consideration for the specific resistant clinical manifestations caused by schistosomiasis. Persistent obstructive uropathy, for example, has been shown to respond well to balloon dilation, but with distal ureteral involvement, techniques such as the Leadbetter-Politano reconstruction may be necessary.[46] Deep bladder ulcers tend to be resistant to fulguration, and partial cystectomy might provide more definitive resolution. Contracted bladders might necessitate augmentation or diversion to provide symptomatic relief.[10] Bladder cancer is treated and monitored with standard resection techniques.

Filariasis

Filariasis is a classification of diseases caused by one of three nematode parasites. While *Wuchereria bancrofti* cause 90% of human lymphatic filarial illness, other organisms such as *Brugia malayi*, of Southeast Asia and the Pacific Isilands, and *Brugia timori* may also be the culprit. The life cycle of these parasites depend upon mosquito vectors that breed in pools of polluted, stagnant water in endemic areas spanning 76 countries, with 40% of the cases occurring in India, affecting over 120 million people worldwide.[50] The larvae dwell in the salivary glands of their mosquito vectors and traverse the bite site, conjunctival or buccal mucosal barriers of their human hosts. From there, adult worms migrate into lymphatic vessels. *W. bancrofti* remains in the central, inguinal, or scrotal channels, while *W. malayi* navigates toward inguinal or distal lymphatics. The female worm will then secrete microfilaria into the lymphatics and blood stream maintaining a constant level. Both cellular and humoral immune responses, likely to dead or dying worms cause local inflammatory and granulomatous responses that damage and obstruct local lymphatic channels.

Clinical Manifestations

Early filarial infection may be asymptomatic, or present with "filarial fever," a clinical syndrome characterized by episodic fever, transient edema, hydroceles, and lymphangitis/lymphadenitis or dermatolymphangioadenitis with cutaneous plaque-like lesions with associated ascending lymphangitis and local adenitis. In contrast, patients may also present with local distinct well-circumscribed nodular areas of local lymphadenitis and lymphangitis with a centrifugal pattern of spread. These may manifest in the nematode's preferred lymphatic distribution or their nesting areas causing "sterile" abscess, funiculoepididymitis or orchitis. Funiculoepididymits causes testicular pain with local edema, hydrocele, and palpable cord-like swelling with possible pampiniform thrombosis. These findings may simulate malignancy, and histological specimen at orchiectomy shows marked eosinophilia and may reveal adult worms. This may resolve spontaneously, or may progress or worsen chronic lymphoedema. These patients will likely not have detectable microfilaremia. As the local inflammation resolves, the local area will be replaced by scar tissue, causing local lymphatic obstruction which initially will be compensated for by local lymphatic collaterals that with repeated chronic infection will further obstruct worsening lymphedema.[10,51]

The most common sequelae of chronic infection are hydroceles. The hydroceles of filariasis present with a milky fluid, often sediment rich and gross specimens may be distinctive with calcium or cholesterol deposits in a fibrous, thick tunica vaginalis. Chronic infections also lead to lymphedema and elephantiasis as the superficial lymphatics obstruct. Secondary bacterial superinfection is a major contributing factor to the worsening and development of severe lymphedema and elephantiasis.[52] As the deep lymphatics obstruct, they rupture spilling chylous fluid into urinary tract resulting in chyluria, the peritoneum causing chylous ascites or into the tunica vaginalis with chylocele.[53]

Diagnosis

The diagnosis of filariasis begins with a thorough history and physical. Transmission of filariasis requires long-term repeated exposure, so patients will have a history of living in endemic areas as well as any of the classical physical findings discussed above. Blood samples may demonstrate microfilaremia, but must be drawn at midnight, the peak of microfilaria release. Histologic specimens that demonstrate adult worms surrounded by graunlomas are definitive, but insensitive.[10] A variety of immunoassays are available including ELISA, the ICT filarial antigen test, antifilarial IgG4 antibody levels, filarial acetylcholinesterase levels, and PCR[51] Choice of methodology will likely be dictated by which resources are available to the diagnosing physician. Finally, suspected filarial diagnosis can be confirmed by ultrasound which demonstrates the "filarial dance sign" with visualization of motile scrotal worms. This may be seen even in otherwise asymptomatic individuals.[54]

Treatment

On an individual level, chemotherapy is the mainstay of treatment (Table 24.2). Several treatment regimens are currently utilized, but currently a single dose of albendazole in combination with either diethylcarbamazine or ivermectin are effective at eradicating microfilaremia.[51,55] Patients must be counseled regarding significant side effects with the use of diethylcarbamazine such as fevers, arthralgias, headache, nausea, and vomiting. This is related to worm death and will be more severe in patients with large worm burdens.[52] In addition to standard chemotherapy regimens, recent study has used concurrent regimens of doxycycline to target endosymbiants such as Wolbachia believed be essential to worm fertility.[56]

In addition to chemotherapy, the sequelae of filariasis such as lymphedema and elephantiasis can be reduced with the use of improved hygiene and antibacterial soaps,[57] as well as treatment of lymphatic and scrotal superinfections believed to be a major contributor to chronic filariasis.[58] Retrograde lymphangiography may be diagnostic and therapeutic. While demonstrating the severe lymphatic obstruction, the contrast material can sclerose lymphatic fistulas in nearly half of patients.[59] Surgical treatment of filariasis is aimed mainly at correcting the anatomic sequelae of filariasis by hydrocele repair or genital reconstruction.

Onchocerciasis

Onchocerciasis is a filarial disease caused by Onchocerca volvulus. Also known as "African River blindness," it affects 17 million people in areas of Africa, Latin America, and Yemen. It is transmitted by the Simulium ssp blackflies. Infected larvae are deposited in the subcutaneous tissue and mature to adult worms within a year, causing subcutaneous nodules. Throughout their 14-year lifespan, the worms release microfilarias, which cause a host inflammatory reaction that leads to the clinical manifestations of chronic dermatitis, skin atrophy, ocular inflammation and blindness, and inguinal lymphadenitis, and scrotal elephantiasis.[60,61] While both filarial diseases may present with elephantiasis and lymphedema, the distinction between onchocerciasis and lymphatic filariasis is important as diethylcarbamazine (Table 24.2), a mainstay of treatment for lymphatic filariasis, causes the Mazzotti reaction in onchocerciasis. This reaction is caused by a severe immune reaction to dead or dying worms characterized by fever, hypotension, tachycardia, adenitis, arthralgia, and pruritis.[62] Thus, Ivermectin is the primary chemotherapeutic agent used to treat onchocerciasis, and requires yearly treatments to maintain amicrofilaridermia. New studies have elucidated the role of endosymbiotic bacteria in the primary pathogenesis of, and severe treatment reactions of onchocerciasis. Wolbachia is a Rickettsia-like bacteria found in the hypodermis, oocytes, and microfilaria of O. Volvulus and appears essential to the fertility of the nematode. In addition, they have endotoxin-like effects that are thought to be one of the primary mechanisms behind the immunologic response behind the nematode's clinical manifestations. In patients treated with doxycycline to eradicate Wolbachia, the absence of microfilaridermia was persistent at 18 months, in contrast to ivermectin alone which allows the resurgence of microfilaridermia at as early as 4 months.[63] These findings may be the beginning of new treatment algorithms and a new understanding of filarial pathogenesis.

References

1. Kauffman CA, Vazquez J, Sobel J, et al. Prospective multicenter surveillance study of funguria in hospitalized patients. Clin Infect Dis. 2000;30:14-18

2. Zaoutis TE, Argon J, Chu J, et al. The epidemiology and attributable outcomes of candidemia in adults and children hospitalized in the United States: a propensity analysis. Clin Infect Dis. 2005;41:1232-1239

3. Hamory BH, Wenzel RP. Hospital associated candiduria: predisposing factors and review of the literature. J Urol. 1978;120:444-448

4. Pappas PG, Rex JH, Lee J, et al. A prospective observational study of candidemia: epidemiology, therapy, and influences on mortality in hospitalized adult and pediatric patients. *Clin Infect Dis.* 2003;37:634-643

5. Wise GJ, Talluri GS, Marella VK. Fungal infections of the genitourinary system: manifestations, diagnosis, and treatment. *Urol Clin N Am.* 1999;26:701-718

6. Lentino JR, Zielinski A, Stachowski M, et al. Prostatic abscesses due to candida albicans. *J Infect Dis.* 1984;149:282

7. Docimo SG, Kang J, Rukstalis D, et al. Candida epididymitis: newly recognized opportunistic epididymal infection. *Urology.* 1993;41:280-282

8. Nassoura Z, Ivatury RR, Stahl WM, et al. Candiduria as an early marker of disseminated infection in critically ill surgical patients. The role of fluconazole therapy. *J Trauma.* 1994;35:290-295

9. Pappas PG. Invasive candidiasis. *Infect Dis Clin N Am.* 2006;20:485-506

10. McAleer SJ, Johnson CW, Johnson WD Jr. In: Wein AJ, Kavoussi LR, et al, editors. Tuberculosis and Parasitic and Fungal infections of the Genitourinary systems. Campbell-Walsh Urology. 9th ed. Philadelphia, PA: W. B. Saunders; 2007. p. 436-470

11. Wise GJ, Silver D. Fungal infections of the genitourinary system. *J Urol.* 1993;148:1377-1388

12. Young RC, Bennett JR, Vogel CL, et al. Aspergillosis. The spectrum of disease in 98 patients. *Medicine.* 1970;49:147

13. Khan ZU, Gopalakrishnan G, Al-Awadi K, et al. Renal aspergilloma due to *Aspergillus flavus. Clin Infect Dis.* 1995;12:210-212

14. Bibler MR, Gianis JT. Acute ureteral colic from an obstructing renal aspergilloma. *Rev Infect Dis.* 1987;9:790-793

15. Shah B, Taylor HC, Pillay I, et al. Adrenal insufficiency due to cryptococcosis. *JAMA.* 1986;256:3247

16. Salyer WR, Salyer DC. Involvement of the kidney and prostate in cryptococcosis. *J Urol.* 1973;109:695

17. Larsen RA, Bozzette S, McCutchan JA, et al. Persistant *Cryptococcus neoformans* infection of the prostate after successful treatment of meningitis. California collaborative treatment group. *Ann Intern Med.* 1989;111:125

18. Eickenberg HU, Amin M, Lich R Jr. Blastomycosis of the genitourinary tract. *J Urol.* 1975;113:650

19. Bergner DM, Kraus SD, Duck GB, et al. Systemic blastomycosis presenting with acute prostatic abscess. *J Urol.* 1981;126:132

20. Craig MW, Davey WN, Green RA. Conjugal blastomycosis. *Am Rev Respir Dis.* 1970;102:86

21. Kuntze JR, Herman MH, Evans SG. Genitourinary coccidioidomycosis. *J Urol.* 1988;140:370

22. Conner WT, Drach GW, Bucher WC Jr. Genitourinary aspects of disseminated coccicioidomycosis. *J Urol.* 1975;113:82

23. Price MJ, Lewis EL, Carmalt JE. Coccidioidomycosis of the prostate gland. *Urology.* 1982;19:653

24. Einstein HE, Johnson RH. Coccidioidomycosis: new aspects of epidemiology and therapy. *Clin Infect Dis.* 1993;16:349-354

25. Sohail MR, Andrews PE, Blair J. Coccicioidomycosis of the male genital tract. *J Urol.* 2005;173: 1978-1982

26. Goodwin RA Jr, Shapiro JL, Thurman GH, et al. Disseminated histoplasmosis: clinical and pathologic correlations. *Medicine.* 1980;59:1

27. Rubin H, Furclow ML, Yates JL, et al. The course and prognosis of histoplasmosis. *Am J Med.* 1959;27:278

28. Wilson DA, Muchmore GH, Tisdal RG, et al. Histoplasmosis of the adrenal gland studied by CT. *Radiology.* 1984;150:779

29. Bartlett JG, John Hopkins antibiotic guide. http://prod. hopkins-abxguide.org/. Accessed March 9, 2009

30. Wise GJ, Marella V. Genitourinary manifestations of tuberculosis. *Urol Clin N Am.* 2003;30(1):111-121

31. Weinberg AC, Boyd SD. Short-course chemotherapy and the role of surgery in adult and pediatric genitourinary tuberculosis. *Urology.* 1988;31:95

32. Small PM, Fujiwara PI. Management of tuberculosis in the United States. *N Engl J Med.* 2001;345:189-200

33. Wise GJ, Shyteynshlyuger A. An update on lower urinary tract tuberculosis. *Curr Prostatic Rep.* 2007;5:87-95

34. Gow JG. The current management of patients with genitourinary tuberculosis. *AUA Update Ser.* 1992;26: 202-207

35. Carl P, Stark L. Indications for surgical management of genitourinary tuberculosis. *World J Surg.* 1997;21: 505-510

36. Premkumar A, Lattimer J, Newhouse JH. CT and sonography of advanced urinary tract tuberculosis. *Am J Rad.* 1987;148:65-69

37. Vijaikumar M, Thappa DM, Kaviarasan PK. Papulonecrotic tuberculide of the glans penis. *Sex Transm Infect.* 2001;77:147

38. Pal DK. Erectile failure and destruction of glans penis by tuberculosis. *Trop Doct.* 1997;27:178

39. Wolf JS Jr, McAninch JW. Tuberculous epididymo-orchitis: diagnosis by fine needle aspiration. *J Urol.* 1991;145:836-838

40. Koukol SC, DeHaven JI, Riggs DR, et al. Drug therapy of bacillus Calmette-Guerin sepsis. *Urol Res.* 1995;22: 373-376

41. Wang LJ, Wong YC, Chen CJ, Lim KE. CT features of genitourinary tuberculosis. *J Comput Assist Tomogr.* 1997;21:254-258

42. Chung JJ, Kim MJ, Lee T, et al. Sonographic findings in tuberculosis epididymitis and epididymo-orchitis. *J Clin Ultrasound.* 1997;25:390-394

43. Fraietta R, Mori MM, De Oliveira JM, et al. Tuberculosis of seminal vesicles as a cause of aspermia. *J Urol.* 2003;169:1472

44. Sheehan G, Sekla L, Harding GKM. Urinary schistosomiasis: a report of four cases and a review. *Can Med Assoc J.* 1984;131:1361-1364

45. Cheever A, Kuntz RE, Moore J, et al. Carcinoma of the urinary bladder in *Schistosoma haematobium* infection. *Am J Path.* 1976;84:673-676

46. Smith MD, Verroust PJ, Morel-Maroger L, et al. A study of the presence of circulating immune complexes in schistosomiasis. *Trans R Soc Trop Med Hyg.* 1977;71: 343-348

47. Smith JH, Kamel IA, Elwi A, et al. A quantitative post mortem analysis of urinary schistosomiasis in Egypt. Pathology and pathogenesis. *Am J Trop Med Hyg.* 1974;23:1054-1071

48. Tsang VC, Wilkins PP. Innumodiagnosis of schistosomiasis. *Immunol Invest.* 1997;26:175-188

49. Jorulf H, Lindstedt E. Urogenital schistosomiasis: CT evaluation. *Radiology.* 1985;157:745-749

50. Michael E, Bundy D. Global mapping of lymphatic filariasis. *Parasitol Today.* 1997;13:472-476

51. Melrose WD. Lymphatic filariasis: new insights into an old disease. *Int J Parasitol.* 2002;32:947-960

52. Dreyer G, Noroes J, Figueredo-Silva J, Piessens WF. Pathogenesis of lymphatic disease in bancroftian filariaisis: A clinical perspective. *Parasitol Today.* 2000;16:544-548

53. Iturregui-Pagan J, Fortuno R, Noy M. Genital manifestations of filariasis. *Urology.* 1976;8:207-209

54. Noroes J, Addiss D, Santos A, et al. Ultrasonic evidence of abnormal lymphatic vessels in young men with adult *Wuchereria bancrofti* infection in the scrotal area. *J Urol.* 1996;156:409-412

55. World Health Organization. Lymphatic filariasis. Fact sheet N 102. 2000. http://www.who.int/mediacentre/factsheets/fs102/en/. Accessed December 7, 2008

56. Hoerauf A. Filariasis: new drugs and new opportunities for lymphatic filariasis and onchocerciasis. *Curr Opin Infect Dis.* 2008;21:673-681

57. Maher D, Ottensen EA. The global lymphatic filariasis initiative. *Trop Doct.* 2000;30:179-9

58. Olszewski WL, Manokaran G, Pani S, et al. Bacteriologic studies of skin, tissue lymph, lymph and lymph nodes in patients with filarial lymphedema. *Am J Trop Med Hyg.* 1997;57:7-15

59. Gandhi GM, Shanker S. Thyroid lymphography. *Am J Surg.* 1976;131:563-565

60. Hoerauf A, Buttner DW, Adjei O, et al. Onchocerciasis. Clinical review. *BJM.* 2003;326:207-210

61. Plaisier AP, Van Oortmarssen GJ, Remme J, et al. The reproductive lifespan of Onchocerca volvulus in west African savanna. *Acta Trop.* 1991; 48:271-284

62. Francis H, Awadzi K, Ottesen EA. The Mazzotti reaction following treatment of onchocerciasis with diethylcarbamazine: clinical severity as a function of infection intensity. *Am J Trop Med Hyg.* 1985;34:529-536

63. Hoerauf A, Mand S, Adjei O, et al. Depletion of Wolbachia endobacteria in Onchocerca volvulus by doxycycline and microfilaridermia after ivermectin treatment. *Lancet.* 2001;357:1415-1416

64. Lehman JS Jr, Smith FZ, Bassily JH et al. Urinary Schistosomiasis in Egypt: clinical, radiological, bacteriological and parasitological correlations. *Am J Trop Med Hyg.* 1973; 67(3): 384-399

25

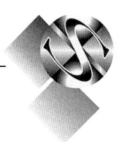

Sexually Transmitted Infections

Tara Lee Frenkl and Jeannette M. Potts

Introduction

The transmission of certain infectious diseases occurs most efficiently via contact of mucous membranes, and therefore, are commonly spread by sexual contact. Early lesions mainly occur on the genitalia and therefore the urologist is the first physician to assess a patient with a sexually transmitted infection (STI). Urologists play an important role in the detection, treatment, and prevention of STIs. If left untreated, STIs may have devastating local and systemic consequences.

CDC estimates that approximately 19 million new infections occur each year.[1] People at high risk for contracting sexually transmitted diseases are young adults between the ages of 15 and 24. Risk factors for contracting an STI include new or multiple sex partners, unprotected sex, illegal drug use, commercial sex work, and previous history of STI. Sexually transmitted infections also rank among the top five risks of international travelers.[2]

STIs Associated with Genital Ulcers

Genital herpes, syphilis, chancroid, and lymphogranuloma venereum (LGV) are often clinically characterized by the genital ulcer that is associated with them. Of these STIs, genital herpes is by far the most common followed by syphilis and chancroid. LGV is rare in the United States but still prevalent in parts of Africa, Asia, South America, and the Caribbean.[3]

The specificity for clinical diagnosis of genital ulcer disease is high (94–98%) but sensitivity is low (31–35%).[4] The differential diagnosis of genital ulcers includes conditions such as Behcet's syndrome, drug reactions, erythema multiforme, Crohn's disease, lichen planus, amebiasis, trauma, and carcinoma. If ulcers do not respond to therapy or appear unusual, a biopsy should be performed. The etiologic agent, classic description of the ulcer, associated lymphadenopathy, and CDC-recommended confirmatory tests are summarized in Table 25.1. CDC-recommended treatment guidelines and other important factors that the treating physician should consider are summarized in Tables 25.2 and 25.3.

Herpes Simplex Virus

Diagnosis

Herpes simplex virus type 2 (HSV-2) is the principle cause of genital herpes although HSV-1 now accounts for at least 50% of first episodes in the United States, Canada, and several European countries.[5] HSV-1 is responsible for common cold sores, but can be transmitted to the genitals through oral secretions during oral-genital sex. It is important to educate patients that asymptomatic viral shedding may account for more than 75% of viral transmission and is more likely during the 3–12 months period following initial clinical presentation.[6]

C.R. Chapple and W.D. Steers (eds.), *Practical Urology: Essential Principles and Practice*,
DOI: 10.1007/978-1-84882-034-0_25, © Springer-Verlag London Limited 2011

Table 25.1. STIs associated with genital ulcers: etiology, lesions, and diagnostic tests

Disease	Etiologic agent	Incubation period	Lesion	Inguinal lymphadenopathy	Diagnostic test
Genital herpes	HSV-2 (principle) HSV-1	1–26 days, usually short (~ 4 days)	Painful shallow, vesicles on an erythematous base, usually multiple	Bilateral, painful	Culture with viral subtyping or antigen test for HSV
Primary syphilis	*Treponema pallidum*	10–90 days	Painless, indurated, clean-based ulcer, usually singular	Bilateral, nontender, rubbery, nonsuppurating	Serology and either darkfield examination or direct immuno-fluorescence for *T. pallidum*
Chancroid	*Haemophilus ducreyi*	1–21 days	Painful, nonindu-rated, shaggy edged, purulent ulcer, single or multiple	Regional, painful, suppurating	Culture PCR assays
Lympho-granuloma venereum	*Chlamydia trachomatis* types L1, L2, and L3	3–30 days	Small painless vesicle or papule that progresses to an ulcer	Large, painful, matted, may ulcerate and develop fistulous tracts	Culture (posi-tive <50% of the time) or compliment-fixation or indirect-fluores-cence antibody titers

Table 25.2. STIs associated with genital ulcers: treatment and other considerations

Disease	Treatment of choice	Alternative treatment	Other considerations
Chancroid	Azithromycin 1 g po × 1 or Ceftriaxone 250 IM × 1	Ciprofloxacin 500 mg po BID × 3 days Erythromycin base 500 mg po TID × 7 days	1. HIV and syphilis screening at diagnosis and 3 months later if negative 2. Examine sexual partner in case of sexual relations within past 2 weeks or during eruption of ulcer
Syphilis primary, secondary or early latent	Benzthiazide Penicillin 2.4 million units IM × 1	Doxycycline 100 mg po BID × 14 days or tetracycline 500 mg QID x 14 days	1. Consider screening for HIV, Hepatitis B and C, gonorrhea, and chlamydia 2. Caution patient about Jarisch-Herxheimer reaction 3. Check nontreponemal anti-body titers at 6 and 12 months
Late latent or late latent of unknown duration	Benzthiazide Penicillin 2.4 million units IM q week × 3 doses	Doxycycline 100 mg po BID × 4 weeks	
Lymphogranuloma venereum	Doxycycline 100 mg po BID × 21 days	Erythromycin base 500 mg po QID × 21 days	1. Examine sexual partner and treat in case of sexual relations within 30 days 2. Inguinal buboes may require incision and drainage to prevent ulceration

Source: Adapted from Sexually Transmitted Diseases Guidelines 2010. MMWR 2010;59(RR-12):19-36.

Table 25.3. CDC-recommended oral treatment for genital herpes

Agent	First clinical episode	Episodic therapy	Suppressive therapy
Acyclovir	400 mg TID for 7–10 days or 200 mg five times per day for 7–10 days	400 mg TID × 5 days or 800 mg TID for 2 days or 800 mg BID for 5 days	400 mg BID
Famciclovir	250 mg TID for 7–10 days	125 mg BID for 5 days or 1000 mg BID x 1 day or 500 mg once, followed by 250 mg BID for 2 day	250 mg BID
Valacyclovir	1 g BID for 7–10 days	500 mg BID for 3 days or 1 g qd for 5 days	500 mg qd or 1 g qd

Source: Adapted from Sexually Transmitted Diseases Guidelines 2010. MMWR 2010;59(RR-12):21-2.

Primary infection manifests with painful ulcers of the genitalia or anus, and bilateral painful inguinal adenopathy. The initial infection is often associated with constitutional flu-like symptoms. A group of vesicles on an erythematous base that does not follow a neural distribution is pathognomonic for herpes simplex. Lesions may be present in the urethra. Sacral radiculomyelopathy is a rare manifestation of primary infection that has a greater association with primary anal HSV. Recurrent episodes are generally less severe than the primary infection and involve only ulceration of the genital or anal area. Genital lesions, especially urethral lesions, may cause transient urinary retention in women. Severe complications of herpes include pneumonitis, disseminated infection, hepatitis, meningitis, and encephalitis.

Diagnosis should be confirmed with laboratory verification because most patients present with atypical lesions. Women especially, may present with fissures, abrasions, or itching.[7] Viral subtyping is important for prognosis and counseling, as HSV-2 will have a greater number of recurrences within the first year than HSV-1. HSV-1 rarely recurs after the first year while the rate of HSV-2 recurrence decreases but slowly.[8] The use of cytologic detection of cellular changes of HSV infection (i.e., Tzanck preparation and Pap smears) is insensitive, nonspecific, and no longer recommended.

Viral culture is generally the preferred method of diagnosis because it is relatively inexpensive and highly specific. To obtain a specimen for viral culture, vesicles should be gently unroofed with a clean needle and then swabbed at the base of the lesion. The specimen should be placed directly into the viral culture media and transported quickly to the laboratory. The sensitivity ranges substantially depending on whether it is the primary infection or a recurrence, and the stage of the lesion. Viral load is highest when the lesion is vesicular and during primary infection. Therefore, viral culture has the highest sensitivity at these times and declines sharply as the lesion heals.

An alternative to viral culture is quantitative real-time polymerase chain reaction (PCR) for HSV DNA. Increasing evidence suggests that PCR is a faster and more sensitive diagnostic method, but its implementation has been limited by concerns over contamination and cost.[9,10]

Type-specific HSV serologic assays identify antibodies to HSV glycoproteins G-1 and G-2.[11] These tests may also be able to identify recently acquired versus established HSV infection based on antibody avidity.[12] They may be useful for patients with recurrent genital symptoms or atypical symptoms with negative HSV cultures; a clinical diagnosis of genital herpes without laboratory confirmation; or for patients with a partner with genital herpes.

Treatment

Oral antiviral therapies approved for treatment include oral acyclovir, valacyclovir, and famciclovir. Topical antiviral medications are not effective. Recurrences can be treated with an episodic or suppressive approach. When used for episodic treatment, treatment must be initiated during the prodrome or within 1 day of the onset of lesions. Daily suppressive therapy has been shown to prevent 80% of recurrences and is an option for patients who suffer from frequent

342

PRACTICAL UROLOGY: ESSENTIAL PRINCIPLES AND PRACTICE

recurrences. Recommended antiviral regimens are listed in Table 25.3.

Chancroid

Diagnosis

Chancroid, caused by *Haemophilus ducreyi*, is the most common STI worldwide, affecting men three times more often than women. The initial lesion at the site of inoculation is a vesicopustule that deteriorates to form a painful, soft ulcer with a friable base covered with a gray or yellow purulent exudate and a shaggy, undetermined border. It is associated with inguinal adenopathy that is typically unilateral, tender, and erythematous that may become fluctuant and fistulize. Four criteria should be considered to corroborate the diagnosis of chancroid: (1) presence of one or more painful ulcers, (2) presence of regional lymphadenopathy, (3) a negative *Treponema pallidum* evaluation or negative serologies at least 1 week after symptoms begin, and (4) a negative HSV culture from the ulcer exudate.[1] HIV and syphilis screening should be done at the time of diagnosis and 3 months after treatment if initially negative.

Culture for *Haemophilus ducreyi* is recommended by the CDC to confirm diagnosis, but requires special media that is not widely available. Gram-stain of a specimen from the undermined edge of the ulcer may identify the gram-negative streptobacilli. PCR assays, available through commercial agencies are sensitive and specific although no PCR test is currently FDA approved.

Treatment

Single-dose treatments consist of azithromycin 1 g orally or ceftriaxone 250 mg intramuscularly. Alternative regimens are listed in Table 25.2. Resistance to ciprofloxacin and erythromycin has been reported in some regions. Ciprofloxacin is contraindicated during pregnancy and lactation.

Subjective improvement should be noted within 3 days and ulcers generally heal completely in 1–2 weeks. Healing may be slower in uncircumcised men with ulcers below the foreskin and in patients with HIV.[13] Patients should be reexamined in 5–7 days and sexual partners should be examined and treated if sexual relations were held within the 2 weeks prior to or during the eruption of the ulcer. Symptomatic relief of inguinal tenderness can be provided by needle aspiration or incision and drainage of the buboes.

Syphilis

Diagnosis

Syphilis is caused by a spirochete, *Treponema pallidum*. Primary syphilis is characterized by a single painless, indurated ulcer that appears about 3 weeks after inoculation and persists for 4–6 weeks. The ulcer is usually found on the glans, corona, or perianal area on men and on the labial or anal area on women. It is often associated with bilateral, nontender inguinal or regional lymphadenopathy. Because the ulcer and adenopathy are painless and spontaneously heal, primary syphilis often goes undetected.

Latent syphilis is defined as seroreactivity with no clinical evidence of disease. Early latent syphilis is latent syphilis acquired within the past year. All other latent syphilis is either referred to as late latent syphilis or latent syphilis of unknown duration.

Secondary syphilis usually develops 4–10 weeks after the ulcer but may present as long as 2 years later. Secondary syphilis manifests with mucocutaneous, constitutional and parenchymal signs and symptoms. Early manifestations frequently include a generalized nontender lymphadenopathy and maculopapular rash on the trunk and arms. After several days or weeks, a papular rash may accompany the primary rash. These papular lesions, commonly seen on the palms and soles, are associated with endarteritis and may become necrotic and pustular. The papules may enlarge and erode to produce condyloma lata which are exceptionally infectious.

Approximately one-third of untreated patients will develop tertiary syphilis. It is very rare in industrialized countries, except for occasional cases reported in HIV patients. Aortitis, meningitis, uveitis, optic neuritis, general paresis, tabe dorsalis, and gummas of the skin and skeleton are just some of the sequalae associated with tertiary syphilis.

Neurosyphilis can occur at any stage of syphilis. Syphilitic uveitis or other ocular manifestations are frequently associated with neurosyphilis. A patient with clinical suggestion of neurologic involvement should have a cerebrospinal fluid examination.

Dark-field microscopy and direct fluorescent antibody (DFA) tests can be performed on specimens obtained from primary or secondary lesions.

Dark-field microscopy is not widely available, but DFA testing of a fixed smear from a lesion is available at many commercial laboratories. Nontreponemal serologic testing with rapid plasma reagin (RPR) or Venereal Disease Research Laboratory (VRDL) are the most common sensitive methods of screening.[14] All positive tests should be confirmed with treponemal testing using *T pallidum* particle agglutination (TP-PA) or florescent treponemal antibody absorbed (FTA-ABS). HIV can cause false-negative results by both treponemal and nontreponemal methods.[15,16]

Positive treponemal antibody tests usually remain positive for life and should not be used to assess response to therapy. Nontreponemal antibody titers, RPR and VDRL, correlate with disease activity. Disease activity should be followed with the same test at the same laboratory as the results are variable among laboratories and are not interchangeable. After treatment, a fourfold decrease in VDRL and RPR titers at 3 months, and an eightfold decrease at 6 months are expected.[17] These tests usually become negative 1 year after treatment.

The U.S. Preventive Services Task Force recommends that pregnant women and people who are at higher risk for syphilis undergo screening.[18] People at higher risk for syphilis include men who have sex with men and engage in high-risk sexual behavior, commercial sex workers, persons who exchange sex for drugs, and those in adult correctional facilities. The CDC recommends that testing for gonorrhea, chlamydia, HIV, hepatitis B and C be considered for all patients with syphilis.

Treatment

Benzthiazide penicillin G (2.4 million units intramuscularly as a single dose) remains the treatment of choice for primary, secondary and early latent syphilis. Other parental preparations or oral penicillin are not acceptable substitutes. Patients should be informed about the Jarisch-Herxheimer reaction, which consists of headache, myalgia, fever, tachycardia, and increased respiratory rate within the first 24 h after treatment with penicillin. Symptoms can usually be managed with bed rest and nonsteroidal anti-inflammatory agents. It may cause fetal distress and preterm labor in pregnant women. If the patient has penicillin allergy, doxycycline 100 mg by mouth twice daily or tetracycline 500 mg by mouth four times a day for 14 days are alternatives.

Late latent syphilis, latent syphilis of unknown duration, or tertiary syphilis, can be treated with benzthiazide penicillin injection repeated weekly for a total of three doses, or doxycycline therapy extended for a total of 4 weeks. In pregnancy, desensitization to penicillin is recommended if the patient has a penicillin allergy because doxycycline is contraindicated.

Neurosyphilis or ocular manifestations are treated with aqueous crystalline penicillin G, 3–4 million units IV every 4 h for 10–14 days; or penicillin G procaine, 2.4 million units IM once daily, plus probenecid, 500 mg orally four times daily, with both drugs given for 10–14 days. Probenecid cannot be used in patients with an allergy to sulfa. The CDC recommends consideration of treatment with benzathine penicillin, 2.4 million units intramuscularly once a week for 3 weeks after completion of the neurosyphilis treatment regimen to provide comparable total duration of therapy to that of late syphilis. Patients should be followed with nontreponemal antibody titers at 6 and 12 months. Patients with neurosyphilis require repeat examination of CSF fluid 3–6 months following therapy and every 6 months afterwards until normal results are observed.

Lymphogranuloma Venereum

Diagnosis

Lymphogranuloma venereum is caused by *Chlamydia trachomatis* types L1, L2, and L3, and is extremely rare in the United States. The initial manifestation is usually a single, painless ulcer on the penis, anus, or vulvovaginal area that goes unnoticed. Patients usually present with painful unilateral suppurating inguinal adenopathy and constitutional symptoms 2–6 weeks after resolution of the ulcer. Significant tissue injury and scarring may lead to labial fenestration, urethral destruction, anorectal fistulas, and elephantiasis of the penis, scrotum, or labia.

The diagnosis is mainly clinical and cultures are positive in only 30–50% of cases. Compliment-fixation or indirect-fluorescence antibody titers can confirm diagnosis. A compliment-fixation titer ≥64 is diagnostic of infection. Other causes of inguinal adenopathy should be excluded.

Treatment

Treatment for LGV is doxycycline 100 mg twice daily or erythromycin 500 mg four times daily for 3 weeks. Doxycycline is contraindicated in pregnant and lactating women. Patients should be followed clinically until symptoms resolve. Sexual partners should be examined, tested for urethral or cervical infection, and treated if sexual relations were held within 30 days of the onset of symptoms.

Aspiration or incision and drainage of buboes may be required to prevent femoral or inguinal ulcerations. Azithromycin, 1 g once a week for 3 weeks may be a potential alternative for treatment, but confirmatory data is insufficient.

STIs that Cause Urethritis, Epididymitis, and Cervicitis

In the setting of STI risk, epididymitis is usually caused by gonorrhea or chlamydia and patients present with a swollen painful scrotum. Palpation may reveal a tender prominent epididymis or a large tense mass that is erythematous, painful, and warm to touch.

The diagnosis of urethritis in men is suggested by mucopurulent urethral discharge with >5 WBC per oil immersion field or first void urine specimen with positive leukocyte esterase or >10 WBC per oil immersion field. Gonococcal urethritis can often be diagnosed by gram stain; however, a negative Gram stain in the setting of urethritis does not rule out gonorrhea.

Cervicitis is characterized by two major diagnostics signs: purulent or mucopurulent endocervical exudate and/or sustained endocervical bleeding that is easily provoked by swabbing the cervical os. Women may complain of post coital bleeding or abnormal vaginal discharge. The following sections will address the most common causes of cervicitis, urethritis, and epididymitis in patients with STI exposure. The etiologic agent, classic manifestations, and CDC-recommended diagnostic tests are summarized in Table 25.4. CDC-recommended treatment

Table 25.4. STIs associated with urethritis, epididymitis, and cervicitis: etiology, lesions, and diagnostic tests

Disease	Etiologic agent	Incubation period	Manifestation	Diagnostic test
Chlamydia	*Chlamydia trachomatis*, serotypes D-K	3–14 days	Majority asymptomatic Men: epididymitis, prostatitis, or urethritis with clear or white discharge Women: vaginal and pelvic discomfort, dysuria, or abnormal vaginal discharge	Endocervical (women) or intraurethral (men) for culture and sensitivity, NAAT, DFA, EIA, or unamplified nucleic acid hybridization If endocervical or intraurethral sample is not feasible, may perform NAAT of urine specimen
Gonorrhea	*Neisseria gonorrhoeae*	2–14 days	Many asymptomatic Men: epididymitis, prostatitis, proctitis, or urethritis with mucopurulent discharge Women: vaginal and pelvic discomfort, dysuria, or abnormal vaginal discharge	Endocervical (women) or intraurethral (men) for culture and sensitivity, NAAT or nucleic acid hybridization test If endocervical or intraurethral sample is not feasible, may perform NAAT of urine specimen
Trichomoniasis	*Trichomoniasis Vaginalis*	4–28 days	Majority asymptomatic Men: transient urethral discharge, urgency and dysuria Women: frothy green or white vaginal discharge, strawberry vulva or cervix, pruritis, erythema and edema, pH > 4.5	Wet mount of vaginal or urethral fluid in normal saline to visualize protozoa standard or commercially available culture kits DNA probes, antigen detection, and PCR available

guidelines and other important factors that the treating physician should consider are summarized in Table 25.5.

Chlamydia

Diagnosis

Chlamydia is caused by *Chlamydia trachomatis*, serotypes D through K. In 2009, it It was the most commonly reported disease to the CDC with over 1.2 million cases and is most prevalent in sexually active adolescents and young adults.[1] The majority of both of men and women are asymptomatic. *C. trachomatis* is the most common cause of epididymitis in young men. Men may also experience lower urinary-tract symptoms and notice a clear or white urethral discharge. Forty percent of women with untreated infection will develop pelvic inflammatory disease (PID) and scarring of the fallopian tubes.[19]

Selective screening has been shown to reduce the incidence of PID.[20] Women should be screened annually until age 25 or if risk factors

such as a new sexual partner are present. Screening tests that may be performed on an intraurethral swab in men or an endocervical swab in women include: (1) nucleic acid amplification test (NAAT), (2) unamplified nucleic acid hybridization test, an enzyme immunoassay (EIA), or direct fluorescent antibody (DFA), or (3) culture.[21] If the performance of a urethral or endocervical swab is not acceptable to the patient, NAAT may be performed on a urine specimen.

Treatment

Azithromycin 1 g by mouth as a single dose or doxycycline 100 mg twice daily for 7 days are equally effective. Alternative therapies are listed in Table 25.5. Doxycycline, erythromycin estolate, levofloxacin, and ofloxacin are contraindicated during pregnancy. Erythromycin base, erythromycin ethylsuccinate, and azithromycin are safe during pregnancy. Another alternative in pregnant women includes amoxicillin 500 mg three times per day for 7 days. Partners should be examined, tested, and treated. Patients should

Table 25.5. STIs Associated with urethritis, epididymitis, and cervicitis: treatment and other considerations

Disease	Treatment of choice	Alternative treatment	Other considerations
Chlamydia	Azithromycin 1 g po × 1 or Doxycycline 100 mg po BID × 7 days	Erythromycin base 500 mg po QID × 7 days or Erythromycin ethylsuccinate 800 mg QID × 7 days or Ofloxacin 300 mg BID or Levofloxacin 500 mg QD × 7 days	1. Women should be screened annually until age 25 or if risk factors present 2. Examine sexual partner and treat 3. Rescreen 3–4 months after treatment
Gonorrhea	Ceftriaxone 250 mg IM × 1 or Cefixime 400 mg po × 1	Ceftizoxime 500 mg IM × 1 or cefoxitin 2 g IM with probenecid 1 g po X1 or Cefotaxime 500 mg IM × 1 For penicillin or cephalosporin allergies Spectinomycin 2 g IM (not available in US) or Azithromycin 2 g po × 1 use should be limited, see text)	1. Women should only be screened if if risk factors present 2. All patients should be treated simultaneously for chlamydia unless chlamydia has been ruled out 3. Sexual partner within the past 60 days should be screened and treated 4. Clinicians and laboratories should report treatment failures or resistant gonococcal isolates to CDC
Trichomoniasis	Metronidazole 2 g po × 1 or Tinidazole 2 g po × 1	Metronidazole 500 mg po BID × 7 days	Examine and treat sexual partners

Source: Adapted from sexually transmitted diseases guidelines 2010. MMWR 2010;59(RR-12):44-55,59.

refrain from sexual intercourse until all parties' treatment is completed or 7 days after single-dose therapy. Reculture for cure is not needed for patients treated with doxycycline or a quinolone, but is recommended 3 weeks after treatment with erythromycin, in pregnant women, or for persistent symptoms. Patients with chlamydia are at high risk for reinfection and should be rescreened 3–4 months after treatment.

Gonorrhea

Diagnosis

Gonorrhea is caused by a gram-negative diplococcus, *Neisseria gonorrhoeae*. Men will usually experience lower urinary-tract symptoms attributed to urethritis, epididymitis, proctitis, or prostatitis, with associated mucopurulent urethral discharge. Women are most often asymptomatic, but may have symptoms of vaginal and pelvic discomfort, dysuria, or abnormal vaginal discharge. Both symptomatic and asymptomatic infections can lead to PID and its subsequent complications. Manifestations of gonococcal dissemination are rare today and include arthritis, dermatitis, meningitis, and endocarditis.

The United States Preventive Services Task Force recommends screenings for gonorrhea to those at increased risk for infection, including women with previous gonorrhea infection, or other STIs, new or multiple sex partners, inconsistent condom use, sex, and drug use; and for women in certain demographic groups and those living in high prevalence areas. Screening may be done by endocervical culture, or can be performed with newer screening tests, including NAAT and nucleic acid hybridization tests using vaginal, urethral (men only), or urine specimens.[33,34] The CDC recommends screening by culture on an endocervical swab specimen in women or an intraurethral swab in men. Culture and sensitivity are important to monitor antibiotic susceptibility and resistance. A positive Gram stain of diplococci on a male urethral swab is highly specific (99%) and sensitive (95%); however, a negative Gram stain does not rule out GC. Gram stain of secretions from the pharynx, cervix, or rectum is insufficient for diagnosis of GC and not recommended. If transport and storage conditions are not conducive to maintaining the viability of *N. gonorrhoeae*, a NAAT or nucleic acid hybridization test can be performed on an intraurethral or endocervical specimen, or on urine. Urine NAATs for *N. gonorrhoeae* have been shown to be less sensitive than endocervical and intraurethral swabs in asymptomatic men.[22]

Treatment

The recommended treatment for gonorrhea is ceftriaxone 250 mg intramuscularly as a single dose. It results in cure in approximately 99% of uncomplicated urogenital, anorectal and pharyngeal cases. An oral alternative is a single oral dose of cefixime 400 mg. Alternative single-dose parenteral agents for uncomplicated urogenital and anorectal gonorrhea are listed in Table 25.4. These agents may not be as effective for pharyngeal infection which often goes undiagnosed. A single 2 g dose of azithromycin is effective in uncomplicated infections, but is not recommended by the CDC because of increasing resistance. It may be an option for uncomplicated infections in patients with a documented severe allergy to penicillins or cephalosporins. Due to emerging resistance, the CDC no longer recommends quinolones for the treatment of GC in any population.[23] Patients infected with gonorrhea are often coinfected with C. trachomatis and should be treated simultaneously for both infections, unless chlamydial infection has been ruled out.

Recent sexual partner (past 60 days) should be evaluated and treated. Sexual activity should be avoided until both partners complete treatment and are symptom free. Persons with persistent symptoms or recurrence shortly after treatment should be re-evaluated by culture for *N. gonorrhoeae* and positive isolates should undergo antimicrobial-susceptibility testing. Clinicians and laboratories should report treatment failures or resistant gonococcal isolates to CDC at 404-639-8373 through state and local public health authorities.

Trichomoniasis

Diagnosis

Trichomoniasis is caused by *Trichomonas vaginalis*, a flagellated protozoan which can inhabit the vagina, urethra, Bartholian glands, Skene's glands, and prostate. It cannot infect the rectum or mouth. Nearly half of women, and most men with *T. vaginalis* infections are asymptomatic. In women, the signs and symptoms of trichomoniasis include vaginal discharge and itching, irritation, odor, edema, erythema, and dysuria. Frothy discharge occurs in about 10% of patients. Colpitis macularis (strawberry cervix) is a specific clinical sign but is rarely detected during routine examination. Men may have short-lived symptoms of urethral discharge, dysuria, and urinary urgency.

Wet mount of the vaginal fluid with normal saline (performed within 20 min of sample collection) or microscopic examination of first void urine sediment in men or women may show motile protozoa, which are one to four times the size of polymorphonuclear cells. The gold standard of diagnosis remains culture of vaginal or urethral swab or urine sediment. The specimens may remain at room temperature for up to 30 min before inoculation on the media and therefore may be performed if the wet preparation is negative. Enzyme immunoassay, nucleic acid amplification, and immunofluorescence techniques are also available for confirmatory testing.

Treatment

Infected individuals and their sexual partners should be treated to prevent recurrence of infection. A single 2 g oral dose of metronidazole is effective in most cases and can be used in the second trimester of pregnancy. Tinidazole is a more expensive alternative but equally effective. Repeat testing at 5–7 days and 30 days should be performed if symptoms fail to resolve and treatment failure is suspected. For nonpregnant treatment failures, a longer course of metronidazole, 500 mg twice daily for 7 days, or 2 g once daily for 3–5 days may be tried. Metronidazole gel for intravaginal application is available; however, it is less than 50% as effective as oral treatment.

Human Papilloma Virus

Diagnosis

Genital warts (condylomata acuminata) are caused by human papilloma virus (HPV). HPV is spread by skin to skin contact usually at sites of microtrauma on the genitalia. Most infections are subclinical and asymptomatic. In women,

HPV may be associated with nonspecific symptoms, such as vulvodynia, pruritis, or a malodorous vaginal discharge. There is a high rate of coinfection with other STIs.

Over 100 types of HPV exist and over 30 types can infect the genital area. Types 6 and 11 HPV most often account for visible external genital warts but patients may be infected with more than one type of HPV.[24] Types 6 and 11 HPV are low risk for conversion to invasive carcinoma of the external genitalia.

Over 99% of cervical cancers and 84% of anal cancers are associated with HPV, most commonly HPV 16 and 18; however, other types have been associated with cervical dysplasia and neoplasm in women and squamous intraepithelial neoplasia in men.[25–27] Smoking may increase the risk of dysplastic progression and malignancy in both men and women.

The diagnosis is made by the visualization or palpation of nontender papillomatous genital lesions. Aceto-whitening with 3–5% acetic acid placed on a towel and wrapped around the genitals may show flat condylomas as whitish areas but is not routinely recommended because of low specificity. The benefit of evaluating and treating asymptomatic sexual partners of women with genital warts or abnormal PAP smears remains unclear. Biopsies of genital warts are not routinely needed, but should be undertaken in all instances of questionable, atypical, pigmented, indurated, fixed, or ulcerated warts, if the lesions persist or worsen after treatment, and in immunocompromised patients.

Treatment

The choice of therapy for genital warts depends on several factors including wart size, number, and location and patient and physician preference. Since genital warts spontaneously resolve with time, observation remains an option. Patient-applied therapies are less expensive and may be more effective than provider-applied therapy.[28,29]

Recommended treatment choices for patient-applied therapy include podofilox 0.5% solution or gel, and imiquimod 5% cream.[30] Podofilox solution should be applied every 12 h for 3 days, then off for 4 days. The treatment cycle may be optionally repeated up to four times. The total volume of solution used should not exceed 0.5 mL/day and the total wart area should not be greater than 10 cm². The first application should be demonstrated in the office. Imiquimod cream should be applied three times per week at bedtime for up to 16 weeks. The area should be thoroughly washed 6–10 min after application. Imiquimod should not be used on vaginal lesions because of a risk of chronic ulceration. Neither medication should be used in pregnancy.

Provider-applied therapy options include cryotherapy with liquid nitrogen, electrosurgery, laser therapy, podophyllin resin 10–25%, trichloroacetic acid (TCA) or bichloroacetic acid (BCA) 80–90%, or surgical excision. Surgical excision, which can be large warts or large areas, may be accomplished by electrocautery or sharply with a tangential incision. Surgical therapies appear to be equally effective with regard to clearance rates.[31] Podophyllin 10–25% in compound tincture of benzoin is applied once and washed thoroughly 1–4 h after treatment. Treatment may be repeated weekly as needed. Podophyllin is contraindicated during pregnancy. TCA and BCA should be carefully applied with a cotton tip applicator only to the warts at 1–2 week intervals. A burning sensation should resolve in 2–5 min. Unreacted acid should be removed with baking soda or talc. TCA and BCA are not preferable for keratinized or large warts. TCA is not absorbed and may be used during pregnancy. Cryotherapy with liquid nitrogen or TCA/BCA is the preferred therapy for vaginal warts.

Large or extensive lesions surrounding the meatus may herald the presence of urethral or bladder condyloma, warranting cystourethroscopy and if seen may be cystoscopically excised. Podophyllin or cryotherapy may be used on urethral meatal warts.

A quadrivalent vaccine against HPV types 6, 11, 16, and 18 and a bivalent vaccine against HPV types 16 and 18 for the prevention of HPV-associated conditions such as cervical cancer and cervical cancer precursors, are available.[32] The CDC's Advisory Committee on Immunization Practices has recommended routine vaccination of females aged 11–12 years with three doses of either the quadrivalent or bivalent HPV vaccine for the prevention of cervical cancer. It may be started at age 9. The quadrivalent vaccine may also be used for the prevention of anogenital warts, and can be administered to boys and men aged 9-26. Although it is preferable that the vaccine be administered prior to sexual activity or known exposure to HPV for optimal benefit, it may also be given to women 13–26 years old who have not been previously vaccinated or who have not completed the series. Vaccination would provide less benefit to females if they have already been infected with the vaccine HPV types; however, it is recommended that these women still be vaccinated.

Scabies

Diagnosis

The mite, Sarcoptes scabiei, causes Scabies. An immune reaction to the mites, their eggs, and feces causes a rash with intense pruritis. The mite burrows appear as undulating, elongated papules. Common areas of involvement include the penile shaft and glans, areolae, finger webs, and auxiliary folds. The diagnosis is confirmed by scraping the burrow with a scalpel blade coated with mineral oil, and viewing under the microscope for eggs and mites.

Treatment

Permethrin cream (5%) should be applied to all areas of the body from the neck down, and washed off 8–14 h later. Lindane (1%) lotion is a second-line alternative and may be applied in a similar fashion and removed after 8 h. Treatment may be repeated in 1 week if necessary. Lindane should not be used after a bath, and is contraindicated in children <2 years of age, pregnant and lactating women, and patients with extensive dermatitis because of increased risk of seizures. An alternative for young children or pregnant/lactating women is sulfur (3–6%) applied on three consecutive nights.

References

1. CDC report. http://www.cdc.gov/std/stats09/trends.htm
2. Mawhorter SD. Travel medicine for the primary care physician. *Cleve Clin J Med*. 1997;64(9):483-492
3. Mabey D. Peeling RW: lymphogranuloma venereum. *Sex Trans Infect*. 2002;357:1831-1836
4. DiCarlo RP, Martin DH. The clinical diagnosis of genital ulcer disease in men. *Clin Infect Dis*. 1997;25(2):292-298
5. Brugha R, Keersmaekers K, Renton A, Meheus A. Genital herpes infection: a review. *Int J Epidemiol*. 1997;26(4):698-709

6. Langenberg AG, Corey L, Ashley RI, et al. A prospective study of new infections with herpes simplex virus type 1 and type 2. Chron HSV Vaccine Study Group. *N Engl J Med.* 1999;341:1432-1438

7. Wald A, Brown Z. ACOG Practice Bulletin No. 57. *Gynecol Herpes Simplex Virus Infect.* 2004;104(5):1111-1117

8. Benedetti J, Corey L, Ashley R. Recurrence rates in genital herpes after symptomatic first-episode infection. *Ann Intern Med.* 1994;121:847-854

9. Filen F, Strand A, Allard A, Blumberg J, Herrmann B. Duplex real-time polymerase chain reaction assay for detection and quantification of herpes simplex virus type 1 and herpes simplex virus type 2 in genital and cutaneous lesions. *Sex Transm Dis.* 2004;31:331-336

10. Ramaswamy M, McDonald C, Smith M, et al. Diagnosis of genital herpes by real time PCR in routine clinical practice. *Sex Transm Infect.* 2004;80:406-410

11. Wald A, Ashley-Morrow R. Serological testing for herpes simplex virus (HSV)-1 and HSV-2 infection. *Clin Infect Dis.* 2002;35(S2):S173-S182

12. Morrow RA, Friedrich D, Krantz E, et al. Development and use of a type-specific antibody avidity test based on herpes simplex virus type 2 glycoprotein G. *Sex Transm Dis.* 2004;31(8):508-515

13. Schmidt GP. Treatment of chancroid. *Clin Infect Dis.* 1999;28(Sup1):S14-S20

14. Hart G. Syphilis tests in diagnostic and therapeutic decision making. *Ann Intern Med.* 1986;104:368-376

15. Hicks CB, Benson PM, Lupton GP, et al. Seronegative secondary syphilis in a patient infected with the human immunodeficiency virus with Kaposi Sarcoma: a diagnostic dilemma. *Ann Intern Med.* 1987;107:492-495

16. Erbelding EJ, Vlahov D, Nelson KE, et al. Syphilis serology in human immunodeficiency virus infection: evidence for false negative fluorescent treponemal testing. *J Infect Dis.* 1997;17:1397-1400

17. Brown ST Zaidi A, Larsen SA, Reynolds GH. Serologic response to syphilis treatment. *J Am Med Assoc.* 1985;253:1296-1299

18. Calonge N. Screening for syphilis infection: recommendation statement. U.S. Preventive Services Task Force. *Ann Fam Med.* 2004;2:362-365

19. Rees E. Treatment of pelvic inflammatory disease. *Am J Obstet Gynecol.* 1980;138:1042-1047

20. Scholes D, Stergachis A, Heidrich FE, et al. Prevention of pelvic inflammatory disease by screening for cervical chlamydial infection. *N Engl J Med.* 1996;334:1362-1366

21. Centers for Disease Control. Laboratory guidelines screening tests to detect *Chlamydia trachomatis* and *Neisseria gonorrhoeae* Infections. *Morb Mortal Wkly Rep.* 2002;51(RR-15):10

22. Van der Pol B, Martin DH, Schachter J, et al. Enhancing the specificity of the COBAS AMPLICOR CT/NG test for *Neisseria gonorrhoeae* by retesting specimens with equivocal results. *J Clin Microbiol.* 2001;39:3092-3098

23. CDC. Update to CDC's Sexually Transmitted Diseases Treatment Guidelines, 2006: fluoroquinolones no longer recommended for treatment of gonococcal infections. *MMWR Morb Mortal Wkly Rep.* April 13, 2007;56(14):332-336

24. Frydenberg M, Malek RS. Human papilloma virus infection and its relationship to carcinoma of the penis. *Urol Ann.* 1993;7:185-198

25. Walboomers JM, Jacobs MV, Manos MM, et al. Human papilloma virus is a necessary cause of invasive cervical cancer worldwide. *J Pathol.* 1999;189:12-19

26. Frisch M, Glimelius B. van deen Brule AJ et al: Sexually transmitted infection as a cause of anal cancer. *N Engl J Med.* 1997;337(19):1350-1358

27. Kulasingham SL, Hughes JP, Kiviat NB, et al. Evaluation of human papillomavirus testing in primary screening for cervical abnormalities: comparison of sensitivity, specificity, and frequency of referral. *J Am Med Assoc.* 2002;288:1749-1757

28. Arican O, Suneri F, Bilgie K, et al. Topical imiquimod 5% cream in external genital warts: a randomized, double-blind, placebo-controlled study. *J Dermtol.* 2004;31(8):627-631

29. Langley PC, Tyring SK, Smith MH. The cost effectiveness of patient applied versus provider administered intervention strategies for the treatment of external genital warts. *Am J Manag Care.* 1999;5(1):69-77

30. Perry CM, Lab HM. Topical Imiquod: a review of its use in genital warts. *Drugs.* 1999;58:375-390

31. Wiley DJ, Doughlas J, Beutner K, et al. External genital warts: diagnosis, treatment and prevention. *Clin Infect Dis.* 2002;35:S210-S224

32. FDA Licensure of Bivalent Human Papillomavirus Vaccine (HPV2, Cervarix) for Use in Females and Updated HPV Vaccination Recommendations from the Advisory Committee on Immunization Practices (ACIP) MMWR 59(20);626-629

33. U.S. Preventative Services Task Force. Screening for gonorrhea: recommendation statement. Ann Fam Med 2005; 3;263-7

34. CDC. Sexually Transmitted Diseases Treatment Guidelines 2010. MMWR 2010. 59(RR-12):49

26

Hematuria: Evaluation and Management

Richard J. Bryant and James W.F. Catto

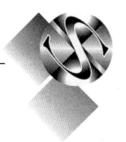

Introduction

Hematuria is the presence of red blood cells in the urine and can be visible to the naked eye (macroscopic), detectable with microscopic analysis or found by dipstick testing of urine. Around 40% of patients with hematuria have a significant underlying cause regardless of the quantity of blood in the urine. As the presence of hematuria is common and there are often no clues as to the underlying cause, this condition comprises a large amount of the urological workload and should be regarded as a manifestation of urological malignancy until proven otherwise.[1] While it is recognized that the contemporary urological approach for the investigation of hematuria may not always be evidence-based medicine,[1] there are numerous high-quality studies confirming the prevalence of disease within patients with this condition.

Classification of Hematuria

The simplest classification of hematuria is according to the extent of blood.

Macroscopic Hematuria

Macroscopic hematuria is the presence of visible blood in the urine and is a common cause of urological referral. Around 2.5% of the community

has macroscopic hematuria[2] and the incidence of underlying cancer has been reported as between 22% and 24.2%.[2,3] The risk of cancer is greater with macroscopic than microscopic hematuria and rises with advancing patient age. Macroscopic hematuria is the commonest presenting symptom for patients with urothelial cell carcinoma (UCC)[3] and investigation of this symptom is considered mandatory in all patients.[4]

Microscopic Hematuria

Microscopic hematuria is the presence of red blood cells (RBCs) within the urine that are visible only with microscopic analysis of centrifuged urinary sediments. Asymptomatic hematuria is common and has a reported prevalence between 0.19% and 21%.[5-7] For example, in British males, the prevalence of microscopic hematuria is around 2.5%.[8] This frequency varies according to the population studied and the definition of hematuria used. The definition of abnormal urinary RBCs is contentious. Traditionally, the upper limit of normal urinary RBC has been between three and five RBCs per high power field (RBC/hpf).[5,9,10] The American Urological Association has recently defined microscopic hematuria as ≥ 3 RBCs/hpf in the urinary sediment from two of three properly collected specimens.[6,11] However, malignancies can be detected in patients with fewer than 3 RBCs/hpf, and therefore, some authors suggest investigating all patients with

C.R. Chapple and W.D. Steers (eds.), *Practical Urology: Essential Principles and Practice*,
DOI: 10.1007/978-1-84882-034-0_26, © Springer-Verlag London Limited 2011

microscopic RBCs within their urine. While persistent hematuria may be more sinister than transient, it is well recognized that the latter can occur with both renal cell carcinoma and UCC.[12] Bladder cancer represents the most commonly diagnosed malignancy in patients with microscopic hematuria[13] and microscopic hematuria is associated with a urological malignancy in up to 10% of adults.[2,14] Microscopic hematuria has a reported prevalence of 0–7.2%[15] in patients under the age of 40 years; however, significant pathology is rare at this age. Younger patients typically have a glomerular cause for their microscopic hematuria and renal referral is often appropriate. The presence of dysmorphic RBCs, red cell casts, significant proteinuria or hypertension suggests that the cause may be glomerular in nature.[5] The risk of a significant underlying cause of microscopic hematuria increases with age.[8]

Dipstick Hematuria

Dipstick hematuria describes the use of reagent strips to chemically detect the presence of blood within the urine. Intact urinary RBCs lyse following contact with the test paper and release hemoglobin. The peroxidase-like activity of hemoglobin oxidises a dipstick-adherent chromogen indicator, which subsequently changes color. The dipstick test can detect RBCs below 3 RBCs/hpf,[12] but it has a low specificity as free hemoglobin, myoglobin, and other oxidizing agents (such as hypochloride bleaches) can give false-positive results. False-negative results can occur in the presence of reducing agents (such as vitamin C). Different commercially available dipsticks vary in their sensitivity to detect blood within urine. Most kits detect around 8 RBCs/hpf and score the concentration as "trace," +, ++, or +++. Recent British guidelines[16] recommend that a trace of dipstick hematuria should be regarded as normal. Routine microscopy for confirmation of dipstick-positive hematuria is now generally deemed unnecessary,[16] although it is often useful to perform microscopy and culture of the urine sample in order to confirm or refute the presence of infection.

Pseudohematuria

Occasionally, macroscopic hematuria may be confused with a red or brown discoloration resulting from the presence of an agent which artificially colors the urine. These may be foodstuffs such as beetroot or blackberries, or drugs such as rifampicin or chloroquine.

Factitious Hematuria

Patients with Munchausen Syndrome may deliberately contaminate their urine samples in order to seek medical examination and investigation.

Menstruation

Menstruation may cause transient false-positive hematuria[17]; therefore, women should not be tested for the presence of dipstick or microscopic hematuria during their menstrual period.

Aetiology

The causes of hematuria may be classified in a number of ways, including anatomical site and pathological process (Table 26.1). Around 40% of patients with hematuria have an identifiable cause, and these are mostly bladder cancer, urinary tract infection (UTI), urinary calculus, or intrinsic renal pathology. The single commonest cause of frank hematuria in patients over the age of 50 years is bladder cancer.

Malignancy

The commonest malignancies causing hematuria are bladder and renal cancer.[2] Some 85% of patients with bladder cancer have either macroscopic or microscopic hematuria.[18,19] Many of the investigations outlined below are aimed at identifying these malignancies. A less common cause of hematuria is UCC arising from the upper urinary tract. Nowadays, prostate cancer rarely presents for the first time with hematuria; however, this malignancy may often be found incidentally in men undergoing hematuria investigations.

Urinary Calculi

Urinary stones commonly cause pain associated with hematuria. Rarely, stones can cause isolated

Table 26.1. Pathological processes causing hematuria stratified for anatomical location

Kidney	Renal cell carcinoma (RCC), Urothelial cell carcinoma (UCC), renal calculi, trauma, infection (e.g., Pyelonephritis, tuberculosis), inflammatory (e.g., Nephritides), vascular (e.g., renal papillary necrosis), genetic (e.g., von Hippel-Lindau disease), congenital (e.g., Renal cystic disease, Pelvi-ureteric junction [PUJ] obstruction)
Ureter	Calculi, UCC, iatrogenic
Bladder	Bladder cancer (TCC, SCC, adenocarcinoma, neuroendocrine), calculi, infection (bacterial hemorrhagic cystitis, parasitic), trauma, decompression hematuria (postcatheterization)
Prostate	Benign prostatic hyperplasia (BPH), prostate cancer, prostatitis, calculi
Urethra	Urethral tumor, calculi, trauma, stricture, iatrogenic
Systemic	Coagulopathies, systemic disorders (e.g., Sickle cell disease)
Drugs	Interstitial nephritis (e.g., penicillin, nonsteroidal anti-inflammatory agents), nephrotoxic drugs (e.g., cyclophosphamide), anticoagulants

macroscopic hematuria, and staghorn calculi may present with either asymptomatic microscopic hematuria or recurrent urinary tract infections. Patients presenting with loin pain and microscopic hematuria are usually investigated in the acute setting with a noncontrast CT; however, if this fails to demonstrate a urinary calculus, then the microscopic hematuria should be investigated further as outlined below.

Infection and Inflammation

The commonest clinical scenario in which microscopic or dipstick-positive hematuria is found is with a UTI.[10] As infection may be a manifestation of other uropathology, the clinician should not ignore the hematuria, and investigate the UTI as appropriate. If hematuria persists after UTI treatment then it requires investigating in its own right.

Noninfective inflammatory conditions such as radiation-induced cystitis and interstitial cystitis may cause hematuria. An associated focal or diffuse erythema may be seen at flexible cystoscopy and this requires rigid cystoscopic evaluation under anesthetic and biopsy in order to distinguish these conditions from carcinoma in situ (CIS).

Benign Prostatic Hyperplasia

An enlarged prostate gland may bleed from tortuous surface veins, and benign prostatic hyperplasia (BPH) is a common cause of frank hematuria in older men. Contact bleeding may occur from these veins during flexible cystoscopy. BPH-related hematuria may be reduced by treatment with 5 alpha reductase inhibitors.

Trauma

Trauma to the urinary tract is an important cause of hematuria. Patients with hematuria secondary to a traumatic cause usually present in an emergency setting rather than to the urology clinic. Their management and investigation is related to the traumatic incident and a detailed discussion is not included here.

Drugs

Numerous medications can cause hematuria.[20,21] Anticoagulants such as warfarin or aspirin may cause hematuria in the presence of pathology, and therefore, these patients should still be investigated for underlying disease.[11]

Nephrological Causes

Renal parenchymal disease is a common cause of hematuria and includes focal glomerular diseases such as membranoproliferative glomerulonephritis, interstitial renal diseases such as drug-induced nephropathy, and systemic conditions such as systemic lupus erythematosis. Some of these conditions may cause frank hematuria. Patients with an absence of a urological cause of their hematuria require referral for a nephrological opinion if they have hypertension, significant proteinuria (defined as a total protein excretion of greater than 1,000 mg/24 h) or other indicators of renal pathology such as red cell casts of dysmorphic RBCs within a fresh urine sample.[6,12] Many of these patients may require a renal biopsy in order to diagnose the nature of the underlying renal parenchymal disease.

Patients with microscopic hematuria in the absence of demonstrable urological or nephrological pathology should be considered at high risk of developing renal disease (mostly IgA nephropathy). These patients should be followed up in a primary care setting and referred to a renal physician if they develop hypertension, renal insufficiency, or significant proteinuria.[6]

Assessment

History

History taking should try to establish the causes of hematuria[22] (Table 26.1), predisposing disease factors, and establish the risk of underlying pathology. For example, macroscopic hematuria has a higher risk of pathology than that detected by dipstick, while the absence of associated pain is a feature of malignancy. The presence of associated symptoms should be established, for example, dysuria may indicate an infective or inflammatory cause while colicky loin pain may indicate an upper tract calculus. Difficulty passing urine in the presence of frank hematuria, particularly if there are associated clots, suggests that the patient is developing clot retention and will require catheterization with a three-way catheter. The timing of hematuria may point to the underlying source: initial hematuria suggests urethral pathology, hematuria throughout the stream suggests an intravesical or upper tract cause, while terminal bleeding suggests that it is from the bladder neck or prostate. The presence of associated clots indicates a significant amount of hematuria and is associated with a greater probability of finding serious underlying pathology such as a malignancy. If the hematuria is microscopic in nature, then it is important to establish whether this is a recurrent finding, as this would indicate a greater chance of finding significant underlying pathology.

The age of the patient is important as patients over the age of 40 years have a greater chance of harboring significant underlying pathology.[5] The history should also focus on identifying the presence of known risk factors for significant disease in patients with hematuria, such as a smoking history, occupational exposure to chemicals or dyes such as benzenes or aromatic amines, previous pelvic irradiation, and a history of irritative urinary symptoms.

It is important to be sure that the bleeding is definitely from the urinary tract, rather than from a colorectal or gynecological cause, and the patient's past medical history and drug history are important.

Examination

Patients with macroscopic hematuria should have their vital signs measured to check if they are hemodynamically stable. Unstable patients may require resuscitation and blood transfusion. Patients should undergo abdominal examination to exclude a renal or bladder mass. In men, genital examination and digital rectal examination to detect the presence of prostatic pathology are required. Female patients should undergo a pelvic examination to exclude a mass. All patients presenting to the hematuria clinic should have their blood pressure checked to exclude hypertension (suggestive of renal pathology as a possible cause of hematuria).

Investigations

The ideal practice is probably a "one-stop" hematuria clinic in which synchronous clinical and radiological evaluation of the patient is performed. This design reduces diagnostic delay and patient anxiety.

Dipstick Urinalysis

A fresh uncontaminated mid-stream urine (MSU) sample should be dipstick tested for blood, protein (renal disease), nitrate (infection), leukocytes (inflammation), and glucose (diabetes). Urine samples should also be sent for microscopy, culture, and sensitivity (MC&S). Patients found to have nitrites on dipstick urinalysis, but asymptomatic for infection, should receive a prophylactic dose of antibiotic at the time of flexible cystoscopic evaluation of the lower urinary tract (see later) followed by a course of antibiotics in order to minimize the risk of precipitating an upper tract or systemic infection. An asymptomatic UTI may be the cause of microscopic hematuria[23]; however, these patients should still undergo urological investigation to exclude concomitant underlying urological pathology. Patients symptomatic of a urinary tract infection should receive a course of antibiotics and the flexible cystoscopy should be postponed for a couple of weeks in order to allow the urinary tract infection to be fully treated.

The use of routine urinalysis as a screening tool for urological malignancy remains the subject of debate. While the detection of microscopic hematuria at urinalysis may predict the development of bladder cancer,[19] there is also evidence that patients testing positive and negative for microscopic hematuria have an equal chance of developing a urological malignancy.[24] A routine screening program for urological malignancy based on urinalysis and the detection of hematuria is therefore not currently advocated.

Cytology

Urine cytology can detect atypical or malignant cells but its sensitivity depends upon numerous factors including the grade of the urothelial malignancy and the experience of the reporting pathologist.[5] It has a high specificity for the detection of high-grade urothelial tumors and CIS,[25] but can be positive with nonmalignant conditions such as chronic infection or inflammation and urinary calculus disease.[23]

Molecular Tests

Recently, numerous molecular tests have been designed to detect urothelial malignancy using urine analysis.[25] The most developed of these are the detection of bladder tumor antigen (BTA),[26-28] nuclear matrix protein 22 (NMP22),[29-32] and fluorescence in-situ hybridization for chromosomal anomalies (UroVysion). The NMP22 test is one of the best evaluated and detects the NMP22 protein which is present at significantly greater concentration in the urine of patients with bladder cancer as compared with normal controls.[25] NMP22 detection has a sensitivity between 58% (specificity 84%) and 91% (specificity 76%) in reported studies.[32-36] Data suggest that it should be used to complement a flexible cystoscopy.

Blood Tests

A full blood count should be considered in patients with heavy or long-standing hematuria to detect anemia, while plasma creatinine and eGFR should also be measured as an indicator of renal impairment.

Flexible Cystoscopy

Flexible cystoscopy under local anesthetic is probably the ideal way to investigate the lower urinary tract for hematuria. It combines good patient tolerability with safety and low cost, and the views are usually as good as those obtained with a rigid instrument.[23] Cystoscopy reportedly has a 5% risk of causing urinary infection.[37] Of note, the ability of flexible cystoscopy to detect CIS of the bladder may be more limited than with rigid instrumentation.[38] If a bladder or urethral tumor is found at flexible cystoscopy, the patient should undergo examination under anesthesia and formal transurethral resection, together with upper tract evaluation (see below) including an intravenous urogram (IVU) or, increasingly commonly, a contrast-enhanced computer tomography urogram (CTU), in order to detect a synchronous urothelial lesion elsewhere within the urinary tract.

Upper Urinary Tract Evaluation

Evaluation of the upper urinary tract is complex and requires a balance between the number of radiological investigations required to detect significant pathology and the low detection rate of each test (Fig. 26.1). This balance varies between institutions (reflecting that no single protocol is ideal), and depends upon the individual patient's pathological risks (established from history and examination) and their medical comorbidity. For example, unfit patients may not benefit from investigations that would not alter their management even if pathology was found. Many urologists adopt a pragmatic approach and utilize a renal ultrasound (USS) scan in order to detect renal parenchymal lesions and a plain abdominal x-ray for calculi. If flexible cystoscopy and these radiological tests are normal, then patients with macroscopic or persistent microscopic hematuria should probably undergo additional upper tract imaging in the form of either an IVU or CTU. If these investigations are negative and the patient continues to have frank hematuria, additional investigations may be required, depending upon the index of suspicion of a malignant cause of hematuria.

Figure 26.1. Algorithm for the investigation of hematuria. In all patients, a full history should be elicited and an abdominal and pelvic examination should be performed in addition to urinary testing (to check for red cells, white blood cells, infection, and atypical cytology). Additional hematological and biochemical blood tests are also usually required. *CTU* CT urogram, *IVU* intravenous urography, *USS* abdominal and pelvic ultrasound, *UTI* urinary tract infection, *LUTS* lower urinary tract symptoms.

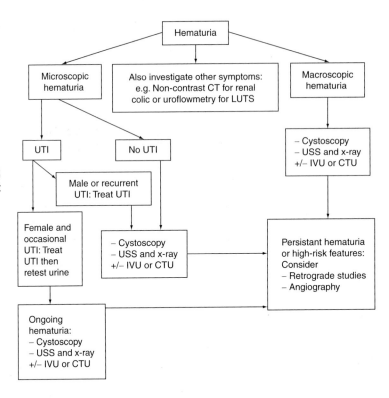

Renal USS

Ultrasound is a relatively cheap, safe, and noninvasive investigation. While it is useful for the detection of renal parenchymal lesions such as renal tumors, characterization of renal cysts, and the detection of hydronephrosis,[39] it has a limited ability to detect solid renal lesions less than 3 cm in size[40] or small tumors within the urinary collecting system. CT is required for the further characterization of complex renal cysts (contrast enhanced) or stones (noncontrast). The ureter is often not well visualized with USS.

KUB Abdominal X-Ray

In many centers, a plain abdominal x-ray is used in the initial assessment of hematuria to detect urinary calculi. This is a pragmatic choice as it avoids the added radiation exposure of an IVU or CT scan, but can miss many urinary stones and doesn't help in ureteric or renal pelvis visualization. Patients with suspected urinary calculi should undergo a noncontrast CT. Patients with features suggesting high malignancy risk (such as advanced age, strong history of smoking or occupational carcinogen exposure, or macroscopic

hematuria) should undergo more thorough upper tract radiological imaging

Intravenous Urography (IVU)

While an IVU is useful for the detection of abnormalities of the upper urinary tract such as UCC,[41] calculi, and hydronephrosis, it exposes the patient to nephrotoxic contrast media and is contra-indicated in renal insufficiency. An IVU has limited sensitivity for detecting small renal masses[42] and is not as accurate as USS at identifying small renal parenchymal lesions.[5] Therefore, an IVU should be used in conjunction with a renal USS. If a mass is detected by IVU, the lesion should be further characterized by either USS or CT. A recent study of 1,930 patients found that 9.4% of the patients with microscopic hematuria had cancer, and that evaluation of the upper urinary tract with one imaging modality alone would miss an upper tract malignancy in 4 patients.[2] In many centres in the United Kingdom and elsewhere USS and IVU have now been replaced by CTU as the first-line investigation of the upper tract in patients with macroscopic hematuria.

Computed Tomography (CT)

CT with contrast delivers optimal visualization of the urinary anatomy while a noncontrast CT is useful if renal calculi are suspected.[42-44] Ideally, several CT phases should be used including (1) noncontrast phase to detect stones, (2) portal venous and arterial phases for renal lesions, and (3) excretory phase for intraluminal pathology (UCC of the ureter or renal pelvis).[45,46] However, a CT is more expensive and carries a higher radiation exposure than an IVU or USS, and thus should be used with caution when looking for disease in patients with a low incidence. The replacement of both USS and IVU by CTU is becoming more widely adopted.

Retrograde Urogram Studies

Retrograde studies usually require anesthesia and involve direct cannulation of the ureteric orifice with retrograde injection of contrast media under radiological screening. This investigation is particularly useful for the evaluation of equivocal filling defects seen on an IVU, and it may be combined with upper urinary tract endoscopy in order to obtain cellular brushings or histology of suspicious upper tract lesions. This procedure is highly invasive and should be reserved for selected cases of hematuria with a sufficient index of suspicion.

Magnetic Resonance Imaging (MRI)

An MRI of the pelvis is indicated if a solid-appearing bladder cancer is visualized at the time of flexible cystoscopy in order to provide radiological staging information. Ideally, the MRI should be performed prior to the transurethral resection of an invasive-looking bladder tumor. If the MRI is performed after transurethral resection, an interval of at least 4 weeks is required between the resection and the MRI scan in order to prevent inaccurate radiological upstaging of the bladder mass as a result of changes occurring as a result of the surgical resection.

Additional Tests and Renal Biopsy

A renal biopsy is indicated when there is evidence of renal parenchymal disease (such as significant proteinuria or hypertension). Serum immunological investigations are indicated if there is a suspicion of an underlying immunological cause of renal disease-related hematuria.

Nonurological/Intrinsic Renal Causes of Hematuria

Intrinsic nephrological causes of hematuria should be considered if urological investigations fail to identify pathology. Nephrological causes are more common in younger patients and those with proteinuria or hypertension. Frank hematuria and concomitant upper respiratory tract infection could suggest glomerulonephritis and it is often appropriate to refer these patients for renal assessment rather than delay with urological investigations.

It is important to measure the patients' blood pressure during their hematuria clinic consultation, and the urinalysis should investigate the presence of proteinuria, while urine should be sent for formal microscopy in order to investigate the presence of urinary casts. Patients with proteinuria on dipstick urinalysis should have urine sent for protein:creatinine ratio (PCR) or albumin:creatinine ratio (ACR) measurement and their glomerular filtration rate (creatinine clearance) measured. Further nephrological evaluation may include a renal biopsy in order to identify an intrinsic renal cause of hematuria.

Intractable Hematuria

Patients with advanced urological malignancy and following radiotherapy may develop intractable hematuria leading to anemia and clot retention. Various palliative options are available to try and ease the hematuria including a "toilet" transurethral resection of their tumor, palliative radiotherapy for malignancy, radiological internal iliac embolization or intravesical instillation of chemicals such as alum or formalin. Palliative cystectomy may be performed as a last resort for intractable hematuria in selected patients. Transurethral resection may also be helpful to reduce hematuria due to advanced prostate cancer. Patients with renal tumors causing intractable hematuria may be successfully palliated with radiotherapy or radiological embolization. Hematuria following radiotherapy should always be investigated with cystoscopy, as in these patients there is an increased risk of malignancy.

Loin Pain Hematuria Syndrome

The term "loin pain hematuria syndrome" is given to describe a condition whereby patients experience loin pain associated with hematuria, but in whom no identifiable cause is found. The condition is commoner in women than men and may persist for many years. No pathological cause is found following full hematuria investigations including renal biopsy and angiography.

Follow-Up for Patients with Hematuria in the Absence of Demonstrable Pathology

Some patients with a negative initial urological evaluation eventually develop significant urological or renal disease; therefore, patients with negative initial investigations require adequate follow-up, usually in a primary care setting. This follow-up is important if the patient has risk factors for the development of urological[47] or renal pathology. Patients with microscopic hematuria should undergo repeat urinalysis and referral to a renal physician should be considered if the patient develops hypertension, significant proteinuria or evidence of renal insufficiency. The development of macroscopic hematuria in a patient who has previously been evaluated for microscopic hematuria warrants referral back to the urologist for further investigations, while patients with ongoing macroscopic hematuria also should be considered for rereferral for additional investigation.

References

1. Rodgers MA et al. Diagnostic tests used in the investigation of adult haematuria: a systematic review. *BJU Int.* 2006;98(6):1154-1160

2. Khadra MH et al. A prospective analysis of 1,930 patients with hematuria to evaluate current diagnostic practice. *J Urol.* 2000;163(2):524-527
3. Nishikawa Y et al. Clinical assessment of patients with microscopic hematuria pointed out by mass screening examination. *Hinyokika Kiyo.* 1992;38(6):647-651
4. Grossfeld GD, Carroll PR. Evaluation of asymptomatic microscopic hematuria. *Urol Clin North Am.* 1998;25(4): 661-676
5. Grossfeld GD et al. Evaluation of asymptomatic microscopic hematuria in adults: the American Urological Association best practice policy–part II: patient evaluation, cytology, voided markers, imaging, cystoscopy, nephrology evaluation, and follow-up. *Urology.* 2001; 57(4):604-610
6. Grossfeld GD et al. Asymptomatic microscopic hematuria in adults: summary of the AUA best practice policy recommendations. *Am Fam Physician.* 2001;63(6): 1145-1154
7. Briganti E, McNeil J, Atkins R. The epidemiology of diseases of the kidney and urinary tract: an Australian perspective. Report to the Board of the Australian Kidney Foundation [online]. http://www.med.monash.edu.au/epidemiology/general_info/disease_kidney.html. 2001
8. Ritchie CD, Bevan EA, Collier SJ. Importance of occult haematuria found at screening. *Br Med J (Clin Res Ed).* 1986;292(6521):681-683
9. Scottish Intercollegiate Guidelines Network. Investigation of asymptomatic microscopic haematuria in adults. www.sign.ac.uk/pdf/sign17.pdf. 1997
10. McDonald MM, Swagerty D, Wetzel L. Assessment of microscopic hematuria in adults. *Am Fam Physician.* 2006;73(10):1748-1754
11. Sokolosky MC. Hematuria. *Emerg Med Clin North Am.* 2001;19(3):621-632
12. Cohen RA, Brown RS. Clinical practice. Microscopic hematuria. *N Engl J Med.* 2003;348(23):2330-2338
13. U.S. Preventive Series Task Force. *Guide to Clinical Preventive Series.* Alexandria, VA: International Medical Publishing; 1996
14. Sultana SR et al. Microscopic haematuria: urological investigation using a standard protocol. *Br J Urol.* 1996; 78(5):691-696; discussion 697-698
15. Benbassat J et al. Symptomless microhaematuria in schoolchildren: causes for variable management strategies. *Q J Med.* 1996;89(11):845-854
16. Renal Association and British Association of Urological Surgeons. Joint consensus statement on the initial assessment of haematuria. 2008
17. Khan MA, Shaw G, Paris AM. Is microscopic haematuria a urological emergency? *BJU Int.* 2002;90(4):355-357
18. Schroeder GL et al. A side by side comparison of cytology and biomarkers for bladder cancer detection. *J Urol.* 2004;172(3):1123-1126
19. Friedman GD et al. Can hematuria be a predictor as well as a symptom or sign of bladder cancer? *Cancer Epidemiol Biomarkers Prev.* 1996;5(12):993-996
20. Mazhari R, Kimmel PL. Hematuria: an algorithmic approach to finding the cause. *Cleve Clin J Med.* 2002;69(11):870, 872-874, 876 passim
21. Feld LG et al. Hematuria: an integrated medical and surgical approach. *Pediatr Clin N Am.* 1997;44(5):1191–1210
22. Rockall AG et al. Haematuria. *Postgrad Med J.* 1997;73 (857):129-136

23. Connelly JE. Microscopic hematuria. In: Black ER, Tape TG, Panzer RJ, eds. *Diagnostic Strategies for Common Medical Problems*. Philadelphia, PA: American College of Physicians; 1999:518-526

24. Hiatt RA, Ordonez JD. Dipstick urinalysis screening, asymptomatic microhematuria, and subsequent urological cancers in a population-based sample. *Cancer Epidemiol Biomarkers Prev*. 1994;3(5):439-443

25. Budman LI, Kassouf W, Steinberg JR. Biomarkers for detection and surveillance of bladder cancer. *Can Urol Assoc J*. 2008;2(3):212-221

26. Pode D et al. Noninvasive detection of bladder cancer with the BTA stat test. *J Urol*. 1999;161(2):443-446

27. Nasuti JF et al. Utility of the BTA stat test kit for bladder cancer screening. *Diagn Cytopathol*. 1999;21(1):27-29.

28. Walsh IK et al. The BTA stat test: a tumor marker for the detection of upper tract transitional cell carcinoma. *Urology*. 2001;58(4):532-535

29. Chahal R et al. Evaluation of the clinical value of urinary NMP22 as a marker in the screening and surveillance of transitional cell carcinoma of the urinary bladder. *Eur Urol*. 2001;40(4):415-420; discussion 421

30. Ponsky LE et al. Screening and monitoring for bladder cancer: refining the use of NMP22. *J Urol*. 2001;166(1):75-78

31. Zippe C, Pandrangi L, Agarwal A. NMP22 is a sensitive, cost-effective test in patients at risk for bladder cancer. *J Urol*. 1999;161(1):62-65

32. Akaza H et al. Evaluation of urinary NMP22 (nuclear matrix protein 22) as a diagnostic marker for urothelial cancer – screening for urothelial cancer in patients with microscopic hematuria. NMP Study Group. *Gan To Kagaku Ryoho*. 1997;24(7):837-842

33. Miyanaga N et al. Urinary nuclear matrix protein 22 as a new marker for the screening of urothelial cancer in patients with microscopic hematuria. *Int J Urol*. 1999; 6(4):173-177

34. Miyoshi Y, Matsuzaki J, Miura T. Evaluation of usefulness of urinary nuclear matrix protein 22 (NMP22) in the detection of urothelial transitional cell carcinoma. *Hinyokika Kiyo*. 2001;47(6):379-383

35. Oge O et al. Evaluation of nuclear matrix protein 22 (NMP22) as a tumor marker in the detection of bladder cancer. *Int Urol Nephrol*. 2001;32(3):367-370

36. Paoluzzi M et al. Urinary dosage of nuclear matrix protein 22 (NMP22) like biologic marker of transitional cell carcinoma (TCC): a study on patients with hematuria. *Arch Ital Urol Androl*. 1999;71(1):13-18

37. Vasanthakumar V et al. A study to assess the efficacy of chemoprophylaxis in the prevention of endoscopy-related bacteraemia in patients aged 60 and over. *Q J Med*. 1990;75(278):647-653

38. Koss LG et al. Diagnostic value of cytology of voided urine. *Acta Cytol*. 1985;29(5):810-816

39. Jaffe JS et al. A new diagnostic algorithm for the evaluation of microscopic hematuria. *Urology*. 2001;57(5): 889-894

40. Jamis-Dow CA et al. Small (< or = 3-cm) renal masses: detection with CT versus US and pathologic correlation. *Radiology*. 1996;198(3):785-788

41. Sutton JM. Evaluation of hematuria in adults. *J Am Med Assoc*. 1990;263(18):2475-2480

42. Gray Sears CL et al. Prospective comparison of computerized tomography and excretory urography in the initial evaluation of asymptomatic microhematuria. *J Urol*. 2002;168(6):2457-2460

43. Sourtzis S et al. Radiologic investigation of renal colic: unenhanced helical CT compared with excretory urography. *Am J Roentgenol*. 1999;172(6):1491-1494

44. Luchs JS et al. Utility of hematuria testing in patients with suspected renal colic: correlation with unenhanced helical CT results. *Urology*. 2002;59(6):839-842

45. Igarashi T et al. Clinical and radiological aspects of infiltrating transitional cell carcinoma of the kidney. *Urol Int*. 1994;52(4):181-184

46. Buckley JA et al. Transitional cell carcinoma of the renal pelvis: a retrospective look at CT staging with pathologic correlation. *Radiology*. 1996;201(1):194-198

47. Carson CC III, Segura JW, Greene LF. Clinical importance of microhematuria. *J Am Med Assoc*. 1979;241(2): 149-150

27

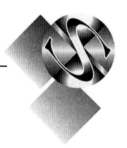

Benign Prostatic Hyperplasia (BPH)

Andrea Tubaro and Cosimo de Nunzio

Historical Background

The first description of the prostate gland goes back to Andreas Vesalius in his book entitled *Tabulae anatomicae* (1538). In 1564, Ambroise Paré, the Renaissance master of French surgery, described obstructive urinary symptoms. Two centuries later, in 1786, John Hunter, the famous British surgeon, related prostatic enlargement to obstructive symptoms, detrusor hypertrophy, and upper urinary tract dilatation. Transurethral instruments to relieve prostatic obstruction were first developed by Jean Civiale in Paris and Enrico Bottini. Eugene Fuller (1858–1930) and Peter Fryer (1852–1921) in Britain and George Goodfellow (1855–1910) in the United States pioneered surgery of BPH. In the twentieth century, new surgical techniques were developed thanks to people like Terence Millin, Hugh H. Young, James Buchanan Brady, George Luys, Maximilian Stern, Joseph McCarthy, and Frederic Foley.[1]

Epidemiology and Natural History

Epidemiology research strictly depends upon the definition of the disease/condition and BPH is not without problem as there is no consensus on a unique definition.[2] Current terminology, as revised by Abrams et al. in 2002, describe the objective finding of a Benign Prostatic Enlargement (BPE), a histological diagnosis (Benign Prostatic Hyperplasia – BPH) and the obstruction that can derive from BPH (Benign Prostatic Obstruction – BPO).[3] Unless the patient suffers complications of BPH such as renal failure, bladder stones or diverticula, recurrent urinary tract infection, and acute or chronic retention and surgery is performed on the enlarged prostate gland, treatment is targeted at reducing lower urinary tract symptoms (LUTS) that can be associated with but are not uniquely due to BPH. This is the reason why, in the lack of a univocal definition of BPE/BPH/BPO, most epidemiological work on BPH is based upon the incidence and prevalence of LUTS with the risk of including patients whose symptoms depend on causes other than BPH. Analysis of the General Practice Research database from the UK suggests that both incidence and prevalence of LUTS increase with age. Incidence values of 5 and 50 per 1,000 person-years were observed in men aged 45–49 and >80 years, respectively. Prevalence increased from 3.5% in the fourth decade to 30% in men of 85 years or older.[4] The increase of LUTS prevalence with age has been confirmed in several studies performed in different countries/populations although slight differences in the absolute age-specific prevalence value were observed.

Although BPH is an androgen-dependent condition (it does not develop in castrated men and families with a 5-alpha reductase deficiency), there is little evidence of an effect of hormone levels on clinical manifestations of the

C.R. Chapple and W.D. Steers (eds.), *Practical Urology: Essential Principles and Practice*,
DOI: 10.1007/978-1-84882-034-0_27, © Springer-Verlag London Limited 2011

disease in population studies. Some degree of association has been found between BPH and growth factors such as Insulin Growth Factor-1 and its binding globulin (IGFBP-3). LUTS have also been correlated with sexual dysfunction and the relation holds true in different studies also after data were adjusted for age although no clear explanation has been found. A weak association between clinical manifestations of BPH and cardiovascular disease has been described. No relation between LUTS and lifestyle factors (namely diet and exercise) has been observed.

Since surgical treatment of BPH was developed, the condition is no longer life-threatening but remains progressive. Studies on the natural history of the disease tell us that an increase of about 0.2 points/year in the IPSS scale is expected; 50–80% of men will remain stable over a 1–5-year period with a 20–50% progression rate also depending on the definition of progression and type of population. The risk of acute urinary retention (AUR) varies from 2 to 18 per 1,000 person-years with lower values observed in community studies (2–6.8%) and higher ones in the placebo arms of clinical trials. Age, symptom severity, and maximum flow rate (Q_{max}) were independent predictors of AUR. In the Olmstead County study, an age-related deterioration of flow rate was observed with a 1.3% decrease per year in men in the 40s and 6.5% decrease in men in their 70s.[5] Longitudinal studies of voiding dynamics are rare. Thomas et al. reported no significant increase of bladder outflow obstruction over a 13.9-year period although decrease of detrusor contractility was found.[6] The prostate gland tends to grow over time; population studies suggested a 1.6–2.0% increase of prostate volume per year.[7,8] A 4.5% increase was observed in the placebo arm of the MTOPS.[9] Using a stricter parameter such as increase of prostate volume of 26% or higher, 22.6% of men progressed over a 4.2-year period in the population-based Krimpen study.[8] PSA concentration is known to be related to age and prostate volume; in the Krimpen study, a 5% increase of serum PSA per year was seen. A shorter PSA doubling time was observed in men with BPH compared to those without it. Asian populations were recently investigated to obtain epidemiological data on LUTS/BPH. Prevalence of LUTS is comparable to that observed in Europe and USA with an 8% increase per decade (from 41.7% in the fifth decade to 65.4% in men of 70 years or older). Although mean prostate volume in Japan community-based studies is lower than in Caucasian-American and Africa-American series, Japanese prostates are more glandular. In Malaysia no difference in Q_{max} and prostate volume was found among Chinese, Malay, and Indian populations.[10]

Pathophysiology

The term "prostatism," suggesting a cohort of symptoms deriving from the enlarging prostate, has been replaced by the term "Lower Urinary Tract Symptoms."[11] LUTS terminology was redefined 8 years later and now includes filling/storage, emptying/voiding, and postvoiding symptoms (Table 27.1).[3] Voiding symptoms are known to be more prevalent than storage ones although these are more bothersome.[12] Frequency with reduced voided volume may be associated with detrusor overactivity, significant post-void residual, bladder neoplasms, fear of urinary retention, and psychogenic causes. A small

Table 27.1. LUTS

Filling/storage	Emptying/voiding	Postvoiding symptoms
Frequency	Hesitancy	Post-micturition dribbling
Urgency	Straining to void	Feeling of incomplete emptying
Nocturia	Poor stream	
Urgency incontinence	Intermittency	
Stress incontinence	Dysuria	
Nocturnal incontinence	Terminal dribbling	
Bladder/urethral pain		
Absent or impaired sensation		

bladder capacity may occur because of fibrosis, noninfectious inflammatory disorders, irradiation, and previous bladder surgery. Frequency with normal voided volume may depend upon polydipsia, osmotic diuresis, or diabetes insipidus. Urgency (the sudden compelling desire to void, which is difficult to defer), urgency incontinence, and overactive bladder indicate neurogenic origin (reduced suprapontine inhibition, damaged axonal paths in the spinal cord, increased afferent input to the lower urinary tract, loss of peripheral inhibition, enhancement of excitatory neurotransmission, in the micturition reflex pathway), myogenic (due to the effect of BOO on smooth muscle fibers) and structural causes. Nocturia, defined as the need to wake up at night to void, is a troublesome symptom that should always be distinguished from nocturnal polyuria. Prevalence of nocturia increases with age and is sometimes considered part of the normal aging process. Voiding symptoms include all symptoms experienced during voiding. There is no pathophysiological correlation between these symptoms and urodynamic parameters of outlet obstruction and this is why the term "obstructive symptoms" has been dropped. The relation between LUTS and BPH is complex particularly when epidemiological data suggested a similar prevalence in women.[12]

Patient Assessment

Patient assessment aims at establishing the pathophysiology of LUTS in the individual subject and include: history taking, frequency–volume charts, and symptom scores; physical examination; urinalysis; biochemical testing; post-void residual urine measurement, imaging, and endoscopy of lower urinary tract (LUT) (Table 27.2, Figs. 27.1 and 27.2).[13]

History and physical examination aims at diagnosing concomitant conditions of the bladder, the central nervous system, or other organs that may be responsible for LUTS beyond benign and malignant disorders of the prostate. Frequency–volume charts are instrumental to analyze day- and night-time frequency, mean voided volume, total urine output, nocturnal urine output, urgency and urgency incontinence episodes. Three- to seven-day charts are used with voided volumes recorded at least for 1 day. The instrument is accurate and inexpensive and its widespread use should be encouraged. Symptom score have been developed to standardize the assessment of symptom severity by using questions that have been psychometrically validated although they can also be used to predict the response to treatment and to assess treatment outcome. Different symptom scores are available and have been validated in several languages (IPSS, ICIQMLUTS, Dan PSS, OABq); they all contain one or more questions about quality of life and symptom bother. Although the IPSS is the most popular symptom score, it does not address urinary incontinence and may therefore be suboptimal whenever continence is impaired. Urinalysis is a recommended test also at the primary level because it allows to diagnose concomitant conditions that may or may not be associated with LUTS such as hematuria, but it is also instrumental in suspecting urinary tract infection, a common cause of LUTS. Although there is no association between BPE, BPH/BPO, and chronic kidney disease, some national guidelines still recommend to measure

Table 27.2. Diagnostic tests

Basic evaluation	Specialized management	
Recommended tests	Recommended tests	Optional tests
History	Detailed quantification of symptoms by validated questionnaires	Transrectal ultrasonography of the prostate
Assessment of symptoms and bother	Uroflowmetry	Ultrasound imaging of the upper urinary tract or intravenous urography
Urinalysis	Post-void residual urine	Endoscopy of the lower urinary tract
Serum prostate-specific antigen (when indicated)	Pressure-flow studies	
Frequency–volume chart (voiding diary)		

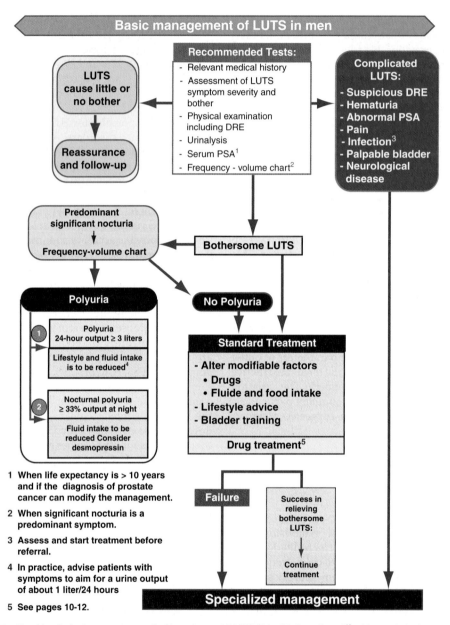

Figure 27.1. Algorithm for basic management of male patients with LUTS (From McConnell et al.[13] with permission).

serum creatinine. Prostate-specific antigen (PSA) is recommended by most guidelines in patients with a life expectancy of 10 years or greater; the test can be used as a screening tool for prostate cancer, is a proxy for prostate volume, and is a good prognostic parameter for BPH progression. Measurement of post-void residual has been recommended as part of the initial evaluation although there is a weak evidence for it. The relation between elevated PVR and UTI is in fact evident in the pediatric and neurogenic populations but scanty in the BPH patient. PVR values below 50–100 mL are considered to be normal and value >300 mL is used to identify patients at risk of unfavorable outcome. Imaging of the LUT includes bladder and prostate. Bladder imaging is usually performed for evaluating PVR but also provides

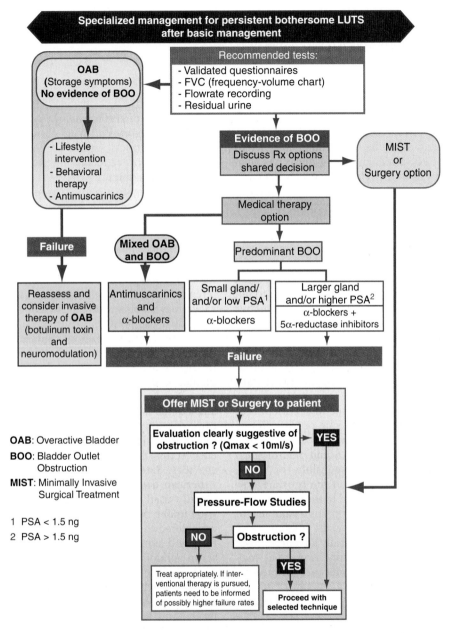

Figure 27.2. Algorithm for specialized management of male patients with persistent LUTS following basic management (From McConnell et al.[13] with permission).

information regarding possible comorbidities (bladder stones, diverticula, neoplasms, etc.), intravesical prostate protrusion, prostate volume, and bladder wall thickness. Transrectal imaging of the prostate cannot be used to diagnose or rule out prostate cancer in patients with LUTS but allows accurate evaluation of prostate volume and gland morphology. Endoscopy is an optional test in all guidelines, because it cannot diagnose BPO although it may rule out concomitant disorders of the urinary bladder and urethra that may be responsible for LUTS. Urodynamics include different tests although uroflowmetry and pressure-flow study are most frequently performed. Uroflowmetry has a good positive predictive value for the diagnosis of BPO and Q_{max} values <10 mL/s have a 70% specificity.[14,15] A weak stream is generally due to BPO although detrusor underactivity cannot be ruled unless pressure-flow study is performed. Voided volumes of 150 mL or higher are associated with a lower variability within the same patient; the test should always be performed in triplicate. Pressure-flow study has the unique capacity to diagnose BPO (although no consensus has been reached yet as to the relation between BPO and the outcome of surgery), detrusor overactivity and detrusor underactivity. Detrusor disorders are considered to be associated with unfavorable outcome following TURP.

Diagnostic tests performed in the assessment of BPH can also be used to predict the outcome of treatment. Patients with elevated PSA and BPO levels have a higher chance to fail watchful waiting.[16] Prostate volume and higher IPSS values are associated with a higher risk of invasive therapy in patients receiving pharmacological treatment.[16,17] Prostate volume was found to influence the success of a trial without catheter in patients suffering acute urinary retention.[18]

Physical examination of the BPH patient is of importance as it allows to rule out conditions such as chronic retention that may require immediate treatment and occult neurological disorders that may be responsible for LUTS. Digital rectal examination of the prostate now plays a minor role compared to the pre-PSA and pre-ultrasound era, but it remains a valid test to diagnose BPE and rule out acute inflammatory disorders of the prostate, locally advanced prostate cancer, neurological conditions that may affect anal sphincter tone, and cancer of the lowermost part of the rectum.

Treatment of BPH

Watchful Waiting

The simple diagnosis of LUTS due to BPH does necessarily trigger treatment. Most national and international guidelines suggest that patients with mild symptoms and no bother can be safely managed in a watchful waiting program.[19-21]

A good number of patients will never progress to pharmacological or surgical treatment.

Drug Therapy

If surgery was the first revolution in the management of BPH, pharmacotherapy was the second one. Four categories of drugs should be considered: plant extracts, alpha1 adrenoceptor (AR) antagonists, 5α- reductase inhibitors (5ARIs), and antimuscarinics.

Phytotherapy is a popular remedy for LUTS due to BPH that falls within the framework of complimentary medicine in most countries although some products are registered as drugs, particularly in Europe. Plant extracts suffer differences in the pharmaceutical preparation as the extraction procedures may differ among different commercial products, so the activity (efficacy, bioavailability, and pharmacodynamics) of individual components is not comparable; furthermore, some preparations contain mixture of different extracts. The origin of phytotherapeutic agents include: American dwarf palm, Saw palmetto, African plum tree, South African star grass, Pine Spruce, Stinging nettle, Rye, Pumpkin, and Cactus flower extracts. Active components comprise: phytosterols (alpha-sitosterol), phytoestrogens, fatty acids (lauric and myristica cid), lectins, flavonoids, plant oils, and polysaccharides. Serenoa repens, extracted from the American dwarf palm is one of the most frequently used products commercialized worldwide under the name of Permixon. The drug is considered to have antiandrogen, antiproliferative, and anti-inflammatory activities. Six of seven randomized studies showed superiority over placebo in reducing LUTS and improving flow rate, and two large comparative trials suggested a similar efficacy among Permixon, finasteride, and tamsulosin. Two meta analyses of Permixon studies performed by P. Boyle suggested a significant improvement of IPSS (−4.7), nocturia (1.0 over placebo), and maximum flow rate (2.2 mL/s over placebo).[22] A different conclusion was reached by a recent meta-analysis published by the Cochrane Library suggesting that Serenoa repens is not more effective than placebo for the treatment of symptoms consistent with BPH.[23] Clinical trials performed using other phytotherapeutics such as Pygeum Africanum (Tadenan) or synthetic polyenes

(Mepartricin) are considered to be insufficient and further research is needed before any recommendation can be made.

AR antagonists are the first-line treatment in the management of BPH because of their speed of action, safety, tolerability, and efficacy. They are considered to act on smooth muscle fibers tone (the so-called dynamic component of BPO). Although most clinical trials were limited to 3- or 6-month treatment, more recent studies such as MTOPS and Combat trials provided 4-year data and CombAT trial will do the same in due time.[9,24] α_{1A}-AR and α_{1D}-Ar subtypes expressed in the prostate, urinary bladder, and spinal cord are considered to be more important than α_{1B}-AR that are more involved in the blood pressure regulation. Diffusion of α_1-AR antagonists into the central nervous system (CNS) is considered to be responsible for dizziness and asthenia although there is no proof of it.

α-1 AR antagonists are known to improve LUTS and flow rate by acting on the receptors expressed in smooth muscle fibers of the prostatic stroma, bladder neck, and urethra. Possible mechanisms of action outside the LUT involving ganglia, spinal, and/or supraspinal structures in the CNS have been hypothesized.[25,26] The positive effect of these drugs on LUTS cannot be explained by the moderate improvement of BPO.[27] The concept of uroselectivity (desired effects on obstruction and LUTS related to adverse effects) was proposed to highlight the low rate of adverse events observed with modern molecules having minimal effect on blood pressure and the CNS.[28] There is no consensus as to the ideal profile of AR subtype selectivity; modern molecules have a high affinity for α_{1A} and α_{1D} AR subtype and low affinity for α_{1B} that seems involved in blood pressure regulation. Slow release, once daily formulations of α_1-AR antagonists were developed to increase patient compliance and tolerability although none of the clinical trials was able to show superiority of the slow release formulation versus the immediate release one so that the clinical relevance of such development remains unclear.[29,30] Distribution of α_1 AR antagonists in the human body is of importance as penetration of the blood–brain barrier may be responsible for some of the side effects. Neither slow release formulation nor difference in lypophilicity among different molecules appeared to provide a clinical advantage to any drug.

Since α_1 AR antagonists are not first-line treatment for arterial hypertension, the use of nonselective antagonists to control hypertension and LUTS at the same time is not encouraged and each condition should be treated independently.[13] Adverse events most frequently involve orthostatic hypotension, dizziness, and asthenia suggesting that AR receptors expressed in blood vessels and CNS are of importance. Multiple, placebo-controlled, randomized, double-blind study of adequate size and duration confirmed the positive effect of α_1 AR antagonists on LUTS.[31-34] Alfuzosin and tamsulosin are known to be equally effective with similar tolerability although tamsulosin is known to cause ejaculatory dysfunction in <10% of patients. Tamsulosin proved to be better tolerated than terazosin.[35-37] Because of the possible additive effect of α_1 AR antagonists and phosphodiesterase inhibitors in lowering blood pressure, the FDA suggested to avoid using sildenafil within 4h of taking an α_1 AR antagonist.[38]

The issue of patient compliance to prescribed medications is of importance as market data suggest that most BPH patients remain on treatment for a few months only. Outcome measures used in clinical trials of drug treatment of BPH are validated parameters that proved to be sensitive to change, but the problem of statistical significance versus clinical one remains open. In particular, little information is available as to the clinical outcome and disease progression in real-life practice.

After the use of antiandrogens and androgen ablation was discontinued, hormonal therapy of BPH is nowadays based on 5α-reductase inhibitors (5ARIs).[39-42] The introduction of 5ARIs opens a new perspective because of the significant effect of these drugs on prostate volume suggesting that the progression of the disease could be somehow halted.[43] The slow onset of the therapeutic effect on LUTS prevented these drugs from being used as first-line treatment for many years. Short-term randomized studies failed to prove advantage of 5ARIs versus placebo.[44-46] A paradigm shift was caused by the results of an independent, long-term study that randomized patients among placebo, doxazosin, finasteride, and their combination using overall disease progression as the primary endpoint.[9] After an average 4.5 years of follow-up, combination treatment proved to be superior to either monotherapy treatments in reducing overall disease progression. Preliminary. Data from the CombAT study, confirm the long-term efficacy and safety of combination treatment with tamsulosin and dutasteride. Post hoc analyses of randomized trials suggest that 5ARIs are more efficacious in patients with enlarged prostates, which are also at a higher risk of disease progression.[47,48] Open label extensions of randomized trials and long-term studies such as the MTOPS provided convincing evidence of a sustained therapeutic effect over time. The aim of 5ARIs treatment is twofold: to reduce parameters of disease severity that are usually associated with a decreased quality of life such as LUTS, and to prevent disease progression. Longterm treatment with 5ARIs as monotherapy or in combination with α-AR antagonists provides a significant improvement of LUTS, maximum flow rate, and post-void residual. Evaluation of 5ARIs arms (monotherapy or combination) of randomized trials show a significant reduction in the overall disease progression and particularly in terms of symptom progression, prostate volume increase, acute urinary retention episodes, and need for surgery compared to placebo. 5ARIs are known to reduce total PSA values by roughly 50%, but accuracy of this marker for early diagnosis of prostate cancer is maintained.[49] Long-term use of 5ARIs proved to be safe and adverse events mainly consist in decreased libido, diminished ejaculation, and impotence. Contrary to α-AR antagonists, the therapeutic effect of 5ARIs takes time to develop and patients should not be reassessed before 3 months of treatment. Randomized trials of 5ARIs in monotherapy or combination show that patients should initiate treatment if they do not commit long-term as clinical benefit over α-AR antagonists needs at least 1 year to develop. Patients with LUTS associated with proven BPE are candidates for combination treatment as post hoc analyses suggest that every male patient with a total PSA of 1.5 ng/mL or greater and a prostate volume of 30 mL or larger is at risk for disease progression.[50]

The use of antimuscarinics in the management of patients with LUTS due to BPH has been recently proposed to manage storage symptoms that may remain following treatment with α-AR antagonists.[51] Evidence from randomized trials confirms that the use of antimuscarinics. In patients with LUTS and symptoms of overactive bladder, α-$_1$ AR antagonists and antimuscarinics can be prescribed in combination at treatment start, alternatively antimuscarinics can be added only in those patients who do not improve sufficiently on α-$_1$ AR antagonists.

Interventional Therapies

The challenge of BPH surgery is in the management of very large prostates as complications of Trans-Urethral Resection of the Prostate (TURP) are known to increase in larger prostates.[54] Open surgery is rapidly fading away from the urologist armamentarium because the outstanding outcome is associated with increased morbidity and high cost compared to TURP. The small number of open prostatectomies performed in urological centers does no longer allow proper training of our residents. Transurethral resection of the prostate TURP evolved significantly over the last decades and the transfusion rate dropped from the two-digit to the single-digit range.[55] Technical improvement in electrocautery units and the availability of bipolar surgery were instrumental in making TURP safer.[56] Although transurethral resection of the prostate remains the gold standard treatment for BPO, several alternative treatments have been developed over the last decade to provide durable improvement with reduced morbidity and side effects. The term "minimally invasive" is a frequently abused one, particularly in BPH treatment and comprises totally different treatments.

Transurethral microwave thermotherapy (TUMT) and transurethral needle ablation of the prostate (TUNA) may be performed as office-based procedures with no anesthesia.[57,58] Long-term data of TUMT series suggest how one in four patients with moderate degree of bladder obstruction and one in three patients with severe BPO required surgery in the long term (8 years).[59] Long-term data on TUNA are not yet available although a large European registry database will provide an answer by 2012. Both techniques provide clinical outcome that is certainly inferior to that produced by surgery although the morbidity is certainly lower.[60]

Laser treatments of BPH are often called "minimally invasive" although both Holmium Laser Enucleation of the Prostate (HoLEP) and Photo Vaporization of the Prostate (PVP) differ from TURP only in terms of reduced bleeding and shorter hospital stay.[61] Each technique has its advantages and disadvantages. HoLEP proved to be effective in the management of very large prostates but usually requires bladder irrigation for a few hours. PVP can be performed in patients on anticoagulants and antiaggregants, requires no bladder irrigation, and can be performed as a day case although proper debulking of large prostates remains a challenge.

Conclusions

The management of patients with LUTS due to BPH evolved significantly over the last 2 decades with the use of pharmacological treatment and the introduction of combination therapy. Following the use of pharmacotherapy, the number of surgical procedures performed in BPH patients dropped dramatically. Patients now tend to receive surgery at an older age and the average prostate volume tends to be larger.[62] The morbidity of BPH surgery was significantly reduced because of the introduction of bipolar and laser surgery. Notwithstanding all the technological developments, proper knowledge of the pathophysiology of lower urinary tract dysfunction and a correct diagnosis remains the mainstay for a successful treatment of patients suffering from LUTS.

References

1. Chapple C, Tubaro A. *Current Therapy of Benign Prostatic Hyperplasia*. London: Martin Dunitz Ltd.; 2000
2. Bosch JL, Hop WC, Kirkels WJ, Schroder FH. Natural history of benign prostatic hyperplasia: appropriate case definition and estimation of its prevalence in the community. *Urology*. 1995;46:34-40
3. Abrams P, Cardozo L, Fall M, et al. The standardisation of terminology of lower urinary tract function: report from the Standardisation Sub-committee of the International Continence Society. *Neurourol Urodyn*. 2002;21: 167-178
4. Logie J, Clifford GM, Farmer RD. Incidence, prevalence and management of lower urinary tract symptoms in men in the UK. *BJU Int*. 2005;95:557-562
5. Gades NM, Jacobson DJ, Girman CJ, Roberts RO, Lieber MM, Jacobsen SJ. Prevalence of conditions potentially associated with lower urinary tract symptoms in men. *BJU Int*. 2005;95:549-553
6. Thomas AW, Cannon A, Bartlett E, Ellis-Jones J, Abrams P. The natural history of lower urinary tract dysfunction in men: minimum 10-year urodynamic follow-up of untreated bladder outlet obstruction. *BJU Int*. 2005; 96:1301-1306

7. Rhodes T, Girman CJ, Jacobsen SJ, Roberts RO, Guess HA, Lieber MM. Longitudinal prostate growth rates during 5 years in randomly selected community men 40–79 years old. *J Urol*. 1999;161:1174-1179
8. Bosch JL, Hop WC, Niemer AQ, Bangma CH, Kirkels WJ, Schroder FH. Parameters of prostate volume and shape in a community based population of men 55-74 years old. *J Urol*. 1994;152:1501-1505
9. McConnell JD, Roehrborn CG, Bautista OM, et al. The long-term effect of doxazosin, finasteride, and combination therapy on the clinical progression of benign prostatic hyperplasia. *N Engl J Med*. 2003;349:2387-2398
10. Teh GC, Sahabudin RM, Lim TC, et al. Prevalence of symptomatic BPE among Malaysian men aged 50 and above attending screening during prostate health awareness campaign. *Med J Malays*. 2001;56:186-195
11. Abrams P. New words for old: lower urinary tract symptoms for "prostatism". *BMJ*. 1994;308:929-930
12. Frymann RJ, Abrams PA. Current diagnosis in the management of men with lower urinary tract symptoms. In: Walsh P, Retik A, Vaughn ED, Wein A, eds. *Campbell's Urology Updates*, Vol 1. Philadelphia: Saunders, Co.; 2000:1-17
13. Abrams P, Chapple C, Khoury S, Roehrborn C, de la Rosette J; International Scientific Committee. Evaluation and treatment of lower urinary tract symptoms in older men. *J Urol*. 2009 Apr;181(4):1779-87
14. Poulsen AL, Schou J, Puggaard L, Torp-Pedersen S, Nordling J. Prostatic enlargement, symptomatology and pressure/flow evaluation: interrelations in patients with symptomatic BPH. *Scand J Urol Nephrol Suppl*. 1994;157:67-73
15. Nielsen KK, Nordling J, Hald T. Critical review of the diagnosis of prostatic obstruction. *Neurourol Urodyn*. 1994;13:201-217
16. Mochtar CA, Kiemeney LA, Laguna MP, et al. Prognostic role of prostate-specific antigen and prostate volume for the risk of invasive therapy in patients with benign prostatic hyperplasia initially managed with alpha1-blockers and watchful waiting. *Urology*. 2005;65:300-305
17. Hong SJ, Ko WJ, Kim SI, Chung BH. Identification of baseline clinical factors which predict medical treatment failure of benign prostatic hyperplasia: an observational cohort study. *Eur Urol*. 2003;44:94-99; discussion 99-100
18. McNeill AS, Rizvi S, Byrne DJ. Prostate size influences the outcome after presenting with acute urinary retention. *BJU Int*. 2004;94:559-562
19. Roehrborn CG, Bartsch G, Kirby R, et al. Guidelines for the diagnosis and treatment of benign prostatic hyperplasia: a comparative, international overview. *Urology*. 2001;50:642
20. de la Rosette JJ, Alivizatos G, Madersbacher S, et al. EAU guidelines on benign prostatic hyperplasia (BPH). *Eur Urol*. 2001;40:256-263; discussion 264
21. Kaplan SA. Update on the American urological association guidelines for the treatment of benign prostatic hyperplasia. *Rev Urol*. 2006;4(8 suppl):S10-S17
22. Boyle P, Robertson C, Lowe F, Roehrborn C. Meta-analysis of clinical trials of permixon in the treatment of symptomatic benign prostatic hyperplasia. *Urology*. 2000;55:533-539

23. Tacklind J, MacDonald R, Rutks I, Wilt TJ. Serenoa repens for benign prostatic hyperplasia. *Cochrane Database Syst Rev.* CD001423; 2009

24. Roehrborn CG, Siami P, Barkin J et al.: The Effects of Combination Therapy with Dutasteride and Tamsulosin on Clinical Outcomes in Men with Symptomatic Benign Prostatic Hyperplasia: 4-Year Results from the CombAT Study. *Eur Urol.* 2010; 57: 123-131

25. Roehrborn CG, Schwinn DA. Alpha1-adrenergic receptors and their inhibitors in lower urinary tract symptoms and benign prostatic hyperplasia. *J Urol.* 2004;171: 1029-1035

26. Michel MC. Potential role of a1-adrenoceptor subtypes in the aetiology of LUTS. *Eur Urol Suppl.* 2002;1:5-13.

27. Kortmann BB, Floratos DL, Kiemeney LA, Wijkstra H, de la Rosette JJ. Urodynamic effects of alpha-adrenoceptor blockers: a review of clinical trials. *Urology.* 2003;62:1-9

28. Andersson KE. The concept of uroselectivity. *Eur Urol Suppl.* 1998;33:7-11

29. Kirby RS, Andersen M, Gratzke P, Dahlstrand C, Hoye K. A combined analysis of double-blind trials of the efficacy and tolerability of doxazosin-gastrointestinal therapeutic system, doxazosin standard and placebo in patients with benign prostatic hyperplasia. *BJU Int.* 2001;87:192-200

30. van Kerrebroeck P, Jardin A, Laval KU, van Cangh P. Efficacy and safety of a new prolonged release formulation of alfuzosin 10 mg once daily versus alfuzosin 2.5 mg thrice daily and placebo in patients with symptomatic benign prostatic hyperplasia. ALFORTI Study Group. *Eur Urol.* 2000;37:306-313

31. Wilt TJ, Howe RW, Rutks IR, MacDonald R. Terazosin for benign prostatic hyperplasia. *Cochrane Database Syst Rev.* CD003851; 2002

32. Wilt TJ, MacDonald R, Nelson D. Tamsulosin for treating lower urinary tract symptoms compatible with benign prostatic obstruction: a systematic review of efficacy and adverse effects. *J Urol.* 2002;167:177-183

33. Milani S, Djavan B. Lower urinary tract symptoms suggestive of benign prostatic hyperplasia: latest update on alpha-adrenoceptor antagonists. *BJU Int.* 2005;95(suppl 4): 29-36

34. Djavan B, Marberger M. A meta-analysis on the efficacy and tolerability of alpha1-adrenoceptor antagonists in patients with lower urinary tract symptoms suggestive of benign prostatic obstruction. *Eur Urol.* 1999;36:1-13

35. Narayan P, Tunuguntla HS. Long-term efficacy and safety of tamsulosin for benign prostatic hyperplasia. *Rev Urol.* 2005;7(suppl 4):S42-S48

36. Na YJ, Guo YL, Gu FL. Clinical comparison of selective and non-selective alpha 1A-adrenoceptor antagonists for bladder outlet obstruction associated with benign prostatic hyperplasia: studies on tamsulosin and terazosin in Chinese patients. The Chinese Tamsulosin Study Group. *J Med.* 1998;29:289-304

37. Lee E, Lee C. Clinical comparison of selective and non-selective alpha 1A-adrenoreceptor antagonists in benign prostatic hyperplasia: studies on tamsulosin in a fixed dose and terazosin in increasing doses. *Br J Urol.* 1997;80: 606-611

38. Barendrecht MM, Koopmans RP, de la Rosette JJ, Michel MC. Treatment of lower urinary tract symptoms suggestive of benign prostatic hyperplasia: the cardiovascular system. *BJU Int.* 2005;95(suppl 4):19-28

39. Wilson JD, Griffin JE, Russell DW. Steroid 5 alpha-reductase 2 deficiency. *Endocr Rev.* 1993;14:577-593

40. Russell DW, Wilson JD. Steroid 5 alpha-reductase: two genes/two enzymes. *Annu Rev Biochem.* 1994;63:25-61

41. Randall VA. Role of 5 alpha-reductase in health and disease. *Baillières Clin Endocrinol Metab.* 1994;8:405-431

42. Andersson S, Berman DM, Jenkins EP, Russell DW. Deletion of steroid 5 alpha-reductase 2 gene in male pseudohermaphroditism. *Nature.* 1991;354:159-161

43. Gormley GJ, Stoner E, Bruskewitz RC, et al. The effect of finasteride in men with benign prostatic hyperplasia the finasteride study group. *N Engl J Med.* 992;327:1185-1191

44. Debruyne FM, Jardin A, Colloi D, et al. Sustained-release alfuzosin, finasteride and the combination of both in the treatment of benign prostatic hyperplasia. European ALFIN Study Group. *Eur Urol.* 1998;34:169-175

45. Lepor H, Williford WO, Barry MJ, et al. The efficacy of terazosin, finasteride, or both in benign prostatic hyperplasia veterans affairs cooperative studies benign prostatic hyperplasia study group. *N Engl J Med.* 1996;335: 533-539

46. Kirby RS, Roehrborn C, Boyle P, et al. Efficacy and tolerability of doxazosin and finasteride, alone or in combination, in treatment of symptomatic benign prostatic hyperplasia: The Prospective European Doxazosin and Combination Therapy (PREDICT) trial. *Urology.* 2003;61:119-126

47. Kaplan SA, McConnell JD, Roehrborn CG, et al. Combination therapy with doxazosin and finasteride for benign prostatic hyperplasia in patients with lower urinary tract symptoms and a baseline total prostate volume of 25 ml or greater. *J Urol.* 2006;175:217-220; discussion 220-221

48. Crawford ED, Wilson SS, McConnell JD, et al. Baseline factors as predictors of clinical progression of benign prostatic hyperplasia in men treated with placebo. *J Urol.* 2006;175:1422-1426; discussion 1426-1427

49. Gormley GJ, Ng J, Cook T, Stoner E, Guess H, Walsh P. Effect of finasteride on prostate-specific antigen density. *Urology.* 1994;43:53-58; discussion 58-59

50. Lowe FC, Batista J, Berges R, et al. Risk factors for disease progression in patients with lower urinary tract symptoms/benign prostatic hyperplasia (LUTS/BPH): a systematic analysis of expert opinion. *Prostate Cancer Prostatic Dis.* 2005;8:206-209

51. Lee JY, Kim HW, Lee SJ, Koh JS, Suh HJ, Chancellor MB. Comparison of doxazosin with or without tolterodine in men with symptomatic bladder outlet obstruction and an overactive bladder. *BJU Int.* 2004;94:817-820

52. Abrams P, Kaplan S, De Koning Gans HJ, Millard R. Safety and tolerability of tolterodine for the treatment of overactive bladder in men with bladder outlet obstruction. *J Urol.* 2006;175:999-1004; discussion 1004

53. Kaplan SA, Roehrborn CG, Rovner ES, Carlsson M, Bavendam T, Guan Z. Tolterodine and tamsulosin for treatment of men with lower urinary tract symptoms and overactive bladder: a randomized controlled trial. *JAMA.* 2006;296:2319-2328

54. Mebust WK, Holtgrewe HL, Cockett AT, Peters PC. Transurethral prostatectomy: immediate and postoperative complications. A cooperative study of 13 participating institutions evaluating 3,885 patients. *J Urol*. 1989; 141:243-247

55. Rassweiler J, Teber D, Kuntz R, Hofmann R. Complications of transurethral resection of the prostate (TURP) – incidence, management, and prevention. *Eur Urol*. 2006;50:969-979; discussion 980

56. Hon NH, Brathwaite D, Hussain Z, et al. A prospective, randomized trial comparing conventional transurethral prostate resection with PlasmaKinetic vaporization of the prostate: physiological changes, early complications and long-term followup. *J Urol*. 2006;176: 205-209

57. Boyle P, Robertson C, Vaughan ED, Fitzpatrick JM. A meta-analysis of trials of transurethral needle ablation for treating symptomatic benign prostatic hyperplasia. *BJU Int*. 2004;94:83-88

58. Wagrell L, Schelin S, Nordling J, et al. Three-year follow-up of feedback microwave thermotherapy versus TURP for clinical BPH: a prospective randomized multicenter study. *Urology*. 2004;64:698-702

59. Vesely S, Knutson T, Damber JE, Dicuio M, Dahlstrand C. TURP and low-energy TUMT treatment in men with LUTS suggestive of bladder outlet obstruction selected by means of pressure-flow studies: 8-year follow-up. *Neurourol Urodyn*. 2006;25:770-775

60. Hoffman RM, MacDonald R, Monga M, Wilt TJ. Transurethral microwave thermotherapy vs transurethral resection for treating benign prostatic hyperplasia: a systematic review. *BJU Int*. 2004;94:1031-1036

61. Naspro R, Bachmann A, Gilling P, et al. A review of the recent evidence (2006–2008) for 532-nm photoselective laser vaporisation and holmium laser enucleation of the prostate. *Eur Urol*. 2009;55:1345-1357

62. Vela-Navarrete R, Gonzalez-Enguita C, Garcia-Cardoso JV, Manzarbeitia F, Sarasa-Corral JL, Granizo JJ. The impact of medical therapy on surgery for benign prostatic hyperplasia: a study comparing changes in a decade (1992–2002). *BJU Int*. 2005;96:1045-1048

28

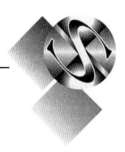

Practical Guidelines for the Treatment of Erectile Dysfunction and Peyronie´s Disease

Christian Gratzke, Karl-Erik Andersson, Thorsten Diemer, Wolfgang Weidner, and Christian G. Stief

Erectile Dysfunction

Introduction

Erectile dysfunction (ED) is defined as persistent inability to attain and/or maintain an erection sufficient for sexual performance.[1,2] It is assumed that 5–20% of men complain of moderate to severe ED[3]; common risk factors are very similar to risk factors of cardiovascular disease and include smoking, hypertension, diabetes, lipidemia, atherosclerosis, and pelvic surgery.[2,4] The introduction of oral drugs has revolutionized the medical treatment of ED; successful intercourse can be achieved with inhibitors of phosphodiesterase 5 (PDE-5) such as sildenafil, tadalafil, and vardenafil in about 75% of patients suffering from ED.[5] However, a considerable amount of men does not respond to PDE-5 inhibitors, particularly patients with diabetes mellitus (DM) or patients having undergone radical prostatectomy. This chapter aims to present a pragmatic approach for the clinical diagnosis and therapy of ED, based on available literature, particularly the guidelines of the European Association of Urology,[6] the American Urological Association[7] as well as the British Society for Sexual Medicine,[5] and on current research and clinical practice.

Diagnosis

Diagnostic steps of patients presenting with ED contain basic tests, which are recommended in all patients, optional and specialized evaluations that should be tailored to the individual patient´s profile.

Basic Evaluation

It is crucial to obtain a thorough medical, sexual and psychosocial history, physical examination, and focused laboratory tests. A detailed patient´s history evaluates the presence of risk factors such as hypertension, diabetes mellitus, myocardial disease, lipidemia, hypercholesterolemia, renal insufficiency, hypogonadism, and neurologic and psychiatric disorders.[8] If possible, the partner should be included. Predisposing, precipitating, and maintaining factors should be obtained (Table 28.1) as well as a detailed description of the quality of morning and erotic or masturbation-induced erections, in terms of rigidity and duration, as well as arousal, ejaculation, and orgasmic problems. Lower urinary tract symptoms and genitourinary (mainly radical prostatectomy) and rectal surgery, as well as many drugs, particularly antihypertensive and psychotropic drugs may cause ED.[9-11] The chronic use of alcohol, marijuana, codeine,

Table 28.1. Pathophysiological causes of ED

Predisposing	Precipitating	Maintaining
Lack of sexual knowledge	New relationship	Relationship problems
Poor past sexual experience	Acute relationship problems	Poor communication between partners
Relationship problems	Family or social pressures	Lack of knowledge about treatment options
Religious or cultural beliefs	Pregnancy and childbirth	
Restrictive upbringing	Other major life events	Ongoing physical or mental health problems
Unclear sexual or gender preference	Partner's menopause	Other sexual problems in the man or his partner
Previous sexual abuse	Acute physical or mental health problems	Drugs
Other sexual problems in the man or his partner	Lack of knowledge about normal changes of aging	
Drugs	Other sexual problems in the man or his partner	
	Drugs	

ED erectile dysfunction.
Source: Reprinted from Hackett et al. 5. With permission from Wiley-Blackwell.

meperidine, methadone, and heroin is also associated with a high percentage of ED.[12]

The use of validated questionnaires, such as the International Index for Erectile Function (IIEF), may be helpful to assess all sexual function domains (erectile function, orgasmic function, sexual desire, ejaculation, intercourse, and overall satisfaction) and also the impact of a specific treatment modality (Grade C – level IV).[13]

A focused physical examination must be performed on every patient, with particular emphasis on the genitourinary, endocrine, vascular, and neurologic systems. All patients should have a focused physical examination. A genital examination is recommended to detect a history of rapid onset of pain, deviation of the penis during tumescence, the symptoms of hypogonadism, or other urological symptoms (past or present). A digital rectal examination of the prostate is not mandatory in ED but should be conducted in the presence of genitourinary or protracted secondary ejaculatory symptoms. Blood pressure, heart rate, waist circumference, and weight should be measured[14] (Grade C – level IV).

Laboratory testing must be tailored to the patient's complaints and risk factors. All patients must undergo a fasting glucose and lipid profile if not assessed in the previous 12 months to rule out diabetes and hyperlipidemia. Hormonal testing must include a morning sample of total testosterone (bioavailable or calculated-free testosterone is more reliable to establish the presence of hypogonadism, i.e., these tests are preferable to total testosterone if available). Additional hormonal tests (e.g., prolactin, follicle-stimulating hormone [FSH], luteinizing hormone [LH]) must be carried out when low testosterone levels are detected (Grade B – level IIa). If any abnormality is observed, further investigation by referral to another specialist may be necessary.[10] Minimal diagnostic evaluation (basic workup) in patients with ED is presented in Fig. 28.1. Serum prostate-specific antigen should be considered if clinically indicated. It should certainly be measured before commencing testosterone and at regular intervals during testosterone therapy (Grade C – level IV).

Cardiovascular System and Sexual Activity

Coronary heart disease (CHD) shares many risk factors with ED[15] since endothelial dysfunction and atherosclerosis affect both coronary arteries and penile vasculature. ED often precedes coronary artery disease.[16] Guidelines for the management of ED in patients with cardiovascular disease have been developed by the Princeton Consensus Panel.[17] Patients with ED

Figure 28.1. Minimal diagnostic evaluation for patients with erectile dysfunction (*ED*). *IIEF* International Index for Erectile Function, *CV* cardiovascular (Reprinted from [6]. Copyright 2006, with permission from Elsevier).

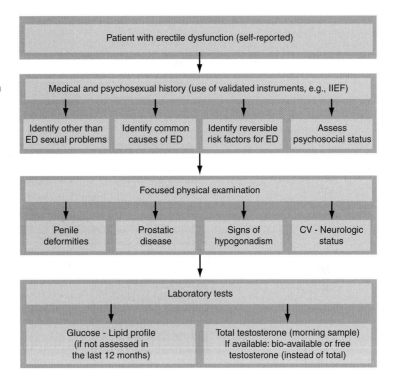

requiring initiating or resuming sexual activity are stratified into three risk categories based on their cardiovascular risk factors. High-risk patients are defined as those with unstable or refractory angina; uncontrolled hypertension; left ventricular dysfunction/congestive heart failure (CHF; New York Heart Association class II); MI or a cardiovascular accident within the previous 2 weeks; high-risk arrhythmias; hypertrophic obstructive and other cardiomyopathies; or moderate-to-severe valvular disease. It is recommended that patients at high risk should not receive treatment for sexual dysfunction until their cardiac condition has stabilized. Patients at low risk may be considered for all first-line therapies. The majority of patients treated for ED are in the low-risk category defined as those who have asymptomatic coronary artery disease and less than three risk factors for coronary artery disease (excluding gender); controlled hypertension; mild, stable angina; a successful coronary revascularization; uncomplicated past MI; mild valvular disease; or CHF (left ventricular dysfunction and/or New York Heart Association class I). Patients whose risk is indeterminate should undergo further evaluation by a cardiologist before receiving therapies for sexual dysfunction. The vast majority of men with CHD can safely resume sexual activity and use ED therapies.[18] Education and appropriate counseling about sex should be given to all men with CHD. There is currently no proof that licensed treatments for ED increase the cardiovascular risk in patients with or without previously diagnosed cardiovascular disease (Grade A – level Ia[5]) (Fig. 28.2).

Optional Tests

Even though most patients do not require further investigations, in certain circumstances, specific test may be required. In order to analyze the etiology of erectile dysfunction, appropriate assessments have to be conducted (Grade C – level IV). Other indications for special investigations include: young patients who have always had difficulty in obtaining and/or sustaining an erection, patients with a history of trauma, if an abnormality of the testes or penis is found on examination, and nonresponders to medical therapy potentially needing surgical treatment.[5-7]

Nocturnal penile tumescence and rigidity assessments measure natural nocturnal and early awakening erections, which are normal physiological events. With the Intracavernous Injection (ICI) test, penile rigidity is evaluated 10 min after injection of prostaglandin E1 into

Figure 28.2. Sexual activity and cardiac risk: the Princeton-II-consensus (Reprinted from Kostis et al. [17] pp. 85–93.

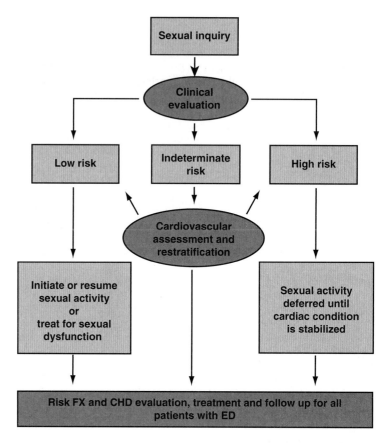

the corpus cavernosum of the penis. It has to be noted that a positive result is found in patients with both normal and mild vascular disease; therefore, results have to be interpreted with caution. Duplex ultrasound of Penile Arteries measures blood flow in order to study penile vasculature in response to an injection of a vasoactive agent.[19] Cavernosometry and cavernosography are highly specialized investigations that are performed only in specific circumstances, while arteriography ought to be performed when an arterial lesion has been found on Duplex Doppler evaluation. Cavernosometry is used to diagnose primary venous pathology in young men. Penile abnormalities such as phimosis, tight frenulum, and penile curvatures have to be treated surgically. Peyronie's disease is discussed further below.

Treatment

Among the various treatment options which include medical, psychosocial, and surgical treatment, it is important to carefully select the most suitable option based on the patient´s individual profile. Treatment modalities should be discussed with the patient and his partner and should be based on the patient´s risk factors and comorbidities after appropriate counseling of the patient.

Important "reversible" causes for ED including lifestyle factors such as obesity, cigarette smoking, alcoholism, or substance abuse have to be managed as well as psychosocial factors such as partner conflicts or any psychosexual dysfunctions. Modification in the comedication such as antihypertensive agents (particularly beta-blockers and diuretics), psychotropic drugs such as antidepressants and antiandrogens, steroids and antiarrhythmics might result in clinical benefits. In case of hypogonadism and hyperprolactinemia, hormone replacement therapy should be offered. However, patients need to be followed closely when receiving androgen therapy. Contraindications include abnormal liver function, hyperlipidemia, polycythemia, prostate cancer, aggressive behavior, and sleep apnea.

In young patients with posttraumatic arteriogenic ED, penile revascularization interventions have shown a 60–70% long-term success rate (Grade B – level IIb).[20] Imaging modalities such as duplex ultrasound and penile pharmacoarteriography have to be used to demonstrate and confirm the lesion. In case of corporal veno-occlusive dysfunction revascularization is contraindicated.[15,16] In patients with veno-occlusive dysfunction, surgical treatment has not shown satisfactory results and is no longer recommended.[18]

Medical Treatment

The majority of patients will seek medical treatment for ED. Treatment strategies depend on the patient´s risks and benefits, the cardiovascular safety (see above), costs, patient´s preferences, and partner issues. Accordingly, treatment will be selected based not only on the efficacy and safety profile of the drugs available, but also on the patient's cultural, religious, and economic background. A treatment algorithm for ED is presented in Fig. 28.3.[6]

Oral Agents

Several agents are approved and available for this indication (selective PDE5 inhibitors, apomorphine and yohimbine). In most patients with ED, PDE5-inhibitors are the gold standard due to their potential benefits and lack of invasiveness.[5-7]

Phosphodiesterase Type 5 (PDE 5) Inhibitors PDE5-inhibitors are associated with the broadest efficacy and highest tolerability in the treatment of ED. Sildenafil, tadalafil, and vardenafil are commercially available potent, reversible, competitive inhibitors of PDE5 (Grade A – level Ia).

All PDE5 inhibitors are nonhydrolyzable analogues to cGMP that prevent the degradation of this cyclic nucleotide by competitive binding to the catalytic site of PDE5. Thus, enhancement of NO-initiated relaxations of cavernous erectile tissue can be obtained.[21] To date, the abundant expression of PDE5 protein in the human corpus cavernosum versus other tissues is considered the main reason for the clinical efficacy of PDE5 inhibitors in the treatment of ED. In turn, this elevated expression of PDE5 in the penis

might be responsible for the low efficacy of NO donor drugs, which have not yet been introduced successfully to the pharmaceutical market.

Superiority has not been proven for any of these substances in spite of existing differences in pharmacokinetic and adverse event profiles (Table 28.2). Sildenafil was approved worldwide in 1998 and vardenafil and tadalafil in 2003. PDE5 inhibitors are effective and well tolerated as demonstrated in controlled clinical trials and clinical practice experience. In general ED, a high level of evidence exists for the efficacy of all three drugs. As side effect, mild transient systemic vasodilation may occur; this effect may be aggravated by alpha-blocking therapies for lower urinary tract symptoms due to bladder outlet obstruction (BOO). PDE5 inhibitors are strictly contraindicated in patients receiving organic nitrates and nitrate donors. The onset of nonarteritic anterior ischemic optic neuropathy (NAION) has not been proven to be associated with the use of PDE5-inhibitors.

Nonresponders to PDE5 Inhibitors In spite of the excellent clinical effects of PDE5-inhibitors, about 20–30% of patients do not respond to PDE5 inhibitors. Particularly, patients suffering from ED associated with diabetes and after radical prostatectomy for prostate cancer are difficult to treat. These patients should receive a minimum of four of the highest tolerated dose of at least two drugs.[5] In case of failure, it is recommended to reinstruct the patient on how to use the drug correctly (Grade B – level Ib), re-evaluate (new) risk factors, treat concurrent hypogonadism (Grade A – level Ib), change to another drug (Grade C – level IIa), and prescribe more frequent dosing regimes (Grade B – level Ib) (Fig. 28.4).

Apomorphine SL Apomorphine SL (sublingual), administered in 2- or 3-mg doses, is a centrally acting nonselective dopamine agonist (mainly D2), improving erectile function by enhancing the natural central erectile signals that usually occur during sexual stimulation.[22] It acts with modest efficacy and good tolerability in mild ED. It is associated with mild to moderate nausea and rare bradycardia/syncopy (vasovagal) syndrome. Apomorphine SL is registered in various countries (not in the US) since 2002. Efficacy rates (erections hard enough for

Figure 28.3. Treatment algorithm for erectile dysfunction (*ED*) (Reprinted from [6]. Copyright 2006, with permission from Elsevier).

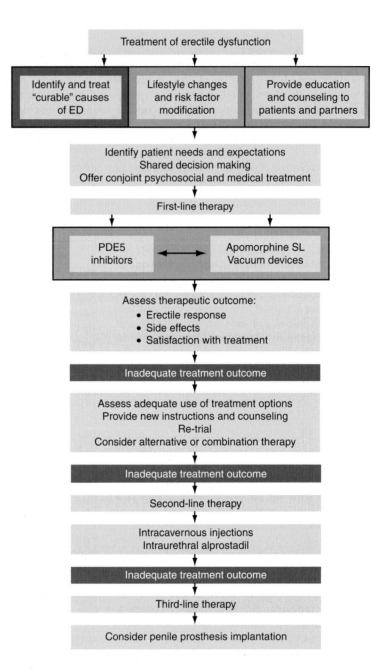

intercourse) range from 28.5% to 55%. The use of apomorphine is mainly recommended for patients suffering from psychogenic causes.

Yohimbine Yohimbine is an indole alkaloid, acting both peripherally and centrally by blocking alpha-2-blocker associated with low level of evidence for efficacy in general ED.[23] Yohimbine is known to cause elevations of blood pressure and heart rate, increased motor activity, irritability, and tremor.

Intracavernosal and Intraurethral Therapy

Intracavernosal Injection (ICI) Therapy Intracavernous drug injection is the most effective nonsurgical treatment for ED. *Alprostadil* represents the synthetic formulation of prostaglandin E1 and

Table 28.2. Pharmacokinetic properties of sildenafil, tadalafil, and vardenafil

Parameter	Sildenafil (100 mg)	Tadalafil (20 mg)	Vardenafil (20 mg)
C_{max}	560 µg/L	378 µg/L	18.7 µg/L
T_{max}	0.8–1 h	2 h	0.9 h
$T_{1/2}$	2.6–3.7 h	17.5 h	3.9 h
AUC	1685 µg/h/L	8066 µg/h/L	56.8 µg/h/L
Protein binding	96%	94%	94%
Bioavailability	41%	NA	15%

Data based on fasted state, higher recommended dose, and information from the European Medicine Evaluation Association statements on product characteristics.

C_{max} maximal concentration, T_{max} time to maximum plasma concentration, $T_{1/2}$ plasma elimination half-time, *AUC* area under curve – serum concentration time curve.

Source: (Reprinted from Wespes et al.[6]. Copyright 2006, with permission from Elsevier).

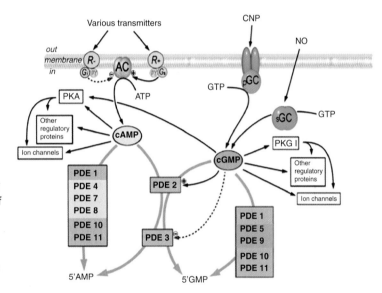

Figure 28.4. Schematic illustration of the pathways involved in regulation of signals mediated by adenosine and guanosine cyclic monophosphates (cAMP and cGMP) in the urogenital tract (Reprinted from Uckert et al.[21]. Copyright 2006, with permission from Elsevier).

is injected into the corpora cavernosa.[24,25] By increasing cyclic AMP levels, it causes smooth muscle relaxation. In spite of high efficacy, alprostadil has a low tolerability due to uncommon adverse events such as penile pain and priapism and, chronically, penile fibrosis or curvature (Grade A – level Ia).

Papaverine hydrochloride alone or in combination with phentolamine or a combination of papaverine, phentolamine, and alprostadil (triple mix) is highly effective and has found frequent use in daily practice; however, it is not approved as standard therapy. Generally, intracavernous injections are contraindicated in patients with sickle cell anemia and with other conditions that predispose to priapism.

Intraurethral Therapy Intraurethral alprostadil therapy is less invasive than intracavernous injections therapies. It offers moderate efficacy and tolerability in the management of general ED. Adverse events resemble intracavernous therapy; in addition, systemic side effects have been observed (Grade A – level Ib).[26]

Vacuum Constriction Devices

Vacuum constriction devices (VCD) are widely available and beneficial for patients who disapprove of medical therapy or those who have any contraindication. Vacuum devices work by creating negative pressure to the pendulous penis, thus drawing blood into the penis, which is then retained by the application of an elastic band at the base of the penis.[6] Penile pain and the tedious use of VCDs limit a wider use.

Surgical Therapy

As ultimate option, malleable (semirigid) or inflatable (two- or three-piece) penile prosthesis may be offered. Prosthesis implantation has one of the highest satisfaction rates (70–87%) among treatment options for ED. Main complications of penile prosthesis implantation are mechanical failures and infection (1–5%). Mechanical failures are now less than 5% in the first year, about 20% at 5 years, and 50% at 10 years.

Conclusion

The majority of patients suffering from erectile dysfunction will benefit from oral PDE5-inhibitors. The selection of the drug has to be based on personal preferences and efficacy of the individual substance. Great emphasis by the practicing physician should be laid on the evaluation of potential risk factors. Due to the evident association of cardiovascular disease and erectile dysfunction, a careful assessment is obligatory. In case of patients not responding to PDE5-inhibitors, optional strategies include intracavernous or intrameatal injection as well as vacuum constricting devices or, ultimately, the implantation of penile prosthesis.

Peyronie´s Disease (PD)

Introduction

Peyronie's disease (PD) is a localized disorder of the connective tissue characterized by the formation of fibrotic plaques in the tunica albuginea of the *corpus cavernosum*. PD appears as an inflammatory lesion in its first stages, but ultimately results in fibrosis and calcification.[27]

The prevalence of PD among men is estimated at 0.4–8.9% usually affecting men between 40 and 70 years of age.[28] Microtraumatic lesions of the tunica represent generally accepted causes of PD resulting in the initiation of a cascade of connective tissue reactions and scarification.[29-31] However, the exact pathophysiology of PD appears to be complex[32,33] and has not been elucidated to date. The unknown pathophysiology of the process has prevented the development of causal therapy strategies, and in fact, most medical approaches towards PD can actually be considered ineffective.[34]

Clinical Appearance and Diagnostic Workup

PD results in a variety of penile symptoms: Penile nodes and plaque formation, penile pain, painful erections, penile angulation, deformity, and erectile dysfunction that is prevalent in up to 60% of all patients.[30,31] Clinical workup in patients includes measurement of plaque dimension, determination of penile length in the flaccid and erectile status, and determination of angulation. Sonography of the plaques is suggested and – in elderly men – erectile hemodynamics should be evaluated by color duplex ultrasound. The IIEF is used for erectile function assessment; however, particularly in patients with high-grade deformity of the penis, IIEF fails to describe erectile function due to the nature of the questions. Patients frequently do not suffer from insufficient erectile status but are unable to perform sexual intercourse due to mechanical reasons, e.g. immission of the penis.[31]

In the early stages, PD appears as an inflammatory disorder of the Tunica albuginea of the corpus cavernosum clinically typified by penile pain and discomfort. Painful erections are seen frequently. This early phase has been termed "inflammatory phase" and usually lasts for 6–12 months. After this interval, patients enter into a stable phase of the disease as indicated by the cessation of penile pain and lack of progression in penile curvature. Surgical corrections are obsolete in the inflammatory phase but are possible and successful in the stable phase of the disease.[30]

Medical and Minimally Invasive Treatment Strategies

Medical therapy of PD in general has been based on a variety of anti-inflammatory drugs that are applied orally or by direct injection into the penile lesion (plaque).

Oral Drug Therapy

Studies on the use of potassium para-aminobenzoate (Potaba™), vitamin E, colchicine, tamoxifen, acetyl-L-carnitine, and propionyl-L-carnitine have been published. A recent survey regarding drug therapy indicated that the majority of patients (76%) are treated by the use of potassium para-aminobenzoate (46%) or vitamin E (29%).[34,35]

Potassium para-aminobenzoate (Potaba™) seems to be useful to stabilize the disorder and prevent progression of penile curvature in patients during the early stage of the disease. Moreover it can reduce plaque size significantly. No significant effect on reduction of pain has been observed.[35]

The use of vitamin E is widely performed. However, there is no evidence that vitamin E has a significant effect on the symptoms of PD. The data on tamoxifen and on colchicine indicate alterations or 'improvements' of the disorder only in the range of the natural history. In recent studies, acetyl-L-carnitine and propionyl-L-carnitine have been investigated with interesting results; however, these studies combined the administration of these substances with other drugs or were uncontrolled.

Intralesional Drug Therapy

Several substances have been applied for intralesional drug therapy of PD: verapamil, interferon-α2a and interferon-α2b, collagenase, corticosteroids, and hyaluronidase.

Following the demand for a significant effect in prospective, randomized, controlled trials, a significant effect could be revealed only for collagenase in cases of mild curvature. For interferon-α and verapamil a positive effect has just been evident in patients with short case history in single-blinded studies, while the only double-blind approach resulted in insignificant effects of verapamil. Corticosteroids are a traditional option in intralesional therapy. However, only one randomized, single-blinded, placebo-controlled study on the use of corticosteroid has been published so far revealing that betamethasone is not effective.[34]

Iontophoresis

The therapy combination using verapamil and dexamethasone has been significantly effective compared to placebo in the reduction of plaque size, curvature, and pain, respectively. Furthermore, iontophoresis appears to be a cost-effective method since the patient can perform this therapy at home using an applicator on loan thus replacing in-office therapy.[36]

Extracorporeal Shock-Wave Therapy (ESWT)

The first noncontrolled studies on ESWT reported amazing results. However, studies with exact documentation of the symptoms before and after the intervention could not reveal significant effects on the most important symptoms that are penile curvature and plaque size. The exploratory meta-analysis of the studies published so far in peer-reviewed journals could not demonstrate a significant effect of ESWT on penile curvature or plaque size. Pain seems to resolve faster after ESWT treatment.[37]

Radiation Therapy

No prospective, randomized, placebo-controlled studies have been published. The majority of recently published studies represent retrospective analyses with narrowly defined study parameters. So far, radiation therapy has not been recommended.

Surgical Therapy

Surgical therapy in patients with angulation and deformities should be delayed until the acute, painful inflammatory phase has been resolved, since early recurrences have been described when surgery had been performed early.[38]

Standardized surgical procedures are intended to lengthen the concavity (excision, incision, grafting with different materials) or to shorten the convexity (Nesbit, plication procedure).[39-41] Wide excision of plaque material from the tunica is not considered "state-of-the-art" anymore due to a variety of subsequent complications. Penile shortening is the main concern for all surgical techniques that involve plication/excision of the tunica contralaterally to the plaque. However, these procedures are still common and the rate of complications is low.[38]

All procedures are well established with a predictable rate of side effects and ideal for men with normal erectile function. In men with ED, surgical correction of penile deviations in combination with the implantation of hydraulic penile implants has been established as the therapy of choice. Depending upon penile deformities, incisions, graftings, or remodeling has been suggested to straighten the penis during surgery.[42,43]

Conclusively, management of PD remains one of the most challenging issues of sexual medicine and reconstructive genital surgery.[42]

References

1. Andersson KE. Pharmacology of penile erection. *Pharmacol Rev.* 2001;53(3):417-450
2. Lue TF. Erectile dysfunction. *N Engl J Med.* 2000;342(24): 1802-1813
3. Kubin M, Wagner G, Fugl-Meyer AR. Epidemiology of erectile dysfunction. *Int J Impot Res.* 2003;15(1):63-71
4. Roumeguere T, Wespes E, Carpentier Y, Hoffmann P, Schulman CC. Erectile dysfunction is associated with a high prevalence of hyperlipidemia and coronary heart disease risk. *Eur Urol.* 2003;44(3):355-359
5. Hackett G, Kell P, Ralph D, et al. British society for sexual medicine guidelines on the management of erectile dysfunction. *J Sex Med.* 2008;5(8):1841-1865
6. Wespes E, Amar E, Hatzichristou D, et al. EAU guidelines on erectile dysfunction: an update. *Eur Urol.* 2006;49(5): 806-815
7. Montague DK, Jarow J, Broderick GA, et al. American urological association guideline on the management of priapism. *J Urol.* 2003;170(4 Pt 1):1318-1324
8. Hatzichristou D, Hatzimouratidis K, Bekas M, Apostolidis A, Tzortzis V, Yannakoyorgos K. Diagnostic steps in the evaluation of patients with erectile dysfunction. *J Urol.* 2002;168(2):615-620
9. Burnett AL, Aus G, Canby-Hagino ED, et al. Erectile function outcome reporting after clinically localized prostate cancer treatment. *J Urol.* 2007;178(2):597-601
10. Lue TF, Giuliano F, Montorsi F, et al. Summary of the recommendations on sexual dysfunctions in men. *J Sex Med.* 2004;1(1):6-23
11. Esposito K, Marfella R, Ciotola M, et al. Effect of a Mediterranean-style diet on endothelial dysfunction and markers of vascular inflammation in the metabolic syndrome: A randomized trial. *J Am Med Assoc.* 2004;292 (12):1440-1446
12. Davis-Joseph B, Tiefer L, Melman A. Accuracy of the initial history and physical examination to establish the etiology of erectile dysfunction. *Urology.* 1995;45(3): 498-502
13. Rosen RC, Riley A, Wagner G, Osterloh IH, Kirkpatrick J, Mishra A. The international index of erectile function (IIEF): a multidimensional scale for assessment of erectile dysfunction. *Urology.* 1997;49(6):822-830
14. Hatzichristou D, Rosen RC, Broderick G, et al. Clinical evaluation and management strategy for sexual dysfunction in men and women. *J Sex Med.* 2004;1(1): 49-57
15. Johannes CB, Araujo AB, Feldman HA, Derby CA, Kleinman KP, McKinlay JB. Incidence of erectile dysfunction in men 40–69 years old: longitudinal results from the Massachusetts male aging study. *J Urol.* 2000;163(2):460-463
16. Montorsi P, Ravagnani PM, Galli S, et al. Common grounds for erectile dysfunction and coronary artery disease. *Curr Opin Urol.* 2004;14(6):361-365
17. Kostis JB, Jackson G, Rosen R, et al. Sexual dysfunction and cardiac risk (the Second Princeton Consensus Conference). *Am J Cardiol.* 2005;96(12B):85M–93M
18. Jackson G, Betteridge J, Dean J, et al. A systematic approach to erectile dysfunction in the cardiovascular patient: A consensus statement – update 2002 *Int J Clin Pract.* 2002;56(9):663-671
19. Meuleman EJ, Diemont WL. Investigation of erectile dysfunction. Diagnostic testing for vascular factors in erectile dysfunction. *Urol Clin North Am.* 1995;22(4): 803-819
20. Jarow JP, DeFranzo AJ. Long-term results of arterial bypass surgery for impotence secondary to segmental vascular disease. *J Urol.* 1996;156(3):982-985
21. Uckert S, Hedlund P, Andersson KE, Truss MC, Jonas U, Stief CG. Update on phosphodiesterase (PDE) isoenzymes as pharmacologic targets in urology: present and future. *Eur Urol.* 2006;50(6):1194-1207; discussion 1207
22. Dula E, Bukofzer S, Perdok R, George M. Double-blind, crossover comparison of 3 mg apomorphine SL with placebo and with 4 mg apomorphine SL in male erectile dysfunction. *Eur Urol.* 2001;39(5):558-553; discussion 564
23. Andersson KE, Stief C. Oral alpha adrenoceptor blockade as a treatment of erectile dysfunction. *World J Urol.* 2001;19(1):9-13
24. Linet OI, Ogrinc FG. Efficacy and safety of intracavernosal alprostadil in men with erectile dysfunction. The alprostadil study group. *N Engl J Med.* 1996;334(14): 873-877
25. Jaffe JS, Antell MR, Greenstein M, Ginsberg PC, Mydlo JH, Harkaway RC. Use of intraurethral alprostadil in

patients not responding to sildenafil citrate. *Urology.* 2004;63(5):951-954

26. Padma-Nathan H, Hellstrom WJ, Kaiser FE, et al. Treatment of men with erectile dysfunction with transurethral alprostadil. Medicated Urethral System for Erection (MUSE) Study Group. *N Engl J Med.* 1997;336(1):1-7

27. Gholami SS, Gonzalez-Cadavid NF, Lin CS, Rajfer J, Lue TF. Peyronie's disease: a review. *J Urol.* 2003;169(4): 1234-1241

28. Schwarzer U, Sommer F, Klotz T, Braun M, Reifenrath B, Engelmann U. The prevalence of Peyronie's disease: Results of a large survey. *BJU Int.* 2001;88(7):727-730

29. Gelbard MK, Dorey F, James K. The natural history of Peyronie's disease. *J Urol.* 1990;144(6):1376-1379

30. Kadioglu A, Akman T, Sanli O, Gurkan L, Cakan M, Celtik M. Surgical treatment of Peyronie's disease: a critical analysis. *Eur Urol.* 2006;50(2):235-248

31. Weidner W, Schroeder-Printzen I, Weiske WH, Vosshenrich R. Sexual dysfunction in Peyronie's disease: an analysis of 222 patients without previous local plaque therapy. *J Urol.* 1997;157(1):325-328

32. Hauck EW, Hauptmann A, Weidner W, Bein G, Hackstein H. Prospective analysis of HLA classes I and II antigen frequency in patients with Peyronie's disease. *J Urol.* 2003;170(4 Pt 1):1443-1446

33. Haag SM, Hauck EW, Szardening-Kirchner C, et al. Alterations in the transforming growth factor (TGF)-beta pathway as a potential factor in the pathogenesis of Peyronie's disease. *Eur Urol.* 2007;51(1):255-261

34. Hauck EW, Diemer T, Schmelz HU, Weidner W. A critical analysis of nonsurgical treatment of Peyronie's disease. *Eur Urol.* 2006;49(6):987-997

35. Weidner W, Hauck EW, Schnitker J. Potassium paraaminobenzoate (POTABA) in the treatment of Peyronie's disease: A prospective, placebo-controlled, randomized study. *Eur Urol.* 2005;47(4):530-535; discussion 535-536

36. Di Stasi SM, Giannantoni A, Stephen RL, et al. A prospective, randomized study using transdermal electromotive administration of verapamil and dexamethasone for Peyronie's disease. *J Urol.* 2004;171(4):1605-1608

37. Hauck EW, Mueller UO, Bschleipfer T, Schmelz HU, Diemer T, Weidner W. Extracorporeal shock wave therapy for Peyronie's disease: exploratory meta-analysis of clinical trials. *J Urol.* 2004;171(2 Pt 1):740-745

38. Hauck EW. Against the motion: surgery is the best choice for Peyronie's disease. *Eur Urol.* 2006;49(6):1128; discussion 1128-1129

39. Lue TF, El-Sakka AI. Venous patch graft for Peyronie's disease part I: technique. *J Urol.* 1998;160(6 Pt 1): 2047-2049

40. El-Sakka AI, Rashwan HM, Lue TF. Venous patch graft for Peyronie's disease part II: outcome analysis. *J Urol.* 1998;160(6 Pt 1):2050-2053

41. Hellstrom WJ, Reddy S. Application of pericardial graft in the surgical management of Peyronie's disease. *J Urol.* 2000;163(5):1445-1447

42. Hauck EW, Weidner W. Francois de la Peyronie and the disease named after him. *Lancet.* 2001;357(9273):2049-2051

43. Montorsi F, Salonia A, Maga T, et al. Reconfiguration of the severely fibrotic penis with a penile implant. *J Urol.* 2001;166(5):1782-1786

29

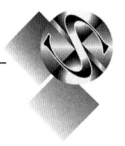

Premature Ejaculation

Chris G. McMahon

Introduction

Over the past 20–30 years, the PE treatment paradigm, previously limited to behavioral psychotherapy, has expanded to include drug treatment.[1,2] Animal and human sexual psychopharmacological studies have demonstrated that serotonin and 5-HT receptors are involved in ejaculation and confirm a role for SSRIs in the treatment of PE.[3-6] Multiple well-controlled evidence-based studies have demonstrated the efficacy and safety of SSRIs in delaying ejaculation, confirming their role as first-line agents for the treatment of lifelong and acquired PE.[7] More recently, there has been increased attention to the psychosocial consequences of PE, its epidemiology, its etiology, and its pathophysiology by both clinicians and the pharmaceutical industry.[8-13]

Epidemiology

Premature ejaculation (PE) has been estimated to occur in 4–39% of men in the general community.[12,14-19] and is often reported as the most common male sexual disorder, despite a substantial disparity between the self-reported incidence of PE in epidemiological studies[19] and that suggested by community-based normative stopwatch intravaginal ejaculation latency time (IELT) studies.[10] However, most epidemiological studies are limited by their reliance on either patients' self-reporting of PE or inconsistent and poorly validated definitions of PE.[11,13,19] A multinational, community-based, age-ranging stopwatch IELT study demonstrated that the distribution of the IELT was positively skewed, with a median IELT of 5.4 min (range, 0.55–44.1 min), decreased with age, and varied between countries.[10] (Fig. 29.1) Using an epidemiological approach to assess PE risk, the authors regarded the 0.5 and 2.5 percentiles as acceptable standards of disease definition in this type of skewed distribution, and proposed that men with an IELT of less than 1 min (belonging to the 0.5 percentile) have "definite" PE, while men with IELTs between 1 and 1.5 min (between 0.5 and 2.5 percentile) have "probable" PE.[20] These normative data support the notion that IELTs of less than 1 min are statistically abnormal compared to men in the general Western population.

Classification of Premature Ejaculation

The population of men with PE is not homogenous. In 1943, Schapiro classified PE as either primary (lifelong) or secondary (acquired).[21] Recently, Waldinger et al. expanded this classification to include lifelong PE, acquired PE, natural variable PE, and premature-like ejaculatory dysfunction (Table 29.1).[22] Lifelong PE is a syndrome characterized by a cluster of core symptoms including early ejaculation at nearly every intercourse within 30–60 s in the majority of

C.R. Chapple and W.D. Steers (eds.), *Practical Urology: Essential Principles and Practice*,
DOI: 10.1007/978-1-84882-034-0_29, © Springer-Verlag London Limited 2011

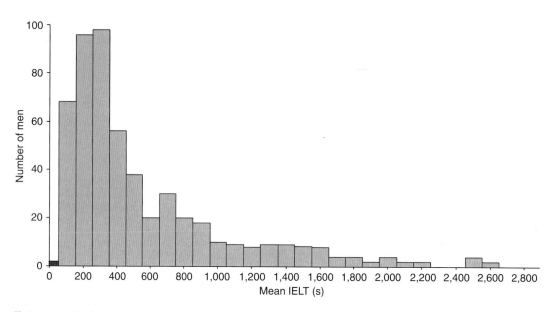

Figure 29.1. Distribution of intravaginal ejaculatory latency times (IELT) values in a random cohort of 491 men (Reprinted from Waldinger et al.[10] Copyright 2005. With permission from Wiley via Copyright Clearance Center Rightslink).

Table 29.1. The four premature ejaculation (PE) syndromes (Data from Waldinger[22])

Variable	Lifelong premature ejaculation	Acquired premature ejaculation	Natural variable premature ejaculation	Premature-like ejaculatory dysfunction
IELT	Very short IELT (<1–1.5 min)	(Very) short IELT (<1.5–2 min)	Normal IELT (3–8 min)	Normal or long IELT (3–30 min)
Frequency	Consistent	(In)consistent	Inconsistent	(In)consistent
Etiology	Neurobiological and genetic	Medical and/or psychological	Normal variation of ejaculatory performance	Psychological
Treatment	Medication with or without counseling	Medication and/or psychotherapy	Psychoeducation, reassurance	Psychotherapy
Prevalence	Low (?)	Low (?)	High (?)	High (?)

IELT intravaginal ejaculation latency time[22].

cases (80%) or between 1 and 2 min (20%), with every or nearly every sexual partner and from the first sexual encounter onwards. Acquired PE differs in that sufferers develop early ejaculation at some point in their life having previously had normal ejaculation experiences. Acquired PE may be due to sexual performance anxiety,[23] psychological or relationship problems,[23] erectile dysfunction (ED),[24] prostatitis,[25] hyperthyroidism,[26] or during withdrawal/detoxification from prescribed[27] or recreational drugs.[28] In a study of 1,326 consecutive men with PE, lifelong PE was present in 736 men (74.4%), and acquired PE was present in 253 men (25.6%).[29] In natural variable PE, the ejaculation time is never consistently rapid but merely coincidental and situational. This type of PE should be regarded as a normal variation in sexual performance and is characterized by inconsistent and irregular early ejaculation, often with reduced ejaculatory control.[30] Men with premature-like ejaculatory dysfunction complain of PE but have a normal ejaculatory latency of 3–6 min. It is characterized by a pre-occupation with a subjective but false perception of PE with an ELT within the normal range but often with reduced ejaculatory control.

Defining Premature Ejaculation

Research into the treatment and epidemiology of PE is heavily dependent on how PE is defined. The medical literature contains several univariate and multivariate operational definitions of PE.[2,20,31-37] Although the most commonly quoted definition, DSM-IV-TR, and other definitions of PE differ substantially, they are all authority based, i.e., expert opinion without explicit critical appraisal,[38] rather than evidence-based and have no support from controlled clinical and/or epidemiological studies. This lack of agreement as to what constitutes PE has hampered clinical research into the etiology and management of this condition, and the development of patient reported outcomes (PROs) to diagnose and assess treatment intervention strategies.[39] The first multivariate evidence-based definition of lifelong PE was recently reported and characterizes lifelong PE as "... ejaculation which always or nearly always occurs prior to or within about one minute of vaginal penetration, the inability to delay ejaculation on all or nearly all vaginal penetrations, and the presence of negative personal consequences, such as distress, bother, frustration and/or the avoidance of sexual intimacy."[40] There is insufficient published evidence to propose an evidenced-based definition of acquired PE.[40]

Intravaginal Ejaculatory Latency Time (IELT)

Operationalization of PE measuring the length of time between penetration and ejaculation with a stopwatch, the intravaginal ejaculatory latency time (IELT), forms the basis of most current clinical studies on PE.[41] There is considerable variance of the latencies used to identify men with PE with IELTs ranging from 1 to 7 min and none of the definitions is based on normative data or offer any supportive rationale for their proposed cut-off time.[42-45]

Several studies suggest that 80–90% of men seeking treatment for lifelong PE ejaculate within 1 min.[29,46,47] Waldinger et al. (1998) reported IELTs <30 s in 77% and <60 s in 90% of 110 men with lifelong PE with only 10% ejaculating between 1 and 2 min.[46] McMahon et al. reported similar results in 1,346 consecutive men with predominant ante portal ejaculation (during foreplay) in 5.6% of men.[29] As such, an IELT cut-off of 1 min captures 90% of treatment-seeking men with lifelong PE. Further qualification of this cut-off to "about 1 min" affords the clinician sufficient flexibility to also diagnose PE in the 10% of PE treatment seeking men who ejaculate within 1–2 min of penetration without unnecessarily stigmatizing the remaining 90% of men who ejaculate within 1–2 min of penetration but have no complaints of PE. In office practice, the IELT can be reliably estimated by men with PE. Several authors report that estimated and stopwatch IELT correlate reasonably well or are interchangeable in assigning PE status when estimated IELT is combined with patient reported outcomes (PROs).[48-50]

Voluntary Control

The ability to prolong sexual intercourse by delaying ejaculation and the subjective feelings of ejaculatory control comprise the complex construct of ejaculatory control. Virtually all men report using at least one cognitive or behavioral technique to prolong intercourse and delay ejaculation, with varying degrees of success, and many young men reported using multiple different techniques.[18]

Several authors have suggested that an inability to voluntarily defer ejaculation defines PE.[51-54] Patrick et al. reported ratings of "very poor" or "poor" for control over ejaculation in 72% of men with PE compared to 5% in a group of normal controls.[11] However, control is a subjective measure that is difficult to translate into quantifiable terms and is the most inconsistent dimension of PE. Grenier and Byers failed to demonstrate a strong correlation between ejaculatory latency and subjective ejaculatory control.[18,55] Several authors report that diminished control is not exclusive to men with PE and that some men with a brief IELT report adequate ejaculatory control and vice versa, suggesting that the dimensions of ejaculatory control and latency are distinct concepts.[11,18]

Contrary to this, several authors have reported a moderate correlation between the IELT and the feeling of ejaculatory control.[11,50,56,57] Rosen et al. report that control over ejaculation, personal distress, and partner distress was more influential in determining PE status than IELT.[50] However, despite conflicting data on the relationship between control and latency, the balance of evidence supports the notion that the inability to delay ejaculation appears to differentiate men with PE from men without PE.[11,57,58]

Sexual Satisfaction

Men with PE report lower levels of sexual satisfaction compared to men with normal ejaculatory latency. However, caution should be exercised in assigning lower levels of sexual satisfaction solely to the effect of PE and contributions from other difficult-to-quantify issues such as reduced intimacy, dysfunctional relationships, poor sexual attraction, and poor communication should not be ignored. This is supported by the report of Patrick et al. that despite reduced ratings for satisfaction with shorter IELTs with "poor" or "very poor" intercourse satisfaction reported by 25.4%, 3.6%, and 2.0% of subjects with an IELT <1 min, >1 min, and >2 min, respectively, a substantial proportion of men with an IELT <1 min report "good" or "very good" satisfaction ratings (43.7%). Current data are limited but suggests that sexual satisfaction is of limited use in differentiating PE subjects from non-PE subjects and has not been included in the ISSM definition of PE.[11]

Distress

Premature ejaculation (PE) has been associated with negative psychological outcomes in men and their partners.[9,11,12,23,57-67] The personal and/or interpersonal distress that result from PE may affect men's quality of life and partner relationships, their self-esteem and self-confidence, and can act as an obstacle to single men forming new partner relationships.[9,11,12,23,57-67] Patrick et al. reported that 64% of men with PE versus 4% of non-PE men reported being "quite a bit" or "extremely" personally distressed. Rowland et al.

showed that men with PE had significantly lower overall health-related quality of life and lower Self-Esteem And Relationship Questionnaire (SEAR) scores with lower confidence and self-esteem compared to non-PE groups (all $p \leq 0.001$).[60] The divergent pattern observed for personal distress suggests that this construct has discriminative validity in diagnosing men with and without PE. The data for satisfaction and interpersonal distress while statistically significant were not as strong.

The Etiology of Premature Ejaculation

Historically, attempts to explain the etiology of PE has included a diverse range of biological and psychological theories. Most of these proposed etiologies are not evidence based and are speculative at best. Psychological theories include the effect of early experience and sexual conditioning, anxiety, sexual technique, the frequency of sexual activity, and psychodynamic explanations. Biological explanations include evolutionary theories, penile hypersensitivity, central neurotransmitter levels and receptor sensitivity, degree of arousability, the speed of the ejaculatory reflex, and the level of sex hormones.

There is little empirical evidence to suggest a causal link between PE and any of the factors thought to cause PE. There is, however, limited correlational evidence to suggest that lifelong PE is genetically determined and related to the inherited altered sensitivity of central 5-HT receptors and acquired PE is due to high levels of sexual anxiety, ED, or lower urinary tract infection.

Ejaculatory latency time is probably a biological variable, which is genetically determined and may differ between populations and cultures, ranging from extremely rapid through average to slow ejaculation. This is supported by animal studies showing a subgroup of persistent rapidly ejaculating Wistar rats,[6] an increased familial occurrence of lifelong PE,[5] and a moderate genetic influence on PE in the Finnish twin study.[68] Hyposensitivity of the 5-HT2C and/or hypersensitivity of the 5-HT1A receptors have been suggested as a possible explanation of lifelong PE.[69,70]

Men with low 5-HT neurotransmission and probable 5-HT2C receptor hyposensitivity may have their ejaculatory threshold genetically "set" at a lower point and ejaculate quickly and with minimal stimulation whereas men with a higher setpoint men can sustain more prolonged and higher levels of sexual stimulation and can exert more control over ejaculation. This is supported by the recent report that genetic polymorphism of the 5-HTT gene determine the regulation of the IELT and that men with LL genotypes have statistically shorter IELTs than men with SS and SL genotypes.[71]

Treatment of Premature Ejaculation

Premature ejaculation treatment strategies include psychosexual counseling, daily or on-demand pharmacotherapy, either alone or in combination as part of an integrated treatment program.

Psychosexual Counseling

The cornerstones of behavioral treatment are the Seman's "stop-start" maneuver and its modification proposed by Masters and Johnson, the squeeze technique. Both are based on the theory that PE occurs because the man fails to pay sufficient attention to pre-orgasmic levels of sexual tension.[1,2] As most men with PE are aware of their anxiety and the sources of that anxiety tend to be relatively superficial, treatment success with these behavioral approaches is relatively good in the short term but convincing long-term treatment outcome data are lacking.[52,72-74] Cognitive behavioral therapy (CBT), especially when combined with pharmacotherapy, is an effective intervention for acquired PE related to sexual performance anxiety and a substantial proportion of men report sustained improvements on ejaculatory latency and control following cessation of pharmacotherapy.[29,36,75] However, men with lifelong PE rarely achieve symptomatic improvement with CBT alone and are best managed with either pharmacotherapy alone or in combination with CBT if there is a significant secondary psychogenic contribution, where cessation of pharmacotherapy invariably results in a return to pre-treatment latency and control within 1–2 weeks.

Pharmacological Treatment

The introduction of the serotonergic tricyclic clomipramine and the SSRIs paroxetine, sertraline, fluoxetine, citalopram, and fluvoxamine, has revolutionized the approach to and treatment of PE. These drugs block axonal re-uptake of serotonin from the synaptic cleft of central and peripheral serotonergic neurons by 5-HT transporters, resulting in enhanced 5-HT neurotransmission and stimulation of post-synaptic membrane 5-HT2C autoreceptors. Although the methodology of the initial drug treatment studies was poor, later double blind and placebo-controlled studies confirmed the ejaculation-delaying effect of clomipramine and SSRIs.

Daily Treatment with Selective Serotonin Reuptake Inhibitors (SSRIs)

Daily treatment with paroxetine 10–40 mg, clomipramine 12.5–50 mg, sertraline 50–200 mg, fluoxetine 20–40 mg, and citalopram 20–40 mg is usually effective in delaying ejaculation (Table 29.2).[77-82] A meta-analysis of published data suggests that paroxetine exerts the strongest ejaculation delay, increasing IELT approximately 8.8-fold over baseline.[77] However, the use of these drugs is limited by the lack of Food and Drug Administration (FDA), European Medicines Agency (EMEA), or other regulatory agency approval and the need to prescribe "off-label." This largely reflects the failure of the pharmaceutical industry to appreciate the prevalence of PE, the unmet treatment need, and the commercial opportunity of an approved drug treatment for PE.[83]

Ejaculation delay usually occurs within 5–10 days of starting treatment, but the full therapeutic effect may require 2–3 weeks of treatment and is usually sustained during long-term use.[29] Although tachyphylaxis is uncommon, some patients report a reduced response after 6–12 months of treatment. Adverse effects are usually minor, start in the first week of treatment, gradually disappear within 2–3 weeks, and include fatigue, yawning, mild nausea, diarrhea, or perspiration. Hypoactive desire and ED is infrequently reported and appear to have a lower incidence in non-depressed PE men compared to depressed men treated with SSRIs.[22] Waldinger et al. have suggested that this may be

Table 29.2. Doses and dosing instructions of drug therapy for PE

Drug	Dose	Dosing instructions	Indication	Comments	Level of evidence[a]
Paroxetine	10–40 mg	Once daily	Lifelong PE Acquired PE		High
Sertraline	50–200 mg	Once daily	Lifelong PE Acquired PE		High
Fluoxetine	20–40 mg	Once daily	Lifelong PE Acquired PE		High
Citalopram	20–40 mg	Once daily	Lifelong PE Acquired PE		High
Clomipramine	12.5–50 mg	Once daily	Lifelong PE Acquired PE		High
	12.5–50 mg	On demand, 3–4 h prior to intercourse	Lifelong PE Acquired PE		High
Terazosin	5 mg	Once daily	Lifelong PE Acquired PE		Low
Tramadol		On demand, 3–4 h prior to intercourse	Lifelong PE Acquired PE	Potential risk of opiate addiction	Low
Dapoxetine	30–60 mg	On demand, 1–3 h prior to intercourse	Lifelong PE Acquired PE	Non-approved investigational drug	High
Topical lignocaine/ priliocaine	Patient titrated	On demand, 20–30 min prior to intercourse	Lifelong PE Acquired PE		High
Alprostadil	5–20 mcg	Patient administered intracavernous injection 5 min prior to intercourse	Lifelong PE Acquired PE	Risk of priapism and corporal fibrosis	Very Low
PDE-5 inhibitors	Sildenafil 25–100 mg Tadalafil 10–20 mg Vardenafil 10–20 mg	On demand, 30–50 min prior to intercourse	Lifelong and acquired PE in men with normal erectile function		Very Low
			Lifelong and acquired PE in men with ED	? improved efficacy if combined with SSRI	Moderate

[a]According to Grading of Recommendations, Assessment and Evaluation (GRADE)[76].

related to the protective effects of increased oxytocin release in men with lifelong PE.[70]

Neurocognitive adverse effects include significant agitation and hypomania in a small number of patients, and treatment with SSRIs should be avoided in men with a history of bipolar depression.[84] Systematic analysis of randomized controlled studies indicates no statistical evidence of an increased risk of suicide with SSRIs in adults.[85,86] However, an FDA meta-analyses of all pediatric randomized clinical trials (RCTs) of antidepressants suggested a small increase in the risk of suicidal ideation or suicide attempts in youth.[86] This effect is quite variable across SSRIs and it is not clear if that variance is a measurement error or represents a real difference between medications. Furthermore, systematic questionnaire data, epidemiological and autopsy studies, recent cohort surveys, and the negligible number of youth suicides taking antidepressants at the time of death do not support the hypothesis that SSRIs induce suicidal acts and suicide, raising concerns over ascertainment artifacts in the AE report method.[85] However, it would seem prudent to not prescribe SSRIs to young men aged 18 years or less, and to men with a depressive disorder particularly when associated with suicidal thoughts. Patients should be advised to avoid sudden cessation or rapid dose reduction of SSRIs which may be associated with a SSRI withdrawal syndrome, characterized by dizziness, headache, nausea, vomiting, and diarrhea, and occasionally agitation, impaired concentration, vivid dreams, depersonalization, irritability, and suicidal ideation.[87,88]

Platelet serotonin release has an important role in hemostasis,[89] and SSRIs especially with concurrent use of aspirin and non-steroidal anti-inflammatory drugs are associated with an increased risk of upper gastrointestinal bleeding.[90,91] Priapism is a rare adverse effect of SSRIs and requires urgent medical treatment.[92-94] Long-term SSRIs may be associated with weight gain and an increased risk of type-2 diabetes mellitus.[95]

Daily Treatment with α1-Adrenoceptor Antagonists

Ejaculation is a sympathetic spinal cord reflex that could theoretically be delayed by α1-adrenergic blockers. Several authors have reported their experience with selective α1-adrenergic blockers, alfuzosin and terazosin, in the treatment of PE. Both drugs are approved only for the treatment of lower urinary tract symptoms (LUTS) in men with obstructive benign prostatic hyperplasia (BPH). In a double blind placebo-controlled study, Cavallini reported that both alfuzosin (6 mg/day) and terazosin (5 mg/day) were effective in delaying ejaculation in approximately 50% of the cases.[96] Similarly, Basar reported that terazosin was effective in 67% of men.[97] However, both studies were limited by the use of subjective study endpoints of patient impression of change and sexual satisfaction and did not evaluate objective endpoints such as IELT. Additional controlled studies are required to determine the role of α1-blockers in the treatment of PE.

On-Demand Treatment with Selective Serotonin Reuptake Inhibitors

Administration of clomipramine, paroxetine, sertraline, and fluoxetine 4–6 h before intercourse is modestly efficacious and well tolerated but is associated with substantially less ejaculatory delay than daily treatment (Table 29.2).[98-101] Following acute on-demand administration of an SSRI, increased synaptic 5-HT levels are downregulated by presynaptic 5-HT1A and 5-HT1B/1D autoreceptors to prevent overstimulation of postsynaptic 5-HT2C receptors. However, during chronic daily SSRI administration, a series of synaptic adaptive processes that may include presynaptic 5-HT1A and 5-HT1B/1D receptor desensitization greatly enhances synaptic 5-HT levels resulting in superior-fold increases in IELT compared to on-demand administration (Fig. 29.2).[69] On-demand treatment may be combined with either an initial trial of daily treatment or concomitant low-dose daily treatment.[98-100]

The assertion that on-demand drug treatment of PE is preferable to daily dosing parallels the rationale for the treatment of ED but is contrary to the results of the only PE drug preference study.[47] The methodology of this trial was not ideal as it involved comparison of preference for daily paroxetine, on-demand clomipramine, or topical anesthetic based only on subject information/questionnaires and not on actual use of the drug. Well-designed preference trials will

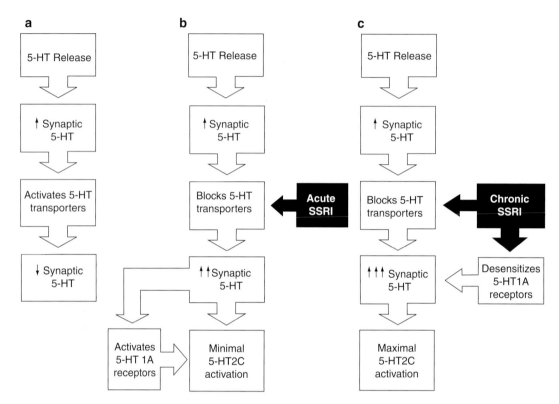

Figure 29.2. (a) Synaptic cleft 5-HT and 5-HT neurotransmission are regulated by somatodendritic 5-HT1A autoreceptors, presynaptic 5-HT1B/1D autoreceptors, and a 5-HT transporters re-uptake system. As 5-HT is released into the synaptic cleft from pre-synaptic axonal vesicles, 5-HT transporters re-uptake and remove 5-HT from the synaptic cleft, preventing overstimulation of the postsynaptic receptors. (b) After blockage of 5-HT transporters by acute administration of SSRI class drugs, synaptic cleft 5-HT increases but is counteracted by activation of 5-HT1A autoreceptors, which inhibit further 5-HT release. (c) Chronic administration of SSRI class drugs results in greatly enhanced 5-HT neurotransmission due to several adaptive processes that may include presynaptic 5-HT1A and 5-HT1B/1D receptor desensitization[4].

provide additional detailed insight into the role of on-demand dosing. While many men suffering from PE who infrequently engage in sexual intercourse may prefer on-demand treatment, many men in established relationships prefer the convenience of daily medication.

On-Demand Treatment with Dapoxetine

Dapoxetine is an investigational SSRI with a pharmacokinetic profile suggesting a role as an on-demand treatment for PE. Dapoxetine has a T_{max} of 1.4–2.0 h and a mean half-life of 0.5–0.8 h with rapidly decline of plasma levels to about 5% of C_{max} at 24 h, ensuring rapid absorption and achievement of peak plasma concentration with minimal accumulation.[102] Both plasma concentration and area under the curve (AUC) are dose dependent up to 100 mg, and are unaffected by repeated daily dosing, food, or alcohol.[103-105] No drug–drug interactions associated with dapoxetine, including phosphodiesterase inhibitors, have been reported.[106]

In randomized, double-blind, placebo-controlled, multicenter, phase III 12-week clinical trials involving 2,614 men with a mean baseline IELT ≤2 min, dapoxetine 30 or 60 mg was more effective than placebo for all study endpoints (Fig. 29.3).[107] Arithmetic mean IELT increased from 0.91 min at baseline to 2.78 and 3.32 min at study end with dapoxetine 30 and 60 mg, respectively, compared to a 1.75 min with placebo. However, as IELT in subjects with PE is distributed in a positively skewed pattern, reporting IELTs as arithmetic means may overestimate the treatment response, and the geometric mean

Figure 29.3. (a) Dapoxetine increased intravaginal ejaculatory latency time (IELT) from 0.91 min at baseline to 2.78 and 3.32 min at study end with dapoxetine 30 and 60 mg, respectively. (b) Percentage of subjects rating control over ejaculation as fair, good, or very good increased from 3.1% at baseline to 51.8% and 58.4% at study end with dapoxetine 30 and 60 mg, respectively. (c) Percentage of subjects rating sexual satisfaction as fair, good, or very good increased from 53.6% at baseline to 70.9% and 79.2% with dapoxetine 30 and 60 mg, respectively (rating scale 0–5 scale, 0 = very poor and 5 = very good) (Reprinted from Pryor et al.[107] Copyright 2006. With permission from Elsevier).

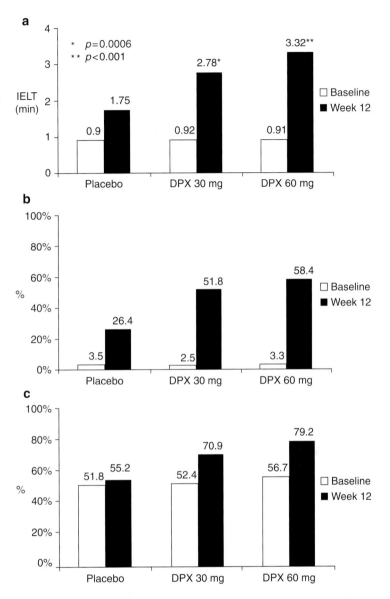

IELT is more representative of the actual treatment effect.[10,29,108-110] Pooled data from four phase III dapoxetine studies confirms this assertion and reports arithmetic and geometric mean IELTs of 1.9 and 1.2 for placebo, 3.1 and 2.0 for dapoxetine 30 mg, and 3.6 and 2.3 for dapoxetine 60 mg, respectively. This represents a 1.6-, 2.5-, and 3.0-fold increase over baseline geometric mean IELT for placebo, and dapoxetine 30 and 60 mg, respectively

Dapoxetine treatment is also associated with significant improvements in patient reported outcomes (PROs) of control, distress, and sexual satisfaction (Fig. 29.3). Mean patient rating of control over ejaculation as fair, good, or very good increased from 2.8% at baseline to 51.8% and 58.4% at study end with dapoxetine 30 and 60 mg, respectively. Treatment-related side effects were uncommon, dose dependent, included nausea, diarrhea, headache, and dizziness, and were responsible for study discontinuation in 4% (30 mg) and 10% (60 mg) of subjects. There was no indication of an increased risk of suicidal ideation or suicide attempts and little indication of withdrawal symptoms with abrupt dapox-etine cessation.[111]

It is likely that dapoxetine, despite its modest effect upon ejaculatory latency, has a place in the management of PE, which will eventually be determined by market forces once the challenge of regulatory approval has been met.

On-Demand Treatment with Tramadol

Tramadol is a centrally acting synthetic opioid analgesic with an unclear mode of action that is thought to include binding of parent and M1 metabolite to μ-opioid receptors and weak inhi-bition of re-uptake of GABA, norepinephrine, and serotonin.[112] The efficacy of on-demand tra-madol in the treatment of PE was recently reported in two RCTs.[113,114] Both studies were poorly designed and although tramadol is reported to have a lower risk of dependence than traditional opioids, its use as an on-demand treatment for PE is limited by the potential risk of addiction.[115] In community practice, depen-dence does occur but appears minimal.[116] Adams et al. reported abuse rates of 0.7% for tramadol compared to 0.5% for non-steroidal anti-inflam-matory drugs and 1.2% for hydrocodone based upon application of a dependency algorithm as a measure of persistence of drug use.[117] Additional flexible dose, long-term follow-up studies to evaluate efficacy, safety and, in par-ticular, the risk of opioid addiction are required.

Topical Anesthetics

The use of topical local anesthetics such as lignocaine and/or prilocaine as a cream, gel, or spray is well established and is moderately effec-tive in retarding ejaculation. They may be asso-ciated with significant penile hypoanesthesia and possible transvaginal absorption, resulting in vaginal numbness and resultant female anor-gasmia unless a condom is used.[118-120] A recent study reported that a metered-dose aerosol spray containing a eutectic mixture of lidocaine and prilocaine (TEMPE®) produced a 2.4-fold increase in baseline IELT and significant improvements in ejaculatory control and both patient and partner sexual quality of life.[121] The physiochemical characteristics of this eutectic mixture and the spray delivery system have been designed to both optimize and limit tissue pen-etration to the mucosa of the glans penis and not the keratinized skin of the penile shaft.[122] Penile hypoanesthesia was reported by 12% of subjects and skin irritation or burning was not observed.

Intracavernous Injection of Vasoactive Drugs

Intracavernous self-injection treatment of PE has been reported but is without any evidence-based support for efficacy or safety.[123] Fein reported an open study of eight men treated with a combination of papaverine and phen-tolamine administered by intracavernous auto-injection where the treatment success was defined as prolongation of erection after ejacu-lation and not by any measure of ejaculatory latency. In the absence of well-controlled stud-ies, treatment of PE by intracavernous auto-injection cannot be routinely recommended but may be of value in treatment refractory informed subjects.

Phosphodiesterase Inhibitors

Phosphodiesterase type-5 isoenzyme (PDE-5) inhibitors, sildenafil, tadalafil, and vardenafil, are effective treatments for ED. Several authors have reported their experience with PDE-5 inhibitors alone or in combination with SSRIs as a treatment for PE.[124-137] The putative role of PDE-5 inhibitors as a treatment for PE is specu-lative and based only upon the role of the NO/cGMP transduction system as a central and peripheral mediator of inhibitory non-adrener-gic, non-cholinergic, nitrergic neurotransmis-sion in the urogenital system.[138]

A recent systematic review of 14 studies ($n = 1,102$) on the PDE5i drug treatment of PE failed to provide any robust empirical evidence to support a role of PDE-5 inhibitors in the treat-ment of PE with the exception of men with PE and co-morbid ED.[139] Only one study fulfilled the contemporary criteria of ideal PE drug trial design,[140,141] and this study failed to confirm any significant treatment effect on IELT.[129] Caution should be exercised in interpreting PDE5i and on-demand SSRI treatment data in inadequately designed studies and their results must be regarded as unreliable.

Premature Ejaculation and Co-morbid ED

Recent data demonstrate that as many as half of subjects with ED also experience PE.[24,142] Subjects with ED may either require higher levels of manual stimulation to achieve an erection or intentionally "rush" intercourse to prevent early detumescence of a partial erection, resulting in ejaculation with a brief latency. This may be compounded by the presence of high levels of performance anxiety related to their ED, which serves to only worsen their prematurity.

There is evidence to suggest that PDE5i's alone or in combination with a SSRI may have a role in the management of acquired PE in men with co-morbid ED.[130,132,136] In 45 men with PE and co-morbid ED treated with flexible doses of sildenafil (50–100 mg) for periods of 1–3 months, Li et al. reported improved erectile function in 40 men (89%) and reduced severity of PE in 27 men (60%).[130] In a group of 37 men with primary or acquired PE and a baseline IIEF EF domain score of 20.9 consistent with mild ED, Sommer et al. reported a 9.7-fold IELT increase and normalization of erectile function (IIEF EF 26.9) with vardenafil treatment as opposed to lesser 4.4-fold IELT increase with on-demand sertraline.[132]

The high level of correlation between improved erectile function with sildenafil and reduced severity of PE reported by Li[130] and the superior IELT fold-increase observed with vardenafil compared to sertraline reported by Sommer et al. indicate that PDE5i-related reduced PE severity is due to improved erectile function.[132] The IELT fold-increase observed by Sommer et al. with on-demand sertraline (4.4) is less than that reported in reviewed studies on men with normal erectile function (mean 5.57, range 3.0–8.5),[124,126,131,136] suggesting that men with PE and co-morbid ED are less responsive to on-demand SSRIs and are best managed with a PDE5i alone or in combination with an SSRI.

The proposed mechanism of action of PDE5i's as monotherapy or in combination with a SSRI in the treatment of acquired PE in men with co-morbid ED includes a reduction in performance anxiety due to better erections, downregulation of the erectile threshold to a lower level of arousal so that increased levels of arousal are required to achieve the ejaculation threshold and reduction of the erectile refractory period,[129,143,144] and reliance upon a second and more controlled ejaculation during a subsequent episode of intercourse.

Premature Ejaculation and Hyperthyroidism

Data from animal studies suggest anatomic and physiological interactions between brain dopamine and serotonin systems and the hypothalamic–pituitary thyroid axis. There is evidence to indicate a link between depression and thyroid hormones.[145,146] Chronic treatment with thyroxine (T4) is an effective therapy of depression.[147-150] The 5-HT2A receptor is upregulated in the cortex of suicide victims,[151] downregulated by antidepressant drugs,[152] and seems to be under TH regulation. Levels of 5-HT2A receptor mRNA in the rat frontal cortex are decreased during thyroxine deficiency and increased during chronic thyroxine treatment, indicating thyroid hormone involvement in 5-HT2A receptor regulation in adult brain.[153,154]

The majority of patients with thyroid hormone disorders experience sexual dysfunction.[26,142] Corona et al. reported a significant correlation between PE and suppressed TSH values in a selected population of andrological and sexological patients.[142] Carani et al. subsequently reported a PE prevalence of 50% in men with hyperthyroidism, which fell to 15% after treatment with thyroid hormone normalization.[26] Waldinger et al. failed to demonstrate an increased incidence of thyroid dysfunction in lifelong PE, consistent with the notion that hyperthyroidism appears to be a cause of only acquired PE.[155] Treatment of acquired PE secondary to hyperthyroidism requires thyroid hormone normalization with anti-thyroid drugs, radioactive iodine, or thyroidectomy. Although occult thyroid disease has been reported in the elderly hospitalized population,[156] it is uncommon in the population who present for treatment of PE and routine TSH screening is not indicated unless clinically indicated.

Premature Ejaculation and Chronic Prostatitis

Acute and chronic lower urogenital infection, prostatodynia, or chronic pelvic pain syndrome (CPPS) is associated with ED, PE, and painful ejaculation. The relationship between chronic prostatitis, CPPS, and premature ejaculation is supported by several recently published studies that focus more on epidemiology and largely ignore treatment. Most of these have are limited by poor study design including inconsistent or absent methodologies of microbiological diagnosis of prostatitis and the lack of a validated questionnaire for combined evaluation of chronic prostatitis and sexual dysfunction.

Painful ejaculation is a common symptom of chronic prostatitis or CPSS and is included in all prostatitis symptom scores. In 3,700 men with benign prostatic hypertrophy (BPH), painful ejaculation was reported by 18.6% and was associated with more severe lower urinary tract symptoms (LUTS), and a 72% and 75% incidence of ED and PE, respectively.[157] Several studies report PE as the main sexual disorder symptom in men with chronic prostatitis or CPPS with a prevalence of 26–77%.[158-162]

Prostatic inflammation and chronic bacterial prostatitis have been reported as common findings in men with both lifelong and acquired PE.[25,163,164] Shamloul and El-Nashaar reported prostatic inflammation and chronic bacterial prostatitis in 64% and 52% of men with PE.[164] The 41.4% incidence of prostatic inflammation in men with lifelong PE parallels that reported by Screponi,[25] but is inconsistent with the proposed genetic basis of lifelong PE, and assumes the presence of prostatic inflammation from the first sexual experience. Although physical and microbiological examination of the prostate in men with painful ejaculation or LUTS is mandatory, there is insufficient evidence to support routine screening of men with PE for chronic prostatitis. The exact pathophysiology of the link between chronic prostatitis, ED, and PE is unknown. It has been hypothesized that prostatic inflammation may result in altered sensation and modulation of the ejaculatory reflex but evidence is lacking.[164]

Although treatment of chronic prostatitis improves LUTS, there is little published data to suggest a parallel improvement in PE and other sexual dysfunction symptoms.[165-167] El-Nashaar and Shamloul reported that antibiotic treatment of microbiologically confirmed bacterial prostatitis in men with acquired PE resulted in a 2.6-fold increase in IELT and improved ejaculatory control in 83.9% of subjects.[167]

The Future of PE Drug Development

Several in vitro and animal studies have demonstrated that the desensitization of 5-HT1A receptors, increased activation of postsynaptic 5-HT2C receptors, and the resultant higher increase in synaptic 5-HT neurotransmission seen in daily dosing of SSRI class drugs can be acutely achieved by blockade of these receptors by administration of an on-demand SSRI and a 5-HT1A receptor antagonist.[168-170] One study reports that PE men refractory to daily paroxetine can be salvaged by the addition of high-dose daily pindolol, a non-selective ß-blocker with partial beta-agonist activity, and a 5-HT1A receptor antagonist.[171]

An increasing number of studies report the involvement of central oxytocinergic neurotransmission in the ejaculatory process. In human males, plasma oxytocin levels are elevated during penile erection and at the time of orgasm.[172,173] Electrical stimulation of the dorsal penile nerve produced excitation in about half of the oxytocin cells in the PVH and SON of rats.[174,175] In a rat model, systematic administration of oxytocin facilitated ejaculation by reducing the number of intromissions required for ejaculation, ejaculation latencies, and post-ejaculation intervals.[176,177] The use of oxytocin or vasopressin receptor antagonists may also have a role but there have been no reports of their efficacy in the treatment of PE.[178]

Drug combinations of on-demand rapid-acting SSRIs and 5-HT1A receptor antagonist and/or oxytocin receptor antagonists, or single agents that target multiple receptors may form the foundation of more effective future on-demand medication.

Surgery

Several authors have reported the use of surgically induced penile hypoanesthesia via selective dorsal nerve neurotomy or hyaluronic acid gel glans penis augmentation in the treatment of lifelong PE refractory to behavioral and/or pharmacological treatment.[179-181] The role of surgery in the management of PE remains unclear until the results of further studies have been reported.

Conclusion

Recent epidemiological and observational research has provided new insights into PE and the associated negative psychosocial effects of this dysfunction. Recent normative data suggest that men with an IELT of less than 1 min have "definite" PE, while men with IELTs between 1 and 1.5 min have "probable" PE. Although there is insufficient empirical evidence to identify the etiology of PE, there is limited correlational evidence to suggest that men with PE have high levels of sexual anxiety and altered sensitivity of central 5-HT receptors.

The off-label use of SSRIs and clomipramine, along with the development of new on-demand drugs for the treatment of PE, has drawn new attention to this common and often ignored sexual problem. Daily administration of an SSRI is associated with superior-fold increases in IELT compared to on-demand administration of SSRIs including dapoxetine due to greatly enhanced 5-HT neurotransmission resulting from several adaptive processes which may include presynaptic 5-HT1a and 5-HT1b/1d receptor desensitization. However, until the neurobiological, physiological, and psychological mechanisms responsible for PE are better understood, ideal treatment outcomes may remain elusive. Drug treatment fails to directly address causal psychological or relationship factors, and data are either lacking or scarce on the efficacy of combined psychosexual counseling and pharmacological treatment, and the maintenance of improved ejaculatory control after drug withdrawal. Drug combinations or single agents that target multiple 5-HT receptors may represent the next stage of PE drug development.

References

1. Semans JH. Premature ejaculation: a new approach. *South Med J.* 1956;49:353-358
2. Masters WH, Johnson VE. *Human Sexual Inadequacy.* Boston, MA: Little Brown; 1970
3. Waldinger MD, Hengeveld M. Neuroseksuologie en seksuele psychofarmacologie. *Tijdschr Psychiatr.* 2000;8: 585-593
4. Olivier B, van Oorschot R, Waldinger MD. Serotonin, serotonergic receptors, selective serotonin reuptake inhibitors and sexual behaviour. *Int Clin Psychopharmacol.* 1998;13:S9-S14
5. Waldinger MD, Rietschel M, Nothen MM, Hengeveld MW, Olivier B. Familial occurrence of primary premature ejaculation. *Psychiatr Genet.* 1998;8:37-40
6. Pattij T, Olivier B, Waldinger MD. Animal models of ejaculatory behavior. *Curr Pharm Des.* 2005;11:4069-4077
7. Waldinger MD, Zwinderman AH, Schweitzer DH, Olivier B. Relevance of methodological design for the interpretation of efficacy of drug treatment of premature ejaculation: a systematic review and meta-analysis. *Int J Impot Res.* 2004;16:369-381
8. Metz ME, Pryor JL, Nesvacil LJ, Abuzzahab F Sr, Koznar J. Premature ejaculation: a psychophysiological review. *J Sex Marital Ther.* 1997;23:3-23
9. Symonds T, Roblin D, Hart K, Althof S. How does premature ejaculation impact a man's life? *J Sex Marital Ther.* 2003;29:361-370
10. Waldinger MD, Quinn P, Dilleen M, Mundayat R, Schweitzer DH, Boolell M. A multinational population survey of intravaginal ejaculation latency time. *J Sex Med.* 2005;2:492-497
11. Patrick DL, Althof SE, Pryor JL, et al. Premature ejaculation: an observational study of men and their partners. *J Sex Med.* 2005;2:58-367
12. Porst H, Montorsi F, Rosen RC, Gaynor L, Grupe S, Alexander J. The Premature Ejaculation Prevalence and Attitudes (PEPA) survey: prevalence, comorbidities, and professional help-seeking. *Eur Urol.* 2007;51: 816-823
13. Giuliano F, Patrick DL, Porst H, et al. Premature ejaculation: results from a five-country European observational study. *Eur Urol.* 2008;53:1048-1057
14. Reading A, Wiest W. An analysis of self-reported sexual behavior in a sample of normal males. *Arch Sex Behav.* 1984;13:69-83
15. Nathan SG. The epidemiology of the DSM-III psychosexual dysfunctions. *J Sex Marital Ther.* 1986;12: 267-281
16. Spector KR, Boyle M. The prevalence and perceived aetiology of male sexual problems in a non-clinical sample. *Br J Med Psychol.* 1986;59:351-358
17. Spector IP, Carey M. Incidence and prevalence of the sexual dysfunctions: a critical review of the empirical literature. *Arch Sex Behav.* 1990;19:389
18. Grenier G, Byers ES. The relationships among ejaculatory control, ejaculatory latency, and attempts to prolong heterosexual intercourse. *Arch Sex Behav.* 1997;26: 27-47
19. Laumann EO, Paik A, Rosen RC. Sexual dysfunction in the United States: prevalence and predictors. *J Am Med Assoc.* 1999;281:537-544

20. Waldinger MD, Zwinderman AH, Olivier B, Schweitzer DH. Proposal for a definition of lifelong premature ejaculation based on epidemiological stopwatch data. *J Sex Med.* 2005;2:498-507

21. Schapiro B. Premature ejaculation, a review of 1,130 cases. *J Urol.* 1943;50:374-379

22. Waldinger MD. Premature ejaculation: definition and drug treatment. *Drugs.* 2007;67:547-568

23. Hartmann U, Schedlowski M, Kruger TH. Cognitive and partner-related factors in rapid ejaculation: differences between dysfunctional and functional men. *World J Urol.* 2005;10:10

24. Laumann EO, Nicolosi A, Glasser DB, et al. Sexual problems among women and men aged 40–80 years: prevalence and correlates identified in the global study of sexual attitudes and behaviors. *Int J Impot Res.* 2005; 17:39-57

25. Screponi E, Carosa E, Di Stasi SM, Pepe M, Carruba G, Jannini EA. Prevalence of chronic prostatitis in men with premature ejaculation. *Urology.* 2001;58:198-202

26. Carani C, Isidori AM, Granata A, et al. Multicenter study on the prevalence of sexual symptoms in male hypo- and hyperthyroid patients. *J Clin Endocrinol Metab.* 2005;90:6472-6479

27. Adson DE, Kotlyar M. Premature ejaculation associated with citalopram withdrawal. *Ann Pharmacother.* 2003;37: 1804-1806

28. Peugh J, Belenko S. Alcohol, drugs and sexual function: a review. *J Psychoactive Drugs.* 2001;33:223-232

29. McMahon CG. Long term results of treatment of premature ejaculation with selective serotonin re-uptake inhibitors. *Int J Impot Res.* 2002;14:S19

30. Waldinger MD, Schweitzer DH. Changing paradigms from a historical DSM-III and DSM-IV view toward an evidence-based definition of premature ejaculation. Part II-proposals for DSM-V and ICD-11. *J Sex Med.* 2006;3:693-705

31. American Psychiatric Association. *Diagnostic and Statistical Manual of Mental Disorders (DSM-IV).* 4th ed. Washington, DC: American Psychiatric Association; 1994

32. World Health Organization. *International Classification of Diseases and Related Health Problems.* 10th ed. Geneva: World Health Organization; 1994

33. Metz M, McCarthy B. *Coping with Premature Ejaculation: How to Overcome PE, Please Your Partner and Have Great Sex.* Oakland: New Harbinber Publications; 2003

34. Montague DK, Jarow J, Broderick GA, et al. AUA guideline on the pharmacologic management of premature ejaculation. *J Urol.* 2004;172:290-294

35. Colpi G, Weidner W, Jungwirth A, et al. EAU guidelines on ejaculatory dysfunction. *Eur Urol.* 2004;46:555-558

36. McMahon CG, Abdo C, Incrocci I, et al. Disorders of orgasm and ejaculation in men. In: Lue TF, Basson R, Rosen R, Giuliano F, Khoury S, Montorsi F, eds. *Sexual Medicine: Sexual Dysfunctions in Men and Women (2nd International Consultation on Sexual Dysfunctions-Paris).* Paris: France Health Publications; 2004:409-468

37. Jannini EA, Lombardo F, Lenzi A. Correlation between ejaculatory and erectile dysfunction. *Int J Androl.* 2005;28(Suppl 2):40-45

38. Centre for Evidence-based Medicine. Oxford Centre for Evidence-based Medicine Levels of Evidence; May 2001.

http://www.cebm.net/index.aspx?o=1025. Accessed February 8, 2008 [cited]

39. Althof SE, Symonds T. Patient reported outcomes used in the assessment of premature ejaculation. *Urol Clin North Am.* 2007;34:581-589

40. McMahon CG, Althof SE, Waldinger MD, et al. An evidence-based definition of lifelong premature ejaculation: report of the International Society for Sexual Medicine (ISSM) ad hoc committee for the definition of premature ejaculation. *J Sex Med.* 2008;5:1590-1606

41. Waldinger MD, Hengeveld MW, Zwinderman AH. Paroxetine treatment of premature ejaculation: a double blind, randomized, placebo controlled study. *Am J Psychiatry.* 1994;151:1377-1379

42. Spiess WF, Geer JH, O'Donohue WT. Premature ejaculation: investigation of factors in ejaculatory latency. *J Abnorm Psychol.* 1984;93:242-245

43. Strassberg DS, Kelly MP, Carroll C, Kircher JC. The psychophysiological nature of premature ejaculation. *Arch Sex Behav.* 1987;16:327-336

44. Kilmann PR, Auerbach R. Treatments of premature ejaculation and psychogenic impotence: a critical review of the literature. *Arch Sex Behav.* 1979;8:81-100

45. Schover L, Friedman J, Weiler S, Heiman J, LoPiccolo J. Multiaxial problem-oriented system for sexual dysfunctions. *Arch Gen Psychiatry.* 1982;39:614-619

46. Waldinger M, Hengeveld M, Zwinderman A, Olivier B. An empirical operationalization of DSM-IV diagnostic criteria for premature ejaculation. *Int J Psychiatr Clin Pract.* 1998;2:287-293

47. Waldinger MD, Zwinderman AH, Olivier B, Schweitzer DH. The majority of men with lifelong premature ejaculation prefer daily drug treatment: an observation study in a consecutive group of Dutch men. *J Sex Med.* 2007;4:1028-1037

48. Althof SE, Levine SB, Corty EW, Risen CB, Stern EB, Kurit DM. A double-blind crossover trial of clomipramine for rapid ejaculation in 15 couples. *J Clin Psychiatry.* 1995;56:402-407

49. Pryor JL, Broderick GA, Ho KF, Jamieson C, Gagnon D. Comparison of estimated versus measured intravaginal ejaculatory latency time (IELT) in Men with and without premature ejaculation (PE). *J Sex Med.* 2005;3:54 (Abstract 126)

50. Rosen RC, McMahon CG, Niederberger C, Broderick GA, Jamieson C, Gagnon DD. Correlates to the clinical diagnosis of premature ejaculation: results from a large observational study of men and their partners. *J Urol.* 2007;177:1059-1064; discussion 64

51. Kaplan HS, Kohl RN, Pomeroy WB, Offit AK, Hogan B. Group treatment of premature ejaculation. *Arch Sex Behav.* 1974;3:443-452

52. McCarthy B. Cognitive-behavioural strategies and techniques in the treatment of early ejaculation. In: Leiblum SR, Rosen R, eds. *Principles and Practices of Sex Therapy: Update for the 1990s.* New York: Guilford; 1988:141-167

53. Vandereycken W. Towards a better delineation of ejaculatory disorders. *Acta Psychiatr Belg.* 1986;86:57-63

54. Zilbergeld B. *Male Sexuality.* Toronto: Bantam; 1978

55. Grenier G, Byers S. Operationalizing premature or rapid ejaculation. *J Sex Res.* 2001;38:369-378

56. Rowland DL, Strassberg DS, de Gouveia Brazao CA, Slob AK. Ejaculatory latency and control in men with premature ejaculation: an analysis across sexual activities

using multiple sources of information. *J Psychosom Res.* 2000;48:69-77

57. Giuliano F, Patrick DL, Porst H, et al. Premature ejaculation: results from a five-country European observational study. *Eur Urol.* October 16, 2007 [Epub ahead of print]

58. Rowland D, Perelman M, Althof S, et al. Self-reported premature ejaculation and aspects of sexual functioning and satisfaction. *J Sex Med.* 2004;1:225-232

59. Dunn KM, Croft PR, Hackett GI. Association of sexual problems with social, psychological, and physical problems in men and women: a cross sectional population survey. *J Epidemiol Community Health.* 1999;53: 144-148

60. Rowland DL, Patrick DL, Rothman M, Gagnon DD. The psychological burden of premature ejaculation. *J Urol.* 2007;177:1065-1070

61. Rosen R, Althof S. Psychological consequences of PE, quality of life and impact on sexual relationships. *J Sex Med.* 2008;5:1296-1307

62. McCabe MP. Intimacy and quality of life among sexually dysfunctional men and women. *J Sex Marital Ther.* 1997;23:276-290

63. Byers ES, Grenier G. Premature or rapid ejaculation: heterosexual couples' perceptions of men's ejaculatory behavior. *Arch Sex Behav.* 2003;32:261-270

64. Riley A, Riley E. Premature ejaculation: presentation and associations. An audit of patients attending a sexual problems clinic. *Int J Clin Pract.* 2005;59:1482-1487

65. Brock GB, Gajewski J, Carrier S, Bernard F, Lee J, Pommerville PJ. The prevalence and impact of premature ejaculation in Canada. Proceedings of Annual Meeting of the American Urological Association; May 19-24, 2007; Anaheim, CA

66. Althof SE. Prevalence, characteristics and implications of premature ejaculation/rapid ejaculation. *J Urol.* 2006;175:842-848

67. Althof S. The psychology of premature ejaculation: therapies and consequences. *J Sex Med.* 2006;3(Suppl 4): 324-331

68. Jern P, Santtila P, Witting K, et al. Premature and delayed ejaculation: genetic and environmental effects in a population-based sample of Finnish twins. *J Sex Med.* 2007;4:1739-1749

69. Waldinger MD, Berendsen HH, Blok BF, Olivier B, Holstege G. Premature ejaculation and serotonergic antidepressants-induced delayed ejaculation: the involvement of the serotonergic system. *Behav Brain Res.* 1998;92:111-118

70. Waldinger MD. The neurobiological approach to premature ejaculation. *J Urol.* 2002;168:2359-2367

71. Janssen PKC, Bakker SC, Réthelyi J, et al. Serotonin transporter promoter region (5-HTTLPR) polymorphism is associated with the intravaginal ejaculation latency time in Dutch men with lifelong premature ejaculation. *J Sex Med.* 2008;6:276-284

72. de Carufel F, Trudel G. Effects of a new functional-sexological treatment for premature ejaculation. *J Sex Marital Ther.* 2006;32:97-114

73. De Amicis LA, Goldberg DC, LoPiccolo J, Friedman J, Davies L. Clinical follow-up of couples treated for sexual dysfunction. *Arch Sex Behav.* 1985;14:467-489

74. Hawton K, Catalan J, Martin P, Fagg J. Long-term outcome of sex therapy. *Behav Res Ther.* 1986;24:665-675

75. Perelman MA. A new combination treatment for premature ejaculation: a sex therapist's perspective. *J Sex Med.* 2006;3:1004-1012

76. Atkins D, Best D, Briss PA, et al. Grading quality of evidence and strength of recommendations. *Br Med J.* 2004;328(7454):1490

77. Waldinger M. Towards evidenced based drug treatment research on premature ejaculation: a critical evaluation of methodology. *J Impot Res.* 2003;15:309-313

78. Atmaca M, Kuloglu M, Tezcan E, Semercioz A. The efficacy of citalopram in the treatment of premature ejaculation: a placebo-controlled study. *Int J Impot Res.* 2002;14:502-505

79. McMahon CG. Treatment of premature ejaculation with sertraline hydrochloride: a single-blind placebo controlled crossover study. *J Urol.* 1998;159:1935-1938

80. Kara H, Aydin S, Yucel M, Agargun MY, Odabas O, Yilmaz Y. The efficacy of fluoxetine in the treatment of premature ejaculation: a double-blind placebo controlled study. *J Urol.* 1996;156:1631-1632

81. Waldinger MD, Hengeveld MW, Zwinderman AH. Paroxetine treatment of premature ejaculation: a double-blind, randomized, placebo-controlled study. *Am J Psychiatry.* 1994;151:1377-1379

82. Goodman RE. An assessment of clomipramine (Anafranil) in the treatment of premature ejaculation. *J Int Med Res.* 1980;8:53-59

83. Waldinger MD. Drug treatment of premature ejaculation: pharmacodynamic and pharmacokinetic paradigms. *Drug Discov Today Ther Strateg.* 2005;2: 37-40

84. Marangell LB, Dennehy EB, Wisniewski SR, et al. Case-control analyses of the impact of pharmacotherapy on prospectively observed suicide attempts and completed suicides in bipolar disorder: findings from STEP-BD. *J Clin Psychiatry.* 2008;69:916-922

85. Mann JJ, Emslie G, Baldessarini RJ, et al. ACNP Task Force report on SSRIs and suicidal behavior in youth. *Neuropsychopharmacology.* 2006;31:473-492

86. Khan A, Khan S, Kolts R, Brown WA. Suicide rates in clinical trials of SSRIs, other antidepressants, and placebo: analysis of FDA reports. *Am J Psychiatry.* 2003;160:790-792

87. Ditto KE. SSRI discontinuation syndrome. Awareness as an approach to prevention. *Postgrad Med.* 2003;114: 79-84

88. Black K, Shea CA, Dursun S, Kutcher S. Selective serotonin reuptake inhibitor discontinuation syndrome: proposed diagnostic criteria. *J Psychiatry Neurosci.* 2000;25:255-261

89. Li N, Wallen NH, Ladjevardi M, Hjemdahl P. Effects of serotonin on platelet activation in whole blood. *Blood Coagul Fibrinolysis.* 1997;8:517-523

90. Weinrieb RM, Auriacombe M, Lynch KG, Lewis JD. Selective serotonin re-uptake inhibitors and the risk of bleeding. *Expert Opin Drug Saf.* 2005;4:337-344

91. Garcia Rodriguez LA, Jick H. Risk of upper gastrointestinal bleeding and perforation associated with individual non-steroidal anti-inflammatory drugs. *Lancet.* 1994;343:769-772

92. Ahmad S. Paroxetine-induced priapism. *Arch Intern Med.* 1995;155:645

93. Rand EH. Priapism in a patient taking sertraline. *J Clin Psychiatry.* 1998;59:538

94. Dent LA, Brown WC, Murney JD. Citalopram-induced priapism. *Pharmacotherapy*. 2002;22:538-541

95. Fava M, Judge R, Hoog SL, Nilsson ME, Koke SC. Fluoxetine versus sertraline and paroxetine in major depressive disorder: changes in weight with long-term treatment. *J Clin Psychiatry*. 2000;61:863-867

96. Cavallini G. Alpha-1 blockade pharmacotherapy in primitive psychogenic premature ejaculation resistant to psychotherapy. *Eur Urol*. 1995;28:126-130

97. Basar MM, Yilmaz E, Ferhat M, Basar H, Batislam E. Terazosin in the treatment of premature ejaculation: a short-term follow-up. *Int Urol Nephrol*. 2005;37: 773-777

98. McMahon CG, Touma K. Treatment of premature ejaculation with paroxetine hydrochloride as needed: 2 single-blind placebo controlled crossover studies. *J Urol*. 1999;161:1826-1830

99. Strassberg DS, de Gouveia Brazao CA, Rowland DL, Tan P, Slob AK. Clomipramine in the treatment of rapid (premature) ejaculation. *J Sex Marital Ther*. 1999;25: 89-101

100. Kim SW, Paick JS. Short-term analysis of the effects of as needed use of sertraline at 5 PM for the treatment of premature ejaculation. *Urology*. 1999;54:544-547

101. Waldinger MD, Zwinderman AH, Olivier B. On-demand treatment of premature ejaculation with clomipramine and paroxetine: a randomized, double-blind fixed-dose study with stopwatch assessment. *Eur Urol*. 2004;46: 510-515

102. Dresser MJ, Lindert K, Lin D. Pharmacokinetics of single and multiple escalating doses of dapoxetine in healthy volunteers. *Clin Pharmacol Ther*. 2004;75:113 (Abstract P1)

103. Dresser M, Modi NB, Staehr P, Mulhall JP. The effect of food on the pharmacokinetics of dapoxetine, a new on-demand treatment for premature ejaculation. *J Sex Med*. 2005;3:25 (Abstract 37)

104. Modi NB, Dresser M, Desai D. Dapoxetine, a new on-demand treatment for premature ejaculation exhibits rapid single and multiple-dose pharmacokinetics. *J Sex Med*. 2006;3:228 (Abstract P-02-162)

105. Modi NB, Dresser M, Desai D, Edgar C, Wesnes K. Dapoxetine has no pharmacokinetic or cognitive interactions with ethanol in healthy male volunteers. *J Clin Pharmacol*. 2007;47:315-322

106. Dresser MJ, Desai D, Gidwani S, Seftel AD, Modi NB. Dapoxetine, a novel treatment for premature ejaculation, does not have pharmacokinetic interactions with phosphodiesterase-5 inhibitors. *Int J Impot Res*. 2006;18:104-110

107. Pryor JL, Althof SE, Steidle C, et al. Efficacy and tolerability of dapoxetine in treatment of premature ejaculation: an integrated analysis of two double-blind, randomised controlled trials. *Lancet*. 2006;368: 929-937

108. Waldinger MD, Hengeveld MW, Zwinderman AH, Olivier B. Effect of SSRI antidepressants on ejaculation: a double-blind, randomized, placebo-controlled study with fluoxetine, fluvoxamine, paroxetine, and sertraline. *J Clin Psychopharmacol*. 1998;18:274-281

109. Waldinger MD, Zwinderman AH, Olivier B, Schweitzer DH. Geometric mean IELT and premature ejaculation: appropriate statistics to avoid overestimation of treatment efficacy. *J Sex Med*. 2008;5:492-499

110. McMahon CG. Clinical trial methodology in premature ejaculation observational, interventional, and treatment preference studies—Part II—Study design, outcome measures, data analysis, and reporting. *J Sex Med*. 2008;5:1817-1833

111. Levine SB, Casey RW, Ramagopal VM, Hashmonay R. Evaluation of withdrawal effects with dapoxetine in the treatment of premature ejaculation (PE). *J Sex Medicine*, Jan 2007;4(Supp 1), 91

112. Frink MC, Hennies HH, Englberger W, Haurand M, Wilffert B. Influence of tramadol on neurotransmitter systems of the rat brain. *Arzneimittelforschung*. 1996;46: 1029-1036

113. Safarinejad MR, Hosseini SY. Safety and efficacy of tramadol in the treatment of premature ejaculation: a double-blind, placebo-controlled, fixed-dose, randomized study. *J Clin Psychopharmacol*. 2006;26:27-31

114. Salem EA, Wilson SK, Bissada NK, Delk JR, Hellstrom WJ, Cleves MA. Tramadol HCL has promise in on-demand use to treat premature ejaculation. *J Sex Med*. 2007;5:188-193

115. Cossmann M, Kohnen C, Langford R, McCartney C. Tolerance and safety of tramadol use. Results of international studies and data from drug surveillance. *Drugs*. 1997;53:50-62

116. McDiarmid T, Mackler L, Schneider DM. Clinical inquiries. What is the addiction risk associated with tramadol? *J Fam Pract*. 2005;54:72-73

117. Adams EH, Breiner S, Cicero TJ, et al. A comparison of the abuse liability of tramadol, NSAIDs, and hydrocodone in patients with chronic pain. *J Pain Symptom Manage*. 2006;31:465-476

118. Berkovitch M, Keresteci AG, Koren G. Efficacy of prilocaine-lidocaine cream in the treatment of premature ejaculation. *J Urol*. 1995;154:1360-1361

119. Xin ZC, Choi YD, Lee SH, Choi HK. Efficacy of a topical agent SS-cream in the treatment of premature ejaculation: preliminary clinical studies. *Yonsei Med J*. 1997;38:91-95

120. Busato W, Galindo CC. Topical anaesthetic use for treating premature ejaculation: a double-blind, randomized, placebo-controlled study. *BJU Int*. 2004;93: 1018-1021

121. Dinsmore WW, Hackett G, Goldmeier D, et al. Topical eutectic mixture for premature ejaculation (TEMPE): a novel aerosol-delivery form of lidocaine-prilocaine for treating premature ejaculation. *BJU Int*. 2006;99:369-375

122. Henry R, Morales A, Wyllie MG. TEMPE: topical eutectic-like mixture for premature ejaculation. *Expert Opin Drug Deliv*. 2008;5:251-261

123. Fein RL. Intracavernous medication for treatment of premature ejaculation. *Urology*. 1990;35:301-303

124. Abdel-Hamid IA, El Naggar EA, El Gilany AH. Assessment of as needed use of pharmacotherapy and the pause-squeeze technique in premature ejaculation. *Int J Impot Res*. 2001;13:41-45

125. Salonia A, Maga T, Colombo R, et al. A prospective study comparing paroxetine alone versus paroxetine plus sildenafil in patients with premature ejaculation. *J Urol*. 2002;168:2486-2489

126. Zhang XS, Wang YX, Huang XY, Leng J, Li Z, Han YF. Comparison between sildenafil plus sertraline and sertraline alone in the treatment of premature ejaculation. *Zhonghua Nan Ke Xue*. 2005;11:520-522, 525

127. Chen J, Mabjeesh NJ, Matzkin H, Greenstein A. Efficacy of sildenafil as adjuvant therapy to selective serotonin reuptake inhibitor in alleviating premature ejaculation. *Urology*. 2003;61:197-200

128. Tang W, Ma L, Zhao L, Liu Y, Chen Z. Clinical efficacy of Viagra with behavior therapy against premature ejaculation. *Zhonghua Nan Ke Xue*. 2004;10:366-367, 370

129. McMahon CG, Stuckey B, Andersen ML. Efficacy of Viagra:Sildenafil Citrate in men with premature ejaculation. *J Sex Med*. 2005;2:368-375

130. Li X, Zhang SX, Cheng HM, Zhang WD. Clinical study of sildenafil in the treatment of premature ejaculation complicated by erectile dysfunction. *Zhonghua Nan Ke Xue*. 2003;9:266-269

131. Lozano AF. Premature ejaculation. Pharmacological treatment. Three years after. *Int J Impot Res*. 2003;15:S11 (Abstract MP-2-6)

132. Sommer F, Klotz T, Mathers MJ. Treatment of premature ejaculation: a comparative vardenafil and SSRI crossover study. *J Urol*. 2005;173:202 (Abstract 741)

133. Mattos RM, Lucon AM. Tadalafil and slow-release fluoxetine in premature ejaculation - a prospective study. *J Urol*. 2005;173:239 (Abstract 880)

134. Erenpreiss J, Zalkalns J. Premature ejaculation: comparison of patroxetine alone, paroxetine plus local lidocaine and paroxetine plus sildenafil. *Int J Impot Res*. 2002;14:S33 (Abstract PS-7-4)

135. Linn R, Ginesin Y, Hardak S, Mertyk S. Treatment of sildenfil as part of the treatment in premature ejaculation. *Int J Impot Res*. 2002;14:S39 (Abstract P-168)

136. Chia S. Management of premature ejaculation – a comparison of treatment outcome in patients with and without erectile dysfunction. *Int J Androl*. 2002;25: 301-305

137. Atan A, Basar MM, Tuncel A, Ferhat M, Agras K, Tekdogan U. Comparison of efficacy of sildenafil-only, sildenafil plus topical EMLA cream, and topical EMLA-cream-only in treatment of premature ejaculation. *Urology*. 2006;67:388-391

138. Mamas MA, Reynard JM, Brading AF. Nitric oxide and the lower urinary tract: current concepts, future prospects. *Urology*. 2003;61:1079-1085

139. McMahon CG, McMahon CN, Leow LJ, Winestock CG. Efficacy of type-5 phosphodiesterase inhibitors in the drug treatment of premature ejaculation: a systematic review. *BJU Int*. 2006;98:259-272

140. McMahon CG. Clinical trial methodology in premature ejaculation observational, interventional, and treatment preference studies – Part I – Defining and selecting the study population. *J Sex Med*. 2008;5: 1805-1816

141. McMahon CG. Clinical trial methodology in premature ejaculation observational, interventional, and treatment preference studies – Part II–Study design, outcome measures, data analysis, and reporting. *J Sex Med*. 2008;5:1817-1833

142. Corona G, Petrone L, Mannucci E, et al. Psychobiological correlates of rapid ejaculation in patients attending an andrologic unit for sexual dysfunctions. *Eur Urol*. 2004;46:615-622

143. Aversa A, Mazzilli F, Rossi T, Delfino M, Isidori AM, Fabbri A. Effects of sildenafil (Viagra) administration on seminal parameters and post-ejaculatory refractory time in normal males. *Hum Reprod*. 2000;15:131-134

144. Mondaini N, Ponchietti R, Muir GH, et al. Sildenafil does not improve sexual function in men without erectile dysfunction but does reduce the postorgasmic refractory time. *Int J Impot Res*. 2003;15:225-228

145. Kirkegaard C, Faber J. The role of thyroid hormones in depression. *Eur J Endocrinol*. 1998;138:1-9

146. Musselman DL, Nemeroff CB. Depression and endocrine disorders: focus on the thyroid and adrenal system. *Br J Psychiatry*, Jun 1996;30:123-128

147. Bauer MS, Whybrow PC. Rapid cycling bipolar affective disorder. II. Treatment of refractory rapid cycling with high-dose levothyroxine: a preliminary study. *Arch Gen Psychiatry*. 1990;47:435-440

148. Bauer M, Heinz A, Whybrow PC. Thyroid hormones, serotonin and mood: of synergy and significance in the adult brain. *Mol Psychiatry*. 2002;7:140-156

149. Bauer M, London ED, Silverman DH, Rasgon N, Kirchheiner J, Whybrow PC. Thyroid, brain and mood modulation in affective disorder: insights from molecular research and functional brain imaging. *Pharmacopsychiatry*. 2003;36(Suppl 3):S215-S221

150. Gitlin M, Altshuler LL, Frye MA, et al. Peripheral thyroid hormones and response to selective serotonin reuptake inhibitors. *J Psychiatry Neurosci*. 2004;29: 383-386

151. Hrdina PD, Demeter E, Vu TB, Sotonyi P, Palkovits M. 5-HT uptake sites and 5-HT2 receptors in brain of antidepressant-free suicide victims/depressives: increase in 5-HT2 sites in cortex and amygdala. *Brain Res*. 1993;614:37-44

152. Eison AS, Mullins UL. Regulation of central 5-HT2A receptors: a review of in vivo studies. *Behav Brain Res*. 1996;73:177-181

153. Kulikov AV, Maksyutova AV, Ivanova EA, Khvorostov IB, Popova NK. The effect of thyroidectomy on the expression of the mRNA of 5-HT2A serotonin receptors in the rat frontal cortex. *Dokl Biochem Biophys*. 2002;383: 116-118

154. Kulikov AV, Zubkov EA. Chronic thyroxine treatment activates the 5-HT2A serotonin receptor in the mouse brain. *Neurosci Lett*. 2007;416:307-309

155. Waldinger MD, Zwinderman AH, Olivier B, Schweitzer DH. Thyroid-stimulating hormone assessments in a Dutch cohort of 620 men with lifelong premature ejaculation without erectile dysfunction. *J Sex Med*. 2005;2:865-870

156. Atkinson RL, Dahms WT, Fisher DA, Nichols AL. Occult thyroid disease in an elderly hospitalized population. *J Gerontol*. 1978;33:372-376

157. Nickel JC, Elhilali M, Vallancien G. Benign prostatic hyperplasia (BPH) and prostatitis: prevalence of painful ejaculation in men with clinical BPH. *BJU Int*. 2005;95:571-574

158. Qiu YC, Xie CY, Zeng XD, Zhang JH. Investigation of sexual function in 623 patients with chronic prostatitis. *Zhonghua Nan Ke Xue*. 2007;13:524-526

159. Gonen M, Kalkan M, Cenker A, Ozkardes H. Prevalence of premature ejaculation in Turkish men with chronic pelvic pain syndrome. *J Androl*. 2005;26:601-603

160. Beutel ME, Weidner W, Brahler E. Chronic pelvic pain and its comorbidity. *Urologe A*. 2004;43:261-267

161. Liang CZ, Zhang XJ, Hao ZY, Shi HQ, Wang KX. Prevalence of sexual dysfunction in Chinese men with chronic prostatitis. *BJU Int*. 2004;93:568-570

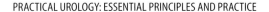
162. Trinchieri A, Magri V, Cariani L, et al. Prevalence of sexual dysfunction in men with chronic prostatitis/chronic pelvic pain syndrome. *Arch Ital Urol Androl.* 2007;79:67-70

163. Xing JP, Fan JH, Wang MZ, Chen XF, Yang ZS. Survey of the prevalence of chronic prostatitis in men with premature ejaculation. *Zhonghua Nan Ke Xue.* 2003;9: 451-453

164. Shamloul R, el-Nashaar A. Chronic prostatitis in premature ejaculation: a cohort study in 153 men. *J Sex Med.* 2006;3:150-154

165. Boneff AN. Topical treatment of chronic prostatitis and premature ejaculation. *Int Urol Nephrol.* 1972;4: 183-186

166. Brown AJ. Ciprofloxacin as cure of premature ejaculation. *J Sex Marital Ther.* 2000;26:351-352

167. El-Nashaar A, Shamloul R. Antibiotic treatment can delay ejaculation in patients with premature ejaculation and chronic bacterial prostatitis. *J Sex Med.* 2007;4:491-496

168. Cremers TI, De Boer P, Liao Y, et al. Augmentation with a 5-HT1A, but not a 5-HT1B receptor antagonist critically depends on the dose of citalopram. *Eur J Pharmacol.* 2000;397:63-74

169. Williamson IJ, Turner L, Woods K, Wayman CP, van der Graaf PH. The 5-HT1A receptor antagonist robalzotan enhances SSRI-induced ejaculation delay in the rat. *Br J Pharmacol Biochem Behav.* 2003;138:PO32

170. de Jong TR, Pattij T, Veening JG, et al. Citalopram combined with WAY 100635 inhibits ejaculation and ejaculation-related Fos immunoreactivity. *Eur J Pharmacol.* 2005;509:49-59 [Epub January 21, 2005]

171. Safarinejad MR. Once-daily high-dose pindolol for paroxetine-refractory premature ejaculation: a double-blind, placebo-controlled and randomized study. *J Clin Psychopharmacol.* 2008;28:39-44

172. Carmichael MS, Humbert R, Dixen J, Palmisano G, Greenleaf W, Davidson JM. Plasma oxytocin increases in the human sexual response. *J Clin Endocrinol Metab.* 1987;64:27-31

173. Uckert S, Becker AJ, Ness BO, et al. Oxytocin plasma levels in the systemic and cavernous blood of healthy males during different penile conditions. *World J Urol.* 2003;20:323-326

174. Honda K, Yanagimoto M, Negoro H, Narita K, Murata T, Higuchi T. Excitation of oxytocin cells in the hypothalamic supraoptic nucleus by electrical stimulation of the dorsal penile nerve and tactile stimulation of the penis in the rat. *Brain Res Bull.* 1999;48:309-313

175. Yanagimoto M, Honda K, Goto Y, Negoro H. Afferents originating from the dorsal penile nerve excite oxytocin cells in the hypothalamic paraventricular nucleus of the rat. *Brain Res.* 1996;733:292-296

176. Arletti R, Bazzani C, Castelli M, Bertolini A. Oxytocin improves male copulatory performance in rats. *Horm Behav.* 1985;19:14-20

177. Arletti R, Benelli A, Bertolini A. Sexual behavior of aging male rats is stimulated by oxytocin. *Eur J Pharmacol.* 1990;179:377-381

178. Gupta J, Russell RJ, Wayman CP, Hurley D, Jackson VM. Oxytocin-induced contractions within rat and rabbit ejaculatory tissues are mediated by vasopressin V(1A) receptors and not oxytocin receptors. *Br J Pharmacol.* 2008;55:118-126

179. Kim JJ, Kwak TI, Jeon BG, Cheon J, Moon DG. Effects of glans penis augmentation using hyaluronic acid gel for premature ejaculation. *Int J Impot Res.* 2004;16:547-551

180. Shi WG, Wang XJ, Liang XQ, et al. Selective resection of the branches of the two dorsal penile nerves for primary premature ejaculation. *Zhonghua Nan Ke Xue.* 2008;14:436-438

181. Kwak TI, Jin MH, Kim JJ, Moon DG. Long-term effects of glans penis augmentation using injectable hyaluronic acid gel for premature ejaculation. *Int J Impot Res.* 2008;20:425-428

30

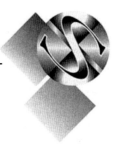

The Role of Interventional Management for Urinary Tract Calculi

Kenneth J. Hastie

The treatment of urinary tract stone disease has been revolutionized over the last 3 decades with the major technological advances of extracorporeal shock wave lithotripsy, percutaneous renal surgery, and ureteroscopy. These have not only made open surgery virtually obsolete but undoubtedly have lowered the threshold for intervention.

The principles and technical aspects of these modern minimally invasive methods for treating calculi are discussed and then how these modalities are applied to specific stone scenarios are described.

Extracorporeal Shock Wave Lithotripsy (ESWL)

The concept of using shock waves to shatter kidney stones was proposed by Chaussy et al. in 1980.[1] As a result of the clinical introduction of this technique in the early part of that decade, the management of urinary tract stone disease was transformed. There are three major types of shock wave generator in common usage: electrohydraulic, piezoelectric, and electromagnetic.

The general principle common to all is the generation of a shock wave in a fluid. Typically, the shock wave is characterized by a rapid positive pressure followed by a shorter and shallower negative pressure component. The first focal point (F1) is at the site of shock wave generation. A focusing device is required to converge the shock waves onto the stone for fragmentation (F2).

Electrohydraulic systems rely on the discharge of a high-voltage current across a spark gap. This results in an expanding gas bubble which creates a shock wave. This is focused by a metallic semiellipsoid which surrounds the generator. The pressures achieved do vary (perhaps by as much as 45%), and the spark gap electrode has a finite life span. There is a risk of cardiac arrhythmias with this shock wave generator and to avoid this ECG gating is required. This ensures that the shock wave occurs after the R wave during the refractory period of the cardiac cycle.

Piezoelectric lithotripters depend on the property that ceramic crystals have a characteristic frequency of resonance. When a high-voltage current is applied, the crystal vibrates producing a shock wave that can be propagated in water. This type of lithotripter has a large number of such elements in a hemispherical array which acts as a self-focusing device. The analgesic requirements are less with this technology and it is accepted that stone fragmentation is slower with a greater retreatment rate.

The basic principle of electromagnetic lithotripsy is the application of an electric current to an electromagnetic coil within a water-filled cylinder. The ensuing magnetic field repels a metallic membrane producing a shock wave which is focused using an acoustic lens. An alternative design is to surround the coil by a membrane in a cylindrical configuration. This in turn is surrounded by a parabolic reflector which focuses the shock wave at F2. This arrangement, as it has a hollow center, lends itself to the addition of in-line ultrasound.

Neither the electromagnetic nor the piezo-ceramic devices require ECG gating.

Coupling of the patient to the shockwave generator is necessary for transmission of the shock wave. With the first Dornier lithotripters, coupling was achieved by fully immersing the patient within a water bath. This has now been refined by the use of cushioned fluid-filled bags which when applied to the skin couple the shock waves to the patient using appropriate jelly to ensure good contact.

Implicit in ESWL is a requirement for targeting. This is achieved by radiographic imaging in two planes or by in-line ultrasound. Clearly, the latter has safety advantages but requires further expertise. Ultrasound is a prerequisite for radiolucent stones.

With modern lithotripters, only simple analgesics such as nonsteroidal anti-inflammatory drugs (NSAIDs) are required in most cases, but children may require general anesthesia.

When a shock wave reaches an interface such as at the surface of the stone the energy is released. A variety of theories have been postulated as to how shock waves cause fragmentation. These include the production of gaseous cavitation bubbles forming as a result of the negative pressure immediately following the shock wave. The positive pressure of the wave may cause fractures at the proximal surface of the stone. There may be reflection of the shock wave within the stone and at the distal surface at the stone/urine interface changing the shock wave to a tensile wave causing stone disintegration by spallation. Studies have suggested that slower shock wave rates at 60 shocks/min are more effective than higher rates of up to 120/min.

Contraindications to ESWL

Certain factors related to patients may preclude ESWL: these include bleeding diatheses and anticoagulation, pregnancy and aortic aneurysm. They can be issues with certain cardiac pacemakers. Caution is required if sepsis is suspected and ESWL is less effective for certain harder stone types (cystine and calcium oxalate monohydrate).

Complications of ESWL

Patients undergoing ESWL for renal stones will have transient hematuria and there is the possibility of a significant perirenal hematoma (0.5%) and obstruction due to stone fragments (steinstrasse) within the ureter. The latter can resolve given time but other interventions such as ureteroscopy or further ESWL to the lead fragment may be required. Prestenting the patient for larger stones (>1.5) can prevent obstruction, but the presence of a stent does not necessarily help the passage of stone fragments and the patient has to accept stent symptoms. The use of alternatives such as PCNL should be considered if the stone burden is large.

Urosepsis is a potential complication as bacteria can be released during treatment and it is advised to treat UTI with antibiotics prior to ESWL.

Long-term concerns following lithotripsy have included suggestions that hypertension and the development of diabetes.[2]

Percutaneous Nephrolithotomy (PCNL)

This technique was first proposed by Ferntrom and Johansson in 1976[3] and became standard practice for renal stones from the 1980s.[4]

The principles of PCNL are access to the pelvicalyceal system allowing passage of a nephroscope and the application of instruments for stone fragmentation and removal.

Prior to planning PCNL, it is recommended that in cases of complex stones, renal function on the affected side is checked with renography to ensure that the level of function warrants treatment of the stone. Serious consideration should be given to nephrectomy if ipsilateral function is less than 15–20% assuming the contralateral kidney is normal.

Positive urine cultures prior to PCNL should be treated and if at the time of surgery, the kidney is found to contain purulent urine, the procedure should be abandoned and a nephrostomy drain left in situ.

PCNL Access

Variations in patient position are described with the commonest being the prone position. The safest and easiest access is via a posterior lower pole calyx, but the route into the pelvicalyceal system will be determined by the configuration of the stone and is also facilitated by knowledge of the anatomy. Intravenous urography does give valuable information for both aspects. However in complex cases (e.g., staghorn calculi), special circumstances such as anatomical variants (e.g., horseshoe kidney) or certain patient types including spina bifida, CT scanning can be invaluable. Pre- and postcontrast CT with reconfiguration allows the access strategy to be planned in advance.

A number of radiological techniques are popular in facilitating access to the pelvicalyceal system for PCNL.

In the first method, a retrograde catheter is passed cystoscopically into the collecting system and this allows injection of a mixture of contrast and visible dye such as methylene blue. The former opacifies the system for x-ray screening and the latter gives the operator visible confirmation that the pelvicalyceal system has been punctured.

The second method depends on direct puncture of the pelvicalyceal system under ultrasound guidance. Third, an intravenous injection of contrast may be given and, after the pelvicalyceal system is opacified by any of these methods, access may proceed.

When the pelvicalyceal system is visible, it is punctured as previously planned, ideally through calyx and a guidewire may then be introduced through the needle into the kidney. It is recommended that every effort should be made to feed the wire into the ureter ideally as far as the bladder to prevent loss of the wire. If this is not possible, the wire is coiled within the collecting system. Some advocate the use of a second safety wire as a precaution in case the first wire is displaced. The tract is then dilated using one of a number of methods: serial dilators, the coaxial metal Alken dilators, and balloon dilatation. The latter has the advantages of speed and possibly less blood loss. However, the tapered configuration of the balloon can leave the dilated tract short of the target in certain circumstances (calyceal diverticulum, complete staghorn), and in these circumstances coaxial dilators have an advantage as they are not tapered. Typically, the tract is dilated to 30 F and access to the system is achieved by placing a 30 F Amplatz sheath over the dilator and leaving it in situ. In complex cases, a second tract may be created.

Refinements such as the mini-PCNL using smaller caliber instruments (15 F access and 12 F Nephroscopes) are proposed for smaller stones and ESWL failures.[5] Other than the potential for reduced complication rates no clear benefit of this technique has been shown. The disadvantages may include a longer operating time and the need to acquire further specialized instruments.

Instrumentation for PCNL

Rigid nephroscopes with an offset lens are standard for PCNL. These have large instrument channels allowing deployment of fragmentation probes and retrieval instruments. Flexible cystoscopes inserted via the Amplatz can also be helpful for cases such as complex staghorns with multiple calyceal extensions and may avoid the need for a second tract. A flexible ureteroscope can also be used antegradely to access calyces and the ureter via a PCNL tract.

Nephrostomy Drains Post PCNL

Leaving a nephrostomy drain post PCNL allows tamponade of the tract to minimize hemorrhagic complications and gives the possibility of facilitating a second-look procedure. Furthermore, if ureteric fragments are causing obstruction, the presence of a tube allows the surgeon to temporize and consider options. The drains are however uncomfortable and there has been interest therefore in tubeless PCNL. The nature of the case will determine if this approach is appropriate and a consequence may be a higher rate of stenting.

Contraindications to PCNL

There are few instances when PCNL may be inappropriate and most are patient related. The procedure can be lengthy and therefore fitness for anesthesia is important. In the morbidly obese, there can be problems in reaching the stone and skeletal problems can make access a challenge in spina bifida patients. Stone in a solitary kidney should not be considered a contraindication.

Complications of PCNL

Leaving aside failed access, there a number of potential complications which warrant mention. PCNL tracts can bleed significantly at the time of surgery or in the immediate postoperative period with a quoted transfusion rate of up to 6%. Acute bleeding is managed by tamponade of the tract with a nephrostomy tube. This can be supplemented by clamping the drain if bleeding persists with the intention of promoting clotting within the system. If these conservative measures fail, vascular radiological intervention with a view to embolization is the next step. Nephrectomy is rare but not unknown. Delayed bleeding (<0.5%) suggests pseudoaneurysm or development of an A–V fistula with vascular embolization being the treatment of choice. The possibility of septicemia should be considered if the patient is unwell in the immediate postoperative period.

Other tract-related complications include pleural injury with hydrothorax or pneumothorax. There is a complication rate of up to 16.3% for upper pole punctures compared to the lower pole approach at 4.5% and the rate is strikingly higher after supra 11th rib punctures at 34.6% compared to 9.7% for the supra 12th rib approach with specific intrathoracic complication rates being 23.1% and 1.4%, respectively. A chest drain will be required for most thoracic complications.[6]

Other adjacent structures may be at risk with colonic injury being the most prevalent. Fortunately, these tend to settle conservatively as the injury is retroperitoneal. The nephrostomy drain often acts as a suitable drainage tube and if there are concerns that there may be a higher than usual chance of this injury, using ultrasound at the time of puncture can be helpful in avoiding bowel. This complication is seen most frequently in thin patients and is commoner on the left side.

Retained fragments of stone can cause problems particularly if they migrate into the ureter where they can obviously cause obstruction.

Semirigid Ureteroscopy

The first retrograde endoscopic examination of the ureter using a specifically designed endoscope was described by Perez-Castro Ellendt and Martinez-Pineiro in 1982.[7]

Modern instruments have evolved with the use of fiber optics allowing finer caliber scopes with working channels to introduce fragmentation and retrieval instruments.

X-ray screening in theater is mandatory for ureteroscopy. Initial placement of a guide wire ensures safety and allows placement of a stent if difficulties ensue. These wires should always be placed under x-ray control. This ensures the wire is taking an appropriate course and if the stone is visible, checks can be made to ensure the stone is not inadvertently pushed proximally. Ideally, the wire should be placed beyond the stone into the renal pelvis. If the wire cannot be negotiated past the stone, then a hydrophilic wire may be tried or a hybrid wire with a hydrophilic tip may be used. If a hydrophilic wire is used, it is recommended that it is changed for a standard wire as soon as possible using an exchange catheter as these wires are notorious for falling out.

A number of techniques are available for negotiating the ureteric orifice with the ureteroscope. With the wire in situ, it may be relatively straightforward to access the ureter. The configuration of some ureteroscopes allows easier insertion if the ureteroscope is rotated through 180 so that the smoother beak glides over the trigone. Pushing the ureteroscope against the wire can tent the ureteric orifice open, but passage of a second wire is extremely useful if the surgeon is struggling. With one wire within the instrument channel and the other wire outside, the ureteroscope is rotated to "separate" the wires and passage is achieved by aiming for the gap between them. This technique is also invaluable to safely negotiate difficult areas with the ureter. A number of ureteric dilatation devices are available commercially, but they are used infrequently due to the narrow caliber of modern ureteroscopes. One of the major principles of ureteroscopy is that whenever resistance is noted, the safest course of action is to insert a ureteric stent and come back another day. This prevents major complications and should never be viewed as a failure. It must be remembered that some ureteroscopes are graduated with a larger caliber nearer the hilt. In a narrow ureter, it is therefore possible for there to be no problem with tightness at the tip of the scope but the proximal scope can be gripped by ureter. The ureter in this area can be concertinaed upward if the ureteroscope is advanced further with the potential for avulsion of the ureter for the unwary. If the operator feels that the scope is not moving freely, stenting is strongly advised.

Flexible Ureteroscopy

Modern flexible ureteroscopes have tip sizes of around 7–8 Fr and working channels of 3 Fr. They have active two-way deflection of a least 180° and secondary passive deflection which increases the potential for deflection further when the scope is deployed within the renal pelvis. All of the upper urinary tract is potentially reachable and a variety of flexible accessories and laser fibers are available to aid stone management.

As with all ureteroscopies, x-ray screening in theater and the use of guidewires are considered standard when using the flexible instrument. Some advocate the use of two wires, one for safety and the other as a working wire. The presence of a second wire can on occasions cause the ureter to become crowded. The introduction of the flexible scope can be a challenge, but access sheaths can be of use particularly if there is a need for repeated reinsertion of the scope. Access sheaths when deployed up to the kidney have the additional advantage of allowing flow of fluid around the scope with a resultant reduction in intrarenal pressure and a better view.[8]

When introducing the access sheath over a guidewire, it is important to position the image intensifier over the bladder in order to ensure that the access sheath does safely negotiate the ureteric orifice. If this step is omitted and the direction of the access sheath is not precise, advancing the sheath into the bladder can inadvertently cause the guidewire to flip out of the ureter. The same advice is appropriate if instead of using an access sheath, the scope is advanced into the ureter over the guidewire. This prevents the ureteroscope coiling into a loop within the bladder.

Intracorporeal Stone Fragmentation Devices

Electrohydraulic Lithotripsy (EHL)

Although largely superseded, EHL has the advantage of excellent efficacy. The shock wave is generated by discharge across a coaxial probe ranging in size from 1.4 Fr to 5 Fr. A gaseous bubble is produced by the spark which vaporizes a small volume of water.

Within the confines of the ureter, however, the EHL device is potentially dangerous as any contact with the urothelium at the time of discharge inevitably leads to ureteric perforation with a complication rate of up to 15%. EHL can similarly damage the optical system of the endoscope.

Ultrasound

Safer than EHL, ultrasound may be used both within the ureter and percutaneously within the kidney. The stone is fragmented by transmission of high-frequency vibration through a rigid metal probe. The transfer of this vibration drills into the stone. This technology has largely been superseded for use within the ureter where the heat generated was an issue, but still has a role in percutaneous surgery where it has the distinct advantage of the sheath permitting suction of small fragments.

Ballistic Lithotripsy

In many ways the safest form of intracorporeal lithotripsy, this technique involves pulses of pressurized air propelling a mobile metal pellet within the handpiece onto a solid metal rod. The probes are produced in a number of sizes including those small enough to be used with modern ureteroscopes. Although efficacious, there is the potential for propulsion of the stone further up the ureter and possible loss of stone into the kidney. There is minimal danger to the urothelium and therefore if a ureteric stone is impacted and surrounded by urothelium, ballistic devices have significant advantages. Used percutaneously, ballistic devices are efficacious and have advantages over other techniques as the fragments generated are larger and more efficiently removed from the kidney.

An alternative to the lithoclast is electrokinetic lithotripsy. The principle is similar but the electromagnet within the handpiece moves the metal bearing.

More recently, a combination instrument has been introduced with both standard ballistic lithotripsy and ultrasound. As the latter has integral suction, this device is particularly useful at PCNL for large renal stones.[9]

Laser Lithotripsy

A number of lasers have been applied to stone fragmentation but the most notable is the Holmium YAG device. With a wavelength of 2,100 nm, this pulsed dye laser fragments stones efficiently using heat. As the energy is rapidly absorbed in water, it is ideal for endourological use. The depth of penetration is of the order of 0.4 mm and although pinpoint damage to the urothelium is easily seen, with care, this device is safe. As the laser fibers are flexible, they lend themselves to use with the flexible ureteroscope and the modern prominence of flexi URS is largely due to its combination with laser technology which has opened up this technique for effective stone management within the kidney. The laser is able to break stones into tiny fragments within the system and it is entirely reasonable to avoid the uses of stone retrieval devices altogether. There is a danger of boring holes through larger stones and the technique advised is to allow the fiber to "dance" across the stone surface to avoid this. The size of fragments and relative slowness makes the holmium device less useful with PCNL, unless flexible scopes have to be deployed to deal with stones in less accessible areas.

Endoscopic Management of Ureteric Stones

The most commonly utilized intracorporeal lithotrites used with the ureteroscope are the Holmium YAG Laser and the lithoclast. Within the ureter, the holmium device (using a 365 μm fiber) has the advantage of reducing the stone to very small fragments with minimal risk of propulsion of the stone. Effectively this energy source will fragment all calculi. If there is considerable edema or mucosal growth around the CALCULUS, ballistic devices using a 0.8 mm probe may be safer. These tend to fragment the stone into larger fragments and there is a risk of retrograde propulsion of the stone. A number of equipment manufacturers market devices which can be deployed within the ureter to prevent the stone floating back into the kidney.

A variety of stone retrieval devices are available. These include an array of stone baskets and grabbers with a range of configurations such as tri-radiate forceps.

Obviously, it may be tempting to basket a stone without any attempt at fragmentation and while this may be appropriate for the smallest of stones, it should be remembered that if stone is too small to pass spontaneously, it may be too large to simply basket. Blind dormia basketing of ureteric stones *via* a cystoscope is inappropriate.

Trying to remove an unrealistic stone with a basket passed runs the potential risk of the major complication of ureteric avulsion which would require open repair. If a basket having engaged a stone becomes stuck, any thoughts of pulling hard must be resisted. The situation is easily resolved by dismantling the basket and removing the ureteroscope. The scope is then reinserted effectively using the basket as a guide wire. Any fragmentation device can then be used to conveniently fragment the stuck stone with the advantage that the basket's presence minimizes any chance of retrograde propulsion. It should be noted that although laser technology is very useful in this circumstance, the Holmium laser will damage the wires of the basket in the same way as it will damage guidewires.

If there is evidence of injury to the ureter during the course of ureteroscopy other than full avulsion then a stent can be placed over the guidewire. If there is doubt about the integrity of the ureter, then radiographic contrast can be injected via the irrigation channel of the instrument to check this. Small perforations, trauma to the urothelium, and small laser burns are easily managed by stenting without any concern for long-term sequelae.

The flexible ureteroscope is a useful addition to the endourologist's armamentarium in managing ureteric stones. An obvious indication for its use is when a ureteric stone is inadvertently allowed to migrate back into the kidney. When a stone lies within a capacious ureter, there can be difficulty in deploying the laser onto the stone with the semirigid instrument and going flexible can help. Other uses include where there has been significant prior reconstructive surgery to the urinary tract, with resulting anatomy precluding passage of the semirigid scope. Laser technology is a prerequisite for stone fragmentation when the flexible ureteroscopes is deployed using a 200 μm fiber.

Ureteric Stents

These are frequently used in a wide range of endourological procedures and are widely utilized for safety after ureteroscopy where they can be invaluable. Although mandatory after a complicated ureteroscopy, routine stenting after all interventions is not advised. Although those complications such as obstruction which may necessitate a further intervention are avoided, in a straightforward case severe postoperative complications are unusual. Stents have significant symptoms for patients with quality of life consequences[10] including frequency, urgency, hematuria, loin pain, and infection. The forgotten stent can be a disaster requiring endourological ingenuity to resolve the consequences. In addition, the presence of a stent does not facilitate ESWL in situ for ureteric stones and will not aid stone passage.[11]

Endoscopic Management of Renal Stones

When approached percutaneously, ballistic devices with probes up to 2 mm are ideal for fragmenting renal stones. As large stone fragments are generated these are efficiently removed with retrieval devices. The temptation to fragment the stones to very small fragments must be resisted. Ultrasound is also recommended particularly because of the added advantage of suction and the hybrid ballistic/ultrasound device has the advantages of both. There is little place for using lasers with the rigid nephroscope as it is not only time consuming but there is a propensity for the laser to bore holes through the stone rather than causing efficient fragmentation.

The flexible ureteroscope is a useful addition to the established techniques of PCNL and ESWL for renal calculi.[11] It is perhaps not the first choice therapy but has a role in the following scenarios.

First, for smaller renal stones which have been refractory to lithotripsy as a result of inability to target or failure to fragment. It can be indicated for larger stones where PCNL is undesirable (e.g., morbid obesity or patient fitness) or to manage multiple scattered renal stones. Clearly a very flexible fragmentation device is required. Fine (1.4 F) EHL probes are available, but the combination with laser technology has popularized flexible ureteroscopy.

Consideration should be given to injecting contrast into the pelvicalyceal system through the ureteroscope to give the operator a road map of the anatomy. There are difficulties in orientation when using the flexible instrument, but this is easily resolved by using the imagine intensifier rather than depending on the endoscopic view to move around the system systematically. The overriding principle of using the laser to fragment renal stones is to keep the instrument straight when introducing the fiber. If this safety maneuver is ignored, the damage to these delicate instruments is inevitable. The only way to be certain that the ureteroscope is straight is to use screening. This means, on occasions, deflecting the scope to locate the stone then losing position to insert the laser and then finding the stone again. The laser fiber does cause some loss of flexibility of the scope and can make fragmentation difficult. Many of these problems can be eased with small stones if they are picked up with grabbers or nitinol tipless baskets and relocated into an easier position in the renal pelvis or upper pole.

These are frequently used in a wide range of endourological procedures and are widely utilized for safety after ureteroscopy where they can be invaluable. Although mandatory after a complicated ureteroscopy, routine stenting after all interventions is not advised. Although those complications such as obstruction which may necessitate a further intervention are avoided, in a straightforward case, severe postoperative complications are unusual. Stents have significant symptoms for patients with quality of life consequences[12] including frequency, urgency, hematuria, loin pain and infection. The forgotten stent can be a disaster requiring endourological ingenuity to resolve the consequences. In addition, the presence of a stent does not facilitate ESWL in situ for ureteric stones and will not aid stone passage.[10]

Outcome of Treatment of Renal Stones

There is still a role for conservative therapy for small (0.5 cm) nonobstructing renal stones. The majority of simple renal stones less than 1.5 cm in size are appropriate for ESWL as first-line therapy with success rates for simple stones in excess of 80%.

Percutaneous surgery has a higher success rate for simple stones than ESWL, but is obviously more invasive; nevertheless, PCNL has been shown to be both effective and safe[13] with the inherent advantage of removal of a large stone burden obviating the need for the patient to pass the fragments generated by other techniques.

With flexible ureterorenoscopy, a successful outcome of over 80% can be expected rising to around 90% for repeat sessions when stones are treated with the combination of flexible ureteroscopy and laser given favorable anatomy and a modest stone burden.

The following categories of stone require endoscopic surgery: Larger stones (>2 cm), staghorn calculi, adverse anatomy (larger lower pole stones, associated pelviureteric obstruction), certain stone compositions (cystine or calcium oxalate monohydrate). To this list should be added ESWL failures and certain patient factors including where ESWL is contraindicated or not feasible (e.g., morbid obesity, bleeding diatheses).

Staghorn Calculi

Guidelines indicate that these complex stones should be treated by PCNL as ESWL monotherapy gives poor stone clearance.[13] Careful planning of the approach enhanced in the modern era by 3D CT reconstruction is helpful and multiple tracts may be required. An upper pole approach can improve the chances of stone clearance with predominantly lower pole staghorn calculi which involve parallel calyces. The increased complication rate has been discussed elsewhere. Supplementary ESWL for unreachable fragments needs to be considered with sandwich therapy (PCNL, ESWL, PCNL) and second look nephroscopy as further options. Refinements in PCNL techniques have however further reduced the role of supplementary ESWL.[13]

Lower Pole Stones

Lower pole anatomy has been thought to be relevant to the success or otherwise of ESWL for lower pole stones. Such parameters as infundibulo-pelvic angle, infundibular width and length are thought to have an influence in stone-free rates.[14]

The Lower Pole Study Group[15] reported a multicentre randomized trial of ESWL versus PCNL for lower pole stones less than 3 cm in size. It was found that overall stone-free rate was far superior for PCNL compared to lithotripsy (95% vs. 37%) and for stones greater than 1 cm the stone-free rate for ESWL was only 21%. This group analyzed the various features of lower pole anatomy, but did not find it to be of relevance in the stone-free rate after ESWL. The advent of flexible ureterorenoscopy has added a further option to the endourologist's armamentarium, but there does remain a role for primary lithotripsy stones of 1 cm or less as shown by a randomized prospective trial of ESWL versus ureteroscopy with results showing equivalent success rates.[16]

Horseshoe Kidneys and Stones

The association between horseshoe kidneys and stones is well recognized. ESWL may be unsuccessful because of failure to target the stones with the kidney lying more anteriorly than usual and there may be concern about drainage issues. Endoscopic surgery especially PCNL usually presents little difficulty although the skin to stone depth can be significantly larger than normal. CT is particularly useful in planning the approach.

Calyceal Diverticula Stones

Stones in calyceal diverticula are very unlikely to be cleared by ESWL, but there is anecdotal evidence of resolution of symptoms. A percutaneous approach requires a precise placement of the tract into the diverticulum. Although this can be a challenge, stone removal is straightforward when access is achieved. Attempts are then made to gain access via the diverticulum into the main collecting system to improve later drainage. Balloon dilatation has been proposed to accomplish this[17] and fulguration of the diverticulum has also been suggested to reduce the chances of recurrence.

The alternative is to use the flexible ureteroscope and the holmium laser. Finding the ostium to the diverticulum can be difficult but is greatly enhanced by careful screening in theater. The ostium may be incised with the laser to introduce the ureteroscope and allow treatment to the stone.

There is also a place for laparoscopic treatment and this may be useful if the parenchyma overlying the diverticulum is thin.

Stones and PUJ Obstruction

The combination of stones in an obstructive system requires careful decision making. The question which requires consideration is whether stones are secondary to congenital obstruction or the cause of the obstruction. In addition the system may be baggy rather than truly obstructed. MAG 3 renography can help in the workup and the presence of multiple small stones does suggest that the underlying problem may be one of primary obstruction. In the presence of drainage problems, ESWL is unlikely to be efficacious. Endoscopic approaches for PUJ obstruction which could be combined with endoscopic management of stone are described, such as pyelolysis and balloon dilatation. The role of laparoscopic pyeloplasty is now established as standard treatment for PUJ obstruction and can be combined with stone removal to treat both problems definitively in one procedure.

Outcome of Treatment of Ureteric Stones

Most small ureteric stones pass spontaneously.[18] In a meta-analysis of over 2,700 cases, Hubner et al.[19] confirmed that the likelihood is inversely proportional to stones size with those <4 and >6 mm passing in 38% and 1.2% of cases, respectively. These stone passage figures are lower than those from historical series and may reflect the lower threshold for intervention in the modern era. The same study reported that stone site was a significant factor too, with passage rates of 12%, 22%, and 45% in the upper, mid, and distal ureter, respectively. Where a conservative approach is considered a follow-up strategy is required. The progress of radio-opaque stones can be monitored by serial plain x-rays. Those with radiolucent stones may end up with serial noncontrast CTs in the monitoring period. Clearly, if symptoms persist prolonged conservative therapy is not appropriate. It has been shown that in 10% of cases with asymptomatic stones irreversible renal loss of function is observed with serial renography.

Medical Treatment of Ureteric Stones

Treatment of Ureteric Colic

Both nonsteroidal anti-inflammatory drugs (NSAIDs) and opioids are in common usage. Although the former class of drugs are usually the agent of first choice (e.g., diclofenac), caution is required due to possible gastrointestinal side effects and the adverse effect on renal function with long-term use or in those patients where kidney function is already impaired. NSAIDs are known to reduce ureteric contractility and have an impact on the prostaglandin pain pathway. If there are problems with potential side effects or lack of efficacy then opioids are given. In addition some advocate the use of spasmolytic agents.

Medical Expulsive Therapy (MET)

The role of medical therapy to enhance spontaneous passage has been the subject of significant interest in the past few years and it has been suggested that this practice is cost-effective over conservative therapy alone.[20,21] A number of agents have been suggested including calcium channel blockers, corticosteroids, and alpha blockers. One randomized study reported increased rates of stone passage with a combination of corticosteroid and tamsulosin than combinations of other drugs with steroids including nifedipine.[22] It seems entirely logical to consider medical expulsive therapy to aid passage of stone fragments generated by ESWL.

The most popular choice for MET in clinical use remains alpha-BLOCKADE and it is postulated that these drugs work because of the number of adrenergic receptors of the lower ureter. Patients do need to be warned about the side effects and it is important to note that this remains an off-license use for this class of drugs.

Intervention for Ureteric Stones

Absolute reasons for intervention include pyonephrosis, persistent symptoms, bilateral ureteric stones causing obstruction, and ureteric stones causing obstruction to a solitary kidney. Relative indications include failure of progression and larger stone size.

Pyonephrosis is an emergency situation and immediate drainage is required. There are advocates of emergency stenting, but this requires anesthesia and there may be concerns about the reliability of stent giving adequate decompression in all cases. Percutaneous nephrostomy drainage has the advantage of avoiding anesthetics and consequent decompression of the system can still lead to spontaneous stone passage when coaptation of the ureter is restored. As there is access to the kidney the facility is there for contrast studies in follow-up. A recent consensus report confirmed agreement in both urological and radiological circles that percutaneous drainage was preferable unless the patient had clotting problems.[23]

Regarding definitive treatment of the stone, ESWL or ureteroscopy can be theoretically applied to calculi at any site particularly with the proliferation of flexible ureteroscopy. Patient or stone factors will determine which modality is most suitable for a given stone scenario. There is no evidence that stenting a patient with a ureteric stone improves the outcome of ESWL. Previous guidelines suggest that ESWL is considered the optimal treatment for upper ureteric stones less than 1 cm in size,[18] whereas in the lower ureter, stone-free rates of ESWL and URS are equal and approach 100%.[18,24] There is no evidence that stenting a patient with a ureteric stone improves the outcome of ESWL. Overall, a recent meta-analysis showed that the stone-free rate was higher, but with a higher complication rate and longer hospital stay for URS compared to ESWL.[25] There is however undoubtedly a role for ureteroscopy when ESWL does not work after a maximum of two treatments.[26,27]

Stone size is a further issue with larger ureteric stones (>1 cm) being better treated endoscopically.[18] Flexible ureteroscopy can be invaluable in the upper ureter particularly if the ureter is dilated or tortuous. When stones are radiolucent, there is no place for ESWL unless the stone is at the very top or bottom of the ureter when ultrasound may be able to assist targeting. For giant ureteric stones there may be a role for laparoscopic surgery. The possibility of utilizing percutaneous antegrade access particularly if there upper ureteric dilatation down to a large impacted stone also warrants consideration.

Stones in Pregnancy

The combination of stone disease and pregnancy presents a challenge in both diagnosis and management. There are issues about exposure to x-rays and imaging will be with ultrasound or MRI will be required. The latter will not identify a stone but will indicate the level of any obstruction. The former will help in the detection of renal stones but may miss ureteric calculi. If present hydronephrosis will be apparent, but this may be related to the pregnancy rather than any primary urological problem. In terms of management of proven stones, ESWL is contraindicated. Ureteroscopy may be considered, but this will be without the safety of radiological screening. Temporizing measures such as nephrostomy drainage or stenting can be considered until the pregnancy reaches term. There are disadvantages with both. Percutaneous drains are uncomfortable and require a collection bag. They will need to be changed at 3-month intervals. Stents will accentuate bladder problems and will require regular changes too and therefore the need for endoscopy and anesthesia.

Morbid Obesity

Patients in this category can present challenges in both radiological diagnosis and management. Ultrasound is difficult in the obese and patients may be too large to fit on the CT scanner. In terms of treatment, ESWL may not be possible because the patient may be too heavy for the table and the depth of the stone from the skin may preclude targeting. The skin to stone distance can make a percutaneous approach impossible too or may require the use of longer instruments. A patient's obesity is less of an issue when approaching a stone endoscopically, but the patient's fitness for anesthesia and comorbidities may be an issue.

References

1. Chaussy C, Brendel W, Schmiedt E. Extracorporeally induced destruction of kidney stones by shock waves. *Lancet.* 1980;2:1265-1268

2. Krambeck A, Gettman M, Rohlinger A, et al. Diabetes mellitus and hypertension associated with shock wave lithotripsy of renal and proximal ureteral stones at 19 years of follow up. *J Urol.* 2006;175:1742-1747

3. Fernstrom I, Johanson B. Percutaneous pyelolithotomy a new extraction technique. *Scand J Urol Nephrol.* 1976;10:257-259

4. Wickham J, Kellett M. Percutaneous nephrolithotomy. *BMJ.* 1981;283:1571-1572

5. Lahme S, Bichler K, Strohmaier W, et al. Minimally invasive PCNL in patients with renal pelvic and calyceal stones. *Eur Urol.* 2001;40:619-624

6. Munver R, Delveccio F, Newman G. Critical analysis of supracostal access for percutaneous renal surgery. *J Urol.* 2001;166:1242-1246

7. Perez-Castro Ellendt E, Martinez-Pineiro JA. Ureteral and renal endoscopy a new approach. *Eur Urol.* 1982;8: 117-120

8. Rehman J, Monga M, Landman J, et al. Ureteral Access sheath: impact on flow of irrigant and intrapelvic pressure. *J Urol Abstract.* 2002;167:A291

9. Haupt G, Sabradina N, Orlovske M, et al. Endoscopic lithotripsy with a new device combining ultrasound and lithoclast. *J Endourol.* 2001;15:929-935

10. Nabi G, Cook J, N'Dow J. Outcomes of stenting after uncomplicated ureteroscopy systematic review and meta-analysis. *BMJ.* 2007;334:572

11. Fabrizio M, Behari A, Bagley D. Ureteroscopic management of intrarenal calculi. *J Urol.* 1998;159:1130-1143

12. Joshi H, Stainthorpe A, Keeley F. Indwelling ureteral stents: evaluation of quality of life to aid outcome nalysis. *J Endourol.* 2001;15:151-154

13. Preminger G, Assimos D, Lingeman J, et al. AUA guidelines on the management of staghorn calculi: diagnosis and treatment recommendations. *J Urol.* 2005;173: 1991-2000

14. Keeley F, Moussa Smith G, et al. Clearance of lower pole stones following shock wave lithotripsy; effect of the infundibulopelvic angle. *Eur Urol.* 1999;36:371-375

15. Albana D, Assimos D, Clayman R, et al. Lower pole 1 A prospective randomised trial of extracorporeal shock wave lithotripsy and percutaneous nephrostolithotomy for lower pole nephrolithiasis: initial results. *J Urol.* 2001;166:2072-2080

16. Pearle M, Lingeman J, Leveille R, et al. Prospective randomised trial comparing shock wave lithotripsy and ureteroscopy for lower pole calyceal calculi 1 cm or less. *J Urol.* 2005;173:2005-2009

17. Auge B, Munver R, Kourambas J, et al. Neoinfundibulotomy for the management of symptomatic calyceal diverticula. *J Urol.* 2002;167:1616-1620

18. Segura J, Preminger G, Assimos D, et al. Ureteric stones clinical guidelines panel. Summary report on the management of ureteral calculi. The American Urological Association. *J Urol.* 1997;158:1915-1921

19. Hubner W, Irby P, Stoller M. Natural history and current concepts for the treatment of small ureteral calculi. *Eur Urol.* 1993;24:172-176

20. Hollingsworth J, Rogers M, Kaufman S, et al. Medical therapy to facilitate urinary stone passage: a meta-analysis. *Lancet.* 2006;368:1171-1179

21. Bensalah K, Pearle M, Lotan Y. Cost effectiveness of medical expulsive therapy using alpha blockers for the treatment of distal ureteral stones. *Eur Urol.* 2008;53: 411-419

22. Dellabella M, Milanese G, Muzzonigro G. Randomised of the efficacy of tamsulosin, nifedipine and phloroglucinol in medical expulsive therapy for distal ureteral calculi. *J Urol.* 2005;175:167-172

23. Lynch M, Anson K, Patel U. Percutaneous nephrostomy and stent insertion for acute renal deobstruction. Consensus based guidance. *Br J Med Surg Urol.* 2008;1:120-125

24. Pearle M, Nadler R, Becowsky E, et al. Prospective randomised trial comparing shock wave lithotripsy and ureteroscopy for the management of distal ureteral calculi. *J Urol.* 2001;160:1255-1260

25. Nabi G, Downey P, Keeley F. Extra-corporeal shock wave lithotripsy (ESWL) versus ureteroscopic management for ureteric calculi *Cochrane Database Syst Rev.* Art No. CD0060029, doi:10.1002/14651858.CD006029.pub2

26. Grasso M, Loisides P, Beaghler M, Bagley D, et al. The case for primary endoscopic management of upper tract calculi. A critical review of 121 extracorporeal shock wave lithotripsy failures. *Urology.* 1995;45:363-371

27. Pace K, Weir M, Tariq N, Honey R. Low success rate of repeat shock wave lithotripsy for ureteral stones after failed initial treatment. *J Urol.* 2000;162:1909-1912

31

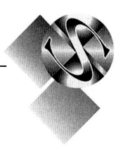

Current Concepts of Anterior Urethral Pathology: Management and Future Directions

Altaf Mangera and Christopher R. Chapple

Anatomy and Function

The male urethra is approximately 20 cm in length and is divided into four sections; the short prostatic and membranous sections form the "posterior" urethra and the longer (approximately 15 cm) bulbar and penile sections form the "anterior" urethra. Therefore, the anterior urethra represents the urethra extending from the external urethral meatus back to the distal end of the distal sphincter mechanism. Commencing at the inferior surface of the perineal membrane, the corpus spongiosum is enlarged forming a "bulb." Having pierced the perineal membrane the urethra enters this bulb and immediately changes direction almost 90° from downward to forward. The bulb narrows back to normal forming the corpus spongiosum on the ventral aspect of the penis. The urethra opens at the external urethral meatus at the tip of the glans penis. The anterior urethra has a segmental blood supply arising chiefly from the internal pudendal arteries, and venous drainage is likewise to the internal pudendal veins. Lymphatic drainage occurs to the internal iliac nodes.

The nerve supply originates from the S2–S4 level (Onuf's nucleus) and provides voluntary control of the external urethral sphincter, lying in the posterior urethra. The posterior urethra is lined by transitional epithelium and the anterior by stratified columnar epithelium. The urethra acts as a sphincter and a conduit allowing passage for urine when appropriate. Therefore, pathology affecting the urethra will have the following two consequences: obstruction to urinary flow due to stricture disease or incontinence due to sphincter deficiency. As there is no sphincter within the anterior urethra this chapter will discuss the management of stricture disease.

Pathophysiology

When dealing with abnormalities of the anterior urethra, it is firstly important to agree upon a terminology which correlates with the underlying pathophysiological abnormality. Narrowing of the urethra or urethral structuring is a consequence of ischemic spongiofibrosis occurring within the urethra.[1] Occasionally, a specific cause may be identified, although the majority are idiopathic. This is extremely important when assessing the size of any stricture. If one just relies on the area of fibrosis seen on imaging, then there is a danger of underestimating the lesion as the underlying ischemic scar may extend more widely.

Much work has gone into providing a means of identifying the extent of the urethral damage and with this in mind it has been suggested one could inject contrast media into the corpus spongiosum[2] or use ultrasound as a diagnostic modality which will identify the extent of the ischemic spongiofibrosis.[3] In fact, neither of these two techniques is widely used and many surgeons will rely upon the visual appearance of

C.R. Chapple and W.D. Steers (eds.), *Practical Urology: Essential Principles and Practice*,
DOI: 10.1007/978-1-84882-034-0_31, © Springer-Verlag London Limited 2011

the urethra based on the findings from surgery. An ischemic urethra looks white or grey, and healthy well vascularized tissue appears pink (Fig. 31.1). Ischemic strictures may also affect the posterior urethra and thus the urethral sphincter mechanism. These pose a difficult problem for surgeons due to the lack of a corpus spongiosum around this portion of the urethra, giving a lack of vascularized tissue upon which to transfer grafts, etc. There is also the foreseeable risk of causing incontinence.

The other form of stenosis of the urethra which occurs is as a consequence of urethral distraction injuries. This is when the ends of the urethra are distracted apart by blunt trauma. As a consequence, there is limited loss of urethral length making direct anastomosis easier, without the need for substitution of the urethra.[2] Distraction injuries are well known to be associated with pelvic fractures affecting the posterior urethra, although approximately 40% of these injuries will occur in the proximal extent of the anterior urethra itself, preserving the distal sphincter mechanism. Urethral distraction injuries are also associated with a fall astride injury affecting the bulbar urethra.

The remainder of this article will deal with true strictures rather than urethral distraction injuries. It is suggested that in many cases there may be a congenital abnormality called a Cop's Ring and this underlies the common finding in the short bulbar stricture in many young men where there is no preceding history.[4] Traumatic strictures are known to occur following any instrumentation of the lower urinary tract. Postinflammatory strictures are seen following genitourinary infections and in the past were even associated with materials used in some of the earlier catheters.

The other major cause of urethral stricture disease is lichen sclerosis or balanitis xerotica obliterans (BXO). First described by Stuhmer in 1928, it is of unknown etiology although it has been suggested that it might have an autoimmune basis.[5] Urethral involvement by BXO was first described by Laymon in 1951.[6] It is recognized that BXO affects a certain epithelial cell type, the stratified columnar epithelium, and therefore does not extend proximal to the urethral sphincter mechanism, transitional cell epithelium. Unfortunately the majority of strictures are idiopathic in origin.

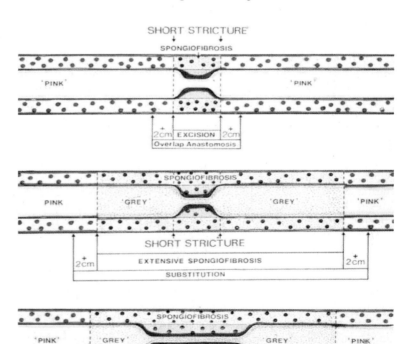

Figure 31.1. Diagrammatic representation of urethral stricture appearance at imaging compared to the actual length of ischemic spongiofibrosis in relation to the length of substitution graft required (Reprinted with permission from Mundy[1]).

Management

There are many management options available for urethral stricture disease: commencing with less invasive urethral dilatation, urethral stenting, urethrotomy and progressing to anastomotic and substitution urethroplasty. There are many techniques and procedures. Each patient must be treated based upon their individual circumstances and with due regard for consent. Below we discuss the evidence for the various options available.

Optical Urethrotomy/Dilatation

Data relating to the prevalence of urethral strictures is rather sparse, but a recent publication reported that in the USA, based on 10 public and private databases between the years 1992 and 2000, there were 5 million office visits per year and more than 5,000 inpatient admissions per year.[7] It was estimated in the year 2000 that the total cost of urethral stricture disease in the USA was $2 million and that this increased healthcare expenditure by $6,000 per insured person.

This leads on to the question as to how anterior urethral strictures are managed. Out of a nationwide survey of 1,262 urologists polled by the American Urology Association, resulting in a response rate of 34%, and from a publication by Bullock et al., 63% of urologists treat between 6 and 20 strictures per year[8] – the most common procedures being dilatation (92.8%), optical internal urethrotomy (85.6%), and endourethral stent insertion (23.4%). Universally, minimally invasive procedures were used much more commonly than urethroplasty, since 57.8% of urologists did not perform urethroplasty surgery. Only 4.2% of urologists performed buccal mucosal grafts and for a long bulbar urethral stricture or a short bulbar urethral stricture refractory to internal urethrotomy, between 20% and 29% of respondents referred to another urologist, while 31–33% continued to manage the stricture by minimally invasive means. It is of note that 74% of urologists believe that urethroplasty should only be performed after repeat failure of endoscopic methods.

It is clear that urethrotomy and dilation are standard procedures which are readily available and minimally invasive. By splitting the stricture via urethrotomy or dilatation, it is presumed healing will occur without re-stenosis.

This is dependent upon adequate vascularity within the underlying corpus spongiosum. There is no compelling evidence in the literature that any particular form of urethrotomy is more effective than another, whether using a cold knife or a laser. A randomized controlled trial reported by Steenkamp and colleagues in 1997 reviewed 210 men of whom 106 underwent dilatation and 104 urethrotomy under local anesthetic.[9] At 1 year there was a success rate of 60% if the stricture was less than 2 cm, 50% if it was between 2 and 4 cm, and 20% if it was more than 4 cm in length. Across the board at 4 years follow-up, for strictures between 2 and 4 cm in length, the success rate of each procedure was 25%. The authors concluded that longer strictures could be appropriately managed in the first instance by urethroplasty, whereas optical urethrotomy or dilatation (both of which seem to be equally effective) were always appropriate for shorter strictures.

In a subsequent publication, Heyns, working on the same dataset, looked at whether repeated dilatation or urethrotomy was useful and noted that after a single treatment, looking at the population group as a whole, 70% would be stricture-free at 3 months, 35–40% would remain stricture free at 48 months, and a secondary procedure was of limited benefit at 24 months, but not at 48 months.[10] A third treatment was of no benefit at all.

It is certainly a perception among urologists working in this area that subsequent urethroplasty is rendered more difficult and is more likely to require a substitution procedure due to lengthening of the stricture as a consequence of trauma due to repeated urethrotomy or dilatation, than if the procedure had been carried out at an earlier stage. The evidence for this is certainly compelling based on the recurrence rate of strictures where a redo procedure has proved to be necessary.[11]

Taking economic analysis into consideration, Greenwell et al. concluded that the use of urethroplasty after failure of initial urethrotomy or dilatation was likely to be the most cost-effective approach.[12] In contrast to this, Rourke and Jordan suggested that treatment of short bulbar strictures by urethroplasty is more cost-effective than urethrotomy.[13] A compromised suggestion from Wright and colleagues suggests that in their view initial urethrotomy followed by urethroplasty is the most cost-effective approach if there is recurrence of the stricture, unless the success rate of urethrotomy as treatment was less than 35%.[14]

Urethral Stents

There has been a great deal of interest in the use of both temporary and permanent stents. Temporary stents can be either absorbable or nonabsorbable, and suffer from all of the disadvantages of a foreign body in the urinary system in terms of encrustation, migration, and act as a nidus for infection. Permanent stents were introduced a number of years ago[15] but unfortunately have not stood the test of time since they have been clearly shown to be associated with complications particularly if they are inserted as management of a failed urethroplasty following a urethral distraction injury.[16,17]

Hussein and colleagues noted by looking at a series of 60 consecutive men treated with permanently implanted stents placed for recurrent bulbar stricture, with a mean age of 58 years, 35 of the 60 men had complications with 27 of them requiring reoperation.[16] The most common surgical interventions required were transurethral resection of obstructing stent hyperplasia (32%), urethral dilatation or urethrotomy for stent obstruction, recurrent stricture, and endoscopic lithalopaxy for stent encrustation or stone (17%). The authors conclude that these permanently implanted stents should only be used in patients who are unfit for, or refuse, a bulbar urethroplasty.

There may be an indication for the use of these stents in exceptional circumstances where all other modalities have proved unsuccessful, for example, in the management of difficult recalcitrant posterior urethral stenosis.[18] It must, however, be borne in mind that failure of a permanently implanted urethral stent represents a significant therapeutic challenge, which often leads to a difficult substitution procedure with consequent limitation of the success of the procedure.[17]

Current consensus in this area is that an urethrotomy or dilatation is certainly a very reasonable first-stage approach, except in the penile urethra where primary urethroplasty may be the most appropriate first line therapy. If an urethrotomy or dilatation fail, then it would seem appropriate if the patient is not keen on urethroplasty (which is suggested as the optimal alternative) to proceed on to further urethrotomy combined with intermittent self-dilatation of the urethra for at least 6 months. Stents should not be used unless there is no viable alternative and therefore should never be considered unless an expert review of the case has been undertaken. In the context of urethral distraction injury, urethrotomy and dilatation is unlikely to be successful and urethroplasty should be considered to be the primary procedure of choice.

Preoperative Assessment

In order to counsel the patient adequately it is important to have a clear anatomical assessment of the site and length of the stricture to be able to give an opinion as to what form of urethral surgery is likely to be necessary. An important aspect which is worth addressing and a question which often arises, relates to the value of the flow rate in assessing patients presenting with stricture or being followed up following stricture surgery. It is well recognized that the majority of men presenting with normal bladder function will usually have a tight stricture at the time of first presentation. Indeed, it was first described in 1968 by Smith[19] that the effective diameter of the unobstructed male urethra was in the order of the size 11F gauge and until the stricture narrowed beyond this point, there would be no significant interference with flow and hence patients would not be necessarily aware that there was a significant problem.

The current standard of care is to use a combined ascending and descending urethrogram to image the urethra. It has been suggested that ultrasonography may be useful.[20] It is our preference to rely upon urethrography supplemented with endoscopic assessment of the urinary tract with a flexible cystoscopy to decide upon the state of the urethra and the length of the stricture. Having obtained this information it is then possible to counsel the patient as to whether an anastomotic or substitution procedure is likely to be necessary.

In deciding upon the management of any stricture, it is important to consider the anatomy of the anterior urethra, bearing in mind that the bulbar urethra has a very thick ventral component and thin dorsal component, whereas in the penile urethra the corpus spongiosum is universally thin. In determining the type of urethroplasty that is appropriate, one has to consider the length of the stricture, its likely cause (in particular if BXO is present), and what previous surgery has been carried out. Traditionally, it is suggested that anastomotic urethroplasty is usually possible with a urethral stricture ranging between 1 and 3 cm in length. Above this length a substitution procedure is more likely. The etiology of a stricture has an influence on any decision since inflammatory strictures and those associated with BXO have a tendency to be longer and in the context of the latter have a tendency to recurrence because of recrudescence of the underlying disease process.

Preoperatively, one must warn the patient about the risks of the procedure mentioning; complications, failure rate, need for additional procedures, need for follow-up, and recurrence. Much is publicized about the risk of erectile dysfunction and three papers have appeared in the literature over the last decade relating to this. Coursey et al. reported in a retrospective study that in experienced hands most men who undergo anterior urethral reconstruction are no more likely to have impaired sexual function than those that undergo circumcision.[21] Clearly, alterations in the penile appearance and sexual performance may occur after anterior urethroplasty, which are usually transient and more likely if the stricture is lengthy, than if it is a short stricture requiring an anastomotic procedure. Anger and colleagues supported this view suggesting that surgery had an insignificant long-term effect on erectile dysfunction and that surgical complexity made no difference to the incidences of erectile dysfunction.[22] Erickson and colleagues (2006) confirmed these findings, both papers however suggesting clearly that there was an increasing risk of erectile dysfunction with increasing age and if there was a preceding history of problems.[23] A prospective study has recently been reported suggesting that there is a risk of erectile dysfunction within the first few months following surgery,[24] which certainly equates with our personal experience, but with time this improves and most men who develop erectile dysfunction of any sort will have full recovery by 7 months. They did note that in some men, persistence of erectile dysfunction was seen, but that long-term follow-up would be necessary before they can categorically provide advice based on this information.

Urethroplasty

The length of a urethral stricture will dictate the complexity of the necessary surgery; longer lesions require more complicated surgery. The spectrum of "urethroplasty" surgery employs the full armamentarium of plastic surgical skills. Ranging from the simplest procedure for short strictures, an anastomotic urethroplasty, where the diseased urethral segment is excised and the two ends anastomosed together; up to a substitution urethroplasty where a longer segment of urethral lumen is replaced by a graft or flap using a one- or two-stage technique. In this chapter we will give an overview of the different techniques in practice and review the evidence base relating to their use.

Anastomotic Urethroplasty

Anastomotic urethroplasty involves excision of the stricture and primary anastomosis of the urethral ends. Traditionally, strictures less than 3 cm only were considered suitable for an anastomotic procedure. However, by freeing up the urethra and separating the corpora (Fig. 31.2a) another few centimeters may be gained in length. Morey et al. when comparing anastomotic procedures carried out for a stricture length ranging from 2.6 to 5.0 cm reported success rates of 91%, as compared to a control group with a stricture length less than 2.5 cm. However, the series only had 11 patients in each group and the mean follow-up period was 22 months.[25] Two large series have recently been reported looking at the success rates of anastomotic urethroplasty – Santucci et al. (2002)[26] and Barbagli et al. (2008),[27] reporting success rates of 95% and 91%, respectively.

The procedure for anastomotic urethroplasty is detailed below: When tackling a bulbar stricture which is one of the commonest types of stricture, a midline skin incision is made in the perineum behind the scrotum. Following dissection through the superficial tissues, the bulbospongiosus muscle is exposed (Fig. 31.2b, c). Division of the bulbospongiosus muscle has been criticized recently by Barbagli et al. who describe a procedure used in 12 patients with bulbar urethral strictures where dissection of the bulbospongiosus muscle off of the corpus spongiosum was avoided, leaving the central tendon of the perineum intact.[28] The majority of surgeons do not feel that it is necessary to preserve the integrity of this muscle and there is only limited expert opinion suggesting that this approach is beneficial.

Thereafter, the next step is to dissect behind the urethra between the corpus spongiosum and the corpora cavernosa, thus freeing the urethra completely (Fig. 31.2d, e). It is important to identify the exact site of the stricture, either using a sound, or as we prefer to do this using an endoscope to precisely identify the stricture, transilluminate its distal end with the cystoscope and then put a stitch directly through at the distal extent of the stricture. By cutting just proximal to the suture which is placed in the stricture, it is possible to transect the urethra accurately without any loss of normal urethra, therefore

minimizing the potential for converting an anastomotic procedure into a substitution procedure by reducing the length of the incised urethra.

In carrying out the anastomotic procedure it is important to spatulate the urethra extending the incision into normal tissue at both ends and to fix the proximal urethra by sutures that pass through

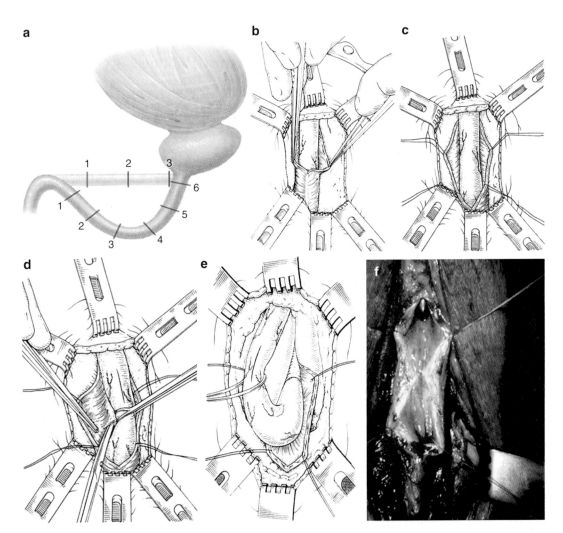

Figure 31.2. (a) Diagrammatic representation of the additional length gained by separation of the corpora cavernosa. Numbers represent approximate length in centimeters (Mundy, BJUI surgical atlas) (b, c) Midline perineal incision, through the superficial tissues exposing and dividing the bulbospongiosus muscle to expose the urethra (Reprinted from Mundy AR, *Urodynamic and Reconstructive Surgery of the Lower Urinary Tract*. Copyright Elsevier, 1993) (d, e) Completely freeing the urethra from the corpora cavernosa (Reprinted from Mundy AR, *Urodynamic and Reconstructive Surgery of the Lower Urinary Tract*. Copyright Elsevier, 1993) (f, g) Spatulating both ends of the urethra to aid anastomosis. Chapple pic, Mundy figure (g – Reprinted from Mundy AR, *Urodynamic and Reconstructive Surgery of the Lower Urinary Tract*. Copyright Elsevier, 1993) (h, i) Completion of the anastomosis, note rotation of the distal urethra by 180° (i – Reprinted from Mundy AR, *Urodynamic and Reconstructive Surgery of the Lower Urinary Tract*. Copyright Elsevier, 1993) (j) Closure of the corpora cavernosa over the bulbar urethral anastomosis (Reprinted from Mundy AR, *Urodynamic and Reconstructive Surgery of the Lower Urinary Tract*. Copyright Elsevier, 1993).

Figure 31.2. (continued)

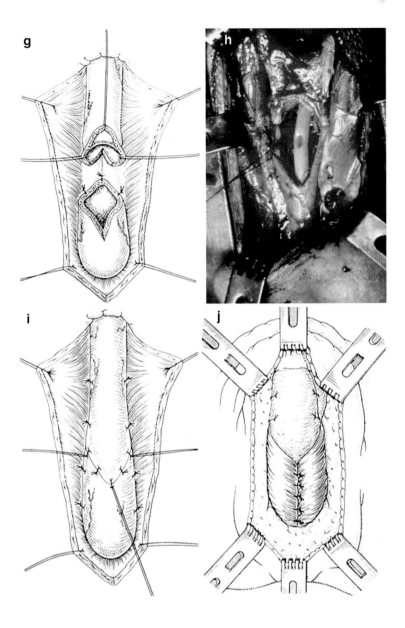

the full thickness of the corpus spongiosum into the tunica albuginea of the corpora cavernosa thereby avoiding contracture at the site of the anastomosis (Fig. 31.2f, g). We usually use a size 32 F sound to check this easily passes through the anastomosis prior to closure. It is also important to bear in mind that one can rotate the distal urethra through 180° to achieve the optimal positioning of the spatulated ends during the subsequent anastomosis (Fig. 31.2h, i).

When closing the urethra we usually use a two-layer anastomosis ventrally, the outer layer should be a running suture as this is important to secure hemostasis of the corpus spongiosum. Careful closure of subcutaneous tissue planes is important to adequately occlude dead space and prevent either hematoma formation or infection from occurring; in our experience using this approach followed by a firm supporting dressing using elasticated knickers for 4 days is important as it prevents hematoma formation. We tend to leave both a urethral and a suprapubic catheter for 12–14 days followed by a contrast study to check that the anastomosis is "watertight." This is followed by removal of the urethral catheter which is in turn followed by removal of the suprapubic catheter.

It is often possible to carry out an anastomotic urethroplasty for strictures longer than 2–3 cm. Foreshortening of the urethral course by separating the two bodies of the corpora cavernosa is an important maneuver since it will lead to straightening of the natural curve of the bulbar urethra and allow an additional 2–4 cm in length depending on local circumstances (Fig. 31.2a). Closure of the urethra can then be accomplished in a standard fashion. The corpora cavernosa can be closed over the bulbar urethral anastomosis (Fig. 31.2l). Clearly, the amount of length that can be gained will depend upon the anatomical circumstances depending on the anatomy of any individual male and this is proportional to the length and the elasticity of the distal urethral segment, and in particular the size of the penis and urethra itself. As we mentioned earlier, it is now clearly established that anastomotic urethroplasty in the bulbar urethra in experienced hands is associated with a success rate of up to 95%.[26,27]

Substitution Urethroplasty

The factors limiting the potential for using anastomotic urethroplasty are the length of the stricture and anatomical considerations. One cannot simply excise a stricture and restore continuity as in the gut, because of the potential for causing a chordee; in fact, it is a useful rule that the bulbar urethra should not be mobilized distal to the penoscrotal junction and therefore if the stricture is lengthy it may be necessary to carry out a substitution procedure. Similarly, it is very uncommon except in the context of a very limited traumatic injury of the penile urethra such as seen with penile rupture injuries to be able to carry out an anastomotic urethroplasty in the penile urethra. A substitution procedure could be either a one-stage or a two-stage procedure.

There are three potential options with a *one-stage* procedure; to excise the stricture and restore a roof strip of native urethra augmented by a patch – an *augmented anastomotic procedure*, to incise the stricture and carry out a patch substitution – a so-called *onlay substitution* procedure, or the third option that we would not recommend is to excise the stricture and put in a circumferential patch – *a tube substitution*. This latter option is associated with a high failure rate, which may be as high as 30%.[29,30] A *two-stage* procedure involves excision of the stricture and the abnormal urethra and reconstruction of a roof strip which is allowed to heal prior to second-stage tubularization.

Grafts Versus Flaps

Prior controversy existed in the field relating to whether one should use a graft or flap, but it is now clearly established from a review of the literature that the re-stenosis rate recorded in the published literature in 1998 was between 14.5% and 15.7% using either a flap or graft, respectively.[31] It can therefore be concluded that there is no advantage of a graft over a flap in terms of re-stenosis rate. Indeed Dubey in a small comparative randomized study confirmed there to be equivalence in terms of success with the two techniques but with higher morbidity for the patients using a flap procedure.[32]

In carrying out a substitution procedure, one has to also consider whether full thickness tissue or partial thickness tissue is used. The importance of this is that partial thickness tissue has a greater propensity to contract than full thickness tissue.

The number of therapeutic options which have been suggested in the past include scrotal skin,[33] extragenital skin,[34] bladder mucosa,[35] and colonic mucosa.[36] In contemporary practice, genital skin or oral mucosa are most commonly used, although there is interest in the future in the potential for tissue engineering.[37] Genital skin flaps are particularly useful when dealing with strictures in the penile urethra where an onlay flap of penile skin can be particularly helpful. However, bear in mind that the use of penile skin in this context is contraindicated if there is any suggestion that BXO is present which tends to recur in skin (either genital or extragenital in origin). Furthermore, Blandy et al. found a scrotal pull through procedure to have a high incidence of complications[38] and to his credit at the end of his career reported on the significant morbidity, in the longer term, associated with the use of scrotal skin. Scrotal skin in our view should not be used except in exceptional circumstances.

A number of different types of flap have been described over the years and these vary in terms of their orientation and whether they have bilateral or unilateral pedicles (Fig. 31.3a–d). A number of eponymous names based on the authors who reported them have been utilized to describe the contemporary flaps which are recognized. We would suggest a more pragmatic approach. When considering a flap, firstly identify an area of hairless penile skin (it is important not to allow the patient to be shaved before coming to the operating room) of adequate length to reconstruct the urethral defect. Next, based on the anatomy of the penis, decide the configuration of the flap, that is, transverse, longitudinal, oblique, etc. Next, determine how to obtain adequate subcutaneous tissue –using a bilateral or unilateral pedicle. Remember that the skin is a "passenger" on the subcutaneous tissues. Ventral onlay skin flaps are particularly useful in the management of penile strictures due to etiologies other than BXO.

When considering the bulbar urethra, the current recognized standard of care is to use a graft in the majority of cases, since the efficacy of grafts and flaps appears to be very similar.[39]

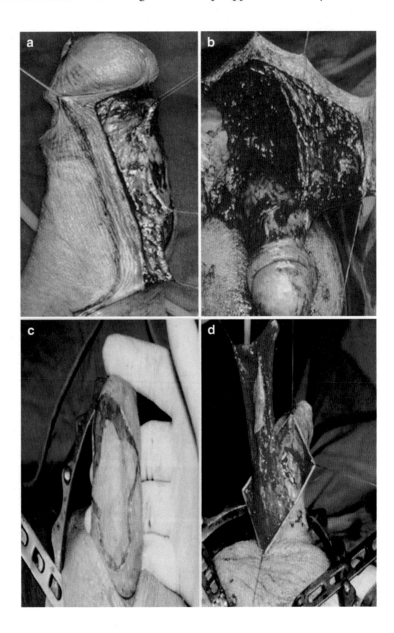

Figure 31.3. (a–d) Various flaps utilized in urethroplasty.

A randomized controlled trial carried out by Dubey, showed that the efficacy of both grafts and flaps was identical, but there was a much higher morbidity with penile skin flaps which were also technically more complex and less likely to be preferred by patients because of the morbidity.[32] Indeed it is well recognized that a number of complications can occur following flap urethroplasty including penile hematoma (Fig. 31.4a), skin necrosis (Fig. 31.4b), fistula formation (Fig. 31.4c), and if one is using a distal flap derived from the prepuce, penile and glans torsion (Fig. 31.4d). In the longer term, flaps are associated with a higher propensity to sacculation formation in the substitution (Fig. 31.4e, f).

Barbagli and colleagues have reviewed their experience using dorsal onlay skin graft

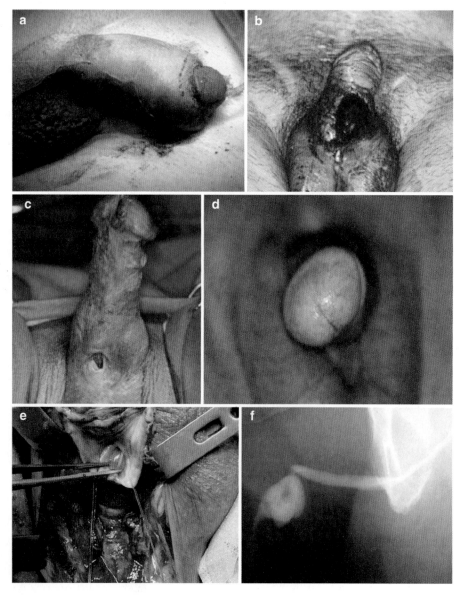

Figure 31.4. (**a–f**) Complications of flap urethroplasty. (**a**) Hematoma, (**b**) skin necrosis, (**c**) fistula, (**d**) glans torsion, (**e, f**) sacculation. (**a–d** – Courtesy of Guido Barbagli).

urethroplasty and reported a series of 38 patients where 65.8% were considered successful over a mean follow-up of 111 months.[40] It is of interest, looking at this series, that the majority of the recurrences occurred within the first year and certainly this has been our first experience[11] in the assessment of patients undergoing substitution urethroplasty who undergo objective assessment using urethrography or endoscopy and where there is no underlying progressive disease condition such as BXO. Certainly, in the longer term it is clear that the recurrence rate after a substitution procedure is far worse than many would otherwise have considered likely based on the existing literature, with a reported recurrence rate of 42% at 15 years for substitution procedures and 14% for anastomotic procedures.[41] However, it needs to be borne in mind that this study reported on a mixed population of cases at a tertiary center and represents a worst case scenario. The complexity of the underlying stricture and whether it is a first time or redo procedure, will obviously dictate the subsequent success rate. We have previously demonstrated that if one utilizes flexible cystoscopy then the majority of recurrences for straightforward strictures, (not complex BXO which has to be considered a potentially progressive disease process), are present within the first 3–6 months following surgery.[11]

Oral Mucosal Grafts

The majority of patients now undergoing substitution urethroplasty, and in particular patients with BXO, are optimally managed by an oral mucosa patch substitution. Oral mucosa was first described in 1941 by Humby[42] and was reintroduced into pediatric urology in 1992 by Berger.[43] It is simple to harvest, tough, resilient, and easy to handle. It is taken as a full thickness graft and there is usually enough of it. It picks up a blood supply very effectively and has a thick epithelium with a thin dermis with a dense subdermal vascular plexus which allows early inosculation. In the majority of cases there is acceptable morbidity at the donor site. This mucosa is used to being wet and is resilient to skin diseases such as BXO, has a privileged immunology, and is also known from preclinical work (in our own laboratory) to have fibroblast behavior which results

in less fibrosis – quite different to that seen with skin. Oral mucosa can be harvested from the cheek (buccal mucosa), from the lip (labial mucosa), or from the tongue (lingual mucosa). If an extensive amount of oral mucosa is being harvested, or the patient has a small mouth then a nasal tube should be utilized for anesthesia, but for most cases this is not essential.

In harvesting buccal mucosa, the landmark to identify is the parotid duct opposite the upper second molar tooth. The length of the oral buccal mucosa that is necessary is then identified using a skin marker; we find infiltration with 1 in 200,000 lignocaine with adrenaline helpful and the buccal mucosa can then be excised with appropriate traction, sticking close to the submucosal layer, in the plane superficial to the underlying muscle. Labial mucosa can be managed in a similar fashion, but in our experience is much thinner and more difficult to handle and associated with greater morbidity.

Clearly, with any surgical procedure, there are potential complications (intraoperative hemorrhage, postoperative infection, pain, swelling, and damage to salivary ducts have all been reported). In some cases, patients do note initial limitation of oral opening, although this is usually transient. Occasionally, there can be loss or altered sensation within the cheek. A permanent palpable scar due to formation of a fibrous band may be noticed by the patient. Particularly, when harvesting tissue from the lower lip, both numbness and deformity have been reported. A recent review of their experience by Barbagli et al. in a survey of 295 patients reported that 98.4% would undergo the surgery again and these authors concluded that harvesting from a single cheek with closure of the donor site was a safe procedure with high patient satisfaction.[44]

Recently, in patients where a greater amount of oral mucosa needs to be harvested, it has been reported that it can be harvested from the tongue (lingual mucosa).[45] The landmarks to be identified are the lingual duct and the lingual nerve. Having done this and having marked the extent of the mucosa necessary, it can be removed in a similar fashion to buccal mucosa. A comparative study of buccal and lingual mucosa is reported by Simmonato and anecdotally the resultant grafts from oral and lingual mucosa appear to be very similar in macroscopic appearance.[46] The initial results using lingual mucosa have been reproduced by others and appear to be equivalent to those seen with buccal mucosa.[46-48]

Having harvested the oral mucosa it is important to excise the excess subcutaneous tissues, and this can easily be achieved, in our experience, by tenting the oral mucosa over a finger and removing the macroscopically evident subcutaneous fat and strands of muscle.

The contemporary evidence is that closure of the donor site is by no means essential – although in our experience gentle apposition may be useful in terms of helping control any bleeding, but other techniques which help achieve this are the use of fibrin glue which can be applied locally (but is very expensive), as well as standard diathermy hemostasis. Certainly, it has been clearly demonstrated that closure of the cheek donor site appears to worsen pain and may result in perioral numbness, difficulty with mouth opening, and alterations in salivary function[49], and this has been confirmed in a randomized study.[50] It is now clearly established that it is wise to avoid harvesting oral mucosa from the lower lip because of the significantly greater long-term morbidity and consequent lower proportion of satisfied patients, due to a long lasting neuropathy of the mental nerve. Certainly with the possibility of using buccal and lingual oral mucosa, there seems little indication for harvesting tissue from the lower lip.[51]

Tissue Engineering

In the future, bioengineered buccal mucosa may be of use, particularly for complex patients where lengthy amounts of oral mucosa are necessary, but this still remains within the realms of ongoing preclinical research.[37,52] Researchers from our own laboratory are working on creating an electrospun polymer matrix capable of hosting fibroblasts and keratinocyes to mimic buccal mucosa. This tissue requires a donation of keratinocyes and fibroblasts obtained from a patient prior to surgery, via a small biopsy carried out under local anesthesia, which are cultured and attached to this matrix to create a lengthy piece of tissue. Longer culture periods allow cells to multiply and potentially generate even larger amounts of tissue. As the cells were donated from the patient, there is no allergenic response as long as the underlying matrix is immunologically inert. At present we have created tissue-engineered buccal mucosa (Fig. 31.5b), which is histologically comparable to buccal mucosa (Fig. 31.5a). The principal problems currently encountered using a biological matrix relate to a marked exudative process and an unpredictable degree of tissue contraction. Work is still continuing on limiting this.

There has been interest in the use of acellular bladder matrix with positive results being reported by El Kassaby (2008) with the proviso

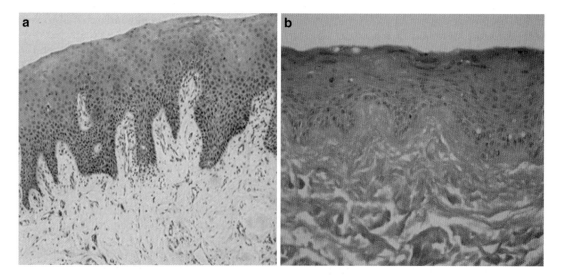

Figure 31.5. (a) Buccal mucosa and (b) tissue-engineered buccal mucosa. H&E stains ×100 magnification.

though that this is a viable option only if there is a healthy well-vascularized urethral bed with limited residual ischemic spongiofibrosis and healthy urethral mucosa at both ends.[53] Regrettably, where there is a lengthy stricture requiring substitution this is not often the case. Positive results had been reported by Fialo and colleagues using small intestinal submucosa (SIS) matrix[54] although a recent update on this suggests that with longer term follow-up the success rate might not have been as good as previously reported.[55] The use of SIS was reported by another group (Hauser et al) as being associated with a poor success rate.[56] It is our perception that any technique which requires the ingrowth of endogenous epithelial and fibroblast cells is unlikely to be applicable to lengthy strictures or strictures where there is extensive spongiofibrosis or ischemia, or a poorly vascularized graft bed, and that the direction for future research should be toward the use of cell seeded matrices.

Graft Position

A question which is often considered is in which position to place the graft. Barbagli and colleagues[57] reported the dorsal free graft urethroplasty initially using skin, but subsequently buccal mucosa (a modification of the Monseur technique).[58] Initially, this was applied in the context of an augmented anastomotic repair. Recently, there has been debate about whether to transect the urethra or not, because of concern over whether this would further damage the blood supply. In our view If there is a severely ischemic area of corpus spongiosum it is unlikely to be important whether the urethra is transected or not as the residual blood flow through that ischemic area is not likely to be significant. In our experience, the dorsal onlay approach with an anastomosis (Fig. 31.6), Mundy[59,60] provides a very effective technique which is easy to use and durable, and the majority of authors in the field[61-63] report success rates in the order of 90%, although a large retrospective analysis by Barbagli[27] suggested a success rate of 70%. Ultimately, as demonstrated previously by Andrich,[41] it is likely that the success rate will depend on the complexity of the cases operated on and the type/duration of follow-up, but a reasonable success rate to quote to patients would be in the order of 85% at 5 years.

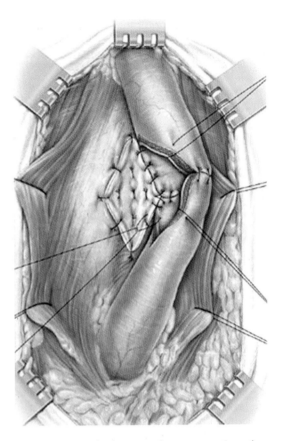

Figure 31.6. Dorsal onlay approach to anastomotic urethroplasty (Mundy, BJUI surgical atlas).

When dealing with an onlay substitution, the options are a ventral, lateral, or dorsal approach (Fig. 31.7a–c) and our preference is for a dorsal or lateral approach, which is certainly supported by Barbagli et al.[64] as the thickness of the corpus spongiosum both dorsally and laterally is far less than ventrally. Therefore, there is likely to be less bleeding from an incision in this plane and potentially less interference with blood supply as one extends into the proximal and distal "more normal" urethra. Barbagli et al. certainly reported comparable success rates of the order of 82–85% using ventral, dorsal, or lateral grafts in a small series of 50 patients. Recently, Kulkarni et al. reported a one-sided anterior dorsal approach, preserving the bulbospongiosus muscle and lateral vascular and nerve supply to the urethra, as having a success rate of 92%.[65] This was from a small series of 24 patients with a short mean follow-up of 22 months.

A review of dorsal or ventral onlay grafting has suggested comparable success rates of

Figure 31.7. (a–c) The different approaches to onlay substitution: (a) ventral, (b) lateral, (c) dorsal (Courtesy of Guido Barbagli).

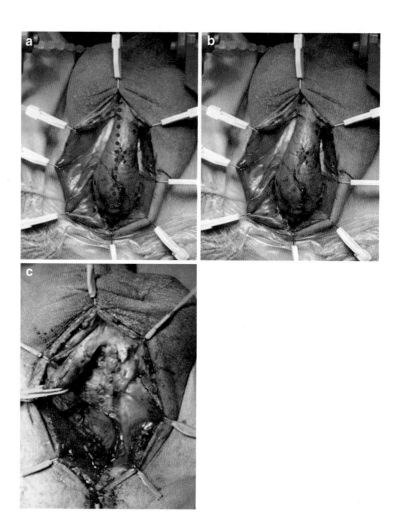

84–88% at 3 years, whichever approach is utilized for the onlay.[29] Asopa in 2001 described a ventral sagittal urethrotomy approach[66] (Fig. 31.7a), with placement of a dorsal inlay graft. This has been reported to produce good success rates, in a study where 58 men underwent treatment with a mean follow up of 42 months with a success rate of 87%.[67] More recently, Palminteri and colleagues have suggested that in addition to placement of a dorsal inlay graft via a ventral sagittal approach, a ventral onlay could be applied as well (Fig. 31.8a–e) reporting a success rate of 89% with a mean follow-up of 22 months, in 48 cases.[68]

As previously noted, one-stage tube repairs should not be used routinely, and it is clear from a review of the literature looking at two-stage procedures that the revision rate for a two-stage

procedure is of the order of 20–25%, which equates well with Greenwell's findings of a 30% failure rate with a tube urethroplasty.[30]

An important indication for a two-stage procedure is in complex retrieval situations after failed previous surgery, for example, to retrieve a situation where there has been inappropriate use of a stent in the penile urethra (Fig. 31.9).

Two-stage reconstruction should certainly be considered to be most appropriate whenever there is concern about the success of any reconstructive procedure in the penile urethra, particularly following failed hypospadic repair or in the presence of severe BXO. The major factors to consider are whether there is an adequate residual roof strip to allow a one-stage reconstruction since a full tube reconstruction

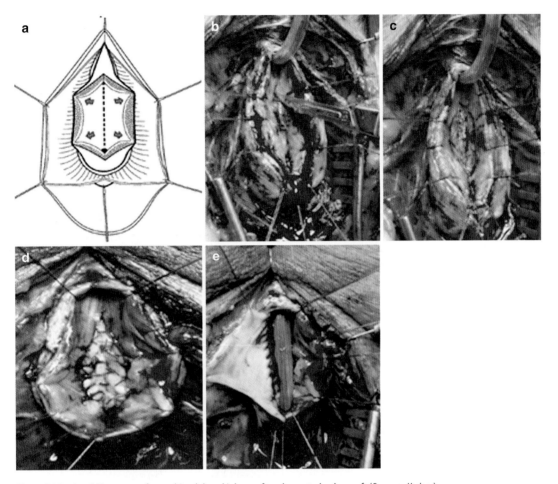

Figure 31.8. (a–e) Placement of a combined dorsal inlay graft and a ventral onlay graft (*European Urology*).

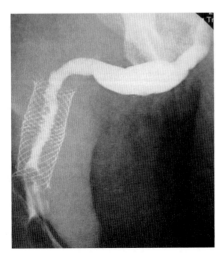

Figure 31.9. Inappropriate placement of a stent resulting in the requirement for a two-stage procedure.

has such a high failure rate and whether there is adequate subcutaneous tissue cover to prevent fistula formation. The two-stage skin reconstruction (Fig 31.10a–d) is very appropriate for the failed hypospadic patient, but clearly for BXO this is not possible and buccal mucosa must be used. There is only a small literature base relating to this[29] and in particular it must be emphasized that there is a 22.5% revision rate in the literature for a first-stage urethroplasty.[69] For one-stage closure, this would have automatically led to a failure. Clearly, with this in mind it is clear why tube substitution procedures have such a high failure rate. Furthermore, when talking about a two-stage procedure, bear in mind that the patient must be warned that the second stage can only be completed when the first stage is adequate for closure. Therefore, if there are

Figure 31.10. (a–d) Second-stage reconstruction of the urethra.

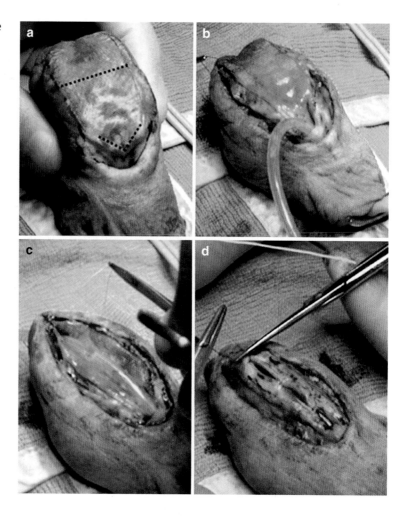

one or more revision procedures, it may in fact be a three- or more-stage procedure.

In carrying out penile surgery, the important factor to bear in mind is the tendency for cordee and use of an artificial erection is advised during the reconstruction. For a two-stage procedure using either skin or buccal mucosa, this is easily accomplished using a standard technique. It must be borne in mind, however, that there are complications following first-stage urethroplasty with 10–39% of patients showing contractual scarring of the initial graft and this requires new grafting techniques.[70] After the first-stage procedure and application of the graft, the wound is smeared with chloramphenicol jelly, dressed with a non-adherent dressing followed by gauze (Fig. 31.11a–c).

Second-stage closure requires tubularization of the first-stage procedure (Fig. 31.12b–d) and it is our practice to try and achieve a roof of 25–30 mm to provide a satisfactory substitution of the urethral lumen allowing for the inevitable contraction that occurs during subsequent healing. It is very important to achieve adequate tissue overclosure of the subsequent anastomosis, with careful attention to the underlying subcutaneous tissue to avoid linear overclosure of the skin subcutaneous tissues and urethra by offsetting the anastomotic line from the overlying skin and subcutaneous closures. If there is inadequate penile tissue then a useful technique is that of mobilizing a flap of scrotum to provide sufficient tissue cover for the urethral reconstruction.

Figure 31.11. (a–c) Application of chloramphenicol jelly, nonadherent dressing and gauze at the end of the first stage.

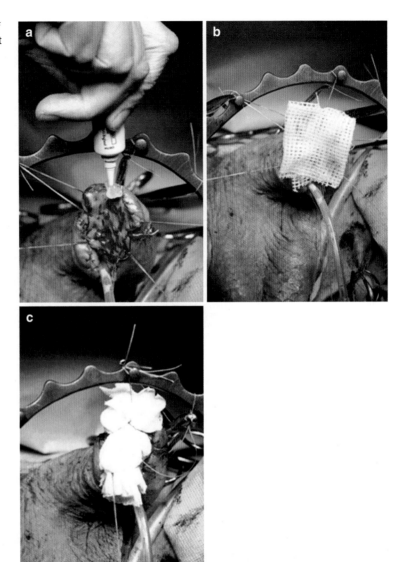

Nevertheless, complications do occur following second-stage urethroplasty with fistula formation, glans dehiscence, and meatal stenosis (Fig. 31.13a–c), all being reported and indeed 30% of patients reported complications following second-stage urethroplasties.[70]

In a follow-up of their experience, Andrich and Mundy reported particularly in BXO patients that there is a tendency to recurrence in the marsupialized segment of the urethra and consideration needs to be given to a perineal urethrostomy as a more reliable management of full length urethral strictures, particularly in the elderly patient.[71] This certainly has been our experience over the last 20 years and Palminteri and Barbagli have also reported this.[72]

Conclusion

The first operation is likely to be the most successful, and as surgeons working in this area we should always consider the simplest

Figure 31.12. (a–d) Second-stage tubularization.

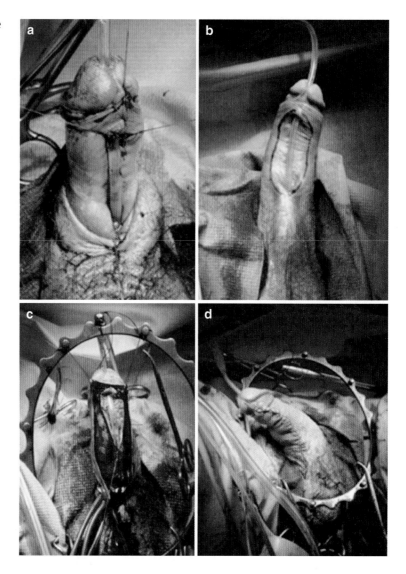

technique, which is likely to be most effective, avoiding substitution wherever possible. As a rule, for bulbar urethral strictures, an initial dilatation or urethrotomy is worth considering, but if this fails then urethroplasty should be offered and if a patient does not wish to follow this path then they should be offered urethrotomy or dilatation followed by intermittent self-dilatation for 3–6 months prior to re-evaluation of the situation. It is unlikely that intermittent self-dilatation in the long term will cure recalcitrant strictures, but will maintain a patent lumen.

If substitution is being considered, then a penile onlay flap for strictures in the urethra is appropriate. Grafts are now more commonly used than flaps for substitution urethroplasty, particularly in the bulbar urethra. Scrotal skin should not be used because of the high morbidity associated with it, now that there are viable and appropriate alternatives. There is a higher morbidity with the use of flaps than grafts, and both have similar efficacy.

433

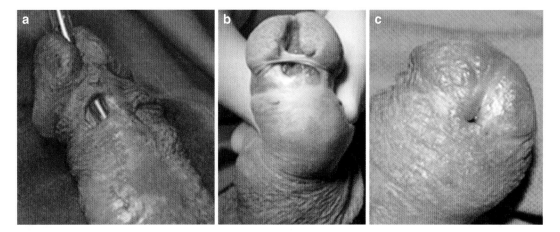

Figure 31.13. (a–c) Complications following second-stage urethroplasty: (a) fistula, (b) glans dehiscence, (c) meatal stenosis (Courtesy of Guido Barbagli).

References

1. Mundy AR. Urethral surgery. In: Warwick RT, ed. *Current Operative Surgery: Urology*. London: Bailliere Tindal; 1988:160-218
2. Chapple C, Barbagli G, Jordan G, et al. Consensus statement on urethral trauma. *BJU Int*. 2004;93:1195-1202
3. Barbagli G, Azzaro F, Menchi I, Amorosi A, Selli C. Bacteriologic, histologic and ultrasonographic findings in strictures recurring after urethrotomy. A preliminary study. *Scand J Urol Nephrol*. 1995;29:193-195
4. Donnellan SM, Costello AJ. Congenital bulbar urethral strictures occurring in three brothers. *Aust N Z J Surg*. 1996;66:423-424
5. Stuhmer A. Balanitis xerotica obliterans (post operationem) and ihre Beziehungen zur "Kraurosis glandis et praeputil penis". *Arch Dermatol Syphil*. 1928;156:613-623
6. Laymon CW, Freeman C. Relationship of Balanitis xerotica obliterans to lichen sclerosis et athrophicus. *Arch Dermatol Syphil*. 1950;42:310-313
7. Santucci RA, Joyce GF, Wise M. Male urethral stricture disease. *J Urol*. 2007;177:1667-1674
8. Bullock TL, Brandes SB. Adult anterior urethral strictures: a national practice patterns survey of board certified urologists in the United States. *J Urol*. 2007;177:685-690
9. Steenkamp JW, Heyns CF, de Kock ML. Internal urethrotomy versus dilation as treatment for male urethral strictures: a prospective, randomized comparison. *J Urol*. 1997;157:98-101
10. Heyns CF, Steenkamp JW, de Kock ML, Whitaker P. Treatment of male urethral strictures: is repeated dilation or internal urethrotomy useful? *J Urol*. 1998;160:356-358
11. Chapple CR, Goonesinghe SK, Nicholson T, and De Nunzio C. The importance of endoscopic surveillance in the follow up of patients with urethral stricture disease. *J Urol*. 25-4-2009;167(suppl 4)
12. Greenwell TJ, Castle C, Andrich DE, MacDonald JT, Nicol DL, Mundy AR. Repeat urethrotomy and dilation for the treatment of urethral stricture are neither clinically effective nor cost-effective. *J Urol*. 2004;172:275-277
13. Rourke KF, Jordan GH. Primary urethral reconstruction: the cost minimized approach to the bulbous urethral stricture. *J Urol*. 2005;173:1206-1210
14. Wright JL, Wessells H, Nathens AB, Hollingworth W. What is the most cost-effective treatment for 1 to 2-cm bulbar urethral strictures: societal approach using decision analysis. *Urology*. 2006;67:889-893
15. Milroy EJ, Chapple CR, Cooper JE, et al. A new treatment for urethral strictures. *Lancet*. 1988;1:1424-1427
16. Hussain M, Greenwell TJ, Shah J, Mundy A. Long-term results of a self-expanding wallstent in the treatment of urethral stricture. *BJU Int*. 2004;94:1037-1039
17. Chapple CR, Bhargava S. Management of the failure of a permanently implanted urethral stent – a therapeutic challenge. *Eur Urol*. 2008;54:665-670
18. Eisenberg ML, Elliott SP, McAninch JW. Preservation of lower urinary tract function in posterior urethral stenosis: selection of appropriate patients for urethral stents. *J Urol*. 2007;178:2456-2460
19. Smith JC. Urethral resistance to micturition. *Br J Urol*. 1968;40:125-156
20. Davies TO. Bulbar urethral reconstruction: does ultrasound add to preoperative planning? McCammon KA, Jordan GH, eds. *J Urol*. 2009;181(4):16
21. Coursey JW, Morey AF, McAninch JW, et al. Erectile function after anterior urethroplasty. *J Urol*. 2001;166:2273-2276

22. Anger JT, Sherman ND, Webster GD. The effect of bulbar urethroplasty on erectile function. *J Urol.* 2007;178: 1009-1011

23. Erickson BA, Wysock JS, McVary KT, Gonzalez CM. Erectile function, sexual drive, and ejaculatory function after reconstructive surgery for anterior urethral stricture disease. *BJU Int.* 2007;99:607-611

24. Erickson BA, Granieri MA, Meeks JJ, Cashy JP, Gonzalez CM. Prospective analysis of erectile dysfunction after anterior urethroplasty: incidence and recovery of function. *J Urol.* 2010;183:657-661

25. Morey AF, Kizer WS. Proximal bulbar urethroplasty via extended anastomotic approach – what are the limits? *J Urol.* 2006;175:2145-2149

26. Santucci RA, Mario LA, McAninch JW. Anastomotic urethroplasty for bulbar urethral stricture: analysis of 168 patients. *J Urol.* 2002;167:1715-1719

27. Barbagli G, Guazzoni G, Lazzeri M. One-stage bulbar urethroplasty: retrospective analysis of the results in 375 patients. *Eur Urol.* 2008;53:828-833

28. Barbagli G, de Stefani S, Annino F, de Carne C, Bianchi G. Muscle- and nerve-sparing bulbar urethroplasty: a new technique. *Eur Urol.* 2008;54:335-343

29. Patterson JM, Chapple CR. Surgical techniques in substitution urethroplasty using buccal mucosa for the treatment of anterior urethral strictures. *Eur Urol.* 2008;53: 1162-1171

30. Greenwell TJ, Venn SN, Mundy AR. Changing practice in anterior urethroplasty. *BJU Int.* 1999;83:631-635

31. Wessells H, McAninch JW. Current controversies in anterior urethral stricture repair: free-graft versus pedicled skin-flap reconstruction. *World J Urol.* 1998;16:175-180

32. Dubey D, Vijjan V, Kapoor R, et al. Dorsal onlay buccal mucosa versus penile skin flap urethroplasty for anterior urethral strictures: results from a randomized prospective trial. *J Urol.* 2007;178:2466-2469

33. Jordan GH. Scrotal and perineal flaps for anterior urethral reconstruction. *Urol Clin North Am.* 2002;29: 411-416. viii

34. Vyas PR, Roth DR, Perlmutter AD. Experience with free grafts in urethral reconstruction. *J Urol.* 1987;137:471-474

35. Kinkead TM, Borzi PA, Duffy PG, Ransley PG. Long-term followup of bladder mucosa graft for male urethral reconstruction. *J Urol.* 1994;151:1056-1058

36. Xu YM, Qiao Y, Sa YL, Zhang J, Fu Q, Song LJ. Urethral reconstruction using colonic mucosa graft for complex strictures. *J Urol.* 2009;182(3):1040-1043

37. Bhargava S, Patterson JM, Inman RD, MacNeil S, Chapple CR. Tissue-engineered buccal mucosa urethroplasty-clinical outcomes. *Eur Urol.* 2008;53:1263-1269

38. Jenkins BJ, Badenoch DF, Fowler CG, Blandy JP. Long-term results of treatment of urethral injuries in males caused by external trauma. *Br J Urol.* 1992;70:73-75

39. Dubey D, Vijjan V, Kapoor R, et al. Dorsal onlay buccal mucosa versus penile skin flap urethroplasty for anterior urethral strictures: results from a randomized prospective trial. *J Urol.* 2007;178:2466-2469

40. Barbagli G, Morgia G, Lazzeri M. Dorsal onlay skin graft bulbar urethroplasty: long-term follow-up. *Eur Urol.* 2008;53:628-633

41. Andrich DE, Dunglison N, Greenwell TJ, Mundy AR. The long-term results of urethroplasty. *J Urol.* 2003;170: 90-92

42. Humby G, Higgins T. A one-stage operation for hypospadias. *Br J Surg.* 2009;29(113):84-92

43. Burger RA, Muller SC, el-Damanhoury H, Tschakaloff A, Riedmiller H, Hohenfellner R. The buccal mucosal graft for urethral reconstruction: a preliminary report. *J Urol.* 1992;147:662-664

44. Barbagli G, Fabbri F, Romano G, De Angelis M, Lazzeri M. Evaluation of early, late complications and patient satisfaction in 300 patients who enderwent oral graft harvesting from a single cheek using a standardised technique in a referral center experience. *J Urol.* 2009; 181 (Suppl 4): Abstract 47

45. Simonato A, Gregori A, Lissiani A, et al. The tongue as an alternative donor site for graft urethroplasty: a pilot study. *J Urol.* 2006;175:589-592

46. Simonato A, Gregori A, Ambruosi C, et al. Lingual mucosal graft urethroplasty for anterior urethral reconstruction. *Eur Urol.* 2008;54:79-85

47. Das SK, Kumar A, Sharma GK, et al. Lingual mucosal graft urethroplasty for anterior urethral strictures. *Urology.* 2009;73:105-108

48. Barbagli G, De Angelis M, Romano G, Ciabatti PG, Lazzeri M. The use of lingual mucosal graft in adult anterior urethroplasty: surgical steps and short-term outcome. *Eur Urol.* 2008;54:671-676

49. Wood DN, Allen SE, Andrich DE, Greenwell TJ, Mundy AR. The morbidity of buccal mucosal graft harvest for urethroplasty and the effect of nonclosure of the graft harvest site on postoperative pain. *J Urol.* 2004;172: 580-583

50. Muruganandam K, Dubey D, Gulia AK, et al. Closure versus nonclosure of buccal mucosal graft harvest site: a prospective randomized study on post operative morbidity. *Indian J Urol.* 2009;25:72-75

51. Kamp S, Knoll T, Osman M, Hacker A, Michel MS, Alken P. Donor-site morbidity in buccal mucosa urethroplasty: lower lip or inner cheek? *BJU Int.* 2005;96:-619-623

52. Bhargava S, Chapple CR, Bullock AJ, Layton C, MacNeil S. Tissue-engineered buccal mucosa for substitution urethroplasty. *BJU Int.* 2004;93:807-811

53. el-Kassaby A, AbouShwareb T, Atala A. Randomized comparative study between buccal mucosal and acellular bladder matrix grafts in complex anterior urethral strictures. *J Urol.* 2008;179:1432-1436

54. Fiala R, Vidlar A, Vrtal R, Belej K, Student V. Porcine small intestinal submucosa graft for repair of anterior urethral strictures. *Eur Urol.* 2007;51:1702-1708

55. Fiala R. Porcine small intestinal submucosa in the treatment of anterior urethral strictures. Vidlar A, Vrtal R, Grpl K, eds. *BJU Int.* 2009;103(Suppl 4): 12-46

56. Hauser S, Bastian PJ, Fechner G, Muller SC. Small intestine submucosa in urethral stricture repair in a consecutive series. *Urology.* 2006;68:263-266

57. Barbagli G, Selli C, Tosto A, Palminteri E. Dorsal free graft urethroplasty. *J Urol.* 1996;155:123-126

58. Monseur J. Widening of the urethra using the supra-urethral layer (author's transl). *J Urol Paris*. 1980;86:439-449

59. Mundy AR. Urodynamic and reconstructive surgery of the lower urinary tract. Churchill Livingstone 1993

60. Mundy AR. BJUI surgical atlas- Anastomotic urethroplasty. 2005 *BJU Int*. 96:921-944

61. El-Kassaby AW, El-Zayat TM, Azazy S, Osman T. One-stage repair of long bulbar urethral strictures using augmented Russell dorsal strip anastomosis: outcome of 234 cases. *Eur Urol*. 2008;53:420-424

62. Abouassaly R, Angermeier KW. Augmented anastomotic urethroplasty. *J Urol*. 2007;177:2211-2215

63. Rourke K, Edmonton AB. Outcomes and complications of urethral reconstruction using dorsal onlay augmented anastomosis with buccal mucosa: is this the evolving gold standard for treatment of the long segment bulbar urethral stricture? *J Urol*. 2009 181 (suppl 4) Abstract 141

64. Barbagli G, Palminteri E, Guazzoni G, Montorsi F, Turini D, Lazzeri M. Bulbar urethroplasty using buccal mucosa grafts placed on the ventral, dorsal or lateral surface of the urethra: are results affected by the surgical technique? *J Urol*. 2005;174:955-957

65. Kulkarni S, Barbagli G, Sansalone S, Lazzeri M. One-sided anterior urethroplasty: a new dorsal onlay graft technique. *BJU Int*. 2009;104:1150-1155

66. Asopa HS, Garg M, Singhal GG, Singh L, Asopa J, Nischal A. Dorsal free graft urethroplasty for urethral stricture by ventral sagittal urethrotomy approach. *Urology*. 2001;58:657-659

67. Pisapati VL, Paturi S, Bethu S, Jada S, Chilumu R, Devraj R, Reddy B, Sriramoju V. Dorsal buccal mucosal graft urethroplasty for anterior urethral stricture by Asopa technique. *Eur Urol*. 2008;56(1):201-205

68. Palminteri E, Manzoni G, Berdondini E, et al. Combined dorsal plus ventral double buccal mucosa graft in bulbar urethral reconstruction. *Eur Urol*. 2008; 53:81-89

69. Andrich DE, Greenwell TJ, Mundy AR. The problems of penile urethroplasty with particular reference to 2-stage reconstructions. *J Urol*. 2003;170:87-89

70. Barbagli G, De AM, Palminteri E, Lazzeri M. Failed hypospadias repair presenting in adults. *Eur Urol*. 2006;49:887-894

71. Andrich DE, Mundy A. Outcome of different management options for full length antreior urethral strictures. *J Urol*. 2009;181(Suppl 4) Abstract 213

72. Peterson AC, Palminteri E, Lazzeri M, Guanzoni G, Barbagli G, Webster GD. Heroic measures may not always be justified in extensive urethral stricture due to lichen sclerosus (balanitis xerotica obliterans). *Urology*. 2004;64: 565-568

32

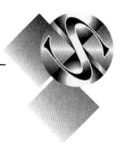

Urinary Incontinence

Priya Padmanabhan and Roger Dmochowski

Urinary incontinence (UI) or the involuntary leakage of urine is a distressing and serious health problem. Its psychosocial and economic burden leads to significant quality of life issues. The prevalence of urinary incontinence (UI) differs by type, etiology, gender, age, and distribution[1] (see Fig. 32.1). The three most common types of UI are stress urinary incontinence (SUI), urge urinary incontinence (UUI), or a combination of both, mixed urinary incontinence (MUI). The International Continence Society (ICS) defines SUI as involuntary leakage on effort or exertion, or on sneezing or coughing. UUI refers to involuntary leakage accompanied or immediately preceded by urgency. MUI is defined as a complaint of involuntary leakage associated with urgency and also with exertion, effort, sneezing, or coughing.[3] UI is a manifestation of different types of injury and disease processes of the lower urinary tract or the nervous system that regulates it.[4] This chapter describes the epidemiology, economics, and pathophysiology of incontinence. The importance of a proper work-up for accurate diagnosis is included. Conservative, pharmacological, and surgical therapy for women and men is delineated.

Epidemiology and Risk Factors

UI cannot be excluded from the discussion of chronic diseases. UI is more prevalent than hypertension, depression, and diabetes.[5-7] While UI is exceedingly prevalent, it is underreported with fewer than half of all patients willing to report their symptoms to their physicians. The incidence of UI is estimated at 2.79 per 1,000 person-years.[8] The prevalence rates are higher with advanced age. Of middle-aged and younger individuals, UI affects 4% of men and 28% of women, whereas in older individuals, UI affects 17% of men and 35% of women.[4] The EPINCONT study, containing a cohort of 27,936 Norwegian women, showed a gradual increase in prevalence until 50 years (30%); a stabilization; slight decline until 70 years; and then an increased prevalence again. Of these women, 50% had SUI, 11% had UUI, and 36% had MUI[9] (Fig. 32.2). Recently, the Boston Area Community Health (BACH) Survey identified the prevalence and

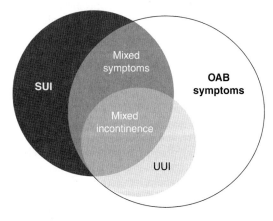

Figure 32.1. Spectrum of urinary incontinence (Reprinted from Wein[2]. Copyright 2006, with permission from Elsevier).

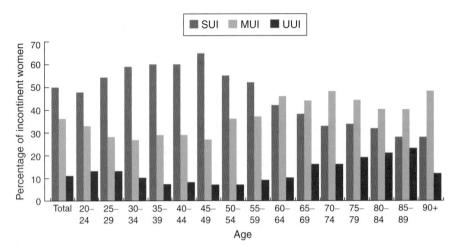

Figure 32.2. Prevalence of incontinence by subtype and age among incontinent women as reported in the EPINCONT survey.[10]

risk factors for UI in racially diverse populations.[11] The survey reported a weekly UI prevalence rate of 8%, 10.4% in women and 5.3% in men. White women were more likely than Black and Hispanic women to report UI (11.7% vs. 9.4% and 14.5%, respectively). White women also reported more SUI (35.4% vs. 9.4% and 14.5%, respectively) and UUI (13.4% vs. 3.3% and 10.8%, respectively). No variability was reported among men based on race or ethnicity.

Aging and age-related changes in bladder function play a significant role in the development of UI. There is an increased frequency of uninhibited detrusor contractions, impaired bladder contractility, abnormal detrusor relaxation, and reduction in bladder capacity.[12] This parallels an age-related increase in nocturnal urine production, increase in prostatic size in men, and urethral shortening and sphincter weakening in women. Elderly are more likely to become incontinent following incontinence-promoting factors, such as constipation, obesity, and polyuria from uncontrolled hypoglycemia, hypercalcemia, or diuretic therapy.[13-16] Other risk factors include cognitive dysfunction, functional impairment, gait abnormality, diuretic therapy, obesity, and coexisting morbidities, i.e., cerebrovascular disease, diabetes radical pelvic surgery, or autonomic neuropathy. The occurrence of cerebrovascular disease doubles the risk for UI in older women. It is clear that UI increases proportionally with a rising BMI. The effects of smoking cannot be underestimated. Smoking-related illnesses, directly or indirectly,

cause increased coughing (chronic obstructive pulmonary disease) and subsequent UI. Female gender alone remains an irreversible predisposing factor for UI. Childbearing (particularly vaginal) and parity are two of the most well-established risk factors among women for developing UI. Genital abnormalities such as hypospadias, epispadias, and ambiguous genitalia can compromise continence.[17-21]

Complications and Consequences

The impact of UI on quality of life in terms of psychosocial and economic burden cannot be understated. UI leads to embarrassment, loss of self-confidence, poor self-esteem,[12] and avoidance of social activities. Sixty percent will develop depressive symptoms. The unpredictability of UI leads to withdrawal and social isolation. Physical limitations of elderly with UI compromise functional status and hasten the progression of their immobility. Sexual relationships are affected due to a fear of involuntary urine loss during sexual intercourse. Sexual dysfunction is independently associated with incontinence in older men.[22-25]

The incidence of falls and consequent fractures increases significantly in women aged over 65 years. Twenty percent to 40% of these age women will fall within 1 year, and 10% of these falls will result in a fracture (usually hip). Thirty percent of women with UI over 65 years will be hospitalized within 1 year. Older men with UI are twice as likely to be hospitalized over a 12-month period. There is a strong association between UI, acute hospitalization, institutionalization, and death. UI is most alarmingly associated with increased mortality.[12,26]

Daily costs associated with UI are not insignificant. Protective garments and bedding are expensive and often not covered by private insurance or Medicare. The productivity of the individual and relative caregiver may be compromised in coping with the unpredictability of UI. UI is the most common cause of institutionalization of elderly with relatives unable to meet their needs. In long-term care facilities, there is an additional $5,000 burden to total health care cost per resident with UI. In 2000, the estimated direct cost of UI in the United States was $19.5 billion.[12,22,27]

Pathophysiology

Classically, the pathophysiology of UI is described as either an overactive detrusor (OAB) or an incompetent urethral sphincter. The underlying pathophysiology of OAB can relate to alterations in any of the reflex cycles in normal micturition or morphological changes in the smooth muscle, nerves, or urothelium. The three main theories for the cause of OAB are: the myogenic or muscle-related theory, neurogenic or nerve-related theory, and the autonomous bladder theory. In the myogenic theory, partial denervation of the detrusor, regardless of etiology, can alter the smooth muscle leading to increased excitability and electrical coupling between cells.[28-30] The neurogenic theory suggests that damage to central inhibitory pathways in the brain or spinal cord or sensitization of peripheral afferent terminals in the bladder can unmask primitive voiding reflexes that trigger detrusor overactivity (DO).[31] The newest of the three theories, autonomous bladder theory, notes that the detrusor is modular (i.e., circumscribed areas of muscle). During normal filling, the autonomous activity with nonmicturition contractions and phasic sensory discharge can become modified. This may lead to excessive excitatory inputs or failure of inhibiting inputs.[32] Either way, the etiology is variable in different individuals and may include one or more of

these theories. In summary, there is damage to afferent or efferent pathways, leading to decreased capacity for increased afferent information, decreased suprapontine inhibition, and increased sensitivity to contraction-mediated transmitters.[33,34]

The micturition reflexes involve several neurotransmitters and transmitter systems which may be targets for drugs aimed at micturition control. Glutamate likely acts as an excitatory transmitter in the supraspinal control circuitry and in the efferent limb of the pontine micturition center and the preganglionic neuron. Other substances, such as GABA, serotonin, dopamine, and norepinephrine, can exert modulatory effects on the glutamatergic mechanisms controlling micturition, and the receptors for these substances may be potential sites for drug intervention. GABA may act as an inhibitory neurotransmitter in the brain and depress excitatory (diencephalon) or inhibitory (mesencephalon and telencephalon) mechanisms for micturition control. The serotonergic input from the raphe nucleus and multiple serotonin 5-HT receptors at afferent and efferent impulse processing sites causes inhibition of bladder contractions. Thus, drugs interfering with serotonin reuptake (i.e., serotonin reuptake inhibitors) may have the opposite effect. Central dopaminergic and noradrenergic pathways may have excitatory and inhibitory effects on bladder function, yet drugs selectively acting at the dopaminergic and adrenoreceptors have not been established.[35]

SUI results from bladder neck/urethral hypermobility and/or neuromuscular defects, i.e., intrinsic sphincter deficiency. This occurs when the intra-abdominal pressure exceeds urethral resistance. Among women, these changes occur due to weak collagen, advanced age, pregnancy, obesity, advanced pelvic prolapse, and chronic obstructive airway disease.[4,36] In men, SUI is due to an iatrogenic cause. A radical prostatectomy can injure the sphincteric mechanism (rhabdosphincter) or cause bladder dysfunction. Suggested mechanisms for sphincteric injury following a radical prostatectomy include: ischemia and immobilization by scar, atrophy, direct pudendal nerve injury, or shortening of urethra below a critical functional length.[37]

Controversy surrounds urethral length as a cause of incontinence. Technical modifications have been made to preserve as much external sphincter as possible following a radical prostatectomy.[38] During a TURP, the verumontanum marks the proximal part of the rhabdosphincter. Resection distal to the verumontanum can lead to sphincteric incompetence. Sphincteric denervation can also occur following other radical pelvic procedures, i.e., abdominoperineal resection, pelvic radiation.

Among postprostatectomy incontinence (PPI) patients, 60% experience detrusor overactivity. The bladder dysfunction leading to UUI must be addressed prior to discussing surgical treatment of SUI.[39] Groutz et al. used urodynamic and clinical evidence to report on 83 men with PPI. Intrinsic sphincter dysfunction was the most common videourodynamic finding and cause of incontinence in 73 (88%) men. Bladder overactivity was the main cause of incontinence among 6 (7.2%) men. Overflow incontinence secondary to a bladder neck contracture was a significant cause of intrinsic sphincter deficiency in 25 (30.1%) patients.[40]

Clinical Assessment of Incontinent Patient

Incontinence can cause tremendous suffering. Hence, it should be assessed thoroughly and treated appropriately. A full and thorough history and physical exam is an important first step in directing appropriate investigations. Providers should examine fluid intake, assess volume of urine lost, number and type of pads used, strength of urinary stream, stress maneuvers or changes in posture associated with urine loss, and if urgency is associated with leakage. Additional information should be collected regarding risk factors and predisposing factors. Medication history, including diuretics or hyperosmolar infusions, anticholinergics, narcotics, sedatives, and hypnotics, is important to document. These may be associated with functional incontinence, especially among the elderly.[12] Physical examination should include a complete neurologic, abdominal, urogenital, pelvic, and rectal examination. Female pelvic exam should make note of urethral pathology, urethral hypermobility, prolapse, and apical support. Anal bulbocavernosus reflexes should be assessed. Urethral sphincteric response to cough or Valsalva should be documented. The basic

assessment should include a urinalysis (urine culture as needed) to exclude infection, hematuria or glucosuria, measurement of postvoid residual to identify possible bladder dysfunction or obstruction, and a quality of life (QoL) questionnaire[34] for assessment of patient-reported outcomes (PRO).

PROs are the best measure of patient health status as directly reported by the patient. They assess outcomes of health-related quality of life (HRQL), symptoms, patient satisfaction, and social, emotional, and physical functioning. The value of these outcomes relies on the validity and reliability of the survey tools being used. PROs require linguistic validation and psychometric evaluation of multiple language versions of a questionnaire. Psychometric characteristics include: internal consistency, reliability, construct validity, and responsiveness. There are multiple International Continence Society (ICS)–validated assessments which are actively utilized for incontinence in men and women, such as the ICS Male Questionnaire, Urogenital Distress Index (UDI-6), or International Consultation on Incontinence Questionnaire (ICIQ). For example, the overactive bladder questionnaire (OAB-q) is a 33-item, self-administered, disease-specific questionnaire to assess symptom bother and HRQL in patients with OAB. This questionnaire was recently validated and shown to have acceptable psychometric characteristics in multiple languages (Danish, German, Polish, Sweden, and Turkish).[41]

Patient-completed voiding diaries are an integral measurement tool for those presenting with complaints of incontinence associated with urgency. Patients are given standard instructions to record micturition events (± voided volumes) and incontinence episodes, while also recording whether the void or leakage episode is associated with a sense of urgency. Brown et al. examined the test-retest reliability and validity of 7-day voiding diaries in the assessment of OAB symptoms. The diary demonstrated excellent reliability with respect to the symptoms of "strong urge," diurnal and nocturnal micturitions, total incontinence, and urgency incontinence episodes.[42] Short voiding diaries have been shown to be just as reliable and valid as traditional 7-day diaries and are less burdensome to patients.[43,44]

Urodynamic studies are not mandatory, but are crucial when a diagnosis is unclear, in considering surgical intervention or in unchanged or worsened incontinence following treatment. They are useful in providing insight into bladder pathophysiology. Urodynamics are strongly encouraged before proceeding with an invasive therapy. In patients with SUI, Valsalva leak point pressure (VLPP) is utilized. This is usually assessed with bladder volumes greater than 150 mL, and repeated every 50 mL until the maximum cystometric capacity is reached.

A methodology for performing VLPP has not been standardized. There can be discrepancies in pressure measurements due to catheter size, patient position, bladder volume, and stress maneuvers.[45] Some feel that VLPP is a measure of the severity of incontinence and can differentiate ISD from urethral hypermobility.[46] In a study of 424 women, no association was found between VLPP and a Q-tip test to assess urethral hypermobility.[47] A majority of men with PPI suffer from ISD, but only 25–50% will have ISD alone on urodynamics.[48] Urodynamics are essential in these cases to identify detrusor overactivity, poor compliance, or bladder dysfunction prior to planning surgery.

There are conflicting opinions on use of preoperative urodynamics in patients with MUI. There is a wide range of variability in bladder sensation of a patient with urgency observed during urodynamic investigation. For example, some patients with detrusor overactivity (DO) demonstrate high-pressure contractions with very little sensation, while others have debilitating urgency with minimal rise in detrusor pressure.[41] In the Stress Incontinence Surgical Treatment Efficacy Trial, including 655 women randomized to either a Burch suspension or autologous sling, there was no difference in outcomes between those with or without detrusor overactivity.[49] Yet, in a series of 144 women with symptomatic MUI undergoing tension-free vaginal tape (TVT), transobturator tape (TOT), or suprapubic arc (SPARC), DO was associated with a three- to fourfold increase in treatment failure.[50]

Urge Incontinence

The International Continence Society (ICS) defines overactive bladder (OAB) as urgency, with or without UUI, usually associated with frequency and nocturia.[3] Treatment of OAB is based on diagnosis after excluding other pathologies, i.e., urinary tract infection, bladder stone, diabetes. Options include conservative management, pharmacotherapy, and invasive/surgical measures. The principles of treatment are to increase voided volumes (thereby reducing frequency and nocturia), decrease urgency, and reduce UUI episodes.[34]

Conservative Treatments

A combination of lifestyle interventions, pelvic floor muscle exercises (Kegel exercises), and bladder training are the initial management options for OAB sufferers. Lifestyle interventions include reduction of fluid intake, avoiding fluid intake prior to bedtime, emptying bladder before leaving home and prior to bedtime, tobacco cessation, weight loss, and caffeine avoidance. Bladder training and pelvic floor muscle exercises are usually complementary. Bladder training aims to regain bladder control by suppressing involuntary detrusor contractions through negative feedback. This in turn increases voided volumes and time interval between voids, which improves voiding pattern. Patients are taught to tighten their pelvic floor during an involuntary contraction and when going from a lying down to sitting or sitting to standing position.[34,51]

Pharmacotherapy

Stimulation of muscarinic receptors in the bladder by acetylcholine leads to the contraction of the detrusor muscle. Therefore, anticholinergic (antimuscarinic) drugs are the pharmacologic choice for OAB. These drugs were believed to act primarily on parasympathetic efferents to the bladder, but there is increasing evidence that there are also important afferent pathways.[52] Additional focus is on sacral reflexes that potentiate detrusor activity. This may help patients with nocturia, many of whom have been largely unresponsive to the mostly efferent changes associated with anticholinergic agents. A major goal with pharmacotherapy is to minimize the side effects associated with anticholinergics in order to avoid the historic, seemingly insoluble problem of noncompliance. New transdermal delivery systems based on patch therapy and depot platforms are being developed and have the major advantage of being long-acting. The transdermal system bypasses first-pass metabolism in the liver and gut, reducing the amount of the metabolite N-desethyloxybutynin (oxybutynin metabolite) in the blood. In 2004, the USA Food and Drug Administration approved four new drugs for the treatment of OAB in men and women: darifenacin, solifenacin, tolterodine, and trospium.

The interaction of widely dispersed muscarinic receptors is poorly understood. The M_1 receptors in the brain and salivary glands have a role in the cognition and production of mucous saliva. The M_2 receptors in the cardiovascular system are involved in heart rate and cardiac output and the M_5 receptors in the eye influence ciliary muscle contraction. The binding of some or all of the antimuscarinics listed with these different receptors leads to the side-effect profile: cognitive impairment, tachycardia, dry mouth, or blurred vision. The classic drug oxybutynin has a high affinity for the M_1 and M_3 receptor subtypes. Darifenacin and solifenacin both are M_3-selective antagonists, with selectivity for the bladder over the salivary glands, thus reducing the characteristic dry mouth seen with oxybutynin. Tolterodine is a specific and potent competitive antagonist of muscarinic receptors, but has no significant selectivity for receptor subtypes. Trospium chloride is a quaternary ammonium compound which does not cross the blood-brain barrier, ideally preventing cognitive effects[4] associated with antimuscarinics.

The Overactive Bladder: Performance of Extended Release Agents (OPERA) Study[53] compared the efficacy and tolerability of extended-release oxybutynin (OER) and extended-release tolterodine (TER). OER was found to be superior in reduction of micturition frequency, while TER was associated with a lower rate of dry mouth. The Solifenacin and Tolterodine as an Active comparator in a Randomized Trial (STAR) Study[54] was a prospective, double-blind, two-arm study comparing the safety and efficacy of solifenacin and TER. There was no difference in reduction in mean number of micturition episodes per 24 h, yet solifenacin was more effective in decreasing daily episodes of urgency, UUI, and incontinence. Haab et al.[55] reported on data from the European trial of darifenacin with 561 patients randomized to once-daily controlled-release darifenacin tablets or placebo. At 12 weeks,

there were significant reductions at 7.5 mg (67.7%) and 15 mg (72.8%) compared to placebo (55.9%) in UUI episodes per week, voiding frequency, urgency, and number of UUI episodes leading to a change in clothing.

Recent interest has focused on resiniferatoxin, a naturally occurring capsaicin-like agent derived from the plant *Euphorbia resinifera*. Capsaicin is a potent neurotoxin that desensitizes the bladder's afferent C-fibers when instilled intravesically. Resiniferatoxin is 1,000 times more potent than capsaicin.[56] In neurologically intact patients, reflex voiding is initiated normally via capsaicin-resistant myelinated A-δ bladder afferent fibers,[57] while in spinal cord injuries, voiding involves stimulation of unmyelinated C-fiber afferents, which are sensitive to neurotoxin.[58,59] Fowler et al.[60] found that intravesical capsaicin caused symptomatic and urodynamic improvement in 60–100% of patients with detrusor hyperreflexia and intractable UUI, lasting up to 1–9 months. No systemic toxic effects were seen. There was a temporary neuronal excitation phase of the primary afferent neurons (temporary acute pain and bladder hyperactivity) following initial capsaicin instillation. Resiniferatoxin is not associated with this initial excitation. In 20 neurologically impaired patients with detrusor hyperreflexia, sequentially increasing intravesical doses of resiniferatoxin were given. Bladder capacity increased and UUI improved in 8 of 13 patients. Bladder discomfort was well tolerated.[61]

Invasive/ Surgical Therapies

Botulinum toxin (BTX) is a potent neurotoxin that inhibits acetylcholine release at the presynaptic cholinergic junction, inducing detrusor muscle relaxation and potentially affecting afferent sensory receptors in the urothelium.[62] Recent evidence supports additional action of BTX on neurotransmitters other than acetylcholine as cause of sensory effects. BTX-A (serotype A toxin) was first investigated 20 years ago for urological indications, i.e., treating detrusor external sphincter dyssynergia following spinal cord injury. Use of BTX-A for neurogenic detrusor overactivity was first described in 1999. All studies to date demonstrating idiopathic detrusor overactivity showed improvement in urodynamic parameters and symptoms with BTX. There were symptomatic improvements in urinary frequency, voided volume, UUI, number of leakage episodes, pad usage, bladder capacity, and quality of life. Literature supports the efficacy of Botox at doses of 10 U per injection site (total of 100–300 U). Procedure-related UTI are the most common side effects. The lowest mean duration of effect for Botox in patients with neurogenic detrusor overactivity was 5.3 months. Duration is typically ≥6 months. Up to 16% of patients with idiopathic detrusor overactivity may need clean intermittent catheterization for several weeks after BTX treatment.[63] In a multi-institutional, randomized, double-blind, placebo-controlled clinical trial comparing 200 U intra-detrusor BTX-A and placebo in women with refractory idiopathic UUI, 60% who received BTX-A had a clinical response. BTX-A was effective and durable, yet 43% experienced a transient increase in postvoid residual.[64]

Sacral nerve stimulation (SNS) or neuromodulation has been approved by the FDA for the treatment of UUI since 1997. The mechanism of action remains unclear, yet numerous studies note long-term success and safety. SNS is usually performed in two stages: first a temporary or permanent external lead is placed into the S3 foramen for external stimulation; and second a subcutaneous impulse pulse generator is implanted. A prospective, multicenter 5-year trial of 163 patients (87% female) was performed to assess the efficacy and safety of SNS. They reported a significant decrease in mean leaking episodes per day (9.6 ± 6 to 3.9 ± 4) and no life-threatening or irreversible adverse events occurred.[65] Sutherland et al. reported on 11 years of experience with SNS performed in 103 patients (87% female). Statistical significant improvement post implantation was noted in leaks per 24 h and pads per 24 h. There was 60.5% improvement based on quality of life.[66]

Central sacral neuromodulation has been successful in treatment of urgency and urge incontinence, yet a significant drawback is that placement of the stimulator is invasive, there is moderate complication rate, and up to 50% require reoperation. Thus, various approaches to minimally invasive, peripheral transcutaneous nerve stimulation (PTNS) have been tested, including stimulation of the posterior tibial nerve and pudendal (dorsal penile/ clitoral) nerves. PTNS like SNS requires a cooperative patient with a morphologically intact urinary tract, normal sacral spinal reflex center, limited degree of peripheral denervation of the pelvic floor striated musculature and the ability to void spontaneously or with self-catheterization (without electrical stimulation). Patient may have transient discomfort at initial skin puncture site, but there is little pain with needle advancement or delayed pain. Initial results of posterior tibial nerve stimulation in 22 patients with primarily urgency and UUI revealed 80% with at least a 75% reduction in incontinence and 45% to be completely dry.

Stress Urinary Incontinence

The International Continence Society (ICS) defines SUI as the complaint of involuntary leakage on effort or exertion, or on sneezing or coughing[3] Unlike men who develop SUI following an iatrogenic cause, SUI in women is an indolent process and may take much longer to present for management.

Male SUI Therapies

Following prostate surgery or radiation, men are encouraged to attempt active conservative management with fluid restriction, medication management (for urgency and UUI related symptoms), and pelvic floor exercises. Parekh et al. reported on pre-op pelvic floor exercises aiding in earlier achievement of urinary continence, yet prolonged conservative management has questionable merit.[67,68] Periurethral bulking agents are a minimally invasive treatment option for male SUI, but have extremely low cure rates, 5–8%.[69-71] Surgical intervention is indicated for treating male SUI that is persistently bothersome despite 12 months of active conservative management. The severity of incontinence and magnitude of the effect on the patient's quality of life is balanced against the risks of surgery. The male sling and artificial urinary sphincter (AUS) are the two most common surgical procedures for the management of PPI. This choice is based on the severity of leakage, comfort with implantation and manipulation of an artificial device, patient physical limitations, and need for continuous intermittent catheterization. There are no prospective, randomized comparisons between these two modalities, yet both techniques have been studied and reported on extensively.[72]

The AUS was first introduced in 1973 and has undergone numerous redesigns to the present date. It circumferentially occludes the urethra (usually bulbar urethra) with continuous compression, controlled by an intra-abdominal pressure regulating balloon (IPG) (with 22 cm^3 of normo-osmotic mixture at 61–70 cm water pressure). During voiding, activation of a scrotal pump diverts the compressive fluid from the cuff to the balloon reservoir, relieving the occlusive effects of the cuff on the urethra. Primary and double-cuff techniques have been utilized, though double cuffs are associated with a higher rate of erosion. Historically abdominal and perineal incisions are made for placement of the IPG, cuff, and pump. There has also been success with single scrotal incision approach for placement of all three parts.[73-77] In cases of an AUS revision for urethral atrophy or erosion, a transcorporeal approach may be used. With the introduction of the narrow back cuff in 1987, the success rates for the AUS are upwards of 90% in modern series for all levels of incontinence. The largest series to date, from the Mayo Clinic, included 323 patients with a mean follow-up of 6 years and reported a 90% success rate. Their revision rate was 17% with a narrow back cuff.[78] Infection and urethral erosion are often related and range from 0% to 25% when reported as a single entity. When reported separately, infection rates with initial AUS surgery is 0–3%, and as high as 10% in patients who underwent radiation therapy or in cases of repeat AUS surgery. Revision rates are approximately 8% and 9% for nonmechanical and mechanical failure and 15–25% for recurrent ISD (from urethral atrophy) at 5 years with the narrow-backed cuff.[72,78]

The male sling was devised in response to the risks of infection and urethral erosion associated with the AUS, and to allow for voiding without device manipulation. The modern male sling has gone through many versions prior to the commonly used transperineal bone-anchored, minimally invasive approach. Six titanium bone screws suspend a piece of silicone-coated polyester mesh to the medial aspect of either descending ramus, creating approximately 60 cm of water compression on the urethra. Two large prospective studies reported success rates of 70–80%. In the first, with a median follow-up of 48 months, symptom score and pad use were significantly improved.[79] Two-thirds were made pad free and 80% were cured

or much improved. Rajpurkar et al. reported satisfaction rates of 70% and 74% improvement in leakage at a median of 24 months.[80] There are no reported cases of prolonged urinary retention or new onset UUI in the literature following a male sling.[70] The infection and erosion rates, 2.1% and 4.2% respectively,[79] are much lower than seen following AUS placement. There is limited published information on a new transobturator male sling. Thus far, reported data indicates a 40% success rate 6 weeks post-op.[81]

The AUS and male sling are both contraindicated for patients requiring transurethral surgery, due to higher risk of erosion and infection. Unlike the AUS, a patient's pre-op detrusor contractility must be considered prior to male sling surgery. Detrusor hypocontractility is a contraindication for the male sling due to the risk of increased outlet resistance leading to upper urinary tract damage. In patients with detrusor hypocontractility, AUS implantation is recommended. In patients with previous AUS or male sling surgery, primary radiation therapy, or severe or total incontinence, the AUS is preferred. The male sling is preferred in patients with poor manual dexterity or insufficient mental faculties to cycle AUS, those patients wanting to spontaneously void without manipulation, and those requiring intermittent catheterization. The male sling is better selected in those patients with mild SUI and good detrusor contractility due to a lower infection and revision rate.[72]

Female SUI Therapies

Patients and physicians can choose between conservative, nonsurgical, pharmacological, and surgical treatment options for female SUI. Conservative therapy is the first-line therapy, especially when the SUI is less severe. Lifestyle modifications such as weight loss, smoking cessation, and fluid intake adjustments are often initially recommended as early measures. Many patients make these changes in order to cope with their condition.[82] In addition, patients are encouraged to perform timed voiding, prompted voiding or bladder training, Kegel exercises, and maintain a voiding diary. These measures ideally help increase effective bladder capacity. Voiding logs are essential in understanding the patient's fluid intake in relationship to their output and the voiding interval. The log therefore can act as a reminder to void (timed voiding) and also provide a schedule to increase their voiding interval. Fantl et al. reported a 57% reduction in incontinence episodes and a 54% reduction in quantity of urine loss in older women attempting conservative measures, which was similar in patients with UUI and SUI.[83] Pelvic floor muscle training (PFMT) incorporates repeated high-intensity, pelvic muscle contractions of both slow- and fast-twitch muscle fibers. PFMT is believed to strengthen the pelvic floor muscles (PFM), particularly the levator ani, and enhance the ability to produce an increase in urethral resistance. Combination therapies involving PFMT and adjuncts, such as vaginal cones, biofeedback, and electrical stimulation, do not have additional benefit, except to assist a woman to learn how to perform a correct PFM contraction.[82,83] A multicenter trial of behavioral measures, PFMT, and combination therapy was conducted in 204 women over 3 months. The combination arm reported significantly fewer incontinence episodes, better quality of life, and greater treatment satisfaction. Yet, 3 months after completion of the trial, there were no differences noted. This confirms the importance of patient compliance and reinforcement in achievement of success.[84] Compliance is in fact the main drawback of conservative therapy.

Nonsurgical, occlusive, or supportive devices are utilized in a group of women for management of SUI. There are some comfort issues related to size, suppleness of device, and patient willingness to manipulate their genitals to utilize these devices. Additionally, a number of the occlusive devices are single or disposable products, making cost substantial. Sexual activity may be affected if the device needs to be removed before or after coitus, resulting in inconvenience and coital incontinence. Extra-urethral, intraurethral and intravaginal (pessaries) supportive devices have been used. The extra-urethral device (Miniguard®, FemAssist®, or CapSure™) must be removed prior to voiding. While subjective and objective (pad test) outcomes have shown slight improvement, there is associated transient vulvar and lower urinary tract irritation, vaginal irritation, and urinary tract infections. Single-use, disposable intraurethral devices (FemSoft®) are inserted directly into the urethra, obstructing the flow of urine into the proximal urethra. They must be removed prior

to urination. There is a meatal plate to prevent migration of the device into the bladder and a string to enhance removal. Adverse effects include hematuria, UTIs, and discomfort.[83,85] Pessaries or intravaginal support devices are often used for symptomatic prolapse, but may be used to treat SUI, especially in those patients with mild to moderate anterior vaginal wall prolapse, associated with hypermobility. Pessaries act by mechanically supporting the bladder neck.[83]

There is no globally used or widely successful pharmacological treatment available for SUI, due to the large variability in success rates and significant adverse effects. Pharmacologic therapy has included: α-adrenergic agonists, imipramine, duloxetine, ß-adrenergic agonists and antagonists, and hormonal therapy. The bladder neck and urethra contain a large number of α-adrenergic receptors that induce muscle contraction and increase outlet resistance. Multiple α-adrenergic agonists (phenylpropanolamine) have been tested with poor cure rates (0–14%) and side effects ranging from 5% to 33%.[86] Caution must be utilized in patients with hypertension, cardiovascular disease, or hyperthyroidism. Phenylpropanolamine was withdrawn from market after an increased risk of hemorrhagic stroke was documented. TCA antidepressants have central and peripheral anticholinergic effects at some sites, block the active transport in presynaptic nerve endings preventing reuptake of norepinephrine and serotonin, and act as a sedative. Imipramine theoretically decreases bladder contractility and increases outlet resistance.[83] In an open label study of imipramine, a 35% cure rate by pad test and additional 25% subjective improvement was reported.[87] TCAs are associated with dry mouth, constipation, retention, orthostatic hypotension, and falls.[33]

Duloxetine was the first widely available pharmacological treatment option licensed for the treatment of SUI. Duloxetine is a combined serotonin and norepinephrine reuptake inhibitor, with no affinity for neurotransmitter receptors. Duloxetine increases the concentration of both serotonin and noradrenaline in the synaptic cleft in Onuf's nucleus, which promotes enhanced activity of the striated urethral sphincter.[83,88] Duloxetine appeared to have great promise on initial use, but has since shown on multiple studies to have high discontinuation rates from adverse effects. Vella et al. reported on 1-year follow-up of duloxetine treatment for SUI in 228 women. Only 9% of patients remained on duloxetine for 1 year and 82% had a tension-free vaginal tape. The majority of women discontinued use due to adverse effects (56%) or lack of efficacy (33%).[89] Adverse effects include nausea, fatigue, dry mouth, insomnia, and suicidal ideation or behavior in individuals under the age of 24 years.[83]

ß-adrenergic agonists (clenbuterol) may have some efficacy through an action agonism resulting in smooth muscle relaxation of the bladder wall. Yasuda et al.[90] reported on results of a double-blind, placebo-controlled trial with clenbuterol in 165 women in Japan and found significant improvement in frequency of incontinence, pads per day, and overall global assessment of treatment. It is presently only approved for SUI use in Japan. ß-adrenergic antagonists theoretically enhance norepinephrine effects on α-adrenergic receptors in the urethra. Propranolol has shown some beneficial effect in uncontrolled small numbers. This has not been reported in randomized, controlled trial.[33,83]

Estrogen receptors are present in the vagina, urethra, bladder, and pelvic floor, yet their role remains controversial. Understanding estrogen's role is based on cytologic and clinical changes observed after menopause and the high incidence of incontinence reported by elderly, post-menopausal women. This literature has been reviewed extensively, and an evidence-based recommendation for the use of estrogens to treat SUI in women is not supported.[4,33,83]

Many surgical procedures have been described, which can be divided into three types: urethral bulking agents (injectables), suburethral sling procedures, and colposuspension. Bulking agents were initially described to treat SUI caused by ISD, but have since been found to have applicability in urethral hypermobility also. Most periurethral agents are injected in a retrograde fashion under direct cystoscopic guidance with local anesthesia. Various agents (GAX collagen, Teflon®, silicone, fat, cartilage, Coaptite®, Durasphere®) have been used to increase outlet resistance. Each of these agents has variable biophysical properties influencing tissue compatibility, tendency for migration, density, durability, and safety. Success rates range from 40% to 86% with continuous decline in efficacy over time. There is low morbidity associated with bulking

agents: UTI, hematuria, and transient elevation of postvoid residuals.[82,83]

Sling procedures can be divided into the classic pubovaginal sling and the minimally invasive mid-urethral polypropylene sling. As opposed to an urethropexy, sling surgery may not only provide a "backboard" of support for the vesicourethral junction, but also create some degree of urethral coaptation or compression. The classic sling is used for women with ISD and may be used as a primary option or in patients who failed initial anti-incontinence surgery. Slings should be tied at the bladder neck (after passage through the endopelvic fascia and behind the pubic bone) with minimal or no tension to prevent bladder outlet obstruction (Fig. 32.3). Historically, autologous rectus fascia and fascia lata are the most commonly used sling materials. Other materials that are used include: vaginal wall, human cadaveric tissue, xenograft, and synthetic materials. Long-term studies note cure rates greater than 80% and rates of improvement of greater than 90%.[92,93] Autologous materials are generally associated with higher cure rates than cadaveric or synthetic materials.[82,83]

In the mid-1990s, the TVT was introduced for treatment of SUI. This is a minimally invasive option mainly used for women with urethral hypermobility. The TVT is passed through the retropubic space and aims to reinforce pubourethral ligaments and secure proper fixation of the mid-urethra to the pubic bone for maintenance of continence. Three small incisions are made (two suprapubic and one on the anterior vaginal wall at the mid-urethra).[82] A prospective study comparing the TVT to the open Burch colposuspension found the same effectiveness (TVT 81% and Burch 80%).[94] Bladder perforation is the most frequent intraoperative complication (intraoperative cystoscopy is required) occurring in 1 in 25 cases. Postoperatively, complications include voiding difficulties, UTI, and de novo detrusor overactivity.[82] The transobturator tape (TOT) was initially marketed to avoid the retropubic space and risk of bladder perforation associated with the TVT. Yet, there are numerous reports of bladder perforation with the TOT, making cystoscopy essential following TOT placement. Three small incisions (two groin incisions lateral to the inferior pubic ramus and one vaginal incision in the mid-urethra) are made with the TOT. The complication and cure rates are similar between the TOT and

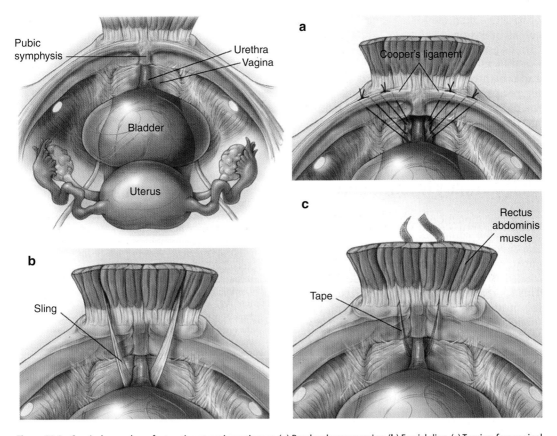

Figure 32.3. Surgical procedures for treating stress incontinence. (**a**) Burch colposuspension, (**b**) Fascial sling, (**c**) Tension-free vaginal tape (Reprinted with permission from Rogers[91]. Copyright © 2008 Massachusetts Medical Society. All rights reserved).

TVT.[95] While avoiding the retropubic space, the passage of the TOT poses risk to the obturator vessel tributary and adductor muscles. The TOT is associated with greater post-op groin/thigh pain (see Fig. 32.3).[96] Recently, FDA-approved single-incision mid-urethral polypropylene slings (MiniArc™, TVT-SECUR™) have been introduced. Short-term data reveals results similar to the TVT or TOT, but long-term efficacy has not been determined.[97]

Transabdominal (retropubic) colposuspension has historically been the standard to correct SUI. The advantages include: familiar retropubic anatomy, exposure, durability, and ability to repair coexisting abdominal pathology. The disadvantages include: large incision, prolonged hospitalization and recovery, and inability to access coexistent vaginal pathology through the same incision. The Marshall-Marchetti-Krantz (MMK), Burch colposuspension, and paravaginal

(Richardson) repairs are the three most common types of open retropubic colposuspension procedures performed.[83] They have excellent long-term success rates, in excess of 80% at 4 years post surgery.[93] In the MMK, the space of Retzius is entered and the anterior bladder and urethra are mobilized. The periurethral fascia anterolateral to the urethra is sutured to the posterior periosteum of the symphysis pubis from mid-urethra to the bladder neck.[83] This procedure is associated with a 2.5% risk of osteitis pubis and more likely to cause urethral obstruction than other anti-incontinence procedures.[98] With Burch colposuspension, the tissue lateral to the bladder neck (paravaginal fascia) is suspended to Cooper's ligaments bilaterally, supporting the vesicourethral junction within the retropubic space (see Fig. 32.3). These sutures are usually more proximal and lateral than the MMK sutures. The Burch procedure is considered less obstructive than the MMK[83] and is usually the colposuspension method of choice. Complications associated with the Burch include voiding difficulties, de novo detrusor overactivity, and prolapse.[92] Paravaginal repairs are reserved for re-approximating the paravaginal fascia to the pelvic sidewall at the level of the tendinous arc when there is detachment of the endopelvic fascia.[83]

Mixed Urinary Incontinence

The International Continence Society describes MUI as the complaint of involuntary leakage associated with urgency and also with exertion, effort, sneezing, or coughing.[3] MUI is often treated as part of the treatment of SUI and UUI. This approach should be individualized, depending on the severity of each component. Epidemiological studies have shown that women with MUI symptoms typically have worse incontinence than women with a pure subtype.[9] Dooley et al. compared the bother of MUI versus pure incontinence subtypes in 551 women. The Urinary Distress Inventory (UDI-6) scores were significantly higher in women with MUI than those with pure SUI or pure UUI.[99] The urgency component is frequently more bothersome and treatment is thus initially focused on this aspect.[4] The efficacy of antimuscarinics in treatment of MUI was studied. Seventy-six percent of patients treated with 8 weeks of an antimuscarinic for urgency (predominantly MUI) reported improvements as compared to a placebo group.[100]

Conclusions

Urinary incontinence carries a greater health, economic, and quality of life burden than most chronic diseases. Aging and female gender are two of the leading risk factors accounting for the large numbers of incontinent individuals. Prompt screening, assessment, and treatment for management of UI will prevent avoidable morbidity and mortality. To effectively treat UI in clinical practice, it is advantageous to differentiate between SUI and UUI. Whether it is UI due to an overactive detrusor, intrinsic sphincter deficiency, urethral hypermobility, or functional limitations, a dynamic, comprehensive management strategy is necessary. Conservative, pharmacological, or surgical measures should bring about an improvement in quality of life and reduction in incontinence episodes.

References

1. Hunskaar S, Arnold EP, Burgio K, et al. Epidemiology and natural history of urinary incontinence. *Int Urogynecol J Pelvic Floor Dysfunct*. 2000;11:301
2. Wein AJ, Rackley RR. Overactive bladder: a better understanding of pathophysiology, diagnosis and management. *J Urol*. 2006;175:S5
3. Abrams P, Cardozo L, Fall M, et al. The standardisation of terminology in lower urinary tract function: report from the standardisation sub-committee of the International Continence Society. *Urology*. 2003;61:37
4. Athanasopoulos A, Perimenis P. Pharmacotherapy of urinary incontinence. *Int Urogynecol J Pelvic Floor Dysfunct*. 2008;20(4):475-482
5. Burt VL, Whelton P, Roccella EJ, et al. Prevalence of hypertension in the US adult population. Results from the third national health and nutrition examination survey, 1988–1991. *Hypertension*. 1995;25:305
6. Silverstein B. Gender difference in the prevalence of clinical depression: the role played by depression associated with somatic symptoms. *Am J Psychiatry*. 1999;156:480
7. Wild S, Roglic G, Green A, et al. Global prevalence of diabetes: estimates for the year 2000 and projections for 2030. *Diab Care*. 2004;27:1047
8. Odeyemi IA, Dakin HA, O'Donnell RA, et al. Epidemiology, prescribing patterns and resource use associated with overactive bladder in UK primary care. *Int J Clin Pract*. 2006;60:949
9. Hannestad YS, Rortveit G, Sandvik H, et al. A community-based epidemiological survey of female urinary incontinence: the Norwegian EPINCONT study. Epidemiology of incontinence in the county of nord-trondelag. *J Clin Epidemiol*. 2000;53:1150
10. Hunskaar S, Burgio K, Diokno AC, et al. Epidemiology and natural history of urinary incontinence. In: Abrams P, Cardozo L, Khoury S, WEin A, eds. *Incontinence*. 2nd ed. Plymouth, UK: Health Publication Ltd.; 2002:165
11. Tennstedt SL, Link CL, Steers WD, et al. Prevalence of and risk factors for urine leakage in a racially and ethnically diverse population of adults: the Boston Area Community Health (BACH) survey. *Am J Epidemiol*. 2008;167:390
12. Wilson MM. Urinary incontinence: selected current concepts. *Med Clin North Am*. 2006;90:825
13. Klauser A, Frauscher F, Strasser H, et al. Age-related rhabdosphincter function in female urinary stress incontinence: assessment of intraurethral sonography. *J Ultrasound Med*. 2004;23:631
14. Lluel P, Deplanne V, Heudes D, et al. Age-related changes in urethrovesical coordination in male rats: relationship with bladder instability? *Am J Physiol Regul Integr Comp Physiol*. 2003;284:R1287

15. Patel MD, Coshall C, Rudd AG, et al. Cognitive impairment after stroke: clinical determinants and its associations with long-term stroke outcomes. *J Am Geriatr Soc.* 2002;50:700

16. Yoshida M, Miyamae K, Iwashita H, et al. Management of detrusor dysfunction in the elderly: changes in acetylcholine and adenosine triphosphate release during aging. *Urology.* 2004;63:17

17. Klausner AP, Vapnek JM. Urinary incontinence in the geriatric population. *Mt Sinai J Med.* 2003;70:54

18. Landi F, Cesari M, Russo A, et al. Potentially reversible risk factors and urinary incontinence in frail older people living in community. *Age Ageing.* 2003;32:194

19. McLoughlin MA, Chew DJ. Diagnosis and surgical management of ectopic ureters. *Clin Tech Small Anim Pract.* 2000;15:17

20. Ouslander JG. Intractable incontinence in the elderly. *BJU Int.* 2000;85(3):72

21. Zunzunegui Pastor MV, Rodriguez-Laso A, Garcia Yebenes MJ, et al. Prevalence of urinary incontinence and linked factors in men and women over 65. *Aten Primaria.* 2003;32:337

22. Bradway C. Urinary incontinence among older women. Measurement of the effect on health-related quality of life. *J Gerontol Nurs.* 2003;29:13

23. Hogan DB. Revisiting the O complex: urinary incontinence, delirium and polypharmacy in elderly patients. *CMAJ.* 1997;157:1071

24. Johansson C, Hellstrom L, Ekelund P, et al. Urinary incontinence: a minor risk factor for hip fractures in elderly women. *Maturitas.* 1996;25:21

25. Saltvedt I, Mo ES, Fayers P, et al. Reduced mortality in treating acutely sick, frail older patients in a geriatric evaluation and management unit. A prospective randomized trial. *J Am Geriatr Soc.* 2002;50:792

26. Baztan JJ, Arias E, Gonzalez N, et al. New-onset urinary incontinence and rehabilitation outcomes in frail older patients. *Age Ageing.* 2005;34:172

27. Miner PB Jr. Economic and personal impact of fecal and urinary incontinence. *Gastroenterology.* 2004;126:S8

28. Brading AF. A myogenic basis for the overactive bladder. *Urology.* 1997;50:57

29. Elbadawi A, Yalla SV, Resnick NM. Structural basis of geriatric voiding dysfunction. III. Detrusor overactivity. *J Urol.* 1993;150:1668

30. Elbadawi A, Yalla SV, Resnick NM. Structural basis of geriatric voiding dysfunction. IV. Bladder outlet obstruction. *J Urol.* 1993;150:1681

31. de Groat WC. A neurologic basis for the overactive bladder. *Urology.* 1997;50:36

32. Drake MJ, Mills IW, Gillespie JI. Model of peripheral autonomous modules and a myovesical plexus in normal and overactive bladder function. *Lancet.* 2001; 358:401

33. Andersson KE, Appell R, Cardozo LD, et al. The pharmacological treatment of urinary incontinence. *BJU Int.* 1999;84:923

34. Hashim H, Abrams P. Overactive bladder: an update. *Curr Opin Urol.* 2007;17:231

35. Andersson KE, Pehrson R. CNS involvement in overactive bladder. *Drugs.* 2003;63:2595

36. Cardozo L. New developments in the management of stress urinary incontinence. *BJU Int.* 2004;94(1):1

37. Mostwin JL. Urinary incontinence. *J Urol.* 1995;153:352

38. Walsh PC, Partin AW, Epstein JI. Cancer control and quality of life following anatomical radical retropubic prostatectomy: results at 10 years. *J Urol.* 1994;152:1831

39. Leach GE, Trockman B, Wong A, et al. Post-prostatectomy incontinence: urodynamic findings and treatment outcomes. *J Urol.* 1996;155:1256

40. Groutz A, Blaivas JG, Chaikin DC, et al. The pathophysiology of post-radical prostatectomy incontinence: a clinical and video urodynamic study. *J Urol.* 2000;163:1767

41. Coyne KS, Margolis MK, Thompson C, et al. Psychometric equivalence of the OAB-q in Danish, German, Polish, Swedish and Turkish. *Int Soc Pharmacoeconomics Outcomes Res ISPOR.* 2008;11(7):1096

42. Brown JS, McNaughton KS, Wyman JF, et al. Measurement characteristics of a voiding diary for use by men and women with overactive bladder. *Urology.* 2003; 61:802

43. Ku JH, Jeong IG, Lim DJ, et al. Voiding diary for the evaluation of urinary incontinence and lower urinary tract symptoms: prospective assessment of patient compliance and burden. *Neurourol Urodyn.* 2004;23:331

44. Nygaard I, Holcomb R. Reproducibility of the seven-day voiding diary in women with stress urinary incontinence. *Int Urogynecol J Pelvic Floor Dysfunct.* 2000;11:15

45. Fletcher SG, Lemack GE. Clarifying the role of urodynamics in the preoperative evaluation of stress urinary incontinence. *ScientificWorld J.* 2008;8:1259

46. Patel AK, Chapple CR. Urodynamics in the management of female stress incontinence – which test and when? *Curr Opin Urol.* 2008;18:359

47. Lemack GE, Xu Y, Brubaker L, et al. Clinical and demographic factors associated with valsalva leak point pressure among women undergoing burch bladder neck suspension or autologous rectus fascial sling procedures. *Neurourol Urodyn.* 2007;26:392

48. Comiter CV. Surgery Insight: surgical management of postprostatectomy incontinence – the artificial urinary sphincter and male sling. *Nat Clin Pract Urol.* 2007; 4:615

49. Nager CW, FitzGerald M, Kraus SR, et al. Urodynamic measures do not predict stress continence outcomes after surgery for stress urinary incontinence in selected women. *J Urol.* 2008;179:1470

50. Paick JS, Oh SJ, Kim SW, et al. Tension-free vaginal tape, suprapubic arc sling, and transobturator tape in the treatment of mixed urinary incontinence in women. *Int Urogynecol J Pelvic Floor Dysfunct.* 2008;19:123

51. Burgio KL. Current perspectives on management of urgency using bladder and behavioral training. *J Am Acad Nurse Pract.* 2004;16:4

52. Andersson KE. Antimuscarinics for treatment of overactive bladder. *Lancet Neurol.* 2004;3:46

53. Anderson RU, MacDiarmid S, Kell S, et al. Effectiveness and tolerability of extended-release oxybutynin vs extended-release tolterodine in women with or without prior anticholinergic treatment for overactive bladder. *Int Urogynecol J Pelvic Floor Dysfunct.* 2006; 17:502

54. Chapple CR, Martinez-Garcia R, Selvaggi L, et al. A comparison of the efficacy and tolerability of solifenacin succinate and extended release tolterodine at treating overactive bladder syndrome: Results of the STAR trial. *Eur Urol.* 2005;48:464

55. Haab F, Stewart L, Dwyer P. Darifenacin, an M3 selective receptor antagonist, is an effective and well-tolerated once-daily treatment for overactive bladder. *Eur Urol.* 2004;45:420

56. Chancellor MB, de Groat WC. Intravesical capsaicin and resiniferatoxin therapy: spicing up the ways to treat the overactive bladder. *J Urol.* 1999;162:3

57. Holzer-Petsche U, Lembeck F. Systemic capsaicin treatment impairs the micturition reflex in the rat. *Br J Pharmacol.* 1984;83:935

58. Kawatani M, Whitney T, Booth AM, et al. Excitatory effect of substance P in parasympathetic ganglia of cat urinary bladder. *Am J Physiol.* 1989;257:R1450

59. Yoshimura N, Erdman SL, Snider MW, et al. Effects of spinal cord injury on neurofilament immunoreactivity and capsaicin sensitivity in rat dorsal root ganglion neurons innervating the urinary bladder. *Neuroscience.* 1998;83:633

60. Fowler CJ, Beck RO, Gerrard S, et al. Intravesical capsaicin for treatment of detrusor hyperreflexia. *J Neurol Neurosurg Psychiatry.* 1994;57:169

61. Kim JH, Rivas DA, Shenot PJ, et al. Intravesical resiniferatoxin for refractory detrusor hyperreflexia: a multicenter, blinded, randomized, placebo-controlled trial. *J Spinal Cord Med.* 2003;26:358

62. Apostolidis A, Popat R, Yiangou Y, et al. Decreased sensory receptors P2X3 and TRPV1 in suburothelial nerve fibers following intradetrusor injections of botulinum toxin for human detrusor overactivity. *J Urol.* 2005; 174:977

63. Dmochowski R, Sand PK. Botulinum toxin A in the overactive bladder: current status and future directions. *BJU Int.* 2007;99:247

64. Brubaker L, Richter HE, Visco A, et al. Refractory idiopathic urge urinary incontinence and botulinum a injection. *J Urol.* 2008;180:217

65. van Kerrebroeck PEV, van Voskuilen AC, Heesakkers JPFA, Nijholt AABL, Siegel S, et al. Results of sacral neuromodulation therapy for urinary voiding dysfunction: outcomes of prospective, worldwide clinical study. *J Urol.* 2007;178:2029

66. Sutherland SE, Lavers A, Carlson A, Holtz C, Kesha J, Siegel SW. Sacral nerve stimulation for voiding dysfunction: one institution's 11-year experience. *Neurourol Urodyn.* 2007;26:19

67. Cooperberg MR, Stoller ML. Posterior tibial nerve stimulation for pelvic floor dysfunction. In: Raz S, Larissa V, eds. *Female Urology.* 3rd ed. Philadelphia, PA: Saunders Elsevier; 2008

68. Parekh AR, Feng MI, Kirages D, Bremner H, et al. The role of pelvic floor exercises on post-prostatectomy incontinence. *J Urol.* 2003;170:130

69. Tiguert R et al. Collagen injection in the management of post-radical retropubic prostatectomy intrinsic sphincteric deficiency. *Neurourol Urodyn.* 1999;18:653

70. Smith DN et al. Collagen injection therapy for postprostatectomy incontinence. *J Urol.* 1998;160:364

71. Sanchez-Ortiz RF et al. Collagen injection therapy for post-radical retropubic prostatectomy incontinence: role of valsalva leak point pressure. *J Urol.* 1997; 158:2132

72. Comiter CV. Surgery insight: surgical management of postprostatecotmy incontinence- the artificial urinary sphincter and male sling. *Nature.* 2007;4:615

73. Montague DK, Angermeier KW. Postprostatectomy urinary incontinence: the case for artificial urinary sphincter implantation. *Urology.* 2000;55:2

74. Litwiller SE et al. Post-prostatectomy iIncontinence and the artificial urinary sphincter: a long-term study of patient satisfaction and criteria for success. *J Urol.* 1996;156(6):1975-1980

75. Petrou SP et al. Artificial urinary sphincter for incontinence. *Urology.* 2000;56:353

76. Fulford SC et al. The fate of the "modern" artificial urinary sphincter with a follow-up of more than 10 Years. *Br J Urol.* 1997;79:713

77. Montague DK. The artificial urinary sphincter (AMS 800): experience in 166 consecutive patients. *J Urol.* 1992;147:380

78. Elliott DS, Barrett DM. May clinic long-term analysis of the functional durability of the AMS 800 artificial urinary sphincter: a review of the 323 cases. *J Urol.* 1998;159:1206

79. Comiter CV. The male perineal sling: intermediate-term results. *Neurourol Urodyn.* 2005;24:648

80. Rajpurkar AD et al. Patient satisfaction and clinical efficacy of the new perineal bone-anchored male sling. *Eur Urol.* 2005;47:237

81. Rehder P, Gozzi C. Transobturator sling suspension for male urinary incontinence including post-radical prostatectomy. *Eur Urol.* 2007;52:860

82. Pesce F. Current management of stress urinary incontinence. *BJU Int.* 2004;94:8

83. Rovner ES, Wein AJ. Treatment options for stress urinary incontinence. *Rev Urol.* 2004;6:S29

84. Wyman JF, Fantl JA, McClish DK, Bump RC. For the continence program for women research group. Comparative efficacy of behavioral interventions in the management of female urinary incontinence. *Am J Obstet Gynecol.* 1998;179:999

85. Wilson PD, Bo K, Hay-Smith J, et al. Conservative treatment in women. In: Abrams P, Cardozo L, Khoury S, Wein A, eds. *Incontinence.* 2nd ed. Plymouth, UK: Health Publication Ltd.; 2002:571-624

86. Agency for Health Care Policy and Research, US Department of Health and Human Services. *Clinical Practice Guidelines: Urinary Incontinence in Adults.* Rockville, MD: Agency for Health Care Policy and Research; 1992. AHCPR Publication 92–0038

87. Lin HH, Sheu BC, Lo MC, Huang SC. Comparison of treatment outcomes for imipramine for female genuine stress incontinence. *Br J Obstet Gynaecol.* 1999; 106:1089

88. Basu M, Duckett J. The treatment of urinary incontinence with Duloxetine. *J Obstet Gynaecol.* 2008;28:166

89. Vella M, Duckett J, Basu M. Duloxetine 1 year on: the long-term outcome of a cohort of women prescribed duloxetine. *Int Urogynecol J*. 2008;19:961

90. Yasuda K, Kawabe K, Takimoto Y, The Clenbuterol Clinical Research Group, et al. A double-blind clinical trial of a ß2-adrenergic agonist in stress incontinence. *Int Urogynecol J*. 1993;4:146

91. Rogers RG. Urinary stress incontinence in women. *N Engl J Med*. 2008;358:1029-1036

92. Abrams P, Cardozo L, Khoury S, Wein A, eds. *Incontinence*. 2nd ed. Plymouth, UK: Health Publication Ltd.; 2002

93. Leach GE, Dmochowski RR, Appell RA, et al. Female stress urinary incontinence clinical guidelines panel summary report on surgical management of female stress urinary incontinence. *J Urol*. 1997;158:875

94. Ward KL, Hilton P. UK and Ireland TVT trial group. A prospective multicenter randomized trial of tension-free vaginal tape and colposuspension for primary urodynamic stress incontinence: 2-year follow-up. *Am J Obstet Gynecol*. 2004;190:324

95. Wang W, Zhu L, Lang J. Transobturator tape procedure versus tension-free vaginal tape for treatment of stress urinary incontinence. *Int J Gynaecol Obstet*. 2009;104(2): 113-116

96. Schulz JA, Chan MC, Farrell SA. The sub-committee on urogynaecology. Midurethral minimally invasive sling procedures for stress. *Urin Incontin*. 2008;213:728

97. Molden SM, Lucente VR. New minimally invasive slings: TVT Secur. *Curr Urol Rep*. 2008;9:358

98. Zimmern PE, Hadley HR, Leach GE, et al. Female urethral obstruction after Marshall-Marchetti-Krantz operation. *J Urol*. 1987;138:517

99. Dooley Y, Lowenstein L, Kenton K, et al. Mixed incontinence is more bother than pure incontinence subtypes. *Int Urogynecol J*. 2008;19:1359

100. Khullar V, Hill S, Laval KU, Schiotz HA, et al. Treatment of urge-predominant mixed urinary incontinence with tolterodine extended release: a randomized, placebo-controlled trial. *Urology*. 2004;64:269

33

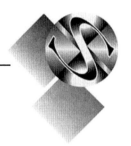

Neurogenic Bladder

William D. Steers

Introduction

When an abnormality of the nervous system triggers changes in continence, micturition, or urinary symptoms, the term "neurogenic bladder" is used. The urinary bladder and its outlet are unique among viscera because of their complex interplay of visceral and somatic systems in regulating the lower urinary tract (LUT) and the ability of emotions to affect visceral function. As might be expected, the neural regulation of the lower urinary tract differs from other organ systems in that these structures, although innervated by the autonomic nervous system, are under voluntary control. This duality of autonomic and somatic innervation is suited for switching from involuntary urine storage to voluntary elimination. This chapter provides a brief overview of the organization of the neural pathways and central sites influencing micturition and continence, catalogs those disorders linked to neurogenic bladder and pathology, and briefly outlines how neurogenic bladder disorders can be diagnosed and treated.

Examination and Diagnostic Tests

History and Physical Examination

Evaluating a patient with neurogenic bladder involves a detailed neurourologic history and focused neurologic exam. In addition to symptom assessment, the onset and duration of symptoms, coexistent sexual and bowel complaints, and previous treatments for the urologic or neurologic condition should be obtained. The urologist can be instrumental in confirming a diagnosis or obtaining baseline LUT function prior to treatment. The neurourologic assessment at a minimum includes evaluating lower extremity motor function, lumbosacral dermatome sensation, and the bulbocavernosus reflex. This is not to exclude an overall neurologic evaluation and an appraisal of mental status which is crucial for designing a treatment regimen. An assessment of blood pressure (BP) should be made especially during symptoms suspicious of autonomic dysreflexia (AD). Supine and upright BPs are recorded to document whether orthostatic hypotension exists which suggests autonomic neuropathy.

Imaging

Imaging of the upper or lower urinary tract in the neurogenic bladder patient is used to assess whether hydronephrosis or calculi are present as well as sites of obstruction or reflux. Serum creatinine may be normal despite upper tract deterioration necessitating periodic renal imaging, especially in patients with clinical or urodynamic findings indicating a high risk for hydronephrosis. Imaging during urodynamics is also crucial to assess structural or functional abnormalities. Most notably, a voiding cystourethrogram can pinpoint the level of obstruction

C.R. Chapple and W.D. Steers (eds.), *Practical Urology: Essential Principles and Practice*,
DOI: 10.1007/978-1-84882-034-0_33, © Springer-Verlag London Limited 2011

at either the bladder neck or external urethral sphincter (EUS) in cases of detrusor intrinsic sphincter dyssynergia (DISD) or detrusor sphincter dyssynergia (DSD). Cystography may also demonstrate vesicoureteral reflux or diverticuli contributing to recurrent infections. Renal scans are occasionally used to assess differential renal function, look for cortical scars, and rule out upper tract obstruction or hydronephrosis.

Advanced imaging modalities of functional BOLD (blood oxygen level dependant) MRI or positron emission scanning (PET) are increasingly used to define sites of involvement in voiding or continence and aberrations with disease.

Urodynamics (UDS)

UDS assess the etiology of symptoms, ascertain the likelihood of complications, and assist treatment planning. Video UDS are especially useful. The urodynamicist needs to be cognizant of additional considerations such as antibiotic prophylaxis for high-risk patients and prevention of AD.

Residual urine must be measured either by catheterization or ultrasound. An uninstrumented flow rate may provide the first hint of loss of coordination between the reflex detrusor contraction and EUS relaxation termed DSD especially if an interrupted stream is documented. Cystometry during medium fill rate assesses sensation, compliance (change in volume/pressure), maximum detrusor pressure, detrusor leak point pressure, and maximum capacity as well as whether involuntary detrusor contractions termed detrusor overactivity (DO) exist. The most important urodynamic parameters to predict future upper tract changes include reduced detrusor compliance <12.5 cm^3/cm H$_2$O and a detrusor leak point pressure (DLLP) over 40 cm H$_2$O at normal resting volumes (Fig. 33.1).[1,2]

UDS provides a framework for treatment and prognosis such that a "hostile bladder" is characterized by either reduced compliance or elevated DLPP. Electromyography (EMG) is essential to document whether dysfunctional voiding versus DSD exists. Although rarely needed and technically difficult, needle electrode electromyography (EMG) can document peripheral neuropathy and help decide between different disorders with similar symptoms. Urodynamic findings for common neurologic disorders are given in Table 33.1.

Evoked Potentials

Rarely, electrical or electromagnetic stimulation of peripheral (dorsal nerve of the penis, clitoris) or central (cortical or sacral) sites with recording from similar sites while measuring latencies, threshold, and conduction velocities is required to document neuropathy.

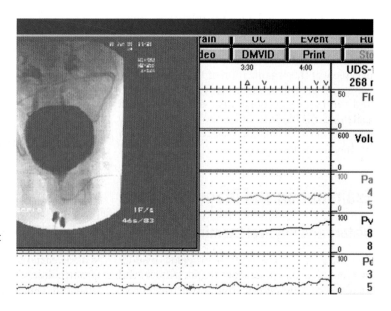

Figure 33.1. Videourodynamic tracing from T10 paraplegic demonstrates poor detrusor leak point pressure of 42 cm^3/cm H$_2$O and compliance of 9 cm^3/cm H$_2$O. Treated with augmentation cystoplasty and catheterizable stoma.

Table 33.1. General urodynamic findings with common neurologic diseases

Disorder	Detrusor overactivity	Detrusor areflexia	Detrusor sphincter dyssynergia	Sensation impaired	Reduced compliance	Intrinsic sphincter deficiency
CVA	+++	+	+?	+/−		
Parkinson's disease	+++++				+	
MSA	+++	+				++
Multiple sclerosis	+++	++	++	+	+	
Huntington's	++					
NPH	++					
Cerebral palsy	++	+				
Cerebellar ataxia	++	+				
Encephalitis	++					
Brain tumors	++					
Cervical disk herniation	++		+++		+	
Lumbosacral disk				+++		
Spinal cord injury	+++	+	+++	+++	++	
Transverse myelitis	+++	++	++			+
Herpetic disease		+++		+++		
Diabetes mellitus	++	+		++		
Pelvic surgery		+++			++	+

Classifications

The most useful classification to plan therapy based on the simple concepts of failure to empty or failure to store urine has been popularized by Wein.[3] Essentially, there are two elements that can have pathology – the bladder or its outlet (Table 33.2). Then there are only two problems each system can exhibit – overactivity or underactivity of the bladder and increased or reduced resistance of the outlet. Combining these four problems for all that is seen with

voiding disorders a total of 14 combinations exist.[4] Therapy either to enhance storage or emptying is directed at reducing DO, bypassing underactivity, reducing resistance, or increasing outlet resistance.

Older terms such as sensory, motor, autonomous, and reflex neurogenic bladder have been abandoned because of the heterogeneous nature of these conditions and their lack of usefulness in planning therapy. Likewise, the terms upper and lower motor neuron bladder, complete, and incomplete represent a theoretical construct limited to SCI patients, and these terms are not relevant to

Table 33.2. Classification based on whether neurogenic vesicourethral dysfunction affects bladder, outlet (urethra, bladder neck, external urethral sphincter), or both

Bladder	Outlet
Overactive	Increased resistance
• Neurogenic detrusor overactivity	• Detrusor sphincter dyssynergia
• Poor compliance	• Detrusor internal sphincter dyssynergia
• High detrusor leak P	
	• Dysfunction voider
Underactive	Reduced resistance
• Impaired contractility	• Uninhibited sphincter relaxation
• Detrusor areflexia	• Intrinsic sphincter deficiency

most other neurologic disorders. The *International Continence Society (ICS) classification* is essentially a urodynamic classification scheme which assumes that every patient undergoes urodynamics.

Autonomic Pathways Innervating the LUT

The parasympathetics innervating the bladder and urethra originate from the sacral parasympathetic nucleus (SPN) located in S2–S4 of the sacral spinal cord to form the pelvic nerve. Preganglionic axons in the pelvic nerve then synapse on postganglionic neurons in pelvic ganglia.

Sensory neuron cell bodies reside in dorsal root ganglia (DRG). Afferents in the bladder and urethra are low threshold myelinated (Aδ) and unmyelinated (C-fibers) fibers that convey mechanical or noxious stimuli to the dorsal horn of the spinal cord via the pelvic and hypogastric nerves. The afferents triggering micturition travel in the pelvic nerve. Bladder afferents containing nitric oxide synthase, glutamate, and a variety of neuropeptides enter the dorsal horn of the spinal cord.[5-7] There, second-order neurons project rostrally to supraspinal sites including the hypothalamus, thalamus, and pons. The hypothalamus is known to coordinate autonomic activity. The thalamus processes nociceptive information. The pons is specifically involved in micturition.

Preganglionic parasympathetic efferents, originating in the SPN, release acetylcholine which activates nicotinic receptors on ganglia in the pelvic plexus or within the bladder/urethral wall. Likewise, postganglionic parasympathetic nerves release acetylcholine that via muscarinic receptor (M3) contract the detrusor, whereas M2 activation turns off intracellular signaling responsible for detrusor relaxation.[8] Thus antimuscarinics are the primary drug treatment of OAB. Nitric oxide (NO) released from parasympathetic efferents relaxes the urethra.[9]

Preganglionic sympathetic fibers in the lower urinary tract in thoracic spinal cord segment T11 to lumbar spinal cord segment L2. Sympathetic postganglionic neurons mostly contain noradrenaline. Exogenous noradrenaline contracts smooth muscle by the stimulation of α1-adrenoceptors predominately 1A in the urethra and 1D in the bladder neck.[9] Therefore, alpha adrenergic antagonists have been useful in reducing outlet resistance in conditions with failure to empty. In contrast, activation of β3-adrenoceptors relaxes smooth muscle in the detrusor.[9] Passive, elastic properties of the bladder body in addition to local neural networks of urothelium and interstitial cells as well as neural mechanisms are involved in accommodation of the bladder to large volumes during urine storage (compliance). Bladder accommodation of urine and contraction is also influenced by the urothelium and interstitial cells although precise mechanisms are unclear.

Somatic Pathways

The neurons innervating the striated muscle of the external urethral sphincter (EUS) and the pelvic floor emerge from the anterior horn of S2–S4. These motoneurons originate in an area termed Onuf's nucleus. The axons travel to the EUS and the periurethral striated muscle in the pudendal nerve.

Afferents from the EUS travel in the pudendal nerve. Neuromodulation by stimulation of sacral nerve roots may work by somatic or non–bladder afferent stimulation causing central inhibition of micturition (for urge urinary incontinence [UI]) or the EUS (for retention). The striated muscles of the lower urinary tract are innervated by somatic cholinergic nerves that arise from the Onuf's nucleus. Acetylcholine acts on nicotinic receptors located at the motor end plate and causes muscle contraction. Botulinum toxin and its various serotypes prevent acetylcholine-containing vesicles from fusing to the prejunctional terminal membrane interfering with the release process. Botulinum toxin A (BoTNA) injections into the EUS have been used for treating DSD.[10] Intravesical BoTNA injections have been useful to treat urinary incontinence due to neurogenic DO.[11]

Central Control of Urine Storage and Release and the Pontine Micturition Center (PMC)

The central regulation of the micturition reflex involves the cerebral cortex, diencephalon, and pons. The command and control center for the bladder is the pons. Stimulation of the dorsomedial pontine center causes urinary bladder contraction and simultaneous EUS inhibition.[12] Stimulation of the dorsolateral pons increases activity of EUS while inhibiting the bladder. Neurons in the dorsomedial pons send axons to the sacral spinal. Onuf's nucleus also receives projections from the dorsolateral pons and the medial hypothalamus as well as axons from a lateral region of the PMC. Other brain regions implicated in bladder control include the central nucleus of the amygdala, bed nucleus stria terminalis, paraventricular nucleus, and locus coeruleus suggesting that stress and alertness could impact on bladder function.[13] Many projections in these pathways contain corticotropin releasing factor (CRF) that when released from the hypothalamus causes ACTH release.[14] Thus it is not surprising that conditions associated with severe stress (posttraumatic stress disorder, abuse) are associated with OAB.[15]

Ascending pathways from neurons arising in the dorsal horn of the spinal cord are involved in transmission of sensory information from the lower urinary tract to the dorsolateral pons including the periaqueductal gray.

To promote bladder distension and urethral sphincter contraction during urine storage, the micturition reflex is inhibited, whereas sympathetic and somatic pathways are activated (Fig. 33.2). During storage, bladder distension initiates low-level afferent activity in the pelvic nerve. Afferent firing originating from the urethra stimulates sympathetic efferent outflow to the bladder base and urethra as well as somatic outflow to the EUS. The storage reflexes are organized at spinal level, whereas the spinal reflex pathways are under influence by a lateral pontine area designated the urine storage center.

During bladder filling, the intravesical pressure remains low and constant (5–10 cm H_2O) until the threshold for inducing voiding is reached. Once this threshold is achieved, the central and peripheral parasympathetic efferent pathways are activated, whereas sympathetic and somatic pathways are inhibited. SCI, MS, cervical disk disease, tumors, or inflammatory processes that interrupt these pathways are associated with loss of coordination between the bladder and its outlet and DSD.

In predicting the impact of neurological conditions on urinary control, it is helpful to envision a hierarchical scheme divided into brain, spine, and periphery, and consider whether pathology exists rostral or caudal to the SPN. However, urodynamic findings and clinical expression of disease do not always clearly fit into known pathophysiological mechanisms. For example, although only lesions between the pons and sacral cord should lead to DSD, sometimes DSD is seen in other conditions either because of multiple levels of pathology or because of erroneous interpretations of UDS. Neuropathology effects both voiding and storage reflexes. Changes in neural connections and transmitter following disease or injury, termed neuroplasticity, alter these pathways sometimes in unpredictable ways.

Brain Lesions

Cerebrovascular Accident (CVA)

LUTS are prevalent in the stroke victim with up to 94% of patients describing at least one urinary symptom with nocturia being the most common complaint.[16] Acute urinary retention is common immediately after a CVA. Bothersome urinary incontinence is seen in 25% of patients at 12 months with a range of UI in the early period of 57–83%. UI following a CVA is the best predictor of future disability.[17]

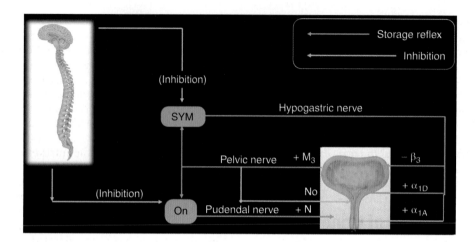

Figure 33.2. CNS control of micturition. Lower urinary tract function works as a switch in the pontine micturition center (PMC) from urine storage to voiding. During voiding, as depicted, sacral mechanisms regulating the external urethral sphincter (EUS), Onuf's nucleus (ON), and sympathetic centers (SYM) are inhibited, whereas preganglionic neurons giving rise to the pelvic nerve are activated. Infrapontine but supraspinal neuropathology may interfere with this switch and cause detrusor sphincter dyssynergia. Acetylcholine released from postganglionic neurons activate M3 receptors expressed by detrusor to contract and NO released in urethra relaxes outlet. During storage, postganglionic sympathetic neurons release norepinephrine which activates α1 receptors in bladder neck and urethra and β3 receptors in bladder body to store urine under low pressure.

Urodynamics studies in stroke patients are variable. In the immediate shock period 21% demonstrate overflow UI secondary to detrusor areflexia (DA). UDS in symptomatic patients revealed 69% had neurogenic DO, 10% hypocontractility, and 22% DSD.[18] The latter finding suggests spinal involvement or misinterpretation due to lack of voluntary relaxation.

Parkinson's Disease (PD)

PD arises from neurodegeneration of dopaminergic neurons in the basal ganglia. An imbalance in activation of excitatory (D2) and inhibitory (D1) dopamine receptors causes LUTs which range from 37% to 71%.[19] Storage symptoms of frequency, urgency, nocturia, and urge UI are most common. Voiding symptoms of slow stream, hesitancy, and double voiding are less frequent and can be confused with symptoms due to benign prostatic hyperplasia (BPH). Sixty-seven to ninety-three percent of CMGs show neurogenic DO, 16% reveal hyporeflexia or DA, 7% have pseudodyssynergia, and 11% demonstrate bradykinesia of the EUS.[19] Abnormal UDS correlate with disease severity. Although pressure flow studies can be useful to diagnose obstruction due to BPH, they fail to accurately predict surgical outcomes with only half of patients undergoing a TURP have an excellent result.[20] Controversy exists whether men with coexistent PD and obstruction should also undergo surgical intervention. Although such procedures may assist evacuation of the bladder, the risk of UI or persistent storage symptoms is substantial.

Multisystem Atrophy (MSA), Olivopontine Cerebellar Degeneration (OPCD), ShyDrager

Urinary complaints are nearly universal in patients with MSA. MSA causes striatonigral degeneration in which Parkinsonian symptoms are predominant. OPCD denotes the condition in which cerebellar signs predominate. Shy Drager describes this neurodegenerative disorder when autonomic failure is present. Neurologic and urinary symptoms in PD and MSA may be identical. But as opposed to PD, neuronal degeneration extends beyond the basal ganglia. In Shy Drager autonomic ganglia and Onuf's nucleus are often involved. In a patient with orthostatic hypotension, UI, retention, and Parkinsonian symptoms, MSA/Shy Drager should be suspected. If physical examination reveals lax anal tone or absent voluntary anal contraction further suspicion of MSA is raised. Nearly a third of MSA patients complain of difficulty voiding, 44% have SUI, a third note urinary frequency, and a third demonstrate urge UI.[21]

Video UDS can differentiate MSA from PD. While up to a third of PD may show an open bladder neck, 46–100% of patients with MSA have this finding.[22] UDS show that more than half the patients lack EUS responses to cough or Valsalva. Sixty-seven percent show DA, a third neurogenic DO, and more than half reduced compliance.[21] Indeed, residual urines greater than 100 cm^3 should lead the clinician to suspect MSA rather than PD. Motor unit responses of the EUS consistent with denervation include polyphasic potentials and increased duration of responses.[23]

For the urologist, the most important reason to differentiate MSA from PD is for the management of a patient in whom bladder outlet obstruction is suspected. Since retention and residuals are common in MSA, these patients more likely to under prostatic surgery to relieve obstruction. Stress urinary incontinence (SUI) occurs either more commonly or exclusively in MSA relative to PD.[24]

Multiple Sclerosis

MS is a demyelinating disorder of axons in the brain and spinal cord. Eighty to ninety percent of MS patients will develop urologic complaints. In a systemic review of UDS in MS patients neurogenic DO was found in 62%, DSD in 25%, and hypocontractility in 20%.[25]

Although upper tract deterioration is unusual in MS, men with lower extremity involvement may be the one group at greater risk and require close monitoring, if not with UDS, than with frequent upper tract imaging.

Huntington's Disease

This autosomal dominant neurodegenerative disorder causes neuronal loss in the cerebral cortex and caudate nucleus. In the rare studies examining urinary complaints, DO was the only finding. In large surveys, LUTS occurred only in late stages (>10 years) of the disease.

Dementias

There is wide variation in UI (11–90%) reported with dementia. UI is more common with Alzheimer's than multi-infarct dementia. Incontinence in patients with dementia is multi-factorial with social factors; such unwillingness to hold urine after first sensation of fullness, cognitive inability to get to toilet, physical inability to reach a toilet, impact of medications, and access are operative. Underlying these limitations are studies demonstrating DO. One study showed that DO was present on CMG in 58% of patients with Alzheimer's disease, 91% with multi-infarct dementia, and 50% who had both.[26] Half of UI patients had DO, whereas none of the continent patients had this urodynamic finding. Another finding in dementia patients is uninhibited sphincter relaxation. Of particular importance is avoiding the use of nonselective antimuscarinics to treat UI in these patients which may exert adverse effects on cognitive function.

Normal Pressure Hydrocephalus (NPH)

Dilated cerebral ventricles and normal cerebrospinal fluid pressure, termed NPH, is associated with gait disturbance, memory defects, and UI. Up to 93% of NPH patients have OAB symptoms with 63–100% demonstrating DO.[27] Some patients demonstrate a PVR urine as well potentially due to aging-related impaired contractile function. In a substantial proportion of patients shunting improves or eliminates LUTS.[28] Care in the use of antimuscarinics is advised due to memory defects.[29]

Cerebral Palsy, Cerebellar Ataxia, Epilepsy

DO has been demonstrated in 31–100% of patients with CP.[30,31] DSD is uncommon(3–19%). UI may be related to underlying bladder dysfunction or social limitations imposed by limited mobility or cognitive function.

Cerebellar ataxia is usually not associated with LUTS unless other neurodegenerative conditions coexist. When present, UI and urgency are typical symptoms. DO in symptomatic patients has been described in 25–53%.[32,33] One study reported that up to 37% had DSD implying spinal involvement.[34] Up to 16% may show DA.

UI can often be preceded with an intense urgency. Rarely, micturition itself can trigger a seizure. It should also be noted that antiepileptics such as gabapentin have been associated with UI.[35]

Encephalitis/Progressive Multifocal Leukoencephalopathy (PML)

PML is an infectious demyelinating disorder of the brain of viral origin occurring in immunosuppressed patients such as those with AIDS. Isolated reports exist of UI and OAB.

Tumors

UI can develop with frontal lobe tumors along with indifference and disinhibition. OAB had been found in 14% of frontal lobe tumors manifesting with behavioral changes.[36]

Psychiatric Disorders

Recent epidemiologic studies implicate depression and anxiety in the pathogenesis of OAB possibly sharing a similar neurochemical background. Often LUTS occurs years after psychiatric symptoms. Urodynamics may reveal DO and a positive ice water test suggestive of C fiber-mediated reflex micturition.[37] Treatment of these disorders fails to eradicate LUTS; conversely, successful treatment of LUTS does not universally relieve depression and anxiety. Interestingly, the tricyclic antidepressants and duloxetine which raise CNS levels of 5-HT and NE have been shown to have some efficacy for OAB or urge UI. Lithium used to treat manic depression can cause diabetes insipidus and urinary frequency.[38]

Spinal Lesions and Pathology

Intervertebral Disk Prolapse

Lumbosacral disk herniation is common and can lead to neurogenic bladder and litigation. With cervical spine disk herniations, neurogenic DO with and without DSD often develop. Thoracic disks although less frequent than at cervical or lumbosacral levels can cause voiding complaints in a quarter to a third of patients. The spinal cord terminates at the level of mid L1 vertebral body in adults. Most disk prolapses occur at either L4/L5 or L5/S1. But at least 75% nerve compression is required to trigger symptoms and bladder dysfunction.[39] Although classically DA is reported in a quarter of patients on UDS, neurogenic DO can occur.[40] Areflexia results from posteriolateral disk protrusion which can injure afferent input necessary to trigger a micturition reflex. Eventually, bladder overdistension can cause changes in compliance and detrusor contractility. DO is likely due to nerve root irritation. Although most patients with cauda equina syndrome exhibit normal bladder compliance, up to 28% have reduced compliance.[41]

Treatment of herniated disks can improve bladder function. The most important predictor of recovery of bladder function is absence of perianal anesthesia though cauda equina syndrome can exist without sacral anesthesia. If detrusor areflexia is found preoperatively, chances of postoperative recovery of bladder function is less even if perianal sensation returns. Regardless, recovery of bladder contractions may take years with only a third in retention resuming voiding.

Spinal Cord Injury (SCI)

The level of SCI provides a guide as to findings on UDS. Injuries rostral to the SPN are often associated with DSD. Injury at the thoracic spine corresponding to the sacral center may lead to DA with an open outlet leading to SUI. Thoracolumbar injury may also lead to detrusor internal sphincter dyssynergia diagnosed by a detrusor contracting against a closed bladder neck on video UDS. Patients with a hostile bladder merit frequent renal ultrasounds (e.g., 3–6 months).

Patients with SCI at or above T6 may develop autonomic dysreflexia (AD) characterized by hypertension, sweating, and bradycardia. Immediate treatment is to empty the bladder. Pharmacologic management with nifedipine (bite and swallow), nitroglycerine ointment above the lesion, or intravenous sodium nitroprusside is required for emergency treatment. Pretreatment or chronic administration of sublingual nifedipine prior to a procedure or oral terazosin is used for recurrent AD.

Transverse Myelitis

Transverse myelitis is an immune disorder that injures the spinal cord. It can be idiopathic or occur as a sequelae of MS or lupus. It is an acute disorder associated with bladder dysfunction in 80–94% of patients.[42,43] DO and DSD are common urodynamic findings. Small studies in children document significant recovery from either retention or urge UI. In adults, numerous small case series highlight difficulties with refractory urge UI and residual urines. Approximately a third of patients recover with no ill effects.[44] Prognostic information gained from MRI findings or cytokine measures are reported.

Peripheral Neuropathies

Infections/Autoimmune Peripheral Neuropathies

Herpes viruses especially varicella-zoster and herpes simplex type 2 can cause neuropathic bladder. Urinary retention occurs in up to 3.5% of patients especially those with sacral dorsal root involvement.[45] Retrograde viral transport to the SPN interferes with the micturition reflex causing detrusor areflexia. If thoracolumbar levels are involved, retention may be due to increased sympathetic outflow to the bladder outlet. Sensation in the afflicted dermatomes is reduced and a bulbocavernosus reflex often weak or absent. Retention develops days to weeks after the skin eruption and lasts for 4–8 weeks.

Late stages of syphilis can trigger detrusor areflexia and reduced bladder sensation causing urinary retention. Rarely, DO has been reported.

Guillain-Barre is an autoimmune disorder that causes demyelination of small- and large-diameter axons. Up to 50% of patients manifest autonomic neuropathy. Detrusor areflexia and reduced bladder sensation leads to large postvoid residual urines or retention. Spontaneous resolution takes at least 6–8 weeks.

Metabolic Neuropathies

Diabetes mellitus can cause an autonomic neuropathy characterized by loss of autonomic fibers and rarely degeneration of spinal centers. UI is more common in diabetics than in nondiabetics.[46] Urinary frequency may be due to DO or osmotic diuresis due to glucosuria. Diabetic cystopathy classically demonstrates reduced bladder sensation with a large capacity bladder and residual urine.[47] UDS more often reveals DO, possibly due to early axonopathy or changes in the detrusor. However in the older patient, coexistent pathology such as BPH or ischemic brain disease may cause DO in diabetics.

Sarcoidosis may involve the central or peripheral nervous system. Neurogenic bladder is rare although DO has been associated with brain lesions, DSD with spinal intramedullary lesions, and DA with subarachnoid granulomas and radiculopathy.

Alcoholic and porphyria-induced peripheral neuropathy can lead to bladder dysfunction. Findings mirror diabetic cystopathy.

Pelvic Surgery

Extensive pelvic surgery can injure the pelvic plexus, pudendal, pelvic, and hypogastric nerves. Historically, the incidence of voiding disorders following abdominal perineal resection varied from 8% to 70%.[48] For anterior resections the incidence of voiding dysfunction is lower at 20–25%.[48] New techniques by colorectal surgeons that avoid dissection beneath the presacral fascia, avoiding levator muscle division, vaginal dissection, and careful dissection near the prostatic apex often spare these nerves and the incidence has fallen. Detrusor hypocontractility, impaired sensation, reduced compliance, and increased capacity are found on UDS. An open bladder neck may be present on video UDS. Postvoid residuals are often found. Although most patients are continent, subsequent surgery on the bladder outlet such as a TURP may result in incontinence secondary to intrinsic sphincter deficiency. Preoperative UDS are usually not helpful in predicting this outcome although reduced compliance and an open bladder neck are worrisome findings.

Radical hysterectomy with removal of uterosacral and cardinal ligaments can cause vesicourethral dysfunction. Reduced compliance and maximal urethral pressures have been measured with hypocontractility causing residual urines. In studies of women with LUTS after simple hysterectomy, 47% have DO, 37% outlet obstruction, and 25% SUI, suggesting both pelvic support injury and changes to the detrusor.[48] Similar to colorectal surgeons, gynecologic oncologists are using nerve-sparing techniques when feasible to avoid creating a neurogenic bladder.

Treatment

Management of patients with neurogenic bladders is complex by nature of the social, economic, overall disability, and cognitive issues beyond urologic considerations. Many of the urologic complications are preventable and arise from lack of monitoring or poor patient compliance with medications, clean intermittent catheterization (CIC), or periodic follow-up with urinalyses/cultures and renal ultrasound. Physicians should strongly counsel patients early in the diagnosis of warning signs, abstinence from smoking because of heightened risk of malignancies, the need for periodic follow-up, and prevention of obesity which may complicate future reconstruction or diversion.

In general, therapies follow a noninvasive and conservative to invasive progression. Issues such as upper tract deterioration or recurrent febrile episodes often require more aggressive intervention. The goals of therapy in order of importance include preventing upper tract deterioration, reducing urinary infections, and improving the quality of life of the patient. It is important to identify family members or care givers who can participate in their care, since coexistent depression and lack of motor or cognitive function may impair the treatment plan.

Table 33.3 outlines therapy in each quadrant of dysfunction. For every functional problem (detrusor overactive/underactive and outlet increased resistance/reduced resistance), a behavioral, pharmacologic device, or surgical approach can be considered.

For overactive detrusor (OAB, urge UI, reduced compliance), pelvic muscle exercises, biofeedback, and time voiding with fluid management represent conservative measures as well as adjustment of medications that may worsen the condition such as diuretics. Antimuscarinics are the mainstay of pharmaco-

Table 33.3. Therapeutic strategies based on underlying bladder or outlet pathology. (A) Drug therapies. (B) Surgeries/devices. Therapies often combined

A.

Bladder	Outlet
Overactive	Increased resistance
• Antimuscarinics	• Alpha-1 antagonists
• Tricyclic	• Dantrolene, benzodiazepines, tizanidine
• Investigational- Botulinum toxin to detrusor	• Botulinum toxin to EUS
Underactive	Reduced resistance
• Bethanechol	• Alpha agonist
	• Tricyclic
	• Duloxetine

B.

Bladder	Outlet
Overactive	Increased resistance
• Interstim, neuromodulation	• Urolume stent
• Augmentation cystoplasty	• Sphincterotomy
• Divert	• TURBN
Underactive	Reduced resistance
• Ileovesicostomy	• Bulking agent
• Mitrofanoff	• AUS
• Divert	• Retropubic suspension/ slings
• Myoplasty	• Closure of bladder neck
	• Tricyclic
	• Duloxetine

logic therapy although tricyclics may have a limited role. Botulinum toxin injections into the detrusor can be tried as a nonapproved therapy. InterStim or other forms of neuromodulation are recommended after failure of antimuscarinics and conservative measures. For refractory cases, especially in whom reduced compliance, low capacity, and high DLLPs lead to upper tract changes, augmentation cystoplasty can be performed. Neurolytic procedures have fallen out of favor in part due to subsequent neuroplasticity leading to worsening or unpredictable LUT changes.

For the underactive detrusor (impaired contractility, areflexia), conservative measures such as double voiding, Valsalva voiding, and pelvic muscle relaxation are often of limited use. The mainstay therapy is CIC. However, if this is not feasible, urinary diversion with an ileal conduit or ileovesicostomy can be performed. Indwelling catheters especially suprapubic tubes are gaining resurgence in popularity since studies are showing relative safety in this era of frequent monitoring, antibiotics, and improved catheter care.[49] However, long-term sequelae decades later may prove that 10-year data is insufficient to make long-term recommendations.

For increased outlet resistance (DSD, DISD) pelvic muscle relaxation is often ineffective but can be tried. Alpha adrenergic antagonists might slightly reduce resistance through local and spinal mechanisms. Antispasmodics such as baclofen, benzodiazepines, and tizanidine are mentioned, but no efficacy data is available for oral administration. Injections of botulinum toxin A into the EUS has a role but requires retreatment and may be insufficient to allow complete emptying. Urethral stents have been used with variable short- and long-term success.[50] Traditional therapy for DSD is a sphincterotomy with a hot knife, resectoscope, or laser. However, long-term efficacy is 50%. In part, failures even with repeated sphincterotomies may be due to inadequate resection due to extensive spasticity and hypertrophy of the entire pelvic floor. Moreover, some preserved outlet resistance may be necessary to trigger a spinal micturition reflex. Paradoxically, complete elimination of outlet resistance may not allow triggering of a sustained or repeated reflex thereby causing increases in residual urine.

For reduced outlet resistance due to intrinsic sphincter deficiency, pelvic muscle exercises can be attempted. Bulking agents, except in women with impaired contractility and ISD, have a limited role. Drugs such as alpha adrenergic agonists are rarely effective and may lead to hypertension or stroke. Duloxetine may also have limited utility to raise outlet resistance.[51] Fascial or midurethral slings can be utilized and for severe ISD a circumferential sling may be needed. Sometimes, closure of the urethra or bladder neck is required with either continent or supravesical diversion.

Summary

The lower urinary tract is a window into the nervous system. Neurologic disease often causes failure to retain urine or empty the bladder, sometimes both. Therapy must be planned to preserve upper tracts, avoid urinary infections, and maintain an acceptable quality of life. Such planning may be complex in view of the social, economic, cognitive, and motor deficits that patients with neurogenic bladder present with. A stepwise approach to management with periodic surveillance offers unique challenges to the urologist.

References

1. Lai HH, Boone TB. Urologic management of spinal cord injury. *AUA Update Ser*. 2008;27:234-243
2. McGuire EJ, Woodside JR, Borden TA. Prognostic value of urodynamic testing in myelodysplasia patients. *J Urol*. 1983;126:205-210
3. Wein A. Classification of neurogenic voiding dysfunction. *J Urol*. 1981;125:605-609
4. Steers WD, Gray M. A simple method for teaching about voiding disorders. *BJU Int*. 2006;97(2):238-242
5. Su HC, Polak JM, Mulderry PK, et al. Calcitonin generated peptide immunoreactivity in afferent neurons supplying the urinary tract: combined retrograde tracing and immunohistochemistry. *Neuroscience*. 1986;18: 727-747
6. Vizzard MA, Erdman SL, de Groat WC. Increased expression of neuronal nitric oxide synthase in bladder afferent pathways following chronic bladder irritation. *J Comp Neurol*. 1996;370:191-202
7. Vizzard MA. Up-regulation of pituitary adenylate cyclase-activating polypeptide in urinary bladder pathways after chronic cystitis. *J Comp Neurol*. 2000;420: 335-348
8. Chess-Williams R. Muscarinic receptors of the urinary bladder: detrusor, urothelial and pre-junctional. *Autonom Autacoid Pharmacol*. 2002;22:133-145
9. Andersson KE, Wein AJ. Pharmacology of the lower urinary tract: basis for current and future treatments of urinary incontinence. *Pharmacol Rev*. 2004;56(4):581-631
10. Schurch B, Hauri D, Rodic B, Curt A, Meyer M, Rossier AB. Botulinum-A toxin as a treatment of detrusor-sphincter dyssynergia: a prospective study in 24 spinal cord injury patients. *J Urol*. 1996;155(3):1023-1029
11. Patel AK, Patterson JM, Chapple CR. Botulinum toxin injections for neurogenic and idiopathic detrusor overactivity: a critical analysis of results. *Eur Urol*. 2006; 50(4):684-710
12. Holstege G, Mouton LJ. Central nervous system control of micturition. *Int Rev Neurobiol*. 2003;56:123-145
13. Nadelhaft PL, Vera JPC, Miselis RR. Central nervous system neurons labelled following the injection of pseudorabies virus into the rat urinary bladder. *Neurosci Lett*. 1992;143:271-274

14. Klausner AP, Streng T, Na YG, et al. The role of corticotropin releasing factor and its antagonist, astressin, on micturition in the rat. *Auton Neurosci.* 2005;123:26-35

15. Link C, Lutfey KE, Steers W, McKinlay JB. Is abuse causally related to urologic symptoms? Results from the Boston Area Community Health (BACH) survey. *Eur Urol.* 2007;52:397-456

16. Tibaek S, Gard G, Klarskov P, Iversen HK, Dehlendorff C, Jensen R. Prevalence of lower urinary tract symptoms (LUTS) in stroke patients: a cross-sectional, clinical survey. *Neurourol Urodyn.* 2008;27:763-771

17. Kolominsky-Rabas PL, Hilz MJ, Neundoerfer B, Heuschmann PU. Impact of urinary incontinence after stroke: results from a prospective population-based stroke register. *Neurourol Urodyn.* 2003;22:322-327

18. Marinkovic S, Badlani G. Voiding and sexual dysfunction after cerebrovascular accidents. *J Urol.* 2001;165:359-370

19. Pavlakis AJ, Siroky MB, Goldstein I, Krane RJ. Neurourologic findings in Parkinson's disease. *J Urol.* 1983; 129:80-83

20. Chandiramani VA, Palace J, Fowler CJ. How to recognize patients with Parkinsonism who should not have urological surgery. *Br J Urol.* 1997;80:100-104

21. Salinas JM, Berger Y, De La Rocha RE, Blaivas JG. Urologic evaluation in the Shy Drager syndrome. *J Urol.* 1986;135:741-743

22. Sakakibara R, Hattori T, Uchiyama T, Yamanishi T. Videourodynamic and sphincter motor unit potential analyses in Parkinson's disease and multiple system atrophy. *J Neurol Neurosurg Psychiatry.* 2001;71: 600-606

23. Palace J, Chandiramani VA, Fowler CJ. Value of sphincter electromyography in the diagnosis of multiple system atrophy. *Muscle Nerve.* 1997;20:1396-1403

24. Sakakibara R, Hattori T, Kita K, Arai K, Yamanishi T, Yasuda K. Stress induced urinary incontinence in patients with spinocerebellar degeneration. *J Neurol Neurosurg Psychiatry.* 1998;64:389-391

25. Litwiller SE, Frohman EM, Zimmern PE. Multiple sclerosis and the urologist. *J Urol.* 1999;161(3):743-757.

26. Mori S, Kojima M, Sakai Y, Nakajima K. Bladder dysfunction in dementia patients showing urinary incontinence; evaluation with cystometry. *Jpn J Geriartr.* 1999; 36:489-494

27. Sakakibara R, Kanda T, Sekido T, et al. Mechanism of bladder dysfunction in idiopathic normal pressure hydrocephalus. *Neurourol Urodyn.* 2008;27:507-510

28. Bech RA, Waldemar G, Gjerris F, Klinken L, Juhler M. Shunting effects in patients with idiopathic normal pressure hydrocephalus: correlation with cerebral and leptomeningeal biopsy findings. *Acta Neurochir Wien.* 1999;141:633-639

29. Lu CJ, Tune LE. Chronic exposure to anticholinergic medications adversely affects the course of Alzheimer disease. *Am J Geriatr Psychiatry.* 2003;11:458-461

30. McNeal DM, Hawtrey CE, Wolraich ML, Mapel JR. Symptomatic neurogenic bladder in a cerebral palsy population. *Dev Med Child Neurol.* 1983;25:612-616

31. Drigo F, Seren W, Artibani AM, et al. Neurogenic vesicourethral dysfunction in children with cerebral palsy. *Ital J Neurol Sci.* 1988;80:151

32. Leach GE, Farsaii A, Kark P, Raz S. Urodynamic manifestations of cerebellar ataxia. *J Urol.* 1982;128:348-350

33. Chami N, Miladi HM, Ben S, et al. Continence disorders in hereditary spinocerebellar degeneration: urodynamic findings in 55 cases. *Acta Neurol Belg.* 1984; 84:194-203

34. Vézina JL, Fox AJ. Double blind study of the toxicity of intrathecal iopamidol and metrizamide in lumbar myelography. *J Can Assoc Radiol.* 1984;35(3):257-258

35. Gil-Nagel A, Gapany S, Blesi K, Villanueva N, Bergen D. Incontinence during treatment with gabapentin. *Neurology.* 1997;48:1467-1471

36. Maurice-Williams RS. Micturition symptoms in frontal tumors. *J Neurol Neurosurg Psychiatry.* 1974; 37:431-436

37. Zorn B, Montgomery H, Gray M, Steers W. Urge urinary incontinence and depression. *J Urol.* 1999; 162:82-84

38. Weiss JP, Blaivas JG. Nocturia. *J Urol.* 2000;163(1):5-12

39. Delamarter RB, Bohlman HH, Bodner D, et al. Urologie function after experimental cauda equine. *Spine.* 1990;15:864-870

40. Fanciullacci F, Sandri S, Politi P, Zanollo A. Clinical, urodynamic and neurophysiological findings in patients with neuropathic bladder. *Paraplegia.* 1989;27:354-358

41. Bartolin Z, Vilendecic M, Derezic D. Bladder function after surgery for lumbar intervertebral disk protrusion. *J Urol.* 1999;161:1885-1887

42. Sakakibara R, Hattori T, Yasuda K, Yamanishi T. Micturitional disturbances in acute transverse myelitis. *Spinal Cord.* 1996;34:481-485

43. Berger Y, Blavis JG, Oliver L. Urinary dysfunction in transverse myelitis. *J Urol.* 1990;144:103-105.

44. Hanus T. Other diseases (transverse myelitis, tropical spastic paraparesis, progressive multifocal leukoencephalopathy, Lyme's disease). In: Corcos J, Schick E, eds. *Textbook of the Neurogenic Bladder.* London: Informa; 2003:312-326

45. Broseta E, Osca JM, Morera J, et al. Urological manifestations of herpes zoster. *Eur Urol.* 1993;24:244-247

46. Anger JT, Saigal CS, Litwin MS. The prevalence of urinary incontinence among community dwelling adult women: results from the National Health and Nutrition Examination Survey. *J Urol.* 2006;175(2):601-604

47. Brown JS, Wessels H, Chancellor MB, et al. Urologic outcomes of diabetes. *Diabetes Care.* 2005;28(1):177-185

48. Kershen RT, Boone TB. Peripheral neuropathies of the lower urinary tract following pelvic surgery and radiation therapy. In: Corcos J, Schick E, eds. *Textbook of the Neurogenic Bladder.* London: Informa; 2003: 246-255

49. Feifer A, Corcos J. Contemporary role of suprapubic cystotomy in the treatment of neuropathic bladder dysfunction in spinal cord injured patients. *Neurourol Urodyn.* 2008;27:475-479

50. Chancellor MB, Gajewski J, Ackman CFD, et al. Longterm followup of the North American multicenter UroLume trial for the treatment of external detrusor-sphincter dyssynergia. *J Urol.* 1999;161:1545-1550

51. Norton PA, Zinner NR, Yalcin I, Bump RC. Duloxetine versus placebo in the treatment of stress urinary incontinence. *Am J Obstet Gynecol.* 2002;187:40-48

34

Pelvic Prolapse

Rashel M. Haverkorn and Philippe E. Zimmern

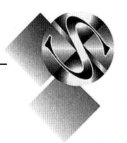

Introduction

Pelvic organ prolapse is a condition in which the pelvic organs are displaced and they protrude by varying degrees into the vaginal canal (ACOG). Affected organs can include the urethra, bladder, rectum, small bowel, uterus, or more commonly, a combination of these pelvic organs. Approximately, 300,000 prolapse surgeries are performed annually in the United States, with an estimated cost of over $1 billion.[1] Several series have estimated that approximately 30–40% of women develop pelvic organ prolapse,[2-4] and the lifetime estimate of surgical risk reaches 11–12% by 80 years of age.[5,6]

In the last few years, this rapidly progressing field has benefited from large-scale studies conducted worldwide, and notably in the United States by the accomplishments of the Pelvic Floor Disease Network (PFDN) of the National Institutes of Health (NIH). Because recurrence is unfortunately common after corrective surgery, with rates approaching 30%, many new techniques using a variety of reinforcing meshes have emerged.[5] A recent FDA warning (October 2008) has reminded patients and physicians alike in cautiously employing mesh until adequate safety and efficacy records are established in randomized trials. While techniques of vaginal repair continue to evolve, newer advances in minimally invasive procedures have become increasingly used widely, with the most recent introduction being the robot. This chapter highlights current areas of controversies and the practical progresses made recently in the field of POP with an emphasis on clinical diagnosis and surgical repair.

Epidemiology

Many factors have been identified as contributing to the development of pelvic organ prolapse, including parity, race, and age (Fig. 34.1). Other medical conditions which are associated with abdominal straining, such as chronic obstructive pulmonary disease and chronic constipation or diseases with connective tissue abnormalities, such as Ehler–Danlos syndrome and Marfan's disease, can lead to greater risk of prolapse.

Prolapse in African American women is less common, while Hispanic females seem to have the highest risk for uterine prolapse.[8] Asian American women are found to have the highest rates of anterior and posterior compartment prolapse.[9,10] A nationwide concern, the trend in obese and overweight adults is increasing. Not only has weight been associated with development of both urge and stress incontinence, but overweight and obese females have been found to have higher risks of prolapse progression as well. Whereas weight loss has been associated with improvement in incontinence, this has not been demonstrated to be true with pelvic organ prolapse.[2,11] Family history plays an important

C.R. Chapple and W.D. Steers (eds.), *Practical Urology: Essential Principles and Practice*,
DOI: 10.1007/978-1-84882-034-0_34, © Springer-Verlag London Limited 2011

Figure 34.1. Model for the development of pelvic floor dysfunction in women (Reprinted from Bump and Norton[7]. Copyright 1998. With permission from Elsevier).

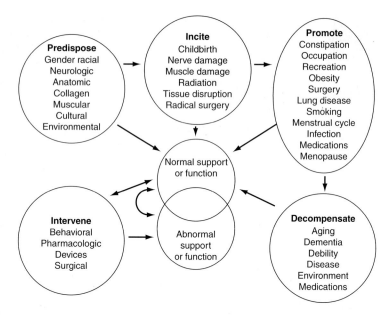

role in many diseases. Positive family history for prolapse was noted in 78% of patients with severe prolapse and 50% of patients with mild prolapse in a study of patients presenting for routine gynecologic care.[12] However, a Swedish twin study examining for the presence of genetic factors in the development of stress incontinence and prolapse noted that genetics may have a contributory role, but that environmental factors remain a strong determinant in the development of prolapse.[13] Occupation may also play a role in prolapse. Several studies have found an association between lower income and less education, with laborers and factory workers having high incidence of severe pelvic organ prolapse.[14] Prior surgery also plays a role with patients having had a previous hysterectomy, particularly by vaginal approach, or prolapse repair at greater risk for developing prolapse.[15]

The strongest associations have been found with advancing age and increased parity. Higher parity confers an 11-fold greater risk in the development of prolapse.[16] Larger babies and number of vaginal deliveries contributed greatly to the presence of prolapse.[3,17] These changes are suspected to be the result of the trauma that occurs during childbirth, characterized by pudendal nerve injury and injury to the muscles, tissues, and nerves of the pelvic floor and perineal body.

Anatomy and Pathophysiology

The pelvic cavity can be divided into anterior, posterior, and apical compartments with respect to the uterus and vagina. The support of the pelvic organs is a result of a combination of the pelvic floor musculature, fascial supports, and suspensory ligaments. The fascial supports and suspensory ligaments are condensations of peritoneum and connective tissues that attach the uterus, cervix, vagina, and urethra at different locations to the fascia of the pelvic sidewall and sacrum, thereby providing distinct levels of support (Fig. 34.2). The uterosacral and cardinal ligaments insert onto the cervix and upper vagina, comprising support at Level I. These ligaments prevent downward descent of the uterus and cervix and are responsible for apical support after hysterectomy. Tears or weakness in Level I support can result in uterine descent or vaginal vault prolapse and apical enterocele. Level II support is comprised of fascial attachments inserting on the midportion of the vagina and urethra, which extend laterally to the obturator internus fascia of the pelvic sidewall at the white line, or arcus tendineus fascia pelvis (ATFP). The lower vagina and urethral tissues are directly attached to surrounding structures, including the perineal body and rectovaginal septum, as Level III support. A defect in Level II or III support results in anterior and/or posterior vaginal wall prolapse, clinically

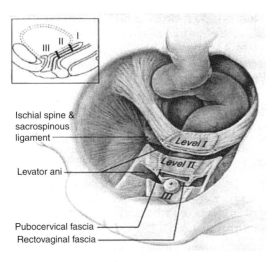

Figure 34.2. Levels of vaginal support (Reprinted from Delancey et al.[18] With permission from Elsevier).

evident as cystocele, rectocele, posterior enterocele, or a combination. The endopelvic fascia and levator ani muscles insert on the perineal body, lifting and supporting the rectum. Detachment or weakness here will produce a mobile and bulging perineum with straining, termed perineocele. Straining can widen the genital hiatus, further decreasing support to the anterior, posterior, and apical compartments, thereby worsening the degree of concomitant prolapse.

The biomechanical properties of connective tissue play an important role in determining the strength of the supporting ligaments and fascia. Smooth muscle, collagen, and elastin are components of connective tissue that impart strength and flexibility to the pelvic fascia and musculature, allowing for changes during pregnancy and childbirth. Dysfunction and alteration of these components are suspected to be contributing factors in the development of prolapse. Surgical biopsies of vaginal epithelium from patients with prolapse have been found to have significantly decreased amounts of smooth muscle in the muscularis layer with increased rates of apoptosis when compared to patients without prolapse.[19] The tensile strength of tissues is the result of its collagen content, with type I collagen primarily responsible for strength and type III collagen responsible for elasticity of the tissues. Alterations in the amount and structure of collagen or in the ratio of types of collagen in pelvic and vaginal tissues account for the

weakness and increased flexibility of pelvic tissues, thereby predisposing to prolapse.[20,21] Additionally, lower elastin expression and altered synthesis has been seen in the vaginal epithelium and uterosacral ligaments.[22,23] Bioengineering of frozen/thawed and fresh vaginal tissues now permits to better understand the deformation of these aging tissues compared to age-comparable controls and to design finite element models of the vaginal wall from which newer reinforcing tissues (biocompatible mesh, tissue engineering) will be developed.[24-26]

Evaluation and Diagnosis

Women with prolapse may complain of a variety of symptoms, including vaginal pressure or fullness, lower back or abdominal pain, incomplete emptying or urinary retention, stress incontinence, constipation or fecal incontinence. Patients with severe pelvic organ prolapse may complain of a vaginal bulge or feeling that something is "falling out" of the vagina. There is no consistent correlation between prolapse symptoms and physical exam findings, other than prolapse 0.5 cm or more beyong the hymen is strongly correlated with bulging symptoms.[27]

The two most employed systems for clinical examination and grading prolapse are the Baden-Walker "half-way" system and the Pelvic Organ Prolapse Quantification (POP-Q). In recent literature, as a result of attempting to reproduce and standardize prolapse grade, the POP-Q has become the predominant grading system. It is a complex system that can be initially challenging to incorporate into practice, but provides detailed information about each compartment that can be useful in patient follow-up.

The Baden-Walker half-way scoring system was introduced in 1972 and consists of a series of stages to quantify vaginal prolapse. It is easy to learn and use, and has good interexaminer reliability. The maximal protruding segment is measured during straining or standing with the reference point being the hymen.

Stage I: the cervix, vaginal apex, anterior or posterior bladder wall descends half-way to the hymen.
Stage II: the cervix, vaginal apex, anterior bladder or posterior wall extends to the lower vagina, but not beyond the hymen.

Stage III: the cervix, vaginal vault, anterior or posterior bladder wall extend beyond the hymen, but is less than half-way completely prolapsed.
Stage IV: the cervix, vaginal vault, anterior or posterior bladder wall extend beyond the hymen, and is more than half-way completely prolapsed.

The Pelvic Organ Prolapse Quantification (POP-Q) system was developed by the International Continence Society (ICS) as an international tool to objectively describe, quantify, and stage pelvic support in women.[28] It divides the vagina into six regions or points measured in centimeters with the reference point being the hymenal ring, consistent and easily identifiable structure that is assigned a measurement of 0. Measurements that are proximal to the hymen are distinguished by negative numbers; likewise, measurements that are distal to the hymen are given positive numbers. Additionally, the genital hiatus, the perineal body, and the total vaginal length are measured to complete the nine points of the system (Figs. 34.3 and 34.4).

Aa: a point in the midline of the anterior vaginal wall that is 3 cm from the hymen
Ba: the point on the anterior vaginal wall which represents the most dependent or prolapsed segment

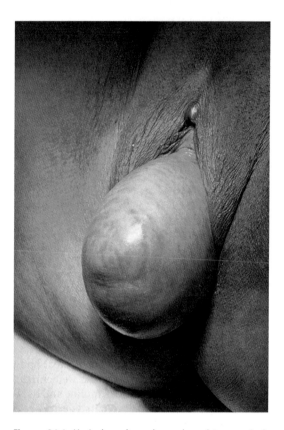

Figure 34.4. Vaginal vault prolapse (complete eversion). According to the POP-Q classification, Aa (point in the midline of the anterior vaginal wall that is 3 cm from the hymen) is approximately 3 cm beyond the hymen. Ap (a point in the midline of the posterior vaginal wall that is 3 cm from the hymen) is also 3 cm beyond the hymen. Point C (the point which represents the most distal surface of the cervix or the vaginal cuff) is approximately 9 cm beyond the hymen. Because point C also represents the most distal prolapsed segments of the anterior and posterior vaginal walls, points Ba and Bp are also assigned values of +9.

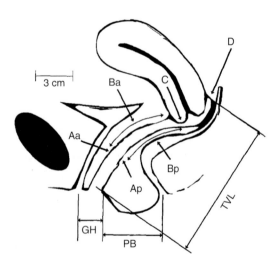

Figure 34.3. Pelvic organ prolapse quantification (POP-Q) scheme. Six points (Aa, Ap, Ba, Bp, C, and D) are labeled. GH represents the genital hiatus, PB represents the length of the perineal body, and TVL represents the total vaginal length (Reprinted from Bump et al.[28] Copyright 1996. With permission from Elsevier).

Ap: a point in the midline of the posterior vaginal wall that is 3 cm from the hymen
Bp: the point on the posterior vaginal wall which represents the most dependent or prolapsed segment
C: the point which represents the most distal surface of the cervix or the vaginal cuff
D: the point which represents the posterior fornix, omitted if the cervix is absent
GH: measured from the external urethral meatus to the midpoint of the posterior hymenal ring
PB: measured from the midpoint of the posterior hymenal ring to the midpoint of the anus
TVL: measured from the hymen to the cervix or vaginal apex in a reduced state

The POP-Q also defines an ordinal staging system for prolapse, which is based upon the maximally protruding segment, and ranges from 0 (no prolapse) to 4 (vaginal eversion). All points must be measured before assigning stage (Table 34.1).

The physical exam should include many of the components of the general exam and should include a thorough pelvic examination and assessment of neurologic status. The pelvic exam is usually performed in dorsal lithotomy position with a full bladder, and may include a standing exam. A bivalved speculum or Sims's retractor is used during the exam to allow inspection of single compartments. Initial exam should include an assessment of inguinal lymph nodes, visual inspection of the external genitalia, assessment of the vaginal mucosa, and notation of estrogen status. The urethral meatus should be inspected for evidence of prolapse or caruncle and the urethra palpated for presence of diverticula or anterior vaginal wall cystic structures. The urethra should also be assessed for hypermobility and for the presence of concomitant stress incontinence. The levator and coccygeus muscles should be palpated for tone and strength of kegel maneuvers evaluated. Examination of the anterior and posterior vaginal walls and cervix/vaginal apex should be performed in a resting state. Each compartment must be examined individually, using the speculum to reduce the other compartments. The compartments are then re-examined individually in a straining state, either during cough or valsalva maneuvers. Sometimes, a rectal exam is necessary to further evaluate for rectocele or posterior enterocele.

Genital sensation should be assessed as part of the neurological evaluation by touch or pinprick. The bulbocavernosus and anal reflexes can be tested by tapping on the clitoris or gently stroking the inside of the thigh and inspecting the anus for subsequent contraction. Anal sphincter tone should be evaluated at the time of rectal exam.

The external components of the POP-Q (genital hiatus, perineal body, and total vaginal length) are measured. Also, notation should be made of vaginal volume particularly if vaginal repairs are considered to avoid narrowing the vaginal vault. Additional assessments can be made using a lubricated Q-tip to quantify urethral hypermobility (degrees at rest and at strain) or by the use of a ring forceps to support the lateral vaginal fornices in evaluating for cystocele (lateral versus central cystocele).

Further imaging or diagnostic testing can be useful to supplement physical exam findings in formulating the diagnosis. Often, urodynamic testing, MRI or CT, fluoroscopic studies, or cystoscopy will be needed to complete the evaluation.

Outcome Measures

Standardization in symptom assessment, physical examination, and outcome measures has been a challenge in the field of female pelvic reconstruction. Despite much effort and attention, there is no uniform system of preoperative or

Table 34.1. States of pelvic organ prolapse. Stages are assigned according to the most severe portion of the prolapsed when the full extent of the protrusion has been demonstrated. (Reprinted from Bump et al.[28] Copyright 1996. With permission from Elsevier)

Stage 0	No prolapse is demonstrated. Points Aa, Ap, Ba, and Bp are all at -3cm and either point C or D is between −TVL cm and −(TVL-2)cm.
Stage I	The criteria for stage 0 are not met, but the most distal portion of the prolpase is >1cm above the level of the hymen (i.e., its quantitation value is <-1cm).
Stage II	The most distal portion of the prolapse is ≤1 cm proximal to or distal to the plane of the hymen (i.e., it quantitation value is ≥−1 cm but ≤+1 cm).
Stage III	The most distal portion of the prolapse is >1cm below the plane of the hymen but protrudes no further than 2cm less than the total vaginal length in cm (i.e., its qunatitation value is >+1cm but <+[TVL-2]cm).
Stage IV	Essentially, complete eversion of the total length of the lower genital tract is demonstrated. The distal portion of the prolapse protrudes to at least (TVL-2)cm (i.e., its quantitation value is ≥+[TVL-2]cm). In most cases, the leading edge of stage IV prolapsed will be the cervix or vaginal cuff scar.

postoperative evaluation in the literature. Progress has been made in adopting the POP-Q grading system for prolapse, but there are many different validated bladder, bowel, and sexual function symptom questionnaires widely in use. Because objective success is often vastly different than patient perception of success, more attention is now being focused on patient symptoms, patient centered goals, and quality of life.

Numerous bladder and bowel specific symptom questionnaires exist, including those which aim to assess related quality of life perception. Most of these questionnaires address voiding symptoms, such as the Urogenital Distress Inventory (UDI) or the Incontinence Impact Questionnaire (IIQ); however, there are questionnaires that are prolapse specific. The Prolapse Quality of Life Questionnaire (P-QOL) is constructed to address the impact of prolapse on several quality of life domains. The Pelvic Floor Distress Inventory (PFDI) and Pelvic Floor Incontinence Questionnaire (PFIQ) incorporate both assessments of prolapse and voiding symptoms and resulting impact on quality of life.

An important part of the initial patient evaluation should be an assessment of patient expectations and goals. Lowenstein et al. evaluated patient goals at initial consultation and repeated an assessment of goals in the same group of patients at follow-up before surgical intervention. The authors found that the "most important" goals changed after the initial visit in 56% of patients from "symptoms," "information," and "treatment" to "treatment" and "emotional" at subsequent visits.[29]

Sexual function is often negatively impacted in patients with pelvic organ prolapse, either as a direct result of the anatomic changes and mechanical difficulties of intercourse or secondarily by coexisting depression. Patients with pelvic organ prolapse are more likely to feel physically and sexually unattractive, more self-conscious, and less confident than their normal counterparts.[30] There are fewer validated sexual function questionnaires, the most commonly employed being the Female Sexual Function Index (FSFI) and the Pelvic Organ Prolapse/Urinary Incontinence Sexual Questionnaire (PISQ). The PISQ addresses bladder and bowel function in addition to sexual function, whereas the FSFI address sexual function alone, examining the domains of desire, arousal, orgasm, and pain.

In identifying objective measures of success, the pad weight test and the voiding diary have often been incorporated as instruments in studies and trials. Both of these measures can be labor intensive and therefore are dependent upon patient compliance. The 3 day voiding diary has been shown to have better patient compliance with more accurate information than the 5 or 7 day diary.[31]

Imaging

A supplement to history and physical exam, pelvic imaging by ultrasound, x-ray studies, or MRI may provide additional anatomic information in prolapse patients, particularly those who have had prior pelvic surgery or prior failed repairs.

The standing cystourethrogram can provide dynamic information in changes in position of the bladder and urethra between rest and straining. It is a readily available modality which requires catheterization with retrograde filling of the bladder with contrast material. Precise measurements of urethal angle and degree/extent of bladder descent can be obtained on lateral views, along with voiding views[32](Figs. 34.5–34.7).

Defecography or culpocystodefecography are specialized imaging techniques requiring instillation of contrast material into the rectum, the bladder, and the vagina. Fluoroscopic images are obtained at rest, at straining, and during defecation/voiding. Interpretation requires a specialized radiologist. Physical examination is not accurate in the detection of rectocele or enterocele, and defecography is used to enhance detection beyond exam.[33] Obstructive defecation correlates well with presence of rectocele on preoperative clinical examination, but not on postoperative exam, and is therefore limited for use in follow-up.[34]

MRI has been recently employed to evaluate the pelvic organs in cases of recurrent or complex prolapse. No standardized technique has been used in performing the study or in measurements/assessment of prolapse; however, MRI has gained wide acceptance thus far (Fig. 34.8). Although the patient is supine and bladder filling is usually not standardized, images can be compared between static and dynamic states and provide exquisite detail of

Figure 34.5. VCUG grading system. Based upon the distance of cystocele descent on lateral cystogram (measured from the inferior edge of the pubic symphysis to inferior edge of the cystocele). (**a**) Stage 0 = inferior edge of cystocele above symphysis; (**b**) stage I = inferior edge <2 cm below inferior edge of symphysis; (**c**) stage II = inferior edge of cystocele 2–5 cm below inferior edge of symphysis; (**d**) stage III = inferior edge of cystocele >5 cm below inferior edge of symphysis.

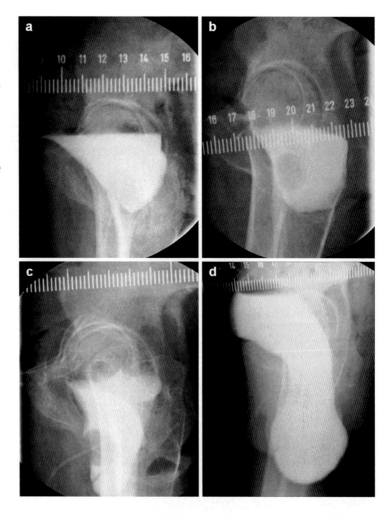

Figure 34.6. Voiding cystoure-throgam (VCUG) for evaluation of prolapse. In addition to staging prolapse, VCUG can give a visual estimate of the size of the pelvic floor defect and resulting pelvic organ herniation. The position of the urethra can also be determined (*left* image is well-supported, *right* image is hypermobile).

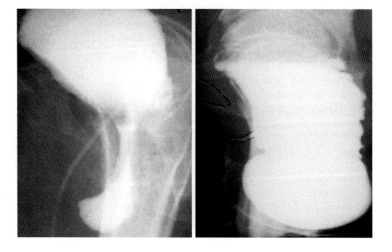

Figure 34.7. VCUG outcome. Preoperative and postoperative voiding views in the same patient documenting resolution of the prolapse and well-supported urethra after repair.

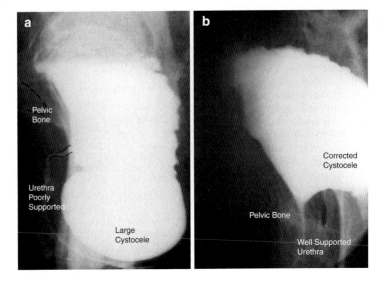

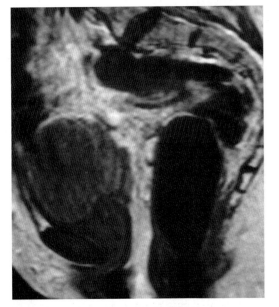

Figure 34.8. MRI of pelvic organ prolapse in a patient complaining of recurrent vaginal bulge, suspected of having a cystocele. The bladder was noted to be well supported by MRI and the bulge represented a large enterocele.

the pelvic organs. MRI is useful in distinguishing the presence of urethral diverticulum or cystic lesions of the urinary or reproductive tracts, as well as in detecting enteroceles, which can be difficult at times to confirm by physical exam alone.

Urodynamics

Urodynamic evaluation in patients with pelvic organ prolapse is aimed at confirming or identifying stress incontinence, which can exist in up to 40% of patients.[35] Stress incontinence is often masked by urethral kinking as a result of the prolapse and may not be detected unless the prolapse is reduced, either on cough stress test or during urodynamics. Obstructive symptoms can also be caused by severe prolapse, with urodynamic parameters demonstrating higher detrusor pressures at peak flow and higher maximum urethral closure pressures.[36] Detrusor overactivity can also be assessed during the filling phase, though the presence of overactivity does not impact the surgical approach employed.

Urodynamic testing should be performed with and without prolapse reduction. Reduction can be effectively achieved using a pessary, ring forceps, a vaginal packing constructed of gauze or swab, or a speculum. The CARE trial demonstrated that the most effective methods of reduction were the forceps, swab, and speculum.[37] Care must be taken to avoid overly aggressive prolapse reduction, which may compress the urethra and prevent demonstration of stress incontinence.

Stress maneuvers should be performed at cystometric capacity for the best chance of eliciting leakage. Urodynamics, using a vaginal pack, unmasked occult stress incontinence in 6–9% of patients with moderate to large cystoceles.[38] However, prior studies have shown that stress incontinence may not be detected by urodynamics in up to 25% of women, and that postoperative stress incontinence may be present as a new finding in 10% of patients after prolapse repair.[39,40] Ballert et al. determined the risk of surgical intervention for anti-incontinence procedure in a patient with no preoperative symptomatic or occult stress incontinence to be 8.3%; the risk of surgical intervention for a patient with clinical stress incontinence not reproduced on urodynamic testing and not receiving a concomitant anti-incontinence procedure at the time of prolapse repair was determined to be approximately 30%.[41] Additionally, the CARE trial noted that a Burch performed at the time of sacrocolpopexy in patients without urodynamically proven leakage significantly reduced postoperative stress incontinence when compared to patients receiving sacrocolpopexy alone.[37]

Indications for Management

Pelvic organ prolapse can be treated in a variety of different ways depending upon symptoms, patient preference, and surgical risk. Approximately, 50% of parous women have prolapse, but most are low grade, asymptomatic or only mildly symptomatic, and only roughly half of the women with symptomatic prolapse desire treatment.[8,15] Pelvic organ prolapse may progress if left untreated; however, many studies document a dynamic state with a process involving both progression and regression over time.[2,4]

Women may base the decision for treatment on severity of symptoms, lifestyle, child-bearing status, sexual activity, or a variety of other reasons. Age, overall health status, and medical comorbidities are other factors that the surgeon should bear in mind when assessing management options. Conservative options or obliterative procedures may be more realistic in a patient who is a borderline or poor surgical candidate with significant symptoms to limit surgical stress and anesthetic time, especially if sexual activity is of no concern. Obesity should not deter from consideration of

an abdominal approach, as a recent randomized trial demonstrated equivalent intermediate term outcomes and perioperative complication rates in obese patients undergoing sacrocolpopexy when compared to nonobese counterparts; however, the difference between these patients lies in exposure and operative time.[42]

Conservative Management of Prolapse

The primary indications for conservative management of pelvic organ prolapse are patient preference for nonsurgical management or comorbidities which make the patient a poor surgical candidate. Pessaries come in a variety of shapes and sizes, and are often constructed of silicone or inert plastic. The pessary is fitted by trial and error and should be comfortable for the patient and retained during valsalva maneuvers and activity. Sexual activity is possible with the pessary in place, depending upon the type of pessary used. Several short-term studies have demonstrated that 75–90% of women were satisfied with a pessary as primary prolapse management.[43,44] Factors associated with unsuccessful pessary placement include hysterectomy, increased parity, prior prolapse procedure, short vaginal length (less than 6 cm), and wide vaginal introitus (four fingerbreadths or more).[44-46] In patients successfully fitted with a pessary, significant improvements in prolapse symptoms, voiding symptoms, and incontinence were noted.[44-46] However, in a study comparing patient-centered goals in patients with prolapse managed surgically versus nonsurgical management, patients treated surgically reported higher satisfaction and goal attainment scores.[47]

Once properly fitted with a pessary, the patient must demonstrate removal and replacement of the pessary. Many patients opt to remove the pessary each evening; however, the pessary may stay in place for up to 6–8 weeks at a time. The pessary should be cleansed with soap and water prior to reinsertion. The patient should be reexamined periodically while using a pessary to evaluate for vaginal abrasions or erosions. If atrophic vaginitis is present, patients should be instructed to use intermittent vaginal estrogen cream to restore the vaginal mucosa. If ulcerations or suspicious lesions are noted, a biopsy should be obtained. Pessary use should be discontinued for noncompliant patients, as, if neglected, severe erosions into the bowel and bladder have been reported.

Additional conservative measures include lifestyle modifications such as weight control and activity limitations, and pelvic floor muscle exercises although no strong conclusive evidence has been demonstrated in the literature to support these measures in managing pelvic organ prolapse. Obese and overweight women do have increased risk of prolapse, noted to be 30–50% higher than their normal-weight counterparts, with the associated risk of prolapse progression in this group of women being increased by 30–70% depending upon prolapsed compartment.[9] Interestingly, a 10% weight loss was not associated with regression.[11] Pelvic floor exercises, or kegel exercises, have been shown to be effective in preventing progression of severe prolapse in one study of elderly Thai women when performed on a daily basis.[48]

Biosynthetics

The application and use of biomaterials and synthetic meshes were introduced to the field of pelvic reconstructive medicine as a response to high rates of prolapse repair failure, seen in up to 30% of cases. Graft materials were employed to augment the repair, in hopes to reinforce and strengthen the affected compartments. The most current literature demonstrates clear advantages in success with the use of mesh grafts in the sacrocolpopexy and midurethral sling for incontinence; however, the evidence supporting use of grafts in anterior and posterior repairs is less compelling.

Grafts can be constructed of a variety of materials, including autografts (rectus fascia or fascia lata), allografts (cadaveric fascia lata, dermis, and dura mater), xenografts (porcine smooth intestinal submucosa and dermis or bovine pericardium and dermis), and synthetic meshes. The success of the graft is dependent upon tissue in-growth and collagen deposition with ensuing complications and failure if the graft is not incorporated or becomes encapsulated.

Xenografts are irradiated or chemically sterilized tissues that are treated to remove their cellular components thereby reducing antigenicity. These materials may be cross-linked to large molecules which stabilize collagen, thereby preventing rapid breakdown by collagenases and cytotoxic host immune responses. However, cross-linking can result in encapsulation of the graft material as tissue in-growth is retarded and the graft is not incorporated. Some of the cross-linked products have pores constructed throughout the graft to aid in host-cell infiltration and collagen deposition. Noncross-linked grafts have better tissue incorporation, but the rapid reaction may cause weakening of the graft. Xenografts and allografts are carefully processed, but carry an estimated one in two million risk of transmitting a viral infection.[49]

Synthetic meshes vary in composition and construction. Pore size and fiber type are physical properties of the mesh that are most important in promoting neovascularization and host cell infiltration, resulting in tissue in-growth. Meshes with pores smaller than 10 μm allow bacterial penetration of the mesh but prevent the entry of macrophages and leukocytes, thereby increasing the risk of infection. Additionally, fibroblasts are unable to traverse the pores and incorporation with collagen deposition is not allowed to occur, placing the material at risk for extrusion. Meshes are constructed from a variety of materials and are available as absorbable, nonabsorbable, monofilament, and multifilament fibers. Multifilament meshes have been found to have more intense lymphoplasmocytic and granulomatous responses with less collagen deposition as compared to monofilament fiber types, reinforcing the idea that monofilament mesh is better incorporated with lower erosion rates.[50] Generally, the monofilament, macroporous polypropylene mesh is the most widely used mesh in pelvic reconstruction due to efficacy and complication rates, with erosion rates estimated at 0–10%.[51]

Synthetic meshes are commercially available for prolapse surgery as sheets of various sizes or as part of a "kit." The prolapse kits are mesh grafts for the anterior or posterior compartments applied transvaginally using a minimally invasive technique. Mesh erosion or infection was the most common complication noted in a systematic review of 3,425 patients undergoing prolapse repair using the mesh kits from 24 studies. Other complications included fistula formation and dyspareunia at rates higher than traditional transvaginal prolapse repairs or sacrocolpopexy.[52] Recently, the FDA has issued a warning regarding the potentially serious

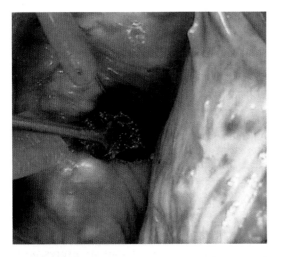

Figure 34.9. Removal of exposed vaginal mesh (extrusion) located under the trigone. This is a difficult location for mesh removal due to potential ureteric injury.

complications of mesh for vaginal surgery. No formal guidelines or recommendations for mesh implantation have followed this warning. It is widely believed that mesh can be beneficial when used in the appropriate, carefully selected, and well-informed patient by an adequately trained surgeon (Fig. 34.9).

Surgical Management

Surgery may be accomplished by a variety of methods according to patient preference and surgeon experience, including vaginal or abdominal approaches, with recent introduction of laparoscopic and robotic assistance furthering the spectrum of minimally invasive techniques available. Concomitant procedures may be performed, as prolapse usually involves more than one compartment and stress incontinence may be addressed in the same setting with sling or suspension techniques. The goal of surgery for pelvic organ prolapse is to restore anatomy, to alleviate prolapse symptoms, and to improve urinary, bowel, and sexual functions.

Anterior Compartment Repair

The approach to cystocele repair depends upon the grade of the prolapse. Higher-grade cystoceles may require additional support from graft or mesh interposition. A variety of techniques exist, each with different approaches to reaching the same goal of restoring anatomy and function. The anterior vaginal wall suspension and the four corner suspension are techniques which allow the vaginal plate itself to act as a support for the bladder base. This addresses concomitant stress incontinence secondary to proximal urethra/bladder neck hypermobility. These techniques are a modification of various bladder neck suspensions, using principles borrowed from the Pereyra and Raz suspension procedures.

Depending upon the defective structure, cystoceles can be classified as either lateral or central/midline. The central or midline cystocele results from weakened or damaged pubocervical fascia, allowing the bladder to prolapse through the anterior vaginal wall. A lateral cystocele forms when the arcus tendineus fascia pelvis (ATFP) is torn or is weakened with subsequent loss of support to the bladder and lateral vaginal fornices, resulting in prolapse through the anterior vaginal wall. Lateral vaginal wall detachments are recognized by loss of the lateral sulci and midline vaginal rugae, as well as elongation of the vaginal wall. The goal of the anterior colporraphy is to eliminate the central defect by reapproximating the pubocervical fascia over the midline and return the bladder to its original anatomic position. It does not address the lateral paravaginal defect and may, in fact, worsen it. The goal of the paravaginal repair is to support the lateral vaginal edges to the arcus tendineus fascia pelvis (ATFP). Mesh may be used to correct cystocele defects or to augment the cystocele repair (Fig. 34.10).

Uterine/Apical Prolapse

Vaginal vault prolapse represents the extreme end of the spectrum in pelvic organ prolapse, rarely but occasionally presenting as total vaginal eversion. Indications for intervention are driven mainly by the severity of symptoms and extent of prolapse. The vaginal mucosa can become irritated and ulcerated due to displacement and friction from undergarments and physical activity. The goal in any vault prolapse repair is to restore the normal axis, position, and function of the vagina. This may

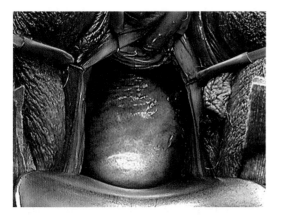

Figure 34.10. Cystocele formation several years after a prior anti-incontinence procedure. Correction of the anterior vaginal wall laxity at the time of the initial incontinence procedure might have avoided this secondary problem.

be accomplished by either transvaginal or abdominal techniques depending upon the degree of prolapse and need for concomitant procedures. The success of surgery is dependent upon securing the vaginal cuff to a fixed point in the pelvis, such as the sacral promontory or the sacrospinous ligament. Apical prolapse can be successfully performed in a transvaginal technique, by suspending the cuff to the sacrospinous or uterosacral ligaments. In those women with high-grade prolapse who have failed prior transvaginal repair or who have foreshortened or narrow vaginas, an

abdominal approach using mesh interposition is indicated. With advances in minimally invasive techniques, the open sacrocolpopexy can be performed using laparoscopic or robotic instruments (Fig. 34.11).

The ideal management of uterine prolapse includes hysterectomy; however, due to age, desire to maintain future fertility, or cultural influences, some women may choose to pursue uterine preservation with suspension. The goals of uterine suspension are identical to those of vaginal vault suspension and aim to restore uterine support and the normal position and function of the vagina, bladder, and bowels. The uterus is suspended from a fixed point in the pelvis by mesh support, as in sacral hysteropexy or to ligamentous structures, as in sacrospinous hysteropexy. These approaches may also be performed vaginally or through an open approach. Older and less commonly performed approaches involve cervical amputation with attachment of ligaments to the remaining uterine segments or plication of the uterine ligaments with suspension to the rectus sheath.

Enterocele Repair

Often associated with other prolapsing compartments, enteroceles are the herniation of omentum or small bowel into the pouch of Douglas. There are four mechanisms for entero-

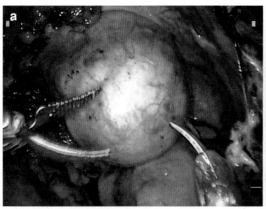 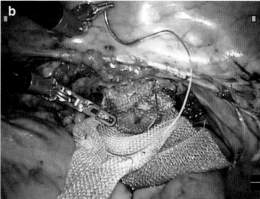

Figure 34.11. (a) Robotic-assisted sacrocolpopexy. While a bowel sizer is inserted into the vagina to easily locate the cuff and place it on tension, the peritoneum overlying the cuff is incised and the bladder and rectum are dissected off the cuff.

(b) Marlex mesh strips are attached to the anterior and posterior surfaces of the vaginal cuff and subsequently to the promontory to suspend the cuff in a tension-free manner.

cele development: congenital, iatrogenic, traction, and pulsion. Congenital enteroceles are the result of failure of the rectovaginal septum to completely fuse, leaving an open cul-de-sac or pouch of Douglas, which fills with small bowel and omentum. Pulsion enteroceles develop in response to conditions leading to chronically elevated intra-abdominal pressures, such as obesity and obstructive airway diseases, particularly after hysterectomy. Contents of the peritoneum may be pulled down along with other prolapsing compartments or the uterus in what is termed a traction enterocele. Iatrogenic enteroceles are due to alterations in the vaginal axis created by surgical procedures for prolapse and incontinence (as in the Burch procedure, for example). The cul-de-sac is left open by the change in vaginal axis, allowing development of the enterocele. This can be addressed in a prophylactic manner at the time of the prolapse or incontinence procedure to prevent enterocele formation from occurring at a later date.

The goals of enterocele repair are to reduce the contents and ligate neck of the herniated peritoneal sac. Therefore, the principles of enterocele repair are: (1) identification of the contents of the enterocele, (2) mobilization of the enterocele with excision of the peritoneal sac, (3) high suture ligation of the peritoneal sac, and (4) closure of the defect by providing support below the peritoneal sac and restoration of the normal vaginal axis[53] (Fig. 34.12). Enterocele repair usually occurs in combination with additional prolapse procedures, and can be effectively performed either by an abdominal or vaginal approach.

Conclusion

Pelvic organ prolapse is a relatively common condition with varying degrees of symptomatology. This chapter is meant to provide an overview of the epidemiology, evaluation, diagnosis (including supplemental studies), and treatment of prolapse. Treatment is generally based upon patient assessment of degree of bother from prolapse, and ranges from conservative options such as pessary and/or pelvic floor muscle therapy to surgical options, with or without the use of mesh grafts. Synthetic mesh has become a hot topic with a recent FDA statement that encourages physicians to exercise caution in regard to mesh implantation due to complications requiring mesh removal and not uncommonly, extensive urinary tract or pelvic floor reconstruction.

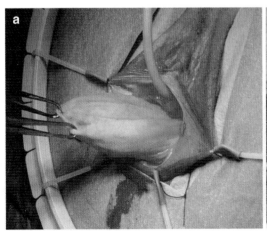 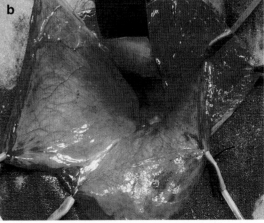

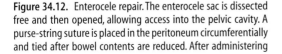

Figure 34.12. Enterocele repair. The enterocele sac is dissected free and then opened, allowing access into the pelvic cavity. A purse-string suture is placed in the peritoneum circumferentially and tied after bowel contents are reduced. After administering IV indigo carmine, cystoscopy is performed to confirm ureteral integrity. Excess sac is excised. Before the vaginal incisions are closed, a vault fixation procedure is performed.

References

1. Subak L, Waetjen L, Eeden Svd, Thom D, Vittinghoff E, Brown J. Cost of pelvic organ prolapse surgery in the United States. *Obstet Gynecol.* 2001;98:646-651

2. Bradley C, Zimmerman M, Qi Y, Nygaard I. Natural history of pelvic organ prolapse in postmenopausal women. *Obstet Gynecol.* 2007;109(4):848-854

3. Nygaard I, Bradley C, Brandt D. Pelvic organ prolapse in older women: prevalence and risk factors. *Obstet Gynecol.* 2004;104(3):489-497

4. Handa V, Garrett E, Hendrix S, Gold E, Robbins J. Progression and remission of pelvic organ prolapse: a longitudinal study of menopausal women. *Am J Obstet Gynecol.* 2004;190:27-32

5. Olsen A, Smith V, Bergstrom J, Colling J, Clark A. Epidemiology of surgically managed pelvic organ prolapse and urinary incontinence. *Obstet Gynecol.* 1997;89(4):501-506

6. Fialkow M, Newton K, Lentz G, Weiss N. Lifetime risk of surgical management for pelvic organ prolapse or urinary incontinence. *Int Urogynecol J.* 2008;19:437-440

7. Bump RA, Norton PA. Epidemiology and natural history of pelvic floor dysfunction. *Obstet Gynecol Clin North Am.* 1998;25(4):723-746

8. Rortveit G, Brown J, Thom D, Eeden SVD, Creasman J, Subak L. Symptomatic pelvic organ prolapse: prevalence and risk factors in a population-based, racially diverse cohort. *Obstet Gynecol.* 2007;109(6):1396-1403

9. Hendrix S, Clark A, Nygaard I, Aragaki A, Barnabei V, McTiernan A. Pelvic organ prolapse in the Women's Health Inititative: gravity and gravidity. *Am J Obstet Gynecol.* 2002;186:1160-1166

10. Sewell C, Chang E, Sultana C. Prevalence of genital prolapse in 3 ethnic groups. *J Reprod Med.* 2007;52(9):769-773

11. Kudish B, Iglesia C, Sokol R, et al. Effect of weight change on natural history of pelvic organ prolapse. *Obstet Gynecol.* 2009;113(1):81-88

12. McLennan M, Harris J, Kariuki B, Meyer S. Family history as a risk factor for pelvic organ prolapse. *Int Urogynecol J.* 2008;19:1063-1069

13. Altman D, Frosman M, Falconer C, Lichtenstein P. Genetic influence on stress urinary incontinence and pelvic organ prolapse. *Eur Urol.* 2008;54:918-923

14. Woodman P, Swift S, O'Boyle A, et al. Prevalence of severe pelvic organ prolapse in relation to job description and socioeconomic status: a multi-center cross-sectional study. *Int Urogynecol J Pelvic Floor Dysfunct.* 2006;17(4):340-345

15. Swift S. The distribution of pelvic organ support in a population of female subjects seen for routine gynecologic health care. *Am J Obstet Gynecol.* 2000;183(2):277-285

16. Mant J, Painter R, Vessey M. Epidemiology of genital prolapse: observations from the oxford family planning association study. *Br J Obstet Gynaecol.* 1997;104:579-585

17. Lukacz E, Lawrence J, Contreras R, Nager C, Luber K. Parity, mode of delivery, and pelvic floor disorders. *Obstet Gynecol.* 2006;107(6):1253-1260

18. Delancey JO et al. Anatomic aspects of vaginal eversion. *Am J Obstet Gynecol.* 1992;166(6 pt 1):1717-1724

19. Badiou W, Granier G, Bousquet P, Monrozies X, Mares P, Tayrac RD. Comparative histological analysis of anterior vaginal wall in women with pelvic organ prolapse or control subjects: a pilot study. *Int Urogynecol J.* 2008;19:723-729

20. Jackson S, Avery N, Tartlton V, Eckford S, Abrams P, Bailey A. Changes in metabolism of collagen in genitourinary prolapse. *Lancet.* 1996;347(9016):1658-1661

21. Moalli P, Talarico L, Sung V, et al. Impact of menopause on collagen subtypes in the arcus tenineous fasciae pelvis. *Am J Obstet Gynecol.* 2004;190:620-627

22. Klutke J, Ji Q, Campeau J, et al. Decreased endopelvic fascia elastin content in uterine prolapse. *Acta Obstet Gynecol.* 2008;87:111-115

23. Karam J, Vazquez D, Lin V, Zimmern P. Elastin expression and elastic fibre width in the anterior vaginal wall of postmenopausal women with and without prolapse. *BJU.* 2007;100:346-350

24. Goh JT. Biomechanical properties of prolapsed vaginal tissue in pre- and postmenopausal women. *Int Urogynecol J Pelvic Floor Dysfunct.* 2002;13(2):76-79; discussion 79

25. Cosson M, Lambaudie E, Boukerrou M, Lobry P, Crepin G, Ego A. A biomechanical study of the strength of vaginal tissues. Results on 16 post-menopausal patients presenting with genital prolapse. *Eur J Obstet Gynecol Reprod Biol.* 2004;112(2):201-205

26. Zimmern PE, Eberhart RC, Bhatt A. Methodology for biomechanical testing of fresh anterior wall vaginal samples from postmenopausal women undergoing cystocele repair. *Neurourol Urodyn.* 2009;28(4):325-329

27. Gutman R, Ford D, Quiroz L, Shippey S, Handa V. Is there a pelvic organ prolapse threshold that predicts pelvic floor symptoms? *Am J Obstet Gynecol.* 2008;6:683.e681-683.e687

28. Bump RC, Mattiasson A, Bo K, et al. The standardization of terminology of female pelvic organ prolapse and pelvic floor dysfunction. *Am J Obstet Gynecol.* 1996;175(1):10-17

29. Lowenstein L, Kenton K, Peirce K, FitzGerald M, Mueller E, Brubaker L. Patients' pelvic goals change after initial urogynecologic consultation. *Am J Obstet Gynecol.* 2007;197:640.e641-640.e643

30. Jelovsek J, Barber M. Women seeking treatment for advanced pelvic organ prolapse have decreased body image and quality of life. *Am J Obstet Gynecol.* 2006;194:1455-1461

31. Dmochowski RR, Sanders SW, Appell RA, Nitti VW, Davila GW. Bladder-health diaries: an assessment of 3-day vs 7-day entries. *BJU Int.* 2005;96(7):1049-1054

32. Showalter P, Zimmern P, Roehrborn C, Lemack G. Standing cystourethrogram: an outcome measure after anti-incontinence procedures and cystocele repair in women. *Urology.* 2001;58:33-37

33. Groenendijk A, Hulst Vvd, Birnie E, Bonsel G. Correlation between posterior vaginal wall defects assessed by clinical examination and by defecography. *Int Urogynecol J.* 2008;19:1291-1297

34. Finco C, Savastano S, Luongo B, et al. Colpocy-stodefecography in obstructed defecation: is it really useful to the surgeon? Correlating clinical and radiological findings in surgery for obstructed defecation. *Colorectal Dis.* 2007;10:446-452

35. Grody M. Urinary incontinence and concomitant prolapse. *Clin Obstet Gynecol.* 1998;41:777-785

36. Long C, Hsu S, Wu T, Sun D, Su J, Tsai E. Urodynamic comparison of continent and incontinent women with severe urogenital prolapse. *J Reprod Med.* 2004;49(1):33-37

37. Brubaker L, Cundiff G, Fine P, et al. Abdominal sacrocolpopexy with Burch colposuspension to reduce urinary stress incontinence. *N Engl J Med.* 2006;354(15):1557-1566

38. Gilleran J, Lemack G, Zimmern P. Reduction of moderate to large cystocele during urodynamic evaluation using a vaginal gauze pack: 8-year experience. *Br J Urol.* 2005;97:292-295

39. Glazener C, Lapitan M. Urodynamic investigations for management of urinary incontinence in children and adults. *Cochrane Database Syst Rev.* 2002; Issue 3, Art. No. CD003195. doi: 10.1002/14651858.CD003195

40. Maher C, Baessler K, Glazener C, Adams E, Hagen S. Surgical management of pelvic organ prolapse in women. *Cochrane Database Syst Rev.* 2007; Issue 3, Art. No. CD004014. doi: 10.1002/14651858.CD004014.pub.3

41. Ballert K, Biggs G, Isenalumhe A, Rosenblum N, Nitti V. Managing the urethra at transvaginal pelvic organ prolapse repair: a urodynamic approach. *J Urol.* 2009;181:679-684

42. Bradley C, Kenton K, Gao X, Zyczynski H, Weber A, Nygaard I. Obestiy and outcomes after sacrocolpopexy. *Am J Obstet Gynecol.* 2008;199(6):690.e691-690.e698

43. Clemons J, Aguilar V, Tillinghast T, Jackson N, Myers D. Patient satisfaction and changes in prolapse and urinary symptoms in women who were fitted successfully with a pessary for pelvic organ prolapse. *Am J Obstet Gynecol.* 2004;190:1025-1029

44. Maito J, Quam Z, Craig E, Danner K, Rogers R. Predictors of successful pessary fitting and continued use in a nurse-midwifery pessary clinic. *J Midwifery Womens Health.* 2006;51:78-84

45. Fernando R, Thakar R, Sultan A, Shah S, Jones P. Effect of vaginal pessaries on symptoms associated with pelvic organ prolapse. *Obstet Gynecol.* 2006;108(1):93-99

46. Clemons J, Aguilar V, Tillinghast T, Jackson N, Myers D. Risk factors associated with an unsuccessful pessary fitting trial in women with pelvic organ prolapse. *Am J Obstet Gynecol.* 2004;190:345-350

47. Barber M, Walters M, Cundiff G. Responsiveness of the Pelvic Floor Distress Inventory (PFDI) and Pelvic Floor Impact Questionnaire (PFIQ) in women undergoing vaginal urgery and pessary treatment for pelvic organ prolapse. *Am J Obstet Gynecol.* 2006;194:1492-1498

48. Piva-Anant M, Therasakvichya S, Leelaphatanadit C, Techantrisak K. Integrated health research program for the Thai elderly: prevalence of genital prolapse and effectiveness of pelvic floor exercise to prevent worsening of genital prolapse in elderly women. *J Med Assoc Thai.* 2003;86(6):509-515

49. Simonds R, Holmberg S, Hurwitz R, et al. Transmission of human immunodeficiency virus type 1 from a sero-negative organ and tissue donor. *N Engl J Med.* 1992;326(11):726-732

50. Riccetto C, Miyaoka R, DeFraga R, et al. Impact of the structure of polypropylene meshes in local tissue reaction: in vivo stereological study. *Int Urogynecol J Pelvic Floor Dysfunct.* 2008;19(8):1117-1123

51. Huebner M, Hsu Y, Fenner D. The use of graft materials in vaginal pelvic floor surgery. *Int J Gynecol Obstet.* 2006;92:279-288

52. Diwadkar G, Barber M, Feiner J, Maher C, Jelovsek J. Complication and reoperation rates after apical vaginal prolapse surgical repair: a systematic review. *Obstet Gynecol.* 2009;113(2):367-373

53. Nichols D, Randall C. *Vaginal Surgery.* 4th ed. Baltimore, MD: Williams & Wilkins; 1996

35

Urinary Tract Fistula

Brett D. Lebed and Eric S. Rovner

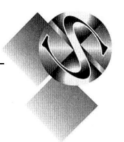

Introduction

A fistula is defined as an extra-anatomic communication between two or more epithelial or mesothelial lined body cavities or the skin surface. Fistula can occur as a result of congenital anomalies, malignancy, inflammation or infection, tissue trauma, or iatrogenic causes, such as surgical injury or radiation. There have been reports of fistula formation since ancient times, involving connections from the urinary tract to a myriad of bodily cavities and organs. Organ systems immediately adjacent to the urinary tract are the most commonly affected, specifically the reproductive, gastrointestinal, and vascular systems. Presenting signs and symptoms of urinary fistula are dependent on the termination point of the fistula, the fistula size, concomitant infection or inflammatory processes, and associated malignancy or other medical conditions.

The principles of general fistula management are applicable to all urinary tract fistulas and should be addressed prior to any planned intervention. Issues of nutrition, infection, and malignancy can significantly alter risk factors for initial fistula formation, the approach to repair, and the risk of recurrence following a given intervention. As most urinary fistulas in the industrialized world are iatrogenic, prevention of fistula development is paramount. Intraoperative and early identification of urinary tract injury allows for immediate management and minimizes the possibility of a fistula.

As a fistula is almost always an unexpected occurrence , the treating physician must also be aware of the potential for medicolegal implications, as well as the considerable physical, emotional, and psychological distress which accompanies the diagnosis.

Once the diagnosis is established, the etiology of the fistula is determined, and complications such as skin breakdown are addressed, definitive therapy is pursued. Although some fistula might respond to conservative management, surgery is often necessary for definitive repair. The principles of management and surgical intervention are outlined in Table 35.1. Surgical repair of urinary fistula is associated with a high rate of success. The finding of a persistent fistula following surgical intervention may suggest the existence of other complicating host factors such as malignancy, nutritional deficiency, poor tissue quality, or surgical factors such as inadequate urinary drainage or relief of obstruction, or technical problems with the actual operation.

Urogynecologic Fistula

Vesicovaginal Fistula

Vesicovaginal fistula (VVF) are the most common acquired fistula of the urinary tract.[1] It is defined as a communication between the bladder and vagina, resulting in continuous urinary

Table 35.1. Principles of treatment and surgical repair of a urinary tract fistula

Nutritional optimization
Elimination of infection
Evaluation for malignancy
Adequate exposure of the fistula tract
Debridement of devitalized or ischemic tissue
Careful dissection to maintain separation of involved organ cavities and hemostasis
Removal of foreign bodies or synthetics
Repair with well-vascularized healthy tissue flaps
Multiple layer closure with nonoverlapping tension-free suture lines
Removal of distal obstruction
Maintain adequate urinary tract drainage
Awareness of medicolegal implications

leakage. Descriptions of vesicovaginal fistulas have been well documented since ancient times, although early attempts at repair met with little success. In 1852, Sims published his method for the surgical treatment of VVF using a transvaginal approach, followed by Trendelenburg in 1888, who successfully performed the transabdominal VVF repair.[2,3]

Etiology and Risk Factors

The etiology and prevalence of VVF differ in various parts of the world. In the industrialized world, the most common cause of VVF is iatrogenic injury during gynecologic, urologic, or other pelvic surgery, accounting for greater than 75% of cases.[2,4,5] Hysterectomy is the most common procedure associated with lower urinary tract injury, with most of the remainder a result of general surgical pelvic procedures, urogynecological procedures such as anterior colporrhaphy, cystocele repair, or incontinence surgery, or other urologic procedures.[6] In a study of 207 VVF repairs by Eilber et al., the cause was reported as 83% from abdominal hysterectomy, 8% from vaginal hysterectomy, 4% from radiation, and miscellaneous in 5%.[7]

The overall rate for iatrogenic bladder injury at the time of hysterectomy is between 0.5% and 1.0%, while the incidence of fistula is approximately 0.1–0.2%.[8,9] The primary risk factor for the development of VVF following hysterectomy appears to be intraoperative injury. Iatrogenic cystotomy, tissue necrosis from cauterization injury, or suture placement through both the bladder and vaginal wall can predispose to postoperative fistula formation. Tissue ischemia and necrosis lead to fibrosis and inflammation between the bladder and vagina, eventually allowing formation of an epithelialized tract. This most commonly occurs at the apex of the vagina at the level of the vaginal cuff.[10] Preoperative risk factors include prior cesarean section or uterine surgery, endometriosis, infection, diabetes, arteriosclerosis, pelvic inflammatory disease, and prior pelvic radiation.[11] Additionally, abdominal hysterectomy is three times more likely to result in bladder injury compared to vaginal hysterectomy.

In the industrialized world, radiation is also a significant cause of complicated urinary tract fistula. The incidence of radiation-induced fistula is dependent on the type, dose, and location of radiation, as well as the specific malignancy undergoing treatment. Urinary fistula rates of 1.6% have been reported following radiation treatment for cervical carcinoma.[12] VVF from radiation may occur as long as several decades following treatment.[13] Biopsy of the fistula tract should be strongly considered prior to any definitive therapy. Malignancy-induced VVFs can occur with locally advanced cervical, vaginal, and endometrial carcinomas and account for approximately 3% of fistulas.[14]

In the developing, nonindustrialized world, VVF most commonly results from complications of childbirth. The incidence of obstetric fistula in developing countries is approximately 0.3–0.4% of deliveries, or between 1 and 4 per 1,000 vaginal deliveries.[15,16] Routine prenatal and perinatal obstetrical care is limited, as is access to general healthcare. Additionally, pelvic size may be small due to poor nutritional status and/or an early age of marriage and conception.[17] Prolonged obstructed labor due to cephalopelvic disproportion can cause pressure necrosis of the anterior vaginal wall, bladder, bladder neck, and proximal urethra. The "obstructed labor injury complex" which occurs in such individuals includes variable degrees of urethral loss, stress incontinence, renal failure, vesicovaginal fistula, rectovaginal fistula, rectal atresia, anal sphincter incompetence, vaginal stenosis, osteitis pubis, and foot drop.[18] Obstetric fistulas tend to be larger than traditional VVF, with necrosis of large parts of the anterior or posterior vaginal wall and/or urethra, distally near the true pelvis and pubis. Repair can be exceedingly complicated due to the large areas of necrosis and poor adjacent tissue quality.

Clinical Factors

Evaluation and Diagnosis

The most common presentation for vesicovaginal fistula is persistent, continuous urinary drainage from the vagina. The amount of drainage is variable and may be directly related to the size of the fistula tract. Pain is uncommon, but can be present in cases with extensive skin irritation or prior radiation. VVF should be distinguished from urinary incontinence due to other causes including stress, urge, and overflow incontinence, as well as ureterovaginal or urethrovaginal fistula.

Iatrogenic VVF from surgical intervention most commonly present 1–3 weeks following the initial procedure, or following removal of the foley catheter. Radiation-induced VVFs can present months to years following therapy. While patients may experience clear or serous vaginal drainage following pelvic procedures, if fistula is suspected, the prolonged discharge can be tested for creatinine and urea. The diagnosis can be established from a thorough history and physical examination, incorporating pelvic examination, endoscopic, and radiologic methods to evaluate the presence, size, and location of the fistula tract (Fig. 35.1).

Pelvic Examination A bimanual pelvic exam and bi-valved speculum evaluation should be performed in cases of suspected VVF. Relevant vaginal anatomy, including depth, prolapse, atrophy, and introital size can affect the decision of surgical approach (Fig. 35.2). The visual and manual assessment of tissue quality, scarring, and inflammation may dictate the timing of repair. For example, acute inflammation and infection at the vaginal cuff may mitigate against an immediate repair until such tissues are treated medically and optimized. Vaginal atrophy should be documented and treated with estrogen cream prior to definitive repair, optimizing the quality of potential vaginal wall flaps. Identification of prior abdominal, perineal, thigh, or vaginal scars are necessary to evaluate for tissues that would provide less favorable reconstructive flaps.

The location of the post-hysterectomy VVF is most commonly on the anterior vaginal wall, near the vaginal cuff. Visualization can occasionally be difficult, as there can be many dimples or folds in the area of the vaginal cuff. Instillation of a vital blue dye, such as indigo

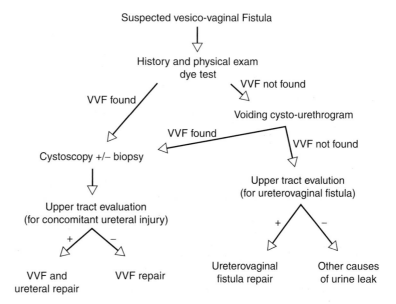

Figure 35.1. Algorithm for diagnosis and management of vesicovaginal fistula.

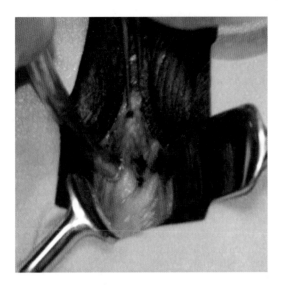

Figure 35.2. Proximal vesicovaginal fistula.

carmine or methylene blue, can assist in identi-fication small or occult fistula tracts (Table 35.2).[19] Double dye or tampon tests may confirm the diagnosis of a urinary fistula and indicate the possibility of primary/concomitant ureterovaginal or urethrovaginal fistula.[20,21]

Cystoscopy An endoscopic evaluation should be performed in all patients with suspected VVF. Immature fistulas are usually surrounded by bullous edema and do not have a distinct ostia.

Mature fistulas are variably sized with smooth, distinct margins. In many cases, especially from iatrogenic VVF, the fistula site will be located at the posterior bladder wall, frequently with multiple pits present, making it difficult to localize the specific tract. In cases where identification of the fistula is difficult, cystoscopic passage of a guide wire via the fistula tract can confirm the exact location of the fistula within the bladder and the vagina.

Imaging Evaluation of VVF should include both bladder and upper tract imaging. A voiding cysto-urethrogram (VCUG) may objectively determine the presence and location of the fistula tract. With bladder filling, the contrast will opacify the vagina, usually best seen in a lateral image projection. Voiding images are occasionally necessary to visualize small VVF, as the increase in intravesical pressure will facilitate fistula drainage. A complete VCUG in the evaluation of VVF includes filling, voiding, and drainage films in multiple projections (A-P, lateral, and oblique). A CT cystogram may be utilized for the evaluation of VVF in certain centers.

Ureteral injury or ureterovaginal fistulas can be present in up to 12% of postsurgical VVF; therefore, upper-tract evaluation is obtained routinely.[22] This can be accomplished easily and successfully with intravenous urography, CT

Table 35.2. Commonly utilized procedures during patient examination for the evaluation of stress urinary incontinence, vesicovaginal fistula, and urethrovaginal fistula

Test	Vaginal packing	Dye	Provacative maneuvers	Diagnosis
Marshall-Bonney	No	Intravesical indigo carmine/methylene blue	Cough	Visualize leak with cough = Stress incontinence
Intravaginal pad test	Yes	Intravesical indigo carmine/methylene blue	None	Distal pad blue = Stress incontinence or urethrovaginal fistula
				Proximal pad blue = VVF
Double dye test	Yes	Intravesical indigo carmine/methylene blue oral pyridium	None	Distal pad blue = stress incontinence or urethrovaginal fistula
				Middle/proximal pad blue = VVF
				Upper pad orange = Uretero-vaginal fistula

urography, or MR urography. Retrograde pyelo-grams may be utilized if the distal ureter is not well visualized, and a concomitant ureterovaginal fistula is suspected but has not been demonstrated on alterative upper urinary-tract imaging.[1,11] Delayed visualization of contrast within the vagina on CT urogram or direct contrast extravasation into the fistula tract on CT cystogram provide alternate means of evaluation, with the added ability to detect additional intra-abdominal pathology.[23]

Treatment

The goal of treatment of VVF should be the timely and complete cessation of urinary leakage with minimal effect on normal urinary and genital function.

Conservative Management　Conservative management of small VVF can be attempted prior to surgical intervention. Although there is some morbidity and discomfort associated with indwelling catheterization, a trial of continuous bladder drainage and anticholinergic medication for 2–3 weeks can be associated with spontaneous healing in properly selected patients.[24] Small epithelialized fistulas may benefit from minimally invasive cystoscopic electrocoagulation of the fistula tract, followed by bladder catheterization. In patients with fistula diameter less than 3.5 mm, 11/15 had successful fistula tract ablation with cauterization and catheter drainage in a study by Stovsky et al.[25] Fibrin sealant has also been utilized with some success to plug the fistula tract, presumably until tissue ingrowth occurs.[26] In general, conservative measures are successful in small fistulas only, less than 2–3 mm in diameter.

Surgical Management　Once the decision has been made by the patient and physician to pursue definitive surgical repair, it is essential to carefully plan an operative approach that will maximize the chance of success. The first attempt at VVF repair is usually the best opportunity for fistula closure, due to later scarring and anatomical distortion. There is no "best" approach for VVF repair as long as the basic principles are followed.

Classic teaching suggests a minimal waiting period of several months after diagnosis for definitive repair; however, delayed management has fallen out of favor over the past few decades. Immediate management, especially in cases of uncomplicated iatrogenic fistula, can minimize patient discomfort and anguish without compromising the surgical repair.[11,27-33] However, in cases of continued infection, obstetric fistula, or radiation-induced fistula, demarcation of inflamed or devascularized tissues may require a waiting period of 1–6 months and 6–12 months, respectively.[18,34,35] Medical factors and wound care also should be addressed and optimized prior to intervention in these and all other fistula cases.

Vesicovaginal fistula can be repaired via a transvaginal or transabdominal approach. Each approach has benefits and drawbacks, but each results in traditionally high rates of successful fistula closure, usually greater than 90% (Table 35.3).[7,36-38] Consideration of factors such as size, location, and need for adjunctive procedures can affect the approach, but

Table 35.3. Surgical management of vesicovaginal fistula. Comparison of transabdominal and transvaginal approaches to repair

Approach	Transabdominal	Transvaginal
Timing	Delayed (3–6 month)	Immediate/delayed
Ureteral involvement	Reimplant possible if indicated	No reimplant possible
Sexual function	No change in vaginal depth	Risk of vaginal shortening
Flaps	Omental, peritoneal	Labial, peritoneal, gluteal, gracilis
Indications	Large fistula, high fistula in narrow vault, radiation, failed vaginal approach, other procedures (augment)	Low fistulas, failed TAFR
Morbidity	High	Low

the most important factor should be surgeon experience and comfort. Surgical mobilization of well-vascularized flaps, followed by a separate water-tight closure of the urinary and genital tracts with nonoverlapping suture lines is the intraoperative goal regardless of the approach.

Transabdominal approaches for fistula repair include supravesical or transvesical approaches, and laparoscopic/robotic techniques. The O'Conor transabdominal VVF repair has been well described.[39] The patient is positioned in a low lithotomy position, with access to the vagina and abdomen. Ureteral catheters may be placed and are recommended if the fistula is near the ureteral orifices or the trigone. A lower midline incision is performed and the bladder is mobilized. The bladder is then bivalved vertically to the level of the fistula, and dissection is continued distally to open the vesicovaginal space, 2–3 cm distal to the fistula site. Following mobilization of the vaginal wall from the bladder wall distal to the fistula tract, the fistula tract is excised, and the vaginal wall is closed with running synthetic absorbable suture (SAS). The bladder is closed in multiple layers with running SAS. An additional layer of tissue can be placed between the suture lines utilizing an omental interposition flap or peritoneal flap. It is important to secure the interpositional flap distally beyond the fistula.

In the transvesical approach, the bladder is opened via a midline cystotomy on the anterior surface of the bladder. The VVF tract is then circumscribed and excised. Following mobilization of the vesicovaginal space surrounding the fistula site, the vaginal and vesical tissues are closed separately. A flap of adjacent bladder tissue may be advanced to avoid overlapping suture lines as described by Gil-Vernet.[40]

The transvaginal approach for fistula repair is shown in Fig. 35.3.[7,41,42] The patient is placed in the dorsal lithotomy position, and a rectal pack is placed. Labial retraction sutures are placed as well as a weighted speculum. A self-retaining ring retractor with hooks is very useful for visualization and retraction. Cystoscopy is performed to localize the fistula tract, and a guide wire is placed though the fistula into the vagina. A 10–12 French foley catheter should be placed though the fistula site, using the previously placed guide wire. This catheter provides traction of the fistula toward the introitus

throughout the case. Ureteral stents are placed if the fistula is in close proximity to the ureteral orifices. A urethral catheter is placed, and a supra-pubic catheter may also be utilized for bladder drainage. An inverted U-shaped incision is made which circumscribes the fistula site. Anterior and posterior vaginal wall flaps are developed after hydro-dissection with sterile saline, and retracted using the ring retractor. Using double-armed SAS, the fistula is closed in an interrupted fashion. The perivesical tissue is then closed over the initial suture line in an interrupted imbricated fashion, 90° in respect to the first layer. A peritoneal flap or a martius flap can be positioned over the imbricated layer of peri-vesical tissue. The posterior vaginal wall flap is advanced over the suture line anteriorly to complete the closure.

Adjacent tissue flaps can be useful in the setting of complex fistula with compromised surrounding tissue, or in patients with prior failed repairs, radiotherapy, obstetric fistula, or large fistula tracts. For patients undergoing a transvaginal approach, a labial fat pad (Martius) or peritoneal flaps are most frequently utilized with success rates of greater than 90%.[7] The Martius graft is harvested from the fibrofatty tissue of the labia majora. It maintains blood supply from the external pudendal artery superiorly and the inferior labial artery inferiorly, allowing rotation and mobilization from either pedicle. Once mobilized via a labial incision, this flap can be tunneled into the vaginal dissection for additional layers of fistula closure. In high VVF repairs from a transvaginal approach, the peritoneum is often encountered during the course of dissection. The peritoneum can be advanced over the fistula repair as an additional layer of closure, with success rates of 91–96%.[7,41] As noted previously, omental interposition flaps are useful adjunctive procedures when performing transabdominal VVF repairs in the manner of O'Conor. Interposition flaps or peritoneal flaps can be incorporated into transabdominal fistula repairs between bladder and vaginal wall suture lines. The omental vascular supply is based on the right and left gastroepiploic arteries. In order to provide sufficient length for the flap to reach the pelvis, the omentum can be mobilized along the greater curvature of the stomach, sacrificing the left gastroepiploic artery and allowing larger right gastroepiploic artery to maintain blood supply.

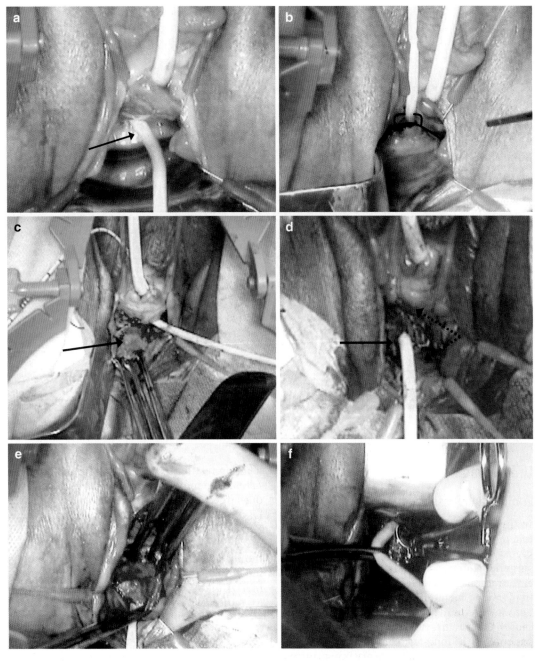

Figure 35.3. (a–j) Transvaginal repair of vesicovaginal fistula. (a) Foley catheter within the urethra and vesicovaginal fistula (*arrow*). (b) Anterior curvo-linear vaginal wall incision (*black line*) incorporating the fistula site. (c) Dissected posterior vaginal wall flap (*arrow*) retracted inferiorly. (d) Perivesical tissue (*solid arrow*) and retracted superior and inferior vaginal wall flaps (*dashed arrow*). (e) Dissection of perivesical tissue from the underlying detrusor muscle to provide an additional layer of closure. (f) Initial suture placement, closing the detrusor and bladder mucosa. (g) Sutures retracted to visualize the initial layer of closure. The foley catheter is then removed from the fistula, and the sutures are tied. (h) Second line of closure with imbricated interrupted sutures to reinforce the initial layer of closure. (i) Third tissue layer of interrupted sutures, bringing together the previously dissected perivesical fascial layers. *Arrows* identify the perivesical tissue flaps. (j) Closure of the vaginal wall (Reprinted from Chapple).

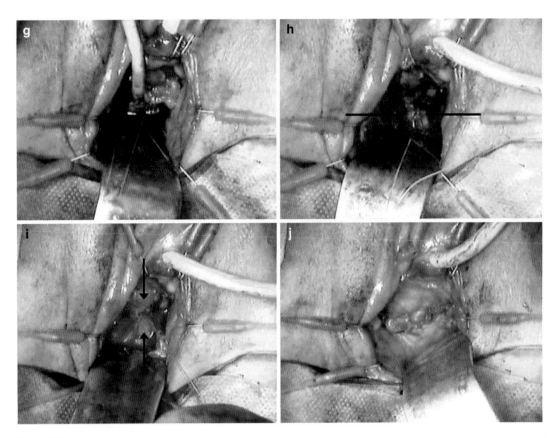

Figure 35.3. (continued)

Urethrovaginal Fistula

Etiology and Presentation

In the industrialized world, urethrovaginal fistula most commonly occurs as a result of transvaginal surgery, including anti-incontinence surgeries, anterior vaginal wall prolapse repair, and urethral diverticulectomy.[43-46] Pelvic radiation, trauma, including pelvic fracture, and vaginal and urethral neoplasms are less common causes of urethrovaginal fistula. In female patients with long-term indwelling urethral catheters and cognitive or sensory impairments, pressure necrosis may cause a traumatic hypospadias and urethrovaginal fistula. In nonindustrialized nations, obstructed labor is the most common etiology of urethrovaginal fistula, usually with concomitant VVF.[47]

Symptoms of urethrovaginal fistula are dependent on the size of the fistula, and the location relative to the urethral sphincter. Large fistulas are more likely to present with continuous large volume incontinence, and small fistulas may produce only a small amount of leakage. Fistulas proximal to the urethral sphincter mechanism, either in the proximal urethra or at the bladder neck, can present with continuous incontinence, similar to VVF. Distal urethrovaginal fistulas, distal to the sphincter, can be asymptomatic or present with a splayed urinary stream. Occasionally, patients will present with vaginal voiding or "pseudo-incontinence," due to accumulation of urine within the vaginal vault. These patients will leak when rising from a seated position after voiding.

Diagnosis and Management

The diagnosis of urethrovaginal fistula can be made based on history, physical exam, and cystourethroscopy, but radiologic imaging can also be helpful in fistula identification and localization. Speculum examination can occasionally identify the fistula tract on the anterior vaginal wall. A thorough pelvic exam is essential to rule out additional pathology, including additional fistula sites more proximal in the vagina. An associated VVF is found in 20% of patients.[48] Vaginal tissues should be inspected for viability, infection, and atrophy, and treated with antibiotics or estrogen cream as needed. Cystourethroscopy is an essential, yet challenging, process due to the short length of the female urethra. Distal compression at the meatus, and a short beak "female" cystoscope or flexible fiberoptic cystoscope can assist in visualization. The bladder neck and bladder should be examined for an additional fistula. If a component of stress or urgency incontinence is suspected, or if the patient has suspected concomitant detrusor dysfunction, videourodynamics can be used to more appropriately characterize the pathology.

Surgical repair of a urethrovaginal fistula can be difficult and requires careful consideration and planning. There may be extensive soft tissue defects and a dearth of viable tissue for a multilayered repair.[9] Surgical approach, including the use of adjacent tissue flaps, is dependent on fistula size, location, and tissue viability. Small fistulas may be managed with a multilayered closure, including interposition grafts such as a Martius flap.[46,49] Large fistulas may require urethral reconstruction and more extensive surgery.[47,50,51] With many urethrovaginal fistulae, soft tissue flaps can provide an additional layer of viable tissue, decreasing the historical high rate of failure with vaginal wall advancement flaps.[9,49,52-57] Labial fat pad flaps (Martius), gracilus and rectus muscle, fibrin glue, myocutaneous flaps, and labial skin grafts have been described to decrease failure rates.[9,46,49,55,57-61] Distal fistulas can be managed conservatively with observation or extended meatotomy if there is no associated incontinence or voiding symptoms.[62] Timing of the operative intervention is controversial, similar to VVF. Preoperative stress incontinence may persist following repair of a proximal or mid-urethral urethrovaginal fistula, and concomitant repair of SUI at the time of initial repair is controversial.[43,46] Concomitant SUI repairs have been reported using Martius flaps interposed between the fistula and the autologous pubovaginal sling.[43]

Ureterovaginal Fistula

Etiology and Presentation

Fistulas from the ureter to the uro-genital tract are uncommon, most frequently involving the proximal vagina and rarely the uterus or fallopian tubes.[63] Risk factors include endometriosis, obesity, pelvic inflammatory disease, radiation therapy, and pelvic malignancy.[64] Iatrogenic injuries during pelvic surgery, specifically gynecologic surgery, are the most common etiologies of ureterovaginal fistulae, with the incidence estimated at 0.5–2.5%.[64,65] Most commonly, UVF result from surgeries for benign disease, during hysterectomy, caesarean section, or cystocele repair[66] rather than oncologic procedures. Risk of injury appears greatest from laparoscopic hysterectomy, followed by abdominal, then vaginal hysterectomy.[67] The ureter is injured in the distal one third or pelvic portion, due to its close proximity to the uterosacral ligaments, uterine artery, and cervix. Direct injury or devascularization with subsequent necrosis can cause urinary extravasation, urinoma formation, and eventual drainage into the vagina at the level of the vaginal cuff.

Patients usually present with clear or serous continuous vaginal discharge 1–4 weeks following surgical intervention.[66] Occasionally, this is associated with a prodrome of flank or abdominal pain, nausea, and low-grade fevers as a result of urinoma formation and/or ureteral obstruction.[48] In contrast to VVF, patients will continue to urinate at normal intervals, as the contralateral kidney maintains cyclic bladder filling.

Diagnosis and Management

Diagnosis of a ureterovaginal fistula can usually be accomplished with a complete history and physical examination, followed by radiologic evaluation with studies, including intravenous urogram (IVU)/CT urogram (CTU), cystoscopy, retrograde pyelography, and cystography (Fig. 35.4). It is imperative to discriminate UVF from VVF and evaluate for concomitant VVF during the course of evaluation. A double dye test may allow differentiation of UVF and VVF in cases of continuous leakage.[21] Once the

Figure 35.4. Algorithm for the diagnosis and management of ureterovaginal fistula.

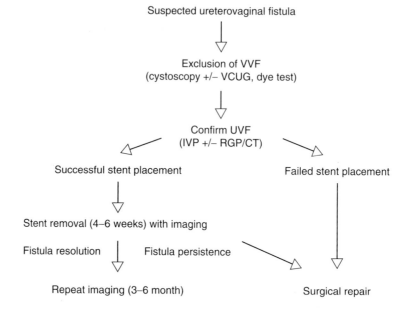

physical exam, cystoscopy, and cystography have ruled out VVF, attention should be turned to upper tract evaluation (Fig. 35.5). The IVU or CT urogram (CTU) will often demonstrate some degree of ureteral dilation or pelviectasis as a result of varying degrees of distal obstruction.[68] Vaginal drainage can be identified on post-void images if the caliber of the fistula is large. CTU can assess ureteral anatomy as well as investigate for abscess, urinoma, or additional intra-abdominal pathology. Retrograde pyelogram may be the best test to diagnose a ureteral injury and can usually identify the fistula site or level of ureteral pathology.[65] If ureteral continuity is established, an attempt at a period of drainage with indwelling ureteral stent is warranted, as some cases may result in resolution of the fistula.

Once the diagnosis of ureterovaginal fistula is confirmed, prompt drainage of the upper tract is essential. Partial obstruction is often present at the level of the fistula, which can lead to progressive renal damage, infection, or sepsis. If retrograde stent placement at the time of retrograde pyelogram is unsuccessful, antegrade stent placement at the time of percutaneous nephrostomy placement can be attempted. Conservative management with ureteral stenting will occasionally result in fistula closure. In a study by Dowling et al., 11 of 23 patients with ureteral injuries recognized postoperatively had fistula closure with

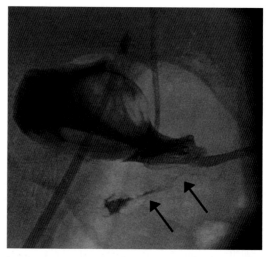

Figure 35.5. Anterograde pyelogram in a patient with bilateral nephro-ureterostomy tubes and indwelling foley catheter. *Arrows* identify the ureterovaginal fistula.

stenting or percutaneous drainage alone.[69] If leakage persists, or complete ureteral occlusion is identified, then formal surgical repair is warranted.

The site of primary injury at the distal ureter is generally surrounded by fibrosis and inflammation, precluding primary uretero-ureterostomy. After dissection from surrounding tissues, division of the ureter just above the level of injury, and confirmation of the viability of the proximal margin, the ureteral length is usually adequate for ureteroneocystotomy. Psoas hitch or Boari flap can provide additional length for a tension free anastomosis. In patients with extensive ureteral damage, trans-ureteroureterostomy, ileal interposition, or renal autotransplant can be an option. If extensive renal injury has already occurred, nephrectomy may be the most expeditious form of management. Successful repair of ureterovaginal fistula occurs in greater than 90% of cases.[11,66]

Vesicouterine Fistula

Etiology and Presentation

Vesicouterine fistula are rare forms of urogynecologic fistula, with less than 100 cases reported in recent literature.[70] Caesarean section is the most common etiology of this type of fistula, with the majority occurring during repeat sections.[71] Numerous case reports of other etiologies include vaginal deliveries after caesarean section, radiation, iatrogenic catheter trauma, or placenta percreta.[72-75] Following uterine rupture during labor, the posterior bladder wall can be torn along the margin of the rupture leading to eventual vesicouterine fistula formation. Unrecognized injury to the bladder at the time of uterine surgery or incorporation of the bladder into a uterine suture line can also result in fistula. The most common location for vesicouterine fistula is from the posterior midline bladder wall to the uterus above the proximal cervical margin. Because the cervical os is generally closed, patients may not present with incontinence. Continuous incontinence can occur in cases of cervical incompetence, or just following vaginal delivery.[70] Patients may also present with menouria and cyclic hematuria in the setting of urinary continence. "Youssef's syndrome" describes the symptom complex of menouria, cyclic hematuria, apparent amenorrhea, infertility, and continence of urine.[70] This must be differentiated from endometriosis of the bladder.

Diagnosis and Management

A history of prior uterine surgery in the setting of compatible symptoms as described above is strongly suggestive of a vesicouterine fistula. Cystoscopy, hysteroscopy, and radiologic imaging can assist in definitive diagnosis. Cystoscopy can visualize the fistula tract along the posterior bladder wall. Urine cytology may reveal endometrial cells during workup of hematuria. Cystogram or hysterosalpingogram can identify the abnormal flow of contrast via the fistula tract from urinary to genital tracts. In cases of continuous incontinence, VCUG and CTU can be utilized to rule out the presence of VVF or ureterovaginal fistula.

Successful treatment of vesicovaginal fistula has been well documented using conservative as well as surgical management. Watchful waiting with spontaneous fistula resolution, urinary diversion with prolonged catheterization, and hormonally induced uterine involution have all been described with successful outcomes.[76-78] Surgical intervention can include hysterectomy with primary closure of the bladder. If the patient desires fertility, uterine sparing surgery can be performed in a technique similar to the O'Conor transabdominal VVF repair with or without omental interposition.

Uro-Enteric Fistula

Vesicoenteric Fistula

Vesicoenteric fistula is most likely to occur in the setting of bowel diseases such as diverticulitis, colorectal carcinoma, and Crohn's disease. Less commonly, radiation, infection, trauma, or iatrogenic surgical injury can result in fistula formation. Approximately 2% of patients with diverticulitis will develop vesicoenteric fistulas secondary to their disease, and these patients account for approximately 70% of all diagnosed colovesical fistulas.[79-81] Ileovesical are more common in Crohn's disease patients, who have a 2% incidence of vesicoenteric fistula formation.[82] Symptoms of vesicoenteric fistula can be gastrointestinal or urologic. Pneumaturia is the most common presenting symptom, occurring in 70% of cases.[83] Persistent or recurrent UTI or cystitis refractory to antibiotic management may suggest colovesical fistula.[84]

Endoscopic and radiologic imaging can be helpful in diagnosis. Cystoscopic examination is sensitive for detecting mucosal abnormalities such as erythema or bullous edema in >90% of cases, but is not definitive for a fistula diagnosis.[85] A biopsy is indicated at the time of endoscopic evaluation to rule out malignancy. CT scan is the most sensitive and specific modality for the diagnosis of colovesical fistula.[80] Identification of the bladder adjacent to a thickened loop of colon, air within the bladder, and colonic diverticula are highly suggestive of a possible fistula.[86] If there is question of a subclinical fistula, the diagnosis can be confirmed by oral administration of activated charcoal, which will appear in the urine as black particles.[87]

Conservative management of vesicoenteric fistula includes bowel rest with total parenteral nutrition and antibiotics in patients with minimal symptoms and no evidence of toxicity.[88] In accordance with the general principles of fistula repair, optimization of nutritional status is important. Surgical intervention can be complicated due to the inflammation and scarring associated with fistula formation. Dissection should continue until viable tissue margins are obtained for bladder closure. An omental flap can be used to prevent overlapping suture lines.[38] If the patient is acutely ill, or abscess or obstruction complicates the procedure, bowel diversion with later reanastomosis (two stage repair) should be considered.[89]

Pyeloenteric Fistula

Pyeloenteric fistula can develop from inflammatory diseases of the kidney, such as xanthogranulomatous pyelonephritis, tuberculosis, chronic pyelonephritis, or inflammatory diseases of the bowel, such as Crohn's disease.[90-92] Iatrogenic trauma from percutaneous nephrolithotomy access and lithotripsy has been associated with an increasing number of fistulas, involving the duodenum during right renal procedures and the colon in left sided intervention.[93] Cryoablation or alternative minimally invasive renal tumor surgery can result in fistula formation.[94] The majority of patients have nonspecific symptoms of malaise, mild GI symptoms, urinary frequency, flank mass, or tenderness; however, many fistulas are diagnosed incidentally on radiographic imaging.[90,95] If there is a suspected pyeloenteric fistula, urinary or GI contrast-based imaging with traditional or CT urography, retrograde pyelogram, nephrostogram, barium swallow, or contrast enema can confirm the diagnosis. Conservative management with large nephrostomy tubes, bowel rest, antibiotics, or internal stenting may result in fistula resolution.[90] Definitive treatment includes open primary repair for nephron sparing or nephrectomy with bowel closure for a poorly functioning renal unit.

Urethrorectal Fistula

Acquired rectourethral or prostatorectal fistula (RUF) has been reported in association with a variety of clinical situations. Fistula can result from prostatic or rectal malignancies, inflammatory disorders of the prostate or bowel, local trauma, or surgical intervention for benign or malignant prostatic or rectal.[38] The most common contemporary etiology of RUF is radical retropubic prostatectomy (RRP) due to an unrecognized bowel injury at the level of the vesicourethral anastomosis. Nevertheless, the overall incidence of fistula following RRP is extremely low, less than 0.2% in one large series.[96] Prior history of pelvic radiation, rectal surgery, or TURP increases the risk of RUF formation following surgical intervention.[96] Fistula formation following alternative therapies for prostatic malignancy such as cryoablation and brachytherapy has also been reported, with an incidence of approximately 0.5% and 0.4%, respectively.[97,98] Salvage cryoablation has a 3.3% incidence of RUF formation following radiation therapy.[99] Larger series of laparoscopic and robotic techniques for radical prostatectomy have similar rectal injury rates when compared to traditional open retropubic radical prostatectomy,[97,100,101] and a 0.1% rate of subsequent fistula formation.[101] Similar to other types of fistula, recognition of an iatrogenic injury and immediate intraoperative repair can decrease the rate of subsequent fistula formation.

Patients may present with urologic complaints of UTI, fecaluria, pneumaturia, hematuria, or gastrointestinal problems such as nausea, vomiting, or peritonitis. Direct visualization via cystoscopy or sigmoidoscopy may identify the fistula tract and provide a means for biopsy in cases of suspected concomitant malignancy. Voiding cystourethrogram or retrograde urethrogram can allow definitive diagnosis and provide details of anatomic location and fistula size (Fig. 35.6). In consideration of surgical intervention, continence must be assessed and discussed as RUF repair may initiate or exacerbate stress incontinence.

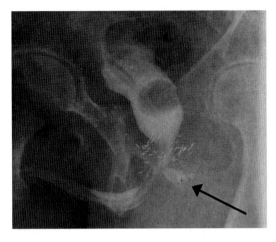

Figure 35.6. Voiding cystourethrogram in a patient with history of brachytherapy for prostate cancer. *Arrow* identifies the rectourethral fistula.

Conservative management with catheter drainage, bowel rest, hyperalimentation, and occasionally fecal diversion can result in spontaneous fistula healing after prostatectomy.[102] In most cases, however, surgical therapy is necessary.[103] Surgical repairs can be performed in single or multiple stages and accessed via transrectal, perineal, or trans-abdominal approaches.

References

1. Gerber GS, Schoenberg HW. Female urinary tract fistulas. *J Urol.* 1993;149:229-236
2. Sims J. On the treatment of vesicovaginal fistula. *Am J Med Sci.* 1852;23:59
3. Trendelenburg F. Discussion zu Halferich Zuganglichmachung der Vorderen Blasenwand. *Dtsch Ges Chir.* 1888;17:101
4. Symmonds RE. Incontinence: vesical and urethral fistulas. *Clin Obstet Gynecol.* 1984;27:499-514
5. Tancer ML. Observations on prevention and management of vesicovaginal fistula after total hysterectomy. *Surg Gynecol Obstet.* 1992;175:501-506
6. Armenakas NA, Pareek G, Fracchia JA. Iatrogenic bladder perforations: longterm followup of 65 patients. *J Am Coll Surg.* 2004;198:78-82
7. Eilber KS, Kavaler E, Rodriguez LV, Rosenblum N, Raz S. Ten-year experience with transvaginal vesicovaginal fistula repair using tissue interposition. *J Urol.* 2003;169:1033-1036
8. Harris WJ. Early complications of abdominal and vaginal hysterectomy. *Obstet Gynecol Surv.* 1995;50:795-805
9. Keettel WC, Sehring FG, de Prosse CA, Scott JR. Surgical management of urethrovaginal and vesicovaginal fistulas. *Am J Obstet Gynecol.* 1978;131:425-431
10. Kursh ED, Morse RM, Resnick MI, Persky L. Prevention of the development of a vesicovaginal fistula. *Surg Gynecol Obstet.* 1988;166:409-412
11. Blandy JP, Badenoch DF, Fowler CG, Jenkins BJ, Thomas NW. Early repair of iatrogenic injury to the ureter or bladder after gynecological surgery. *J Urol.* 1991;146:761-765
12. Alert J, Jimenez J, Beldarrain L, Montalvo J, Roca C. Complications from irradiation of carcinoma of the uterine cervix. *Acta Radiol Oncol.* 1980;19:13-15
13. Zoubek J, McGuire EJ, Noll F, DeLancey JO. The late occurrence of urinary tract damage in patients successfully treated by radiotherapy for cervical carcinoma. *J Urol.* 1989;141:1347-1349
14. Rovner E. Vesicovaginal and urethrovaginal fistulas. *AUA Update Ser.* 2006;25:45-55
15. Danso KA, Martey JO, Wall LL, Elkins TE. The epidemiology of genitourinary fistulae in Kumasi, Ghana, 1977–1992. *Int Urogynecol J Pelvic Floor Dysfunct.* 1996;7:117-120
16. Margolis T, Elkins TE, Seffah J, Oparo-Addo HS, Fort D. Full-thickness Martius grafts to preserve vaginal depth as an adjunct in the repair of large obstetric fistulas. *Obstet Gynecol.* 1994;84:148-152
17. Margolis T, Mercer LJ. Vesicovaginal fistula. *Obstet Gynecol Surv.* 1994;49:840-847
18. Arrowsmith SD. Genitourinary reconstruction in obstetric fistulas. *J Urol.* 1994;152:403-406
19. Drutz HP, Mainprize TC. Unrecognized small vesicovaginal fistula as a cause of persistent urinary incontinence. *Am J Obstet Gynecol.* 1988;158:237-240
20. Moir JC. Vesico-vaginal fistulae as seen in Britain. *J Obstet Gynaecol Br Commonw.* 1973;80:598-602
21. Raghavaiah NV. Double-dye test to diagnose various types of vaginal fistulas. *J Urol.* 1974;112:811-812
22. Goodwin WE, Scardino PT. Vesicovaginal and ureterovaginal fistulas: a summary of 25 years of experience. *J Urol.* 1980;123:370-374
23. Kuhlman JE, Fishman EK. CT evaluation of enterovaginal and vesicovaginal fistulas. *J Comput Assist Tomogr.* 1990;14:390-394
24. Davits RJ, Miranda SI. Conservative treatment of vesicovaginal fistulas by bladder drainage alone. *Br J Urol.* 1991;68:155-156
25. Stovsky MD, Ignatoff JM, Blum MD, Nanninga JB, O'Conor VJ, Kursh ED. Use of electrocoagulation in the treatment of vesicovaginal fistulas. *J Urol.* 1994;152:1443-1444
26. Pettersson S, Hedelin H, Jansson I, Teger-Nilsson AC. Fibrin occlusion of a vesicovaginal fistula. *Lancet.* 1979;1:933
27. Badenoch DF, Tiptaft RC, Thakar DR, Fowler CG, Blandy JP. Early repair of accidental injury to the ureter or bladder following gynaecological surgery. *Br J Urol.* 1987;59:516-518
28. Blaivas JG, Heritz DM, Romanzi LJ. Early versus late repair of vesicovaginal fistulas: vaginal and abdominal approaches. *J Urol.* 1995;153:1110-1112; discussion 1112-1113
29. Collins CG, Collins JH, Harrison BR, Nicholls RA, Hoffman ES, Krupp PJ. Early repair of vesicovaginal fistula. *Am J Obstet Gynecol.* 1971;111:524-528

30. Cruikshank SH. Early closure of posthysterectomy vesicovaginal fistulas. *South Med J.* 1988;81:1525-1528

31. Kostakopoulos A, Deliveliotis C, Louras G, Giftopoulos A, Skolaricos A. Early repair of injury to the ureter or bladder after hysterectomy. *Int Urol Nephrol.* 1998;30: 445-450

32. Persky L, Herman G, Guerrier K. Nondelay in vesicovaginal fistula repair. *Urology.* 1979;13:273-275

33. Wang Y, Hadley HR. Nondelayed transvaginal repair of high lying vesicovaginal fistula. *J Urol.* 1990;144:34-36

34. Waaldijk K. The immediate surgical management of fresh obstetric fistulas with catheter and/or early closure. *Int J Gynaecol Obstet.* 1994;45:11-16

35. Wein AJ, Malloy TR, Carpiniello VL, Greenberg SH, Murphy JJ. Repair of vesicovaginal fistula by a suprapubic transvesical approach. *Surg Gynecol Obstet.* 1980;150:57-60

36. Tancer ML. The post-total hysterectomy (vault) vesicovaginal fistula. *J Urol.* 1980;123:839-840

37. Motiwala HG, Amlani JC, Desai KD, Shah KN, Patel PC. Transvesical vaginal fistula repair: a revival. *Eur Urol.* 1991;19:24-28

38. Rovner E. Urinary tract fistula. In: Wein AJ, ed. *Campbell-Walsh Urology*, vol. 3. Philadelphia: W.B. Saunders; 2007:2322-2360

39. O'Conor VJ Jr. Review of experience with vesicovaginal fistula repair. *J Urol.* 1980;123:367-369

40. Gil-Vernet JM, Gil-Vernet A, Campos JA. New surgical approach for treatment of complex vesicovaginal fistula. *J Urol.* 1989;141:513-516

41. Raz S, Bregg KJ, Nitti VW, Sussman E. Transvaginal repair of vesicovaginal fistula using a peritoneal flap. *J Urol.* 1993;150:56-59

42. Zimmern PE, Hadley HR, Staskin DR, Raz S. Genitourinary fistulae. Vaginal approach for repair of vesicovaginal fistulae. *Urol Clin North Am.* 1985;12:361-367

43. Blaivas JG. Vaginal flap urethral reconstruction: an alternative to the bladder flap neourethra. *J Urol.* 1989;141: 542-545

44. Glavind K, Larsen EH. Results and complications of tension-free vaginal tape (TVT) for surgical treatment of female stress urinary incontinence. *Int Urogynecol J Pelvic Floor Dysfunct.* 2001;12:370-372

45. Henriksson C, Kihl B, Pettersson S. Urethrovaginal and vesicovaginal fistula. A review of 29 patients. *Acta Obstet Gynecol Scand.* 1982;61:143-148

46. Webster GD, Sihelnik SA, Stone AR. Urethrovaginal fistula: a review of the surgical management. *J Urol.* 1984;132:460-462

47. Elkins TE. Surgery for the obstetric vesicovaginal fistula: a review of 100 operations in 82 patients. *Am J Obstet Gynecol.* 1994;170:1108-1118; discussion 1118-1120

48. Lee RA, Symmonds RE, Williams TJ. Current status of genitourinary fistula. *Obstet Gynecol.* 1988;72:313-319

49. Leach GE. Urethrovaginal fistula repair with Martius labial fat pad graft. *Urol Clin North Am.* 1991;18: 409-413

50. Tehan TJ, Nardi JA, Baker R. Complications associated with surgical repair of urethrovaginal fistula. *Urology.* 1980;15:31-35

51. Wang Y, Hadley HR. The use of rotated vascularized pedicle flaps for complex transvaginal procedures. *J Urol.* 1993;149:590-592

52. Birkhoff JD, Wechsler M, Romas NA. Urinary fistulas: vaginal repair using a labial fat pad. *J Urol.* 1977;117:595-597

53. Bruce RG, El-Galley RE, Galloway NT. Use of rectus abdominis muscle flap for the treatment of complex and refractory urethrovaginal fistulas. *J Urol.* 2000;163:1212-1215

54. Davis RS, Linke CA, Kraemer GK. Use of labial tissue in repair of urethrovaginal fistula and injury. *Arch Surg.* 1980;115:628-630

55. Fall M. Vaginal wall bipedicled flap and other techniques in complicated urethral diverticulum and urethrovaginal fistula. *J Am Coll Surg.* 1995;180:150-156

56. Patil U, Waterhouse K, Laungani G. Management of 18 difficult vesicovaginal and urethrovaginal fistulas with modified Ingelman-Sundberg and Martius operations. *J Urol.* 1980;123:653-656

57. Rangnekar NP, Imdad Ali N, Kaul SA, Pathak HR. Role of the martius procedure in the management of urinary-vaginal fistulas. *J Am Coll Surg.* 2000;191:259-263

58. Candiani P, Austoni E, Campiglio GL, Ceresoli A, Zanetti G, Colombo F. Repair of a recurrent urethrovaginal fistula with an island bulbocavernous musculocutaneous flap. *Plast Reconstr Surg.* 1993;92:1393-1396

59. Krogh J, Kay L, Hjortrup A. Treatment of urethrovaginal fistula. *Br J Urol.* 1989;63:555

60. McKinney DE. Use of full thickness patch graft in urethrovaginal fistula. *J Urol.* 1979;122:416

61. Tolle E, Schmandt W, Beizai S, Drepper H. Closure of large vesico – urethra – vaginal defect with pedicled myocutaneous gracilis flap (author's transl). *Urologe A.* 1981;20:274-7

62. Lamensdorf H, Compere DE, Begley GF. Simple surgical correction of urethrovaginal fistula. *Urology.* 1977;10: 152-153

63. Billmeyer BR, Nygaard IE, Kreder KJ. Ureterouterine and vesicoureterovaginal fistulas as a complication of cesarean section. *J Urol.* 2001;165:1212-1213

64. Symmonds RE. Ureteral injuries associated with gynecologic surgery: prevention and management. *Clin Obstet Gynecol.* 1976;19:623-644

65. Payne C. Ureteral injuries in the female: fistulas and obstruction. In: Raz S, ed. *Female Urology.* Philadelphia: W.B. Saunders; 1996:507-520

66. Mandal AK, Sharma SK, Vaidyanathan S, Goswami AK. Ureterovaginal fistula: summary of 18 years' experience. *Br J Urol.* 1990;65:453-456

67. Harkki-Siren P, Sjoberg J, Tiitinen A. Urinary tract injuries after hysterectomy. *Obstet Gynecol.* 1998;92:113-118

68. Selzman AA, Spirnak JP, Kursh ED. The changing management of ureterovaginal fistulas. *J Urol.* 1995;153: 626-628

69. Dowling RA, Corriere JN Jr, Sandler CM. Iatrogenic ureteral injury. *J Urol.* 1986;135:912-915

70. Tancer ML. Vesicouterine fistula – a review. *Obstet Gynecol Surv.* 1986;41:743-753

71. Jozwik M, Jozwik M, Lotocki W. Vesicouterine fistula – an analysis of 24 cases from Poland. *Int J Gynaecol Obstet.* 1997;57:169-172

72. Futter NG, Baker K. A vesicouterine fistula caused by catheterization during delivery. *Can J Urol*. 1995;2: 107-108

73. Gil A, Sultana CJ. Vesicouterine fistula after vacuum delivery and two previous cesarean sections. A case report. *J Reprod Med*. 2001;46:853-855

74. Krysiewicz S, Auh YH, Kazam E. Vesicouterine fistula associated with placenta percreta. *Urol Radiol*. 1988;10:213-215

75. Memon MA, Zieg DA, Neal PM. Vesicouterine fistula twenty years following brachytherapy for cervical cancer. *Scand J Urol Nephrol*. 1998;32:293-295

76. Graziotti P, Lembo A, Artibani W. Spontaneous closure of vesicouterine fistula after cesarean section. *J Urol*. 1978;120:372

77. Jozwik M, Jozwik M. Spontaneous closure of vesicouterine fistula. Account for effective hormonal treatment. *Urol Int*. 1999;62:183-187

78. Novi JM, Rose M, Shaunik A, Ramchandani P, Morgan MA. Conservative management of vesicouterine fistula after uterine rupture. *Int Urogynecol J Pelvic Floor Dysfunct*. 2004;15:434-435

79. Hafner CD PJ, Brush BE. Genitourinary manifestations of diverticulitis of the colon. *J Am Med Assoc*. 1962; 179:76

80. Najjar SF, Jamal MK, Savas JF, Miller TA. The spectrum of colovesical fistula and diagnostic paradigm. *Am J Surg*. 2004;188:617-621

81. Mileski WJ, Joehl RJ, Rege RV, Nahrwold DL. One-stage resection and anastomosis in the management of colovesical fistula. *Am J Surg*. 1987;153:75-79

82. Gruner JS, Sehon JK, Johnson LW. Diagnosis and management of enterovesical fistulas in patients with Crohn's disease. *Am Surg*. 2002;68:714-719

83. Solem CA, Loftus EV Jr, Tremaine WJ, Pemberton JH, Wolff BG, Sandborn WJ. Fistulas to the urinary system in Crohn's disease: clinical features and outcomes. *Am J Gastroenterol*. 2002;97:2300-2305

84. Rao PN, Knox R, Barnard RJ, Schofield PF. Management of colovesical fistula. *Br J Surg*. 1987;74:362-363

85. Morse FP 3rd, Dretler SP. Diagnosis and treatment of colovesical fistula. *J Urol*. 1974;111:22-24

86. Labs JD, Sarr MG, Fishman EK, Siegelman SS, Cameron JL. Complications of acute diverticulitis of the colon: improved early diagnosis with computerized tomography. *Am J Surg*. 1988;155:331-336

87. Geier GR Jr, Ujiki G, Shields TW. Colovesical fistula. *Arch Surg*. 1972;105:347-351

88. Dudrick SJ, Maharaj AR, McKelvey AA. Artificial nutritional support in patients with gastrointestinal fistulas. *World J Surg*. 1999;23:570-576

89. McConnell DB, Sasaki TM, Vetto RM. Experience with colovesical fistula. *Am J Surg*. 1980;140:80-84

90. Desmond JM, Evans SE, Couch A, Morewood DJ. Pyeloduodenal fistulae. A report of two cases and review of the literature. *Clin Radiol*. 1989;40:267-270

91. Majeed HA, Mohammed KA, Salman HA. Renocolic fistula as a complication to xanthogranulomatous pyelonephritis. *Singapore Med J*. 1997;38:116-119

92. Yildiz M, Atan A, Aydoganli L, Cengiz T, Akalin Z. Renocolic fistula secondary to chronic pyelonephritis. *Int Urol Nephrol*. 1993;25:229-233

93. LeRoy AJ, Williams HJ Jr, Bender CE, Segura JW, Patterson DE, Benson RC. Colon perforation following percutaneous nephrostomy and renal calculus removal. *Radiology*. 1985;155:83-85

94. Vanderbrink BA, Rastinehad A, Caplin D, Ost MC, Lobko I, Lee BR. Successful conservative management of colorenal fistula after percutaneous cryoablation of renal-cell carcinoma. *J Endourol*. 2007;21:726-729

95. Culkin DJ, Wheeler JS, Nemchausky BA, Fruin RC, Canning JR. Percutaneous nephrolithotomy: spinal cord injury vs. ambulatory patients. *J Am Paraplegia Soc*. 1990;13:4-6

96. McLaren RH, Barrett DM, Zincke H. Rectal injury occurring at radical retropubic prostatectomy for prostate cancer: etiology and treatment. *Urology*. 1993;42:401-405

97. Long JP, Bahn D, Lee F, Shinohara K, Chinn DO, Macaluso JN Jr. Five-year retrospective, multi-institutional pooled analysis of cancer-related outcomes after cryosurgical ablation of the prostate. *Urology*. 2001;57:518-523

98. Theodorescu D, Gillenwater JY, Koutrouvelis PG. Prostatourethral-rectal fistula after prostate brachytherapy. *Cancer*. 2000;89:2085-2091

99. Chin JL, Pautler SE, Mouraviev V, Touma N, Moore K, Downey DB. Results of salvage cryoablation of the prostate after radiation: identifying predictors of treatment failure and complications. *J Urol*. 2001;165:1937-1941; discussion 1941-1942

100. Menon M, Tewari A, Peabody JO, et al. Vattikuti Institute prostatectomy, a technique of robotic radical prostatectomy for management of localized carcinoma of the prostate: experience of over 1100 cases. *Urol Clin North Am*. 2004;31:701-717

101. Guillonneau B, Gupta R, El Fettouh H, Cathelineau X, Baumert H, Vallancien G. Laparoscopic [correction of laproscopic] management of rectal injury during laparoscopic [correction of laproscopic] radical prostatectomy. *J Urol*. 2003;169:1694-1696

102. Rassweiler J, Seemann O, Schulze M, Teber D, Hatzinger M, Frede T. Laparoscopic versus open radical prostatectomy: a comparative study at a single institution. *J Urol*. 2003;169:1689-1693

103. Bukowski TP, Chakrabarty A, Powell IJ, Frontera R, Perlmutter AD, Montie JE. Acquired rectourethral fistula: methods of repair. *J Urol*. 1995;153:730-733

36

Urologic Trauma

Bradley D. Figler and Viraj A. Master

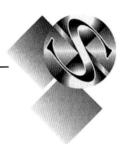

It is the urologist who will have to share the burden of the ultimate disability with the patient when the thoracic, and abdominal, and even orthopedic aspects are probably long forgotten.

—Richard Turner-Warwick, 1977[1]

Introduction

Injury is a major cause of death and disability worldwide and the leading cause of death among young people in the USA. However, fatalities represent only a small fraction of those injured – of the 2.5 million patients who were hospitalized for injuries in 2003, only 148,000 died of their injuries.[2,3] Urogenital injuries, though common, are often not life-threatening and are easily overlooked during the initial stabilization of the trauma patient, resulting in significant morbidity.

Great strides have been made over the last 2 decades in the diagnosis and management of genitourinary trauma. Injuries that were once managed surgically are now being observed, with predictable decreases in morbidity. Advances in imaging have improved detection and staging of injuries, and endovascular techniques have earned a definitive role in the management of renal trauma. Finally, endoscopic techniques, the hallmark of urology, have become routine in the management of certain injuries. Here, we review the essential components of the presentation, workup, and initial management of the most common injuries to the genitourinary tract resulting from external violence. Finally, a section on imaging highlights its importance in the management of GU trauma and serves as a quick-reference guide for some of the most commonly performed techniques in the trauma setting.

Kidney

The kidneys are relatively well protected from external trauma by the spine and large musculature posteriorly and by abdominal viscera anteriorly. Nonetheless, the kidneys are the most commonly injured part of the genitourinary tract, with blunt trauma responsible for 80–90% of these injuries.[4,5] A thorough history and physical are essential to the workup of a patient with suspected renal injury, but the most reliable sign of injury to the kidney is hematuria. Hematuria is usually classified as gross or microscopic (>5 RBC/HPF). Typically, the first voided specimen is analyzed because subsequent specimens may be diluted with resuscitative fluid. If the patient cannot void and suspicion for a urethral injury is low (absence of blood at the meatus and no pelvic fracture), a lubricated catheter can be gently placed in the bladder to obtain a specimen.

Flank tenderness or ecchymosis as well as lower rib fractures are suggestive of underlying renal injury. In penetrating trauma, entry and exit wounds may be a helpful indicator that the

C.R. Chapple and W.D. Steers (eds.), *Practical Urology: Essential Principles and Practice*,
DOI: 10.1007/978-1-84882-034-0_36, © Springer-Verlag London Limited 2011

kidney has been injured. Among the most important aspects of the history is the presence of a rapid deceleration injury, as occurs in MVA or fall from height, as these can lead to renal pedicle avulsion and may not result in hematuria.[5]

Guidelines for imaging patients with suspected renal trauma are given in Fig. 36.1. Importantly, though renal injury resulting from penetrating trauma often presents with hematuria, there is no correlation between severity of injury and the degree of hematuria.[6] Therefore, patients with penetrating trauma and any degree of hematuria should undergo radiologic evaluation. Following blunt trauma, imaging should be reserved for those with gross hematuria, microscopic hematuria and a single SBP < 90 mmHg, or rapid deceleration injuries; these criteria will detect greater than 99% of significant (grade 2 or greater) renal injuries.[5]

Renal injuries are graded according to a system developed by the American Association for the Surgery of Trauma Organ Injury Scaling Committee,[7] represented graphically in Fig. 36.2. Grade 1 injuries include contusion (defined as microscopic or gross hematuria with normal urologic studies) and hematoma (subcapsular

and nonexpanding without parenchymal laceration). Grade 2 injuries include hematoma (nonexpanding and perirenal; confined to renal retroperitoneum) and laceration (<0.1 cm parenchymal depth with no urinary extravasation). Grade 3 injuries are lacerations >0.1 cm without injury to the collecting system or urinary extravasation. Grade 4 includes lacerations extending through the renal cortex, medulla, and collecting system or vascular injury to the main renal artery or vein with contained hemorrhage. Grade 5 injuries include shattered kidney (laceration) or avulsion of the renal hilum (vascular). Grade is advanced by one for bilateral injuries up to grade 3.

Nonoperative management has traditionally been favored for those with minor (grade 1 and 2) renal lacerations following blunt trauma, and now a number of trauma centers have demonstrated that patients with major renal lacerations from blunt[8,10] and penetrating[11,12] trauma, with or without urinary extravasation, can be managed nonoperatively with no apparent increase in acute or long-term morbidity[13].

Nonoperative management of grade 5 renal parenchymal injuries has been reported,[14] but we

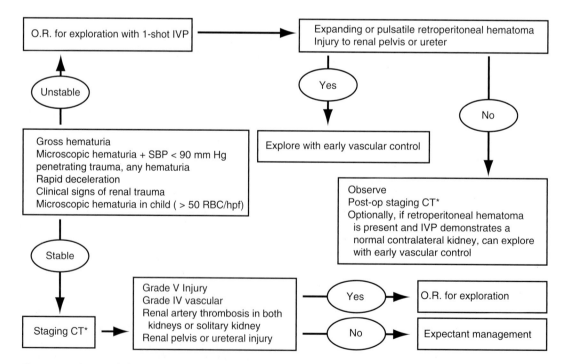

Figure 36.1. Suggested algorithm for the conservative management of renal parenchymal injuries. *SBP* systolic blood pressure, *O.R.* operating room. *Staging CT = CT of abdomen and pelvis with and without IV contrast and with delayed images.

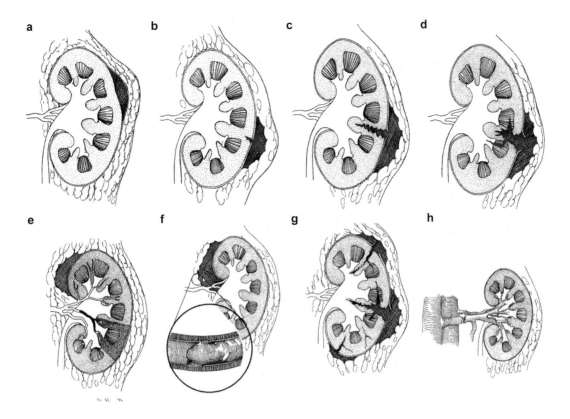

Figure 36.2. American Association for the Surgery of Trauma organ injury severity scale for the kidney (a) Grade 1 injury. (b) Grade 2 injury. (c) Grade 3 injury. (d) Grade 4 parenchymal injury. (e) Grade 4 vascular injury (note that the parenchyma subtended by the injured segmental artery is ischemic). (f) Grade 5 vascular injury (renal artery thrombosis, which generally results from intimal disruption, is demonstrated in the close-up of the figure). (g) Grade 5 parenchymal injury ("shattered kidney"). (h) Grade 5 vascular injury (avulsion of the renal pedicle). (Used from McAninch and Master[9]. With permission).

strongly caution overinterpreting these results, as many reported grade 5 renal injuries simply represent multiple grade 3 or 4 renal lacerations to the same kidney. These injuries, which represent a very different injury pattern than a shattered kidney, can often be managed nonoperatively. However, renal pedicle avulsion or a shattered kidney typically results in massive bleeding and nephrectomy is usually required.[15,16]

Absolute indications for renal exploration are an expanding retroperitoneal hematoma, hemodynamic instability believed to be from the kidney, or injuries to the renal pelvis or ureter. Furthermore, a retroperitoneal hematoma in a patient that has not been properly staged should be explored (see below). Traditional indications for exploration, such as urinary extravasation or concomitant bowel or pancreas injury, may no longer apply.[15]

Expectant Management

Despite the clear benefits of non-operative management in terms of reducing complications and nephrectomies, complications requiring delayed intervention can be expected to occur. Aggressive monitoring during and after the hospitalization is essential to identifying the subset of patients who will require further intervention. Bed rest is recommended until the gross hematuria resolves. For grade 4 injuries with large amounts of urinary extravasation, follow-up imaging is recommended at 48–72 h to evaluate degree of ongoing extravasation. If there is no decrease in the extravasation after 72 h, a stent should be placed. When a stent is in place, a Foley catheter should – at least initially – be used to maximize drainage. Serial hematocrits should be checked until the patient has been able to ambulate for at least 24 h.

Endovascular Therapy

Angio-embolization is an effective therapy for select patients with renal hemorrhage.[17] The following criteria have been proposed for angio-embolization: Persistent bleeding from a renal segmental artery; unstable condition with grade 3–4 injury; arteriovenous fistula or pseudoaneurysm; persistent gross hematuria and/or rapidly decreasing hematocrit requiring 2 U blood.[18] Patients with shattered kidney or injury to the main renal artery or vein should be surgically treated, as embolization does not seem to be effective in these patients and can delay appropriate treatment in an unstable patient, leading to significant morbidity or even mortality. Endovascular stenting is not generally useful in the trauma patient, as it requires anticoagulation, which is typically contraindicated in the patient with multiple organ-system injury.

Operative Intervention

The patient who requires operative intervention following renal trauma is usually unstable and rushed to the operating room without adequate imaging. However, it remains essential to radiographically stage the injury. Though IVP is much less reliable than CT – especially for parenchymal injuries[11] – a one-shot IVP is simple to perform (for technique, see "Imaging" section), does not typically prolong the procedure, and may identify an injury that would otherwise be missed, leading to potentially life-threatening complications postoperatively. Most importantly, the IVP will identify the presence or absence of a contralateral kidney, which cannot be accurately determined by palpation.[19] When there is a high index of suspicion, especially in the case of penetrating trauma where the trajectory is suggestive of injury to the collecting system or ureter, it is reasonable to inject 1–2 cc of dilute methylene blue into the renal pelvis. One or more laparotomy pads can be placed into the retroperitoneum to identify the source, and the ureter can be occluded to further help identify an occult leak from the kidney.

Technique: Renal Exploration and Repair

The goals of operative intervention for renal trauma are to control hemorrhage, adequately repair defects to the collecting system, and preserve as much renal function as reasonably possible. Though principles of damage control and preservation of renal function may initially be at odds, it is clear that early control of the renal hilum is rapid, easily accomplished, and reduces the need for nephrectomy.[20,21] Thus, we believe that renal exploration should only be approached with early control of the renal pedicle.

In select patients who may not tolerate repair, it is reasonable to pack the retroperitoneum and return 24 h later for exploration and repair.

Renal exploration should be approached transperitoneally through a midline incision, which should be carried up to the xiphoid process in order to permit adequate exposure of the upper retroperitoneum. The peritoneum is incised over the aorta from the level of the IMA to the level of the left renal vein. If the aorta is obscured by a retroperitoneal hematoma, the incision can be made medial to the IMV, which is usually readily identified. The left renal vein is secured with a vessel loop and then the left renal artery, right renal vein, and right renal artery are secured in that order. If there is uncontrolled bleeding, the vessel loops can be used to occlude the artery, though often manual compression of the kidney is sufficient.

Principles of renal reconstruction in the trauma setting include exposure of the entire kidney, early vascular control, debridement of nonviable tissue, meticulous hemostasis, watertight closure of the collecting system, careful reapproximation of the parenchymal edges or coverage of the parenchymal defect, and drain placement.[22] Individual vessels should be suture-ligated with 4-0 chromic suture, and collecting system tears should be oversewn with running 4-0 chromic suture. Typically, large parenchymal defects are approximated in a tension-free manner over a bolster made of thrombin-soaked Gelfoam that is tied at 1 cm intervals with an absorbable suture. In the setting of contamination from bowel or pancreatic injuries, pledgets should be made from absorbable material, such as vicryl mesh or peritoneum.

Operative Management: Follow-up

If the drain output is minimal, it should be removed after 48–72 h. If output is high, the drain fluid creatinine should be checked. If consistent with serum, it can be removed, but if consistent with urine then a more prolonged period of drainage is necessary. Placement of a ureteral stent is rarely necessary, but if it is placed, a Foley catheter is necessary to ensure adequate decompression of the collecting system.

Reno-Vascular Injuries

Injury to the renal pedicle or segmental renal vessels typically occurs during rapid deceleration injuries and can result in avulsion, laceration, or occlusion from thrombosis or dissection. Major injury to or avulsion of the renal pedicle usually requires immediate exploration for hemorrhage. Less acute injuries should be managed nonoperatively, as revascularization – even when technically successful – is unlikely to result in a functioning renal unit or prevent the development of hypertension.[23] Our practice has been to treat the initial injury non-operatively, with delayed nephrectomy if intractable hypertension develops. The exception is patients with bilateral renal artery occlusion or unilateral occlusion in a solitary kidney, as up to 50% of these patients can avoid long-term dialysis if revascularization is performed.[24]

Pediatric Renal Injuries

Children have a high catecholamine output after trauma and can sustain a normal blood pressure until approximately half of the blood volume has been lost. Therefore, shock is a poor indicator of significant renal injury in children. Furthermore, gross hematuria is frequently absent.[25] In an effort to limit diagnostic workup in children without significant injuries, it has been suggested that only children with hematuria (>50 RBC/HPF following blunt trauma or >5 RBC/HPF following penetrating trauma) or clinical signs of injury, such as abdominal, flank or pelvic pain, ecchymosis, or a history of rapid deceleration injury undergo CT. When this protocol was followed, grade II or greater injuries were detected with a sensitivity of 98% after blunt trauma and 95% after penetrating trauma.[26]

Adrenal

Significant adrenal injuries are rare. Adrenal hematomas have been reported in approximately 2% of patients undergoing CT for blunt abdominal trauma. They occur more commonly on the right and typically in association with major abdominal and retroperitoneal injuries.[27] Radiographically, the hematoma is usually round or ovoid, with periadrenal stranding present in the vast majority of patients. Adrenal injuries are thought to result from severe hyperextension and compression against the spine and rarely occur as a result of penetrating injury. Though operative management has been reported, the majority of these patients can be managed conservatively with respect to the adrenal injury. Long-term sequelae, specifically adrenal insufficiency, have not been reported.[28,29]

Ureter

Injuries to the ureter resulting from external trauma are rare, representing less than 1% of all genitourinary injuries from violent trauma. They typically result from gunshot wounds, with blunt trauma and stab wounds responsible for less than 20% of ureteral injuries. Diagnosis of ureteral injury requires a high index of suspicion, because except for entrance and exit wounds there are usually no other physical signs of injury. Hematuria (gross or microscopic) is unreliable, as it is absent in about 26% of cases.[30] Furthermore, patients with ureteral injuries typically have multiple associated injuries, and complications resulting from a missed ureteral injury could be fatal in this patient population.

Diagnosis

Retrograde pyelography is the gold standard for diagnosing ureteral injury, but is often impractical in the trauma patient. CT with delayed images is an acceptable alternative, but clinical suspicion is paramount and if injury is suspected, further diagnostic or therapeutic management should occur.

When inspecting the ureter, it should be mobilized along its course and inspected for continuity, hemorrhage, and contusion. Indigo carmine or methylene blue can be given intravenously (typically 5 cc), or 1–2 cc of dilute dye can be directly injected into the renal pelvis to assist with identification of an occult injury. Ureteral injuries are graded according to a system developed by American Association for the Surgery of Trauma Organ Injury Scaling Committee,[31] which has been prospectively validated[32] and correlates with complexity of repair, number of associated injuries, and mortality. Grade I is a hematoma; grade II is a laceration with <50% transection; grade III is a laceration with >50% transection; grade IV is a complete transection with 2 cm or less of devascularized tissue; and grade V is an avulsion with more than 2 cm of devascularization.

Treatment

The ureter has a tenuous blood supply, and treatment of ureteral injuries is generally focused on minimizing disruption of blood flow and avoiding complications related to anastamotic breakdown from ischemia. The ureter is perfused by an anastomotic network of arteries within the adventitia that is supplied by the renal arteries in the upper ureter; by the aorta and iliac arteries in the mid-ureter; and by the superior vesical, vaginal, middle hemorrhoidal, and uterine arteries in the lower ureter. As a result of this tenuous blood supply, even small contusions or proximity gunshot wounds can result in stricture or leak as a result of microvascular damage and should be stented. We typically stent these patients for at least 8 weeks in order to allow adequate time for healing.

For more severe injuries, formal repair – either at the time of diagnosis or delayed – is required. Principles of ureteral repair include: careful mobilization; adequate debridement of nonviable tissue to bleeding edges; spatulated, tension-free, water-tight anastomosis over a stent; use of fine, nonreactive suture; retroperitoneal drainage; and omental interposition wrap when possible.

It is important to note that microvascular damage following gunshot wound or thermal injury can extend for up to 2 cm beyond evidence of gross injury.[33] Historically, high-velocity gunshot wounds have been thought to impart greater tissue damage than low-velocity gunshot wounds, thereby requiring wider debridement. However, this is likely an oversimplification and may result in debridement of unnecessary tissue in certain cases.[34] Therefore, ureteral injuries resulting from gunshot wounds or thermal injuries should be debrided to bleeding edges, but not further. Examination of the ureter with a Wood's lamp after injection of intravenous fluorescein (5 cc, 10% solution) may help identify devascularized areas,[35] though it

must be emphasized that this has not been well studied.

Injuries to the upper and middle two thirds of the ureter can usually be primarily repaired according to the principles outlined above. The ureter will usually need to be mobilized in order to acquire enough length; if necessary, the kidney can be mobilized downward and fixed to the psoas tendon with 0 prolene. For lower ureteral injuries, the ureter can usually be reimplanted directly into the bladder, with or without a psoas hitch. When possible, the anastomosis should be nonrefluxing, which is accomplished by creating a submucosal tunnel that is at least three times as long as the ureter is wide. Psoas hitch is performed by dividing the contralateral inferior pedicle and tacking the bladder to the psoas muscle with nonabsorbable suture. Psoas hitch following ureteral injury has an excellent success rate and is relatively quick and easy to accomplish. An indwelling stent should be placed following all attempts at ureteral repair and left in place for 8 weeks.

A number of other techniques have been described for bridging longer defects in the trauma patient, such as bowel interposition, autotransplant, and Boari flap, but these are time-consuming and in these situations delayed repair may be most appropriate. In certain situations – such as severe hemorrhagic shock, uncontrolled intraoperative bleeding, or severe associated injuries – damage control is an acceptable alternative to definitive repair. If the repair is likely to occur within 24 h, no intervention is necessary. If a delayed repair is planned, the ureter can be tied off with a long silk tie (to aid in dissection during the second-stage repair) and the kidney can be drained percutaneously, though this is best performed postoperatively because open nephrostomy placement can be too time-consuming in an unstable patient.

Delayed Diagnosis

Delayed diagnosis of ureteral injuries is common. Signs and symptoms of a possible missed injury include prolonged ileus, high output from drains, persistent flank or abdominal pain, urinary obstruction, elevated creatinine or BUN, and flank mass.[36] When a delayed diagnosis is recognized, it is usually best managed by percutaneous nephrostomy and, when possible, antegrade ureteral stent (retrograde ureteral stent is difficult and often unsuccessful in this situation). Urinomas can be effectively managed by placing a percutaneous drain. Complications of nondiagnosed ureteral injuries include fistulas, urinomas, and abscesses.

Bladder and Posterior Urethra

In the adult, the bladder lies in the true pelvis and, when not grossly distended, is well protected from injury. As it fills, the dome, which is covered by peritoneum, rises into the abdomen and is no longer protected by the bony pelvis. Therefore, injuries to the bladder from blunt abdominal trauma in an adult nearly always result from a direct blow to the abdomen in the presence of a distended bladder, or from compression of the pelvic contents following pelvic fracture. In the child, the bladder is almost entirely an abdominal organ and is much more susceptible to injury from penetrating and blunt trauma than the adult bladder. The posterior urethra is also well protected by the bony pelvis, but can be partially or completely transected in adults and children following pelvic fracture. Early diagnosis and proper initial management of bladder and posterior urethral injuries is critical to avoiding life-threatening acute complications and potentially debilitating long-term complications.

Gross hematuria is the hallmark sign of injury to the bladder, present in greater than 95% of bladder ruptures from both blunt and penetrating injury[37]; clinical findings can include suprapubic pain, dysuria, ileus, or an acute abdomen. The triad of urinary retention, blood at the meatus, and high-riding prostate is the classic presentation of patients with injuries to the posterior urethra, present in 91%, 87%, and 64% of these patients, respectively.[38] DRE is useful for detecting rectal injuries, which are associated with 5% of pelvic fractures and may affect management of an associated bladder injury, but is less useful in diagnosing urethral injury, as swelling and edema can obscure the exam. When urethral or bladder injury is suspected in a female, a full pelvic exam should be performed to rule out vaginal and rectal injuries. Computed tomography, which is routinely performed on patients with pelvic fracture, has an increasingly important role in screening

for urethral injury: the finding of an inferomedial pubic bone fracture or symphysis diastasis predicts urethral injury with a sensitivity of 92% and specificity of 64%.[39]

An algorithm for the diagnosis and treatment of bladder and urethral injuries is presented in Fig. 36.3. It should be emphasized that CT with delayed images is inadequate for the diagnosis of bladder injuries: when bladder injury is suspected, a cystogram is mandatory.[40] Because coincident upper and lower tract injuries are rare (occurring in 0.4% of all trauma patients) and bladder injury from blunt abdominal trauma is associated with pelvic fracture in the vast majority of cases, it has been suggested that a cystogram should be reserved for those with gross hematuria and concomitant pelvic fracture or clinical signs of bladder injury.[37]

Others have suggested that patients with pelvic fractures that are known to be associated with bladder injury (e.g., diastasis of the pubic symphysis or SI joint and sacral fractures) should also be evaluated with a cystogram, even in the absence of hematuria.[41] Cystogram is recommended in all cases of gross or microscopic hematuria following penetrating trauma to the bladder region. The 2002 Consensus Statement on Bladder Injuries[42] categorizes these injuries based on appearance of the cystogram: contusion (usually a mucosal or muscularis injury without extravasation), intraperitoneal rupture, extraperitoneal rupture, and combined intra- and extraperitoneal rupture.

All patients with suspected urethral injury should undergo retrograde urethrogram (RUG). There are a number of classification schemes for urethral injury, most of which are modifications of the system proposed in 1977 by Colapinto and McCallum.[43] However, these have proven to be complex and of minimal clinical utility, and in 2004, a consensus panel on urethral trauma[44] proposed a new classification system (Table 36.1).

The essential information to be obtained from the RUG (reflected in this new scheme) is the location of the injury (anterior or posterior), extent of the injury (partial or complete), and whether the bladder neck is involved, as up to half of these patients have no functional distal sphincter at follow-up and presumably rely on the bladder neck for continence.[45] As concomitant bladder injuries occur in 10–20% of patients with posterior urethral injuries, all patients with

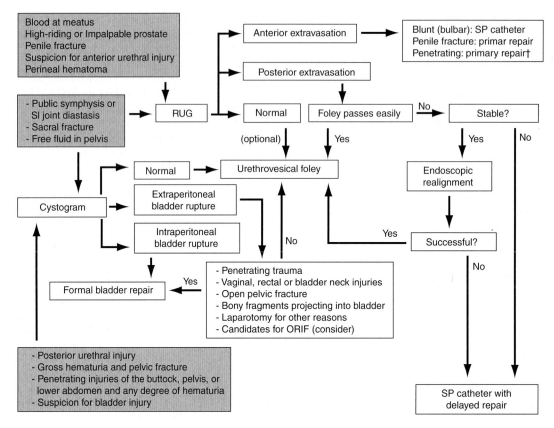

Figure 36.3. Algorithm for the management of traumatic injuries to the bladder and urethra. Gray boxes indicate presenting features. †Large or multiple defects should be repaired in a delayed fashion.

Table 36.1. Staging of urethral injuries according to the 2004 consensus panel on urethral trauma

Anterior urethra	
1	Partial disruption
2	Complete disruption
Posterior urethra	
3	Stretched but intact
4	Partial disruption
5	Complete disruption
6	Complex (involves bladder neck/rectum)

Reprinted from Chapple et al.[44] (with permission of Wiley-Blackwell).

injury to the posterior urethra should undergo antegrade cystoscopy or cystogram through the suprapubic tube to evaluate for bladder injury, specifically injury to the bladder neck.[46]

Bladder Injuries: Initial Management

All penetrating injuries to the bladder should be explored and repaired. Intraperitoneal injuries are often much larger than suggested on cystogram, are unlikely to heal spontaneously, and should be formally repaired.[47] Extraperitoneal bladder ruptures can be managed nonoperatively in select cases, but the incidence of complications such as fistulas, persistent leak, clot retention, and sepsis seem to be lower with open repair than with non-operative management. Therefore, formal repair is indicated if there are any complicating features, such as the presence of vaginal or rectal injuries, injury to the bladder neck, open pelvic fracture, or bony fragments projecting into the bladder.[48,49] Furthermore, if the patient is to undergo laparotomy for any reason, extraperitoneal injuries should be repaired, as these patients may be prone to development of vesicocutaneous fistulas if not repaired.[48] If internal fixation of the pelvic fracture is being considered, then open repair of the bladder at the same setting should be strongly considered in order to minimize the potential for infected hardware as a result of extravasated urine.[50]

Maintenance of adequate bladder drainage and minimization of infectious complications are critical to successful nonoperative management. The patient should be started immediately on prophylaxis for gram-positive and gram-negative organisms, and the bladder should be drained with a large bore Foley catheter, preferably 22-fr or greater. If there is difficulty maintaining reliable drainage after the first 24–48 h, the patient should undergo exploration and formal closure.

Bladder Injuries: Formal Repair

In all cases, the bladder should be approached through a midline incision, with careful inspection of the peritoneal contents for associated injuries[51] or penetrating injuries; the tract should be carefully inspected and all foreign bodies should be removed. The bladder should be inspected for other injuries and repaired transvesically. Intraperitoneal injuries typically have large rents, which can be widened in order to adequately inspect the remainder of the bladder. For penetrating and extraperitoneal injuries, we typically make a large longitudinal incision in the anterior bladder.

Following penetrating trauma, it is essential to visualize efflux of clear urine from each ureteral orifice; if this is not possible, or if efflux is bloody, retrograde pyelography is indicated to assess for ureteral injury. Bone fragments, foreign bodies, and devitalized tissue should be removed, and injuries to the bladder neck and vagina should be repaired. Pelvic hematomas should not be entered. The bladder should be closed in 2 layers with 3-0 absorbable suture. Bladder drainage can be safely accomplished with a large suprapubic tube placed through a separate stab incision or alternatively with a large urethral Foley.[52]

If internal fixation is being considered, suprapubic drainage should be avoided because of the risk of wound infection and subsequent hardware infection.[50,53] Drains are not necessary. The suprapubic tube or Foley catheter can be removed 5–7 days after repair of intraperitoneal rupture or penetrating trauma. For extraperitoneal bladder ruptures, a cystogram should be performed at 7–10 days, as up to 15% may have a persistent leak at that time.[54] If there is no leak, the catheter should be removed; if there is a leak, the cystogram can be repeated every 3–4 days.

Posterior Urethral Disruption: Immediate Management

Patients who suffer posterior urethral distraction injuries typically have a number of associated life-threatening injuries and as many as 50% of these patients will die of related injuries during the initial hospitalization. Therefore, the primary objective of the urologist is to establish prompt, reliable drainage of the bladder so as to avoid potentially fatal complications related to urinary extravasation and to facilitate stabilization of associated injuries.[48] This is best accomplished with immediate placement of a suprapubic catheter, though a single attempt at passing a well lubricated urethral catheter is reasonable. The urethral defect can be treated in a delayed fashion or with early endoscopic realignment.

In one large study that is consistent with several similar but smaller studies, 100% of patients who did not undergo endoscopic realignment developed clinically significant strictures and 47% eventually required perineal urethroplasty. Among patients who underwent early endoscopic realignment, 49% developed stricture and 25% eventually required perineal urethroplasty. The early realignment group required fewer procedures (1.6 vs 3.1) and experienced a slightly lower incidence of impotence and incontinence than the delayed reconstruction group. Though there is a clear selection bias in these studies (stable patients were more likely to undergo early realignment), it is clear that early endoscopic realignment is worthwhile in stable patients with posterior urethral distraction injuries.[38]

Posterior Urethral Disruption: Endoscopic Realignment

Endoscopic realignment can be performed as soon as the patient is stabilized and associated intraabdominal or pelvic injuries have been addressed. The patient should be warm, and any coagulopathies should be corrected. Positioning is typically determined by the extent of pelvic, lower extremity, and lumbar spine fractures. Antibiotics should be administered prior to the procedure. Antegrade access is secured through the existing suprapubic site with a sheath large enough to accommodate the flexible cystoscope. The bladder is inspected with the flexible cystoscope and then the antegrade cystoscope is used to guide a retrograde cystoscope into the bladder.

Through-and-through access is obtained with a guide wire, and an 18-fr council-tip urethral catheter is placed over the wire. When the retrograde cystoscope cannot be guided into the bladder, a wire can be passed through the antegrade cystoscope into the rupture site, and can usually be grasped with alligator forceps and pulled out of the urethra, establishing through-and-through access.

Postoperatively, suprapubic drainage should be continued for 3–4 days. Pericatheter retrograde urethrogram can be performed at 3 weeks after realignment by placing an 18-gauge angiocath alongside the catheter. Alternatively, if suspicion of leak is low, VCUG can be performed at 6 weeks with discontinuation of the catheter if the study is negative. In either case, if a leak is demonstrated, the catheter should be left in place and pericatheter RUG should be repeated in 2–4 week intervals until there is no leak. Close follow-up is necessary to assess for signs of developing stricture.

Anterior Urethral Trauma

The anterior urethra is more commonly injured than the posterior urethra, usually due to the blunt trauma of saddle injury. The mobility of the penis provides excellent protection against both blunt and penetrating injury, but injuries from gunshot wounds do occur and are believed to be increasing in incidence. Finally, the urethra is injured in 10–20% of penile fractures. In all cases, immediate management of the injury is necessary to avoid long-term morbidity, which is mainly due to urethral stricture disease.

All patients suspected of having a urethral injury should undergo retrograde urethrography. Anterior urethral injuries, as discussed previously and summarized in Table 36.1, are classified as partial or complete disruptions. Most penetrating injuries to the anterior urethra can be managed with primary spatulated end-to-end anastomosis over a Foley catheter after adequate irrigation and debridement, though some restraint is advisable during debridement.[55] If the defect is large or there are multiple defects, delayed repair is recommended. Blunt trauma, such as straddle injuries where the immobile bulbar urethra is compressed against the underside of the pubic symphysis, are probably best treated with suprapubic cystotomy and delayed repair,[56] though some advocate immediate endoscopic realignment.[57]

Fractured Penis

Penile fracture, or rupture of the tunica albuginea as a result of blunt trauma to the erect penis, classically occurs during intercourse when the penis is vigorously thrust against the pubic symphysis or perineum, though a number of other causes have been reported. The diagnosis is usually made based on the history and physical exam, which typically reveals the classic "eggplant" sign in which a hematoma develops deep to Buck's fascia. The penis is usually deviated away from the side of injury, and occasionally a blood clot or defect in the tunica can be palpated.

Retrograde urethrography is recommended to assess for concomitant urethral injury. Most authorities recommend early surgical repair of the defect as the most reliable way to decrease morbidity from this injury, which is mostly due to acquired penile angulation and potentially debilitating pain. The tunica defect should be closed with interrupted 2-0 or 3-0 absorbable suture. Complete urethral transections should be formally repaired over a catheter, whereas partial disruptions can be treated with primary repair, suprapubic cystotomy, or urethral catheter.

Penile Amputation

Initial management should focus on resuscitation of the patient and preservation of the penis. The penis should be rinsed in saline solution, wrapped in saline-soaked gauze, and placed in a sealed sterile bag, which is then suspended in ice-slush so as to limit direct contact of ice with the penile skin. Though reimplantation with nonmicrosurgical techniques has been reported, there is increased likelihood of skin loss, urethral stricture, and poor sensation with this approach. Therefore, every attempt should be made to transfer the patient to a tertiary care center with expertise in microsurgery such that the reimplant can occur within 16 h.

Scrotal and Testicular Trauma

Traumatic injuries to the scrotum and its contents are rarely life-threatening, but require prompt management in order to avoid long-term morbidity related to fertility, pain, and cosmesis. The most common scrotal injury is testicular rupture, a tear in the tunica albuginea that most commonly results from blunt trauma during sporting events. Testicular rupture can also occur as a result of MVA, straddle injury, or penetrating trauma from a gunshot or stab wound. It is well accepted that immediate intervention reduces the incidence of testicular loss, chronic pain, infection, and infertility. Therefore, when testicular rupture is suspected prompt surgical intervention is mandatory.[58,59]

The history and physical are essential to the diagnosis of testicular rupture. Typically, the patient reports acute onset of pain or edema associated with nausea and vomiting. The similarities in presentation between this and other acute scrotal conditions call for a broad differential diagnosis, including testicular torsion, torsion of the appendix testis, hematocele or hydrocele, and hematoma of the epididymis or spermatic cord.

Ultrasound is highly sensitive in detecting testicular rupture[60] and can be used when the diagnosis is not clear, but clinical judgment in this case is paramount and exploration should never be delayed in order to perform an ultrasound. In the absence of testicular rupture, small hematoceles, epididymal hematomas, and contusions of the testis can generally be managed non-operatively, though large hematomas should be explored and debrided. The testicle can be approached through a transverse or midline longitudinal incision. The tunica albuginea should be incised and necrotic tubules should be debrided. The tunica albuginea is then closed with 3-0 or 4-0 running absorbable suture. Dartos and skin are closed with 3-0 and then 4-0

chromic and a penrose is placed. The drain can be removed after 24 h, and antibiotics should be administered for 7 days.

Imaging

Imaging is an essential part of the evaluation of trauma to the genitourinary tract, and a thorough understanding of each imaging modality, including indications, techniques, and interpretation, is critical to the effective management of the trauma patient. Here, we discuss the most commonly used imaging modalities in genitourinary trauma and techniques for performing them.

CT-IVP (CT with Delayed Images)

CT is more sensitive than IVP in the diagnosis of renal and ureteral injuries and has largely replaced IVP in the workup of the trauma patient. Delayed images are essential for proper evaluation of the collecting system and ureters, but are inadequate for diagnosis of bladder injuries.

Technique

The study should be performed in three phases: an initial, unenhanced phase; a nephrogenic phase performed 90–100 s after the administration of nonionic contrast material (100–150 mL of 300 mg/mL Iodine at a rate of 2–4 mL/s); and a delayed phase, typically obtained 10 min following contrast administration. Because ureteral injuries often manifest with absence of contrast in the ureter on delayed images, it is essential to trace both ureters throughout their entire course. If the original study did not adequately demonstrate the ureters, a KUB can be performed to assess for delayed drainage.

Cystogram

Cystogram is the most accurate test for bladder rupture. It is critical to adequately distend the bladder: contrast opacification of the bladder following CT, even if the Foley catheter is clamped, is inadequate[40]. Both conventional radiography and CT are adequate, but CT is superior as it allows for identification of the location of many bladder injuries and may allow for identification of bladder neck injury.

Technique

After placing a Foley catheter, a scout film is obtained. The bladder should be distended via gravity; a useful technique is to remove the central piston from a 60 mL catheter-tip syringe, connect the catheter-tipped end to the Foley, and pour contrast into the syringe. The bladder should be filled to capacity: 400 mL in a person older than 11 years, or estimated by the formula "(age in years + 2)*30". If the patient cannot tolerate this amount, the bladder should be filled to capacity and then 50 mL of contrast should be injected by hand. For conventional radiography, half-strength contrast is used (Cystografin 30 diluted with normal saline), and AP and oblique images are necessary to identify lateral or posterior injuries. For CT, contrast should be diluted to 3–5% (approximately 1:6) in order to avoid artifact; the entire pelvis should be imaged, and postdrainage films are not necessary.

Retrograde Urethrogram (RUG)

RUG is the preferred method for evaluation of a suspected urethral injury, and must be performed prior to Foley catheter placement if an injury is suspected. Proper positioning is essential to an adequate exam.[61]

Technique

The patient should be positioned in the 25–35° oblique position, with the bottom leg flexed at the hip and knee such that the femur is outside the exposed field. In patients with pelvic fractures, it may be difficult to achieve this position; in these cases supine or oblique films without flexion at the hip are acceptable, though not ideal. A nonlubricated 14- or 16-French Foley catheter is placed into the urethra, just beyond the meatus. The balloon is inflated with 1–2 cc to ensure a good fit within the fossa navicularis. We typically tie an unfolded 4 × 4 around the glans to prevent leakage of contrast around the catheter and out the meatus, as this can obscure the exam. After obtaining a scout film, approximately 50–60 mL of half-strength Cystografin 30 is gently injected through the catheter, preferably during real-time fluoroscopy. If there is no extravasation, the catheter can be advanced to the bladder in order to perform a cystogram.

Retrograde Pyelogram (RPG)

Though often not practical in the acute trauma patient, RPG is the gold standard imaging modality for suspected ureteral injury.

Technique

A scout radiograph is obtained. The ureteral orifice is visualized cystoscopically and after removing air from the injection catheter and syringe, the ureteral orifice is intubated with a whistle-tip catheter and 5–10 cc of half-strength Renografin 60 is gently injected under real-time fluoroscopy. The entire collecting system and ureter should be visualized. Delayed images can be obtained to assess for drainage, but this is often not necessary in the trauma patient.

One-Shot IVP

In patients who are too unstable for abdominal CT, intraoperative one-shot IVP is a rapid, safe, and accurate tool for guiding decision-making following suspected renal and ureteral injury.

Technique

A bolus of 2 mL/kg Renografin 60 is given intravenously, either during resuscitation in the trauma bay or during laparotomy. A single plain abdominal radiograph is taken 10 min after injection. An additional plain film can be taken 20–30 min later if hypotension prevented adequate uptake by the kidneys or if ureteral opacification was incomplete.

References

1. Turner-Warwick R. A personal view of the immediate management of pelvic fracture urethral injuries. *Urol Clin North Am.* 1977;4:81
2. Traffic Safety Facts 2005. U.S. Department of Transportation http://www-nrd.nhtsa.dot.gov/pubs/tsf2005.pdf
3. 10 Leading Causes of Death by Age Group, United States – 2004. Office of Statistics and Programming, National Center for Injury Prevention and Control, CDC http://www.cdc.gov/injury/wisqars/LeadingCauses.html
4. Alsikafi NF, McAninch JW, Elliott SP, Garcia M. Nonoperative management outcomes of isolated urinary extravasation following renal lacerations due to external trauma. *J Urol.* 2006;176(6 Pt 1):2494-2497

5. Miller KS, McAninch JW. Radiographic assessment of renal trauma: our 15-year experience. *J Urol*. 1995;154 (2 Pt 1):352-355

6. Cass AS. Renovascular injuries from external trauma. *Urol Clin North Am*. 1989;16:213-220

7. Moore E, Shackford S, Packter H, et al. Scaling: spleen, liver, and kidney. *J Trauma*. 1989;29:1664-1666

8. Matthews LA, Smith EM, Spirnak JP. Nonoperative treatment of major blunt renal lacerations with urinary extravasation. *J Urol*. 1997;157:2056-2058

9. McAninch JW, Master VA. Genitourinary tract trauma. In: *Mastery of Surgery*. Philadelphia, PA: Lippincott Williams & Wilkins; 2007:1781

10. Moudouni SM, Hadj Slimen M, Manunta A, et al. Management of major blunt renal lacerations: is a nonoperative approach indicated? *Eur Urol*. 2001;40: 409-414

11. Thall EH, Stone NN, Cheng DL, et al. Conservative management of penetrating and blunt type III renal injuries. *Br J Urol*. 1996;77:512-517

12. Velmahos GC, Demetriades D, Cornwell EE 3rd, et al. Selective management of renal gunshot wounds. *Br J Surg*. 1998;85:1121-1124

13. Santucci RA, Fisher MB. The literature increasingly supports expectant (conservative) management of renal trauma – a systematic review. *J Trauma*. 2005;59(2):493-503; review

14. Altman AL, Haas C, Dinchman KH, Spirnak JP. Selective nonoperative management of blunt grade 5 renal injury. *J Urol*. 2000;164(1):27-30

15. Santucci RA, Wessells H, Bartsch G, et al. Evaluation and management of renal injuries: consensus statement of the renal trauma subcommittee. *BJU Int*. 2004;93(7):937-954

16. McAninch JW. Editorial comment. *J Urol*. 2000;164(1): 30-31

17. Sofocleous CT, Hinrichs C, Hubbi B, et al. Angiographic findings and embolo-therapy in renal arterial trauma. *Cardiovasc Intervent Radiol*. 2005;28:39

18. Breyer BN, McAninch JW, Elliott SP, Master VA. Minimally invasive endovascular techniques to treat acute renal hemorrhage. *J Urol*. 2008;179(6):2248-2252; discussion 2253

19. Morey AF, McAninch JW, Tiller BK, et al. Single shot intraoperative excretory urography for the immediate evaluation of renal trauma. *J Urol*. 1999;161(4):1088-1092

20. McAninch JW, Carroll PR. Renal trauma: kidney preservation through improved vascular control – a refined approach. *J Trauma*. 1982;22(4):285-290

21. Carroll PR, Klosterman P, McAninch JW. Early vascular control for renal trauma: a critical review. *J Urol*. 1989;141(4):826-829

22. Meng MV, Brandes SB, McAninch JW. Renal trauma: indications and techniques for surgical exploration. *World J Urol*. 1999;17(2):71-77; review

23. Haas CA, Dinchman KH, Nasrallah PF, Spirnak JP. Traumatic renal artery occlusion: a 15-year review. *J Trauma*. 1998;45(3):557-561

24. Lohse JR, Botham RJ, Waters RF. Traumatic bilateral renal artery thrombosis: case report and review of literature. *J Urol*. 1982;127:522-525

25. Stein JP, Kaji DM, et al. Blunt renal trauma in the pediatric population: indications for radiographic evaluation. *Urology*. 1994;44(3):406-410

26. Buckley J, McAninch JW. Pediatric renal injuries: management guidelines from a 25-year experience. *J Urol*. 2004;172:687-690

27. Rana AI, Kenney PJ, Lockhart ME, et al. Adrenal gland hematomas in trauma patients. *Radiology*. 2004;230(3): 669-675

28. Gomez RG, McAninch JW, Carroll PR. Adrenal glandtrauma: diagnosis and management. *J Trauma*. 1993;35:870

29. Gabal-Shehab L, Alagiri M. Traumatic adrenal injuries. *J Urol*. 2005;173(4):1330-1331

30. Elliott SP, McAninch JW. Ureteral injuries from external violence: the 25-year experience at San Francisco General Hospital. *J Urol*. 2003;170(4 Pt 1):1213-1216

31. Moore EE, Cogbill TH, Jurkovich GJ, et al. Organ injury scaling. III: chest wall, abdominal vascular, ureter, bladder, and urethra. *J Trauma*. 1992;33(3):337-339

32. Best CD, Petrone P, Buscarini M, et al. Traumatic ureteral injuries: a single institution experience validating the American Association for the Surgery of Trauma-Organ Injury Scale grading scale. *J Urol*. 2005;173(4): 1202-1205

33. Amato JJ, Billy LJ, Gruber RP, et al. Vascular injuries. An experimental study of high and low velocity missile wounds. *Arch Surg*. 1970;101(2):167-174

34. Santucci RA, Chang YJ. Ballistics for physicians: myths about wound ballistics and gunshot injuries. *J Urol*. 2004;171(4):1408-1414

35. Kirchner KA, MacMillan RA, Krueger RP, Raju S. Fluorescein sodium injection for evaluation of ureteric vasculature prior to cadaveric renal transplantation. *Transplantation*. 1982;33(1):100-101

36. Brandes S, Coburn M, Armenakas N, McAninch J. Diagnosis and management of ureteric injury: an evidence-based analysis. *BJU Int*. 2004;94(3):277-289; review

37. Brewer ME, Wilmoth RJ, Enderson BL, Daley BJ. Prospective comparison of microscopic and gross hematuria as predictors of bladder injury in blunt trauma. *Urology*. 2007;69(6):1086-1089

38. Mouraviev VB, Coburn M, Santucci RA. The treatment of posterior urethral disruption associated with pelvic fractures: comparative experience of early realignment versus delayed urethroplasty. *J Urol*. 2005;173(3):873-876

39. Basta AM, Blackmore CC, Wessells H. Predicting urethral injury from pelvic fracture patterns in male patients with blunt trauma. *J Urol*. 2007;177(2):571-575

40. Doyle SM, Master VA, McAninch JW. Appropriate use of CT in the diagnosis of bladder rupture. *J Am Coll Surg*. 2005;200(6):973

41. Voelzke BB, McAninch JW. Is genitourinary imaging necessary in patients who have microscopic hematuria after trauma? *Nat Clin Pract Urol*. 2007;4(11):590-591

42. Gomez RG, Ceballos L, Coburn M, et al. Consensus statement on bladder injuries. *BJU Int*. 2004;94(1):27-32; review

43. Colapinto V, McCallum RW. Injury to the male posterior urethra in fractured pelvis: a new classification. *J Urol*. 1977;118(4):575-580

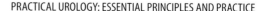
44. Chapple C, Barbagli G, Jordan G, et al. Consensus statement on urethral trauma. *BJU Int.* 2004;93(9):1195-1202; review

45. Whitson JM, McAninch JW, Tanagho EA, et al. Mechanism of continence after repair of posterior urethral disruption: evidence of rhabdosphincter activity. *J Urol.* 2007; 179:1035-1039

46. Carlin BI, Resnick MI. Indications and techniques for urologic evaluation of the trauma patient with suspected urologic injury. *Semin Urol.* 1995;13:9-24

47. Lucey DT, Smith MJ, Koontz WW Jr. Modern trends in the management of urologic trauma. *J Urol.* 1972;107(4): 641-646

48. Kotkin L, Koch MO. Morbidity associated with nonoperative management of extraperitoneal bladder injuries. *J Trauma.* 1995;38(6):895-898

49. Franko ER, Ivatury RR, Schwalb DM. Combined penetrating rectal and genitourinary injuries: a challenge in management. *J Trauma.* 1993;34(3):347-353

50. Taffet R. Management of pelvic fractures with concomitant urologic injuries. *Orthop Clin North Am.* 1997;28(3): 389-396

51. Elliott SP, McAninch JW. Extraperitoneal bladder trauma: delayed surgical management can lead to prolonged convalescence. *J Trauma.* 2009;66:274-275

52. Volpe MA et al. Is there a difference in outcome when treating traumatic intraperitoneal bladder rupture with or without a suprapubic tube? *J Urol.* 1999;161(4):1103-1105

53. Parry NG, Rozycki GS, Feliciano DV, et al. Traumatic rupture of the urinary bladder: is the suprapubic tube necessary? *J Trauma.* 2003;54(3):431-436

54. Corriere JN Jr, Sandler CM. Management of the ruptured bladder: seven years of experience with 111 cases. *J Trauma.* 1986;26(9):830-833

55. Monga M, Moreno T, Hellstrom WJ. Gunshot wounds to the male genitalia. *J Trauma.* 1995;38(6):855-858

56. Park S, McAninch JW. Straddle injuries to the bulbar urethra: management and outcomes in 78 patients. *J Urol.* 2004;171(2 Pt 1):722-725

57. Ying-Hao S, Chuan-Liang X, Guo-Qiang L, et al. Urethroscopic realignment of ruptured bulbar urethra. *J Urol.* 2000;164:1543

58. Kukadia AN, Ercole CJ, Gleich P, et al. Testicular trauma: potential impact on reproductive function. *J Urol.* 1996; 156(5):1643-1646

59. Morey AF, Metro MJ, Carney KJ, et al. Consensus on genitourinary trauma: external genitalia. *BJU Int.* 2004;94(4): 507-515

60. Breyer BN, Cooperberg MR, McAninch JW, Master VA. Improper retrograde urethrogram technique leads to incorrect diagnosis. *J Urol.* 2009 Aug;182(2):716-7

61. Micallef M, Ahmad I, Ramesh N, Hurley M, McInerney D. Ultrasound features of blunt testicular injury. *Injury.* 2001 Jan;32(1):23-6

37

Bladder Cancer

Evelyne C.C. Cauberg, Jean J.M.C.H. de la Rosette, and Theo M. de Reijke

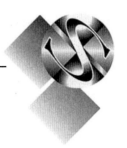

Who Should Be Investigated?

Epidemiology

In Europe, 110,500 cases of bladder cancer were diagnosed in 2008[1] and an estimated 70,530 will be diagnosed in the USA in 2010,[2] making it the fourth most common cancer in men and twelfth most common cancer in women. The incidence is around three to four times higher among men than women and two times higher among white than black populations.[3] It has been demonstrated that bladder cancer is one of the most expensive cancers in terms of lifetime costs per patient, mainly due to the lifelong need for follow-up and high recurrence rates in nonmuscle-invasive disease requiring multiple treatments.[4]

Risk Factors

Several risk factors for bladder cancer have been identified. Cigarette smoking is the most important risk factor, resulting in a two- to fourfold increased risk for bladder cancer. Although cessation of smoking reduces the risk, the risk level will always remain higher compared to non-smoker.[5] Occupational exposure to urothelial carcinogens is another important risk factor. Workers in the chemical, dye, and rubber industries (aromatic amines) or aluminum, coal, and roofing industries (polycyclic aromatic hydrocarbons) have an increased risk of developing bladder cancer, as well as painters and hairdressers.[5] Furthermore, exposure to pelvic radiotherapy or antecedent treatment with cyclophosphamide, a drug used in the management of lymphoproliferative and myeloproliferative diseases, increases the risk for bladder cancer.[5] This risk is proportional to the duration of exposure or received dose. Consumption of coffee or artificial sweeteners has been suggested as risk factor; however, this has never been confirmed in large series.[5] While the aforementioned risk factors may lead to the development of urothelial cell carcinomas (UCC), chronic urinary tract infection (e.g., due to indwelling bladder catheter) and Schistosomiasis infection are both associated with an increased risk of developing squamous cell carcinoma of the bladder.[6] Schistosomiasis (also known as bilharziasis) is a parasitic disease which is highly endemic in Egypt, but also to a lesser degree in other parts of Africa, in the Middle East, the Caribbean, South America, and East Asia. The eggs of *S. haematobium* cause a chronic inflammatory response, resulting in changes in the urothelium that may ultimately lead to a squamous cell carcinoma. The time between onset of schistosomiasis infection and subsequent development of squamous cell carcinoma is around 30 years.[7]

Of all bladder cancers, UCC is the most common subtype (>90%). Squamous cell carcinoma and adenocarcinoma account for 5% and 1% of bladder cancers, respectively. Very rare subtypes of bladder cancer are small cell carcinoma, sarcoma, and metastases.[5]

Role of Screening

The goal of screening for bladder cancer is to detect the disease at an earlier stage, in order to improve the chances of curative treatment or to prolong nonmetastatic disease status. The population to be screened is not yet known, although high-risk patients probably would benefit most. Which test to be used is also not clear, and most research has focused on hematuria detection by simple urinalysis or urine cytology. The diagnostic accuracy of the currently available urinary markers does not (yet) allow them to be used as a primary screening tool.[4] To date, there is no evidence that bladder cancer screening results in better outcomes and no nation-wide programs have been started.

Signs and Symptoms

The most common presenting symptom is painless hematuria, either microscopic or macroscopic, which occurs in 85–90% of patients with bladder cancer. Furthermore, voiding symptoms such as urgency, frequency, or dysuria can indicate the presence of carcinoma in situ (CIS). Physical examination is often unremarkable, especially in nonmuscle-invasive bladder cancer (NMIBC). Rarely, patients present with flank pain (ureteral obstruction), edema of the legs, a palpable pelvic mass, weight loss, or abdominal or bone pain (distant metastases).

Which Investigations Should Be Done?

Imaging

Transabdominal ultrasound of the bladder may reveal bladder wall thickening or a tumor protruding into the bladder lumen. Hydronephrosis may be seen on ultrasound of the kidneys in case of a ureteral tumor or a bladder tumor obstructing the ureteral orifice. Although the incidence of simultaneous bladder and upper urinary tract tumors (UUT) is low (1.8%),[8] detecting an UUT will significantly change management. Several techniques are available for evaluation of the upper urinary tract. Intravenous urography (IVU), CT-urography, and MRI-urography all combine intravenous administration of a contrast agent with imaging in order to detect filling defects in the upper urinary tract and bladder, indicating the presence of tumor. Nowadays, IVU has been replaced by CT-urography in many centers. CT-urography does not require bowel preparation, has a high diagnostic accuracy, and also provides information on possible extravesical growth of the bladder tumor, lymph nodes, and renal parenchyma. Disadvantages of CT-urography are its high radiation dose and high costs.[9] Another, however, invasive technique for evaluation of the upper urinary tract is retrograde uretero-pyelography, a combination of cystoscopic administration of a contrast agent via the ureteral orifices and abdominal x-ray. Which investigation has the highest sensitivity is unknown. At the moment, it is questioned whether imaging of the upper urinary tract should be performed and if so, which modality should be used. The European Association of Urology (EAU) guidelines recommend IVU or CT-urography in selected cases such as tumors located in the trigone and in case of a muscle-invasive bladder cancer.[10] The American Urological Association (AUA) guidelines recommend UUT imaging in all patients with hematuria, especially those without evidence of infections, stones, or other causative factors.

Cystoscopy

White light cystoscopy is the gold standard for detection of bladder cancer in combination with urinary cytology. Cystoscopy enables direct visualization of the urothelium and can be performed in the office. Tumor characteristics such as appearance, number, location, and size as well as mucosal abnormalities should be described and preferably be drawn in a bladder diagram and documented if flexible video-cystoscopy is performed (Fig. 37.1). Most UCCs present as papillary lesions, but solid lesions or a mixed type can also be seen. The cystoscopic appearance of the base of the tumor, either pedunculated or sessile, should also be described. Most low-grade UCCs are pedunculated. CIS is often not visible macroscopically, but it can present as mucosal velvety red spots, although these could be confused with sequelae of urinary tract infections or intravesical instillations.

Flat lesions (e.g., CIS) or small papillary lesions can be missed during white light cystoscopy. Therefore, new techniques have been

Figure 37.1. Example of a bladder diagram and documentation of a papillary bladder tumor (pTaG2) with indication of the anatomic location.

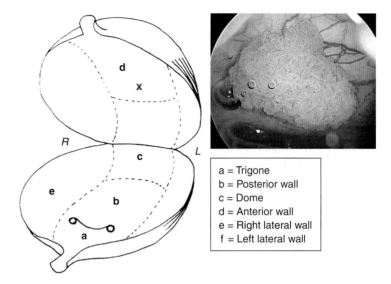

a = Trigone
b = Posterior wall
c = Dome
d = Anterior wall
e = Right lateral wall
f = Left lateral wall

developed to improve the diagnostic accuracy of cystoscopy. Photodynamic diagnosis (PDD), also referred to as fluorescence cystoscopy, is a cystoscopic technique using fluorescence to indicate malignant bladder tissue based on differences in fluorescent capacities between benign and malignant bladder tissue. Prior to cystoscopy, a fluorescent agent is administered intravesically, and when illuminating the bladder wall with light of a specific wavelength (blue light), malignant tissue appears pink/red on a blue background. Several studies have shown that PDD outperforms white light cystoscopy when it comes to sensitivity, especially for CIS.[11] However, the relatively low specificity of this technique and the costs remains a problem. Another more recently developed technique is Narrow Band Imaging (NBI). This technique uses light of narrow wavelengths with center wavelengths in the blue and green spectrum of light to enhance contrast of mucosal surface and microvascular structures without the use of dyes. Only two studies in bladder cancer have been published to date.[12,13] It has some advantages over PDD (e.g., it is immediately applicable, does not cause any side effects, is not restricted in time by photobleaching, and avoids the extra costs of an intravesical agent), but its clinical applicability has to be established in larger series.

During cystoscopy, no information on histopathological diagnosis is obtained, which makes discrimination of inflammatory lesions and CIS often difficult, since they both can present as mucosal red spots. Furthermore, estimation of the grade or stage of a bladder tumor at cystoscopy, even by an experienced urologist, is often not accurate. Therefore, new techniques like Raman spectroscopy and Optical Coherence Tomography (OCT) have been developed that aim at providing an objective histopathological diagnosis during cystoscopy in a minimally invasive way. While Raman spectroscopy can estimate the molecular composition of tissue, OCT can produce cross-sectional images with high resolutions comparable to histopathology.[14] Both methods show promising preliminary results, but more research still has to be conducted before any of the techniques can be implemented in the management of bladder cancer.

Urine Tests

Urinalysis can detect microscopic hematuria, which is most often defined as more than three erythrocytes per high-power field. Since hematuria can be intermittent, repeat testing increases the chance to find hematuria. No clear correlation is found between the degree of hematuria and the aggressiveness of the disease.

Urinary cytology is based on a pathologist's interpretation of morphological changes of urothelial cells. It is an important tool for detection and follow-up of bladder cancer and can be performed on freshly voided urine or on a bladder barbotage specimen. Voided urine can contain malignant cells from the complete urinary tract, while a bladder barbotage only contains cells from the bladder mucosa. Specificity of urine cytology is very high and for high-grade tumors, sensitivity is also high (>90%). However, for low-grade tumors, sensitivity is limited to 30–65%. Thus a negative result cannot exclude the presence of a low-grade cancer. Another limitation of cytology is its high inter- and intraobserver variability.[15] Cytological evaluation can be hampered if the number of cells present in the specimen is low. This is more likely to occur on voided urine specimen, which usually contains fewer cells and cells with a poorer quality, compared to a barbotage specimen.[16] Furthermore, interpretation can be difficult in case of concomitant urinary tract stones, infection, or intravesical therapy.

Urinary bladder tumor markers have been developed in an attempt to provide a noninvasive, objective urine test with high diagnostic accuracy for bladder cancer. These tests detect tumor-associated molecules, altered gene expression, or chromosomal alterations. They are designed to be used for screening of bladder cancer, to replace cystoscopy in the follow-up, or to serve as prognosticators. Several markers exist to date, among which BTA stat, BTA-TRAK, NMP-22, BLCA-4, BLCA-1, Quanticyt, Survivin, FGFR3, and UroVysion test (FISH). Most of these markers have a significantly higher sensitivity than cytology, and some can detect tumors before they are visible at cystoscopy. However, specificity still is lower than of cytology. At the moment, no single urine test can replace cystoscopy for diagnosis and in the field of prognosis more research is needed.[16]

What Is the Primary Treatment in Case a Bladder Tumor Is Detected?

TUR

Transurethral resection (TUR) is the primary treatment for bladder tumors and has both a diagnostic and therapeutic objective: to obtain tissue for histopathological diagnosis and to completely remove all visible tumors. TUR starts with a thorough cystoscopy in order to identify all lesions to be resected. Like in diagnostic cystoscopy, tumor characteristics such as appearance, number, location, and size as well as mucosal abnormalities should be described and preferably be drawn in a bladder diagram. Subsequently, all visible tumors are resected and/or areas suspect for CIS are biopsied. In case of positive urine cytology and negative cystoscopy, random bladder biopsies including biopsies of the prostatic urethra in the male should be taken in order to exclude CIS. During resection, it is important to resect deep enough in order to obtain sufficient muscularis propria, which is essential for correct pathological staging. Cauterization has to be avoided as much as possible since this might hamper pathological examination. Furthermore, overdistension of the bladder should be avoided since this increases the risk of bladder wall perforation.

A bimanual examination should also be performed when the patient is under anesthesia, especially when a muscle-invasive tumor is suspected. It should be performed both before TUR (to estimate if there is suspicion of muscle-invasive growth) and after TUR (to estimate if the resection has been complete).

Performing a complete TUR is important to reduce the risk of recurrence. However, the quality of TUR varies widely among institutions. This was found in a multicenter EORTC GU group study that assessed the recurrence rate at first follow-up cystoscopy after TUR in 2,410 patients. The variance of recurrence rate among the different institutions (3–41%) could not be explained by disease-related factors, suggesting that quality of TUR (thus the urologist) was the only responsible factor.[17]

PDD-Assisted TUR

As mentioned in the previous section, small or flat bladder tumors may be missed during white light cystoscopy, leading to early "recurrences." Using PDD during TUR can be helpful in accomplishing a more complete tumor resection and prevent overlooking tumors. This was investigated in prospective, randomized studies by comparing the residual tumor rate at repeat-TUR 6 weeks after the initial TUR with white light only versus PDD-assisted TUR. All studies showed a statistically significant lower residual tumor rate if resection was performed using PDD. Residual tumor rates varied from 25% to 53.1% for white light resection and 4.5–32.7% for PDD-assisted resection.[18-20] The benefit of PDD in terms of progression rates and survival still has to be established in larger randomized trials.

Immediate Postoperative Intravesical Chemotherapy

Administration of a single intravesical instillation of chemotherapy after TUR decreases the risk of tumor recurrence by 39% in patients with Ta or T1 bladder cancer and is therefore recommended in all patients with NMIBC.[21]

Mitomycin C (MMC) and Epirubicin are most commonly used and are comparable with regard to efficacy. Timing is important though; the instillation should preferably be administered within 24 h following TUR. In case of bladder perforation or extensive TUR, it should not be administered due to the risk of local and systemic complications. The rationale behind the immediate postoperative instillation is to eradicate microscopic tumor left behind or to destroy circulating tumor cells that could implant at sites where the urothelium has been damaged, both factors that are believed to be responsible for early recurrences.

Pathology

Pathologic stage is one of the most important prognostic factors for bladder cancer. Accurate staging is therefore essential, since this highly influences patient management. The 2002 TNM classification proposed by the Union International Contre le Cancer (UICC) is the most frequently used system for staging of bladder cancer (Table 37.1).[22] Stage Ta, T1, and Tis (CIS) are grouped as NMIBC, whereas stages T2, T3, and T4 are grouped as muscle-invasive bladder cancer. The old terminology of "superficial" bladder cancer suggests a non-aggressive biology and should be avoided since some NMIBCs do behave aggressively. CIS is a flat, high-grade noninvasive UCC and is a highly malignant entity. Of all primary UCCs, approximately 70–80% presents as NMIBC and the remainder as muscle-invasive disease. Among the NMIBC, 70% present as Ta lesions, 20% as T1, and 10% as CIS.

Another important prognostic factor, besides stage, is grade. The 1973 World Health Organisation (WHO) grading system is most commonly used for this.[23] This system discriminates well differentiated (G1), moderately differentiated (G2), and poorly differentiated (G3) UCC. In 2004, the WHO and International Society of Urological Pathology (ISUP) published a new grading system in an attempt to reduce the interobserver variability, frequently encountered in the 1973 system.[24] This system differentiates between papillary urothelial neoplasms of low malignant potential (PUNLMP) and low-grade or high-grade UCC. The PUNLMP lesions lack the cytological features of malignancy, but the cells do show a papillary configuration. Until the system is validated by more clinical trials, it is recommended to use it together with the 1973 system. The two systems are compared in Fig. 37.2.

Re-TUR

It has been demonstrated that bladder tumors may be understaged based on the specimen obtained from the initial TUR[25] and there is a substantial risk of residual tumor after the initial TUR.[17] To improve pathologic accuracy and to increase local tumor control, a second or re-TUR can be performed.[25] Re-TUR should be considered in case of incomplete first resection, for example, in multiple or large tumors or when muscular tissue was not present in the pathology specimen. Furthermore, it is recommended in case of high grade Ta or any T1 bladder tumor(s).[10] Preferably, the re-TUR should be performed 2–6 weeks after the initial TUR. It has been shown that by doing so, the recurrence-free survival can be increased.[26]

NMIBC and Risk Groups

After primary treatment, approximately 15–70% of patients with NMIBC will develop recurrent disease in the first year and 7–40% will progress to muscle-invasive disease in the first 5 years.

Many studies have been conducted to identify prognostic factors for recurrence and progression to muscle-invasive disease in patients with NMIBC, with sometimes conflicting results. The EORTC-GU group has conducted a multivariate analysis on prognostic factors in 2,596 patients

Table 37.1. 2002 TNM classification of urinary bladder cancer

Primary tumor (T)		
TX	Primary tumor cannot be assessed	
T0	No evidence of primary tumor	
Ta	Noninvasive papillary carcinoma	
Tis	Carcinoma in situ: "flat tumor"	
T1	Tumor invades subepithelial connective tissue	
T2	Tumor invades muscle	
	T2a	Tumor invades superficial muscle (inner half)
	T2b	Tumor invades deep muscle (outer half)
T3	Tumor invades perivesical tissue	
	T3a	Microscopically
	T3b	Macroscopically
T4	Tumor invades any of the following: prostate, uterus, vagina, pelvic wall, abdominal wall	
	T4a	Tumor invades prostate, uterus, or vagina
	T4b	Tumor invades pelvic wall or abdominal wall
Regional lymph nodes (N)		
Regional nodes are those within the true pelvis; all others are distant lymph nodes.		
NX	Regional lymph nodes cannot be assessed	
N0	No evidence of regional lymph node metastasis	
N1	Metastasis in a single lymph node 2 cm or less in greatest dimension	
N2	Metastasis in a single lymph node, more than 2 cm but not more than 5 cm in greatest dimension; or multiple lymph nodes, none greater than 5 cm in greatest dimension	
N3	Metastasis in a lymph node, more than 5 cm in greatest dimension	
Distant metastasis (M)		
MX	Distant metastasis cannot be assessed	
M0	No evidence of distant metastasis	
M1	Distant metastasis	

Source: Reprinted from *AJCC Cancer Staging Handbook*, 6th ed, p. 369.

with primary NMIBC in order to develop tables to calculate the risk of recurrence and progression in an individual patient.[27] This analysis revealed that the most important prognostic factors for recurrence were number of tumors, tumor size, and prior recurrence rate, whereas the most important prognostic factors for progression were stage, presence of concomitant CIS, and grade. A scoring system was developed based on these six factors, in order to calculate the total scores for recurrence and progression

in an individual patient (Table 37.2). These total scores correspond to a certain risk for recurrence and progression at 1 and 5 years (Table 37.3). Based on these risk tables, low-, intermediate-, and high-risk groups can be defined (last column of Table 37.3). These individualized risk tables can help the urologist in making management decisions. However, these risk tables have not yet been validated externally. Furthermore, 20% of patients from the analysis initially received no treatment, less than

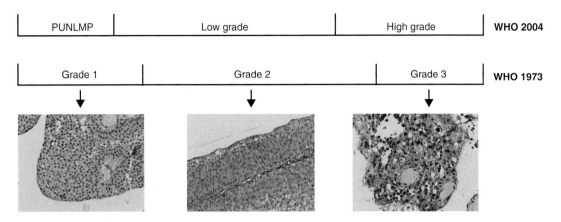

| PUNLMP | Low grade | High grade | **WHO 2004** |

| Grade 1 | Grade 2 | Grade 3 | **WHO 1973** |

Figure 37.2. Histologic spectrum of UCC, comparison of the WHO 1973 and WHO 2004 grading systems.

Table 37.2. EORTC Risk tables for NMIBC: weights used to calculate the recurrence and progression scores

Factor	Recurrence	Progression
Number of tumors		
Single	0	0
2–7	3	3
≥8	6	3
Tumor size		
<3 cm	0	0
≥3 cm	3	3
Prior recurrence rate		
Primary	0	0
≤1 recurrence/year	2	2
>1 recurrence/year	4	2
T category		
Ta	0	0
T1	1	4
CIS		
No	0	0
Yes	1	6
Grade		
G1	0	0
G2	1	0
G3	2	5
Total score	0–17	0–23

10% received an immediate instillation of chemotherapy, a re-TUR was not performed in high-risk patients, and BCG was given without maintenance instillations. Therefore, the predicted recurrence and progression rates of the risk tables might be higher compared to current clinical practice.

Who Needs Adjuvant Therapy in NMIBC?

The need for adjuvant intravesical instillations depends on the patient's risk of recurrence and progression to muscle-invasive disease. In patients with a low risk of recurrence and progression, no further adjuvant treatment is recommended following one immediate adjuvant instillation following TURB. In patients with a high risk of progression, that is, those with a high-grade tumor or CIS, further adjuvant treatment with intravesical immunotherapy is recommended. For the remaining intermediate-risk patients, either further intravesical chemotherapy or immunotherapy is recommended.[10,28]

Intravesical Chemotherapy

Adjuvant intravesical chemotherapy reduces the risk of recurrence with 14–26%, but not the risk of progression or survival.[29] There are no differences in efficacy between the available intravesical chemotherapeutic agents whereas side-effects are mostly mild and transient (Table 37.4). Despite the large amount of research on adjuvant

Table 37.3. EORTC Risk tables for NMIBC: probability of recurrence and progression according to total score

Recurrence score	Prob recurrence 1 year (95% CI)	Prob recurrence 5 years (95% CI)	Risk group
0	15% (10–19%)	31% (24–37%)	Low
1–4	24% (21–26%)	46% (42–49%)	Intermediate
5–9	38% (35–41%)	62% (58–65%)	Intermediate
10–17	61% (55–67%)	78% (73–84%)	High
Progression score	Prob progression 1 year (95% CI)	Prob progression 5 years (95% CI)	Risk group
0	0.2% (0–0.7%)	0.8% (0–1.7%)	Low
2–6	1.0% (0.4–1.6%)	6% (5–8%)	Intermediate
7–13	5% (4–7%)	17% (14–20%)	High
14–23	17% (10–24%)	45% (35–55%)	High

intravesical chemotherapy, the optimal dose, schedule, and duration of treatment have not yet been determined. It seems that long-term instillations, for example, during more than 1 year, only outperform short-term instillations when an immediate postoperative instillation was not administered.[35]

Intravesical Immunotherapy

Intravesical administration of bacille Calmette-Guérin (BCG), a live attenuated strain of Mycobacterium bovis, causes an inflammatory immunologic response in patients with NMIBC.[36] In bladder cancer patients at high risk of tumor recurrence, intravesical BCG instillations reduce recurrence risk significantly (31% reduction compared to MMC). In patients at low risk of recurrence, this effect was not observed.[37] In all patients with CIS, Ta, and T1 bladder cancer, BCG instillations reduce the risk of progression to muscle-invasive disease equally (a reduction of 37% in the odds of progression), but only when a form of maintenance instillations has been given.[38] Compared to intravesical chemotherapy, BCG induces greater toxicity[37] (Table 37.4). Of all patients receiving BCG instillations, approximately 11% have to stop treatment due to mild side effects (irritative bladder symptoms, hematuria) and approximately 5% due to severe side effects (fever, BCG-induced lung infection, liver toxicity, sepsis).[32] The optimal dose of BCG has not yet been defined, nor the optimal schedule of

instillations. An induction course of 6 weekly instillations is advised, but the maintenance schedules vary widely. The South-West Oncology Group proposed maintenance schedule of 3 weekly instillations at[3,6,12,18,24,35] and 36 months is generally used. BCG is indicated in patients at high risk of progression and is the first-line treatment in patients with CIS. In intermediate-risk patients either BCG or chemotherapy can be administered.[10]

Immediate Cystectomy and CIS

Cystectomy is the treatment of choice for patients with CIS not responding to adequate BCG treatment.[10] The timing of cystectomy remains a challenge and is still controversial. There are no prospective trials comparing immediate cystectomy with BCG, but for some patients immediate cystectomy will be overtreatment.[39] Immediate cystectomy after TUR as *primary* treatment option for CIS patients is advised especially in case of concomitant high-grade papillary tumors.

New Developments: Intravesical Chemotherapy

Gemcitabine, a chemotherapeutic agent applied systemically for muscle-invasive disease, has been studied for intravesical instillation in patients with NMIBC. The drug is well tolerated

BLADDER CANCER

Table 37.4. Overview of side effects of the most common used intravesical chemo- and immunotherapeutic agents

Intravesical agent	Side effects	Incidence	Recommendations for management
Epirubicin[30]	Chemical cystitis	13–56%	Consider anticholinergics, if severe postpone instillation
Mitomycin C[30,31]	Chemical cystitis	3–40%	Consider anticholinergics, if severe postpone instillation
	Eczema-like desquamation of the skin (mainly palms, soles, perineum, chest, face)	4–16%	Careful cleaning of hands/genitalia after voiding (prevention) Stop further instillations
BCG[30,32-34]	Local:		
	BCG-induced cystitis	6–95%	Consider acetaminophen and anticholinergics , postpone instillation and consider prophylactic ofloxacin[a]
	Bacterial cystitis	26%	Antibiotics, postpone instillation
	Urinary frequency	31%	Consider anticholinergics or prophylactic ofloxacin[a]
	Macroscopic hematuria	1–40%	Postpone instillation until hematuria resolves
	Contracted bladder	<1%	Stop further BCG, hydrodistention
	Systemic:		
	Fever (≥39°C)	2–17%	Antipyretics, postpone instillation until resolution of symptoms consider BCG dose reduction + prophylactic INH[b]
	Influenza-like symptoms	23%	Antipyretics, postpone instillation until resolution of symptoms
	Skin rash and/or joint pain	0.3–3.3%	Antihistamins and/or NSAIDs, postpone instillation until resolution of symptoms, consider BCG dose reduction + prophylactic INH[b]
	BCG-induced lung infection	<1%	Hospitalization, fluids, INH[b], RFP[c] and ethambutol[d] for at least 6 months. Stop further BCG
	Liver toxicity	<1%	Hospitalization, fluids, INH[b], RFP[c] and ethambutol[d] for at least 6 months. Stop further BCG
	BCG sepsis	<1%	Hospitalization, INH[b], RFP[c] and ethambutol[d] for at least 6 months, prednisolone. Stop further BCG

[a] Ofloxacin: 200 mg.
[b] INH (isoniazid): 300 mg once daily.
[c] RFP (rifampicin): 600 mg once daily.
[d] Ethambutol: 1,200 mg once daily.

and efficacy varies with the highest reported response rate at 56%. Although to be confirmed in larger series, the preliminary results are promising.[40]

Apaziquone (EOquin), a derivative of MMC, is another new agent under investigation for its potential in the treatment of NMIBC. It requires activation by cellular reductase enzymes, which are found in higher concentration in tumor tissue compared to normal tissue, suggesting selective therapy. Intravesical use is shown to be safe, with side effects comparable to the other chemotherapeutic agents. The first marker lesion study has shown promising efficacy and more trials are ongoing.[41,42]

New Developments: Device-Assisted Therapy

The combination of bladder wall hyperthermia and intravesical chemotherapy is a relatively new treatment modality, also known as thermochemo-therapy (Synergo® system, medical enterprises Ltd, Amsterdam, the Netherlands). It has been used both as ablative therapy and prophylactic treatment. The hyperthermia of 42.5–43.5°C is established by a microwave applicator inserted in the bladder through a specially developed intra-vesical catheter which also enables temperature measurements and chemotherapy instillation. Although local side effects appear to be worse compared with intravesical chemotherapy alone, the preliminary clinical results seem promising.[43]

Electromotive drug administration is another technique in development aiming at increasing the drug diffusion across the bladder wall by using intravesical chemotherapy in combination with an external electrical source to tempo-rarily breach the urothelial barrier of the bladder.[40] One randomized clinical trial (212 patients) demonstrated that intravesical admin-istration of sequential BCG and electromotive mitomycin in patients with high-risk NMIBC improved disease-free interval, recurrence, and progression rate with 48 months, 16.0%, and 12.6%, respectively, compared to BCG alone. Side effects of this treatment were comparable to BCG alone.[44]

Although these techniques show hopeful pre-liminary results, more evidence is needed before these can be implemented in the management of NMIBC.

What Is the Preferred Treatment in Patients with Muscle-Invasive Bladder Cancer?

Muscle-invasive bladder cancer is a lethal dis-ease warranting aggressive therapy. If untreated, up to 85% of patients die within 2 years of the diagnosis.[45] Radical cystectomy with pelvic lymph node dissection is the treatment of choice for muscle-invasive bladder cancer.[46] Nowadays, several bladder-preserving treatment modali-ties are being performed, though only in selected cases. The choice of primary therapy is mainly influenced by the age of the patient and his/her comorbidity.[47]

Radical Cystectomy with Pelvic Lymph Node Dissection

Radical cystectomy includes the removal of the bladder and adjacent organs: in male the pros-tate and seminal vesicles, in female the uterus and adnexa. Removal of the complete urethra is advised in case of positive intraoperative frozen section of the urethral margin, if the bladder tumor is located at the trigone (women) or if it infiltrates into the prostatic stroma.[48] Despite the aggressive approach toward muscle-invasive bladder cancer, nearly 25% of patients already have positive lymph nodes at the time of cystec-tomy.[46] Bilateral pelvic lymphadenectomy pro-vides important histopathological information which can be used to indicate patients who might benefit from adjuvant therapy. Additionally, it might have impact on recurrence and survival.[49] Controversy exists on the extent of lymph node dissection; some data showed that an extended lymph node dissection (including the distal para-aortic, para-caval, and presacral lymph nodes) improved survival in patients with muscle-invasive disease.[48] It is suggested that lymph node density (represented by the number of positive nodes divided by the number of lymph nodes removed) might be a useful prog-nostic variable.[48] In most large, contemporary series, mortality of radical cystectomy varies between 3% and 7%.[46] The pathologic stage and presence of lymph node metastases are the most important predictive factors regarding survival. In one of the largest radical cystectomy series for muscle-invasive bladder cancer to date, the overall survival at 5 and 10 years was 60% and 43%, respectively.[46]

Nowadays, in some clinics and in selected cases, radical cystectomy with pelvic lymph node dissection is also performed either completely (robot) laparoscopic or laparoscopic hand-assisted. Peri-operative complications and functional outcomes seem to be comparable to open radical cystectomy, but long-term oncologic results are still awaited.[50]

Urinary Diversion Following Cystectomy

Three modalities can be used to divert the urine: an incontinent stoma (e.g., uretero-ileo (colonic)-cutaneostomy), a continent urinary reservoir to be catheterized or controlled by the anal sphincter (e.g., ileal or colonic pouch, ureterosigmoidstomy), or an orthotopic bladder substitution.[51] The latter is used increasingly during the last decade: in some series up to 90% of patients who undergo a cystectomy.[52] An advantage of an incontinent stoma is that it is easy to construct and that it does not require patient compliance for good function, thus upper urinary tracts are "safe." However, with orthotopic bladder substitution (and to a lesser degree also with continent diversion) the body image is not changed, which can have clear psychological benefits.[52] When choosing for a type of diversion, one has to take into consideration the patient's age, comorbidity, previous surgery, and wishes.[52] Several segments of the intestinal tract can be used for urinary diversion: ileum, colon, ileocaecal, and appendix. For all types of diversion, early and late complications are described. Among these are urine leakage, pouch rupture, stomal stenosis, stone formation, bacteriuria, and metabolic complications (acidosis, vitamin B12 deficiency).

Sexual Function-Preserving Techniques

A maximum of 40–60% of patients still have normal sexual function after radical cystectomy, even when the operation is performed by experienced surgeons. Therefore, a modification of cystectomy has been developed, with preservation of the vas deferens, prostate or prostatic capsule and seminal vesicles (men) or all internal genitalia (women). This should be performed only in highly selected patients, e.g., relatively young patients with organ-confined disease. Overall, this technique seems effective, with reported preservation of sexual function in 75–100% of patients. Long-term follow-up studies are required to determine oncological outcomes.[53]

Bladder-Preservation Treatments

Bladder preservation therapies have been developed for patients wishing to preserve their bladder and/or patients who are poor candidates for radical surgery. Single modality, organ-preserving therapy can either consist of complete TUR of the primary tumor, systemic chemotherapy, or external beam or interstitial radiotherapy. Compared to radical cystectomy, the recurrence-free and long-term survival outcome of patients with a muscle-invasive bladder cancer treated with single modality therapy have been disappointing.[54] Therefore, these single modality therapies should only be considered in highly selected patients, unfit for radical surgery or multimodality treatment. In a group of highly selected patients (solitary T1–T3 tumors, <5 cm, good bladder capacity), single modality treatment using external beam radiotherapy followed by interstitial radiotherapy produced good results.[55]

Multimodality treatment combines the three aforementioned single modality interventions in an attempt to improve survival outcome. The combination of systemic chemotherapy (mostly cisplatin, methotrexate, and vinblastine (CMV)) and radiotherapy aims at eradicating micrometastases whereas complete TUR aims at controlling local disease. The long-term survival rates of multimodality therapy series seem to be comparable to radical cystectomy series. However, these two treatment modalities have never been compared in a randomized study and it is suggested that the encouraging outcomes of the multimodality studies are due to selection bias, e.g., mainly inclusion of patients with favorable pathological characteristics.[54] Multimodality treatment requires compliant patients, good interdisciplinary cooperation, and thorough follow-up.

Partial cystectomy is another bladder-preserving treatment that can be an alternative to radical cystectomy in highly selected cases. Data on this treatment modality are sparse and there are no studies directly comparing it with radical cystectomy. The location and size of the tumor are important factors in selecting patients for partial cystectomy. Small tumors located in the dome or in a diverticulum seem suitable, whereas tumors located in the lateral wall or trigone seem less appropriate. Patients with multifocal tumors are at high risk for nonmuscle-invasive recurrence and the presence of CIS or lymph node metastases is associated with recurrence of advanced disease.[56]

Is There a Role for (Neo) Adjuvant Chemotherapy in Muscle-Invasive Bladder Cancer?

With radical cystectomy as solitary treatment, the 5 year survival rates range from 27% to 67%, depending on the histopathological stage.[57] In order to improve outcome, in 1985 the chemotherapy regimen of methotrexate, vinblastine, doxorubicin, and cisplatin (MVAC) was introduced in the management of muscle-invasive bladder cancer.[57] Since then, several chemotherapeutic regimens have been evaluated, either in neoadjuvant and adjuvant setting.

Neoadjuvant Chemotherapy

Administering chemotherapy before surgery has some advantages. The local response to the agent can be evaluated during surgery, which is a prognostic important issue. Furthermore, surgery might be more effective after shrinkage of the tumor. The delay to systemic therapy is less than in the adjuvant setting and the tolerability is expected to be better.[57] Several randomized clinical trials have assessed the value of neoadjuvant chemotherapy for muscle-invasive bladder cancer, with conflicting outcomes. Therefore, three meta-analyses have been undertaken, each including 11 trials and more than 2,600 patients. All show a statistically significant improvement in survival of 5–6.5% at 5 years in the cisplatin-containing combination chemotherapy trials, irrespective of the type of definitive treatment.[58-60] The question remains whether these results may be generalized to the whole population, since some trials mainly included relatively young patients (median age of 63–65 years),

with an excellent performance status and good renal function.[61]

Adjuvant Chemotherapy

Administering chemotherapy after surgery also has its benefits. Since the histopathological stage is known at that time, patients at risk for recurrence/progression who might benefit from adjuvant treatment can be identified, thus reducing overtreatment. Furthermore, there is no needless delay in surgical treatment, which may occur in patients not responding to neoadjuvant chemotherapy.[57] One meta-analysis on adjuvant chemotherapy for muscle-invasive bladder cancer has been published to date based on 6 trials with only 491 patients available for survival analysis in total. All trials used cisplatin-based chemotherapy after cystectomy. An improvement of 9% on survival at 3 years was found (95% CI: 1–16%). The authors state that a definitive conclusion on the effect of adjuvant chemotherapy cannot be drawn due to the limited number of trials and patients and they highlight the need for further appropriately sized randomized clinical trials.[62]

Preoperative Radiotherapy

The aim of radiotherapy prior to cystectomy is to eradicate microscopic extravesical disease and to prevent seeding of tumor cells during surgery. There is a lack of evidence for the standard use of preoperative radiotherapy. Only a few randomized trials have been conducted, most of them with a limited number of patients.[63]

How Should Bladder Cancer Patients Be Followed-up?

Follow-up After TUR in NMIBC

The high number of recurrence, and progression of NMIBC, even in the long term, demand meticulous follow-up. Assessment should include a history with special focus on voiding symptoms and hematuria, cystoscopy, and cytology. There is no role for urinary markers in the follow-up since no urinary marker available to date meets the requirements to replace cystoscopy. Early recurrences are a very important prognostic factor and therefore, the first follow-up cystoscopy should be performed 3 months after the TUR in every patient with NMIBC. Further follow-up schemes are based on the risks of recurrence and progression. The following schedule for follow-up is proposed by the EAU. In patients with low-risk tumors and no recurrence on cystoscopy at 3 months, the next follow-up assessment can be performed 9 months later and then yearly up to 5 years. In patients with high-risk tumors, assessment should be performed every 3 months following TUR for the first 2 years, every 4 months in the third year, every 6 months up to the fifth year, and annually thereafter. For patients with an intermediate-risk tumor, the schedule lies in between.[10] The AUA recommends a likewise schedule with assessment every 3 months in the first 2 years, every 6 months for the subsequent 2–3 years, and annually thereafter.[28] The risk of upper urinary tract tumors increases in patients with multiple and high-risk tumors. Therefore, it is advised to evaluate the upper urinary tract every year in high-risk patients.[10]

Follow-up in Muscle-Invasive Bladder Cancer

Patients with muscle-invasive bladder cancer treated with radical cystectomy are at risk of developing local or distant recurrence. Contemporary series demonstrate a 5–15% chance of local recurrence and 50% chance of distant recurrence, depending on stage and lymph node status at time of cystectomy. The most common sites of local recurrence are vaginal wall, rectum, or pelvic lymph nodes not removed during surgery. Symptoms of local recurrence are pelvic, perineal, or lower extremity pain, bleeding, lower extremity or penile edema, bowel obstruction, constipation, and priapism. The most common sites of distant recurrence are lung, liver, and bones. Furthermore, recurrence may occur at the urethra (8–17%) or upper urinary tract (2–4%).[64]

Follow-up schedules should be modeled to the patient's risk for tumor recurrence. At every visit, a history and physical examination should be performed including digital rectal or vaginal examination to search for a palpable pelvic mass. Blood chemistry should be performed focusing on liver and kidney tests. With regard to imaging, MRI or CT of the abdomen and pelvis is advised for evaluation of local recurrence and chest X-ray for evaluation of lung metastasis. Cytological examination of urethral washings or voided urinary cytology is advised to monitor urethral recurrence. For evaluation of the upper urinary tracts, CT-urography or IVP and upper tract urinary cytology are advised.[64,65] A recommended follow-up scheme includes imaging of the upper tract yearly and CT/MRI of the pelvis and abdomen, chest X-ray, and cytology (both urethral washing and upper tract) half-yearly for the first 2 years and yearly thereafter.[64]

It is also important to look for functional complications after urinary diversion. Blood chemistry should be performed regularly: electrolytes, base excess, Vitamin B12 for metabolic complications, and creatinin for kidney function. Furthermore, imaging of the diversion and upper urinary tract is required to detect urinary stones or upper tract dilatation.[64]

References

1. Ferlay J, Parkin DM, Steliarova-Foucher E. Estimates of cancer incidence and mortality in Europe in 2008. *Eur J Cancer.* 2010;46:765-781
2. Jemal A, Siegel R, Xu J, Ward E. Cancer statistics, 2010. *CA Cancer J Clin.* 2010;60:277-300
3. Grasso M. Bladder cancer: a major public health issue. *Eur Urol Suppl.* 2008;7:510-515
4. Madeb R, Golijanin D, Knopf J, Messing EM. Current state of screening for bladder cancer. *Expert Rev Anticancer Ther.* 2007;7:981-987
5. Colombel M, Soloway M, Akaza H, et al. Epidemiology, staging, grading and risk stratification of bladder cancer. *Eur Urol Suppl.* 2008;7:618-626
6. Kirkali Z, Chan T, Manoharan M, et al. Bladder cancer: epidemiology, staging and grading, and diagnosis. *Urology.* 2005;66:4-34
7. Shokeir AA. Squamous cell carcinoma of the bladder: pathology, diagnosis and treatment. *BJU Int.* 2004;93: 216-220
8. Palou J, Rodriguez-Rubio F, Huguet J, et al. Multivariate analysis of clinical parameters of synchronous primary superficial bladder cancer and upper urinary tract tumor. *J Urol.* 2005;174:859-861
9. Stacul F, Rossi A, Cova MA. CT urography: the end of IVU? *Radiol Med.* 2008;113:658-669
10. Babjuk M, Oosterlinck W, Sylvester R, Kaasinen E, Bohle A, Palou-Redorta J. EAU Guidelines on non-muscle-invasive urothelial carcinoma of the bladder. *Eur Urol.* 2008;54:303-314
11. Jocham D, Stepp H, Waidelich R. Photodynamic diagnosis in urology: state-of-the-art. *Eur Urol.* 2008;53:1138-1150
12. Bryan RT, Billingham LJ, Wallace DM. Narrow-band imaging flexible cystoscopy in the detection of recurrent

urothelial cancer of the bladder. *BJU Int.* 2008;6: 702-705

13. Herr HW, Donat SM. A comparison of white-light cystoscopy and narrow-band imaging cystoscopy to detect bladder tumour recurrences. *BJU Int.* 2008;9:1111-1114

14. Crow P, Stone N, Kendall CA, Persad RA, Wright MP. Optical diagnostics in urology: current applications and future prospects. *BJU Int.* 2003;92:400-407

15. Engers R. Reproducibility and reliability of tumor grading in urological neoplasms. *World J Urol.* 2007;25: 595-605

16. Lokeshwar VB, Habuchi T, Grossman HB, et al. Bladder tumor markers beyond cytology: International Consensus Panel on bladder tumor markers. *Urology.* 2005;66:35-63

17. Brausi M, Collette L, Kurth K, et al. Variability in the recurrence rate at first follow-up cystoscopy after TUR in stage Ta T1 transitional cell carcinoma of the bladder: a combined analysis of seven EORTC studies. *Eur Urol.* 2002;41:523-531

18. Daniltchenko DI, Riedl CR, Sachs MD, et al. Long-term benefit of 5-aminolevulinic acid fluorescence assisted transurethral resection of superficial bladder cancer: 5-year results of a prospective randomized study. *J Urol.* 2005;174:2129-2133

19. Denzinger S, Burger M, Walter B, et al. Clinically relevant reduction in risk of recurrence of superficial bladder cancer using 5-aminolevulinic acid-induced fluorescence diagnosis: 8-year results of prospective randomized study. *Urology.* 2007;69:675-679

20. Kriegmair M, Zaak D, Rothenberger KH, et al. Transurethral resection for bladder cancer using 5-aminolevulinic acid induced fluorescence endoscopy versus white light endoscopy. *J Urol.* 2002;168:475-478

21. Sylvester RJ, Oosterlinck W, van der Meijden AP. A single immediate postoperative instillation of chemotherapy decreases the risk of recurrence in patients with stage Ta T1 bladder cancer: a meta-analysis of published results of randomized clinical trials. *J Urol.* 2004;171: 2186-90

22. Sobin LH, Wittekind Ch. *TNM Classification of Malignant Tumors.* 6th ed. New York: Wiley Liss; 2002:196-198

23. Epstein JI, Amin MB, Reuter VR, Mostofi FK. The World Health Organization/International Society of Urological Pathology consensus classification of urothelial (transitional cell) neoplasms of the urinary bladder. Bladder Consensus Conference Committee. *Am J Surg Pathol.* 1998;22:1435-1448

24. Eble JN, Sauter G, Epstein JI, Sesterhenn IA. *WHO Classification of Tumours. Pathology and Genetics of Tumours of the Urinary System and Male Genital Organs.* Lyon: IARCC Press; 2004

25. Herr HW. Surgical factors in the treatment of superficial and invasive bladder cancer. *Urol Clin North Am.* 2005;32:157-164

26. Divrik RT, Yildirim U, Zorlu F, Ozen H. The effect of repeat transurethral resection on recurrence and progression rates in patients with T1 tumors of the bladder who received intravesical mitomycin: a prospective, randomized clinical trial. *J Urol.* 2006;175:1641-1644

27. Sylvester RJ, van der Meijden AP, Oosterlinck W, et al. Predicting recurrence and progression in individual patients with stage Ta T1 bladder cancer using EORTC risk tables: a combined analysis of 2596 patients from seven EORTC trials. *Eur Urol.* 2006;49:466-5

28. Hall MC, Chang SS, Dalbagni G, et al. Guideline for the management on nonmuscle invasive bladder cancer (stages Ta, T1, and Tis): 2007 update. *J Urol.* 2007;178: 2314-2330

29. Pawinski A, Sylvester R, Kurth KH, et al. A combined analysis of European Organization for Research and Treatment of Cancer, and Medical Research Council randomized clinical trials for the prophylactic treatment of stage TaT1 bladder cancer. European Organization for Research and Treatment of Cancer Genitourinary Tract Cancer Cooperative Group and the Medical Research Council Working Party on superficial bladder cancer. *J Urol.* 1996;156:1934-40

30. Koya MP, Simon MA, Soloway MS. Complications of intravesical therapy for urothelial cancer of the bladder. *J Urol.* 2006;175:2004-2010

31. Bolenz C, Cao Y, Arancibia MF, Trojan L, Alken P, Michel MS. Intravesical mitomycin C for superficial transitional cell carcinoma. *Expert Rev Anticancer Ther.* 2006;6: 1273-1282

32. van der Meijden AP, Sylvester RJ, Oosterlinck W, Hoeltl W, Bono AV. Maintenance Bacillus Calmette-Guerin for Ta T1 bladder tumors is not associated with increased toxicity: results from a European Organisation for Research and Treatment of Cancer Genito-Urinary Group Phase III Trial. *Eur Urol.* 2003;44:429-434

33. Rischmann P, Desgrandchamps F, Malavaud B, Chopin DK. BCG intravesical instillations: recommendations for side-effects management. *Eur Urol.* 2000;37(suppl 1): 33-36

34. Rischmann P, Nicolas L, Malavaud B, Chopin D, Saint F, Colombel M. The effect of ofloxacin on bacillus Calmette-Guerin induced toxicity in patients with superficial bladder cancer: results of a randomized, prospective, double-blind, placebo controlled, multicenter study. *J Urol.* 2006;176:935-939. and the ITB01 study group

35. Sylvester RJ, Oosterlinck W, Witjes JA. The schedule and duration of intravesical chemotherapy in patients with non-muscle-invasive bladder cancer: a systematic review of the published results of randomized clinical trials. *Eur Urol.* 2008;53:709-719

36. Herr HW, Morales A. History of bacillus Calmette-Guerin and bladder cancer: an immunotherapy success story. *J Urol.* 2008;179:53-56

37. Shelley MD, Wilt TJ, Court J, Coles B, Kynaston H, Mason MD. Intravesical bacillus Calmette-Guerin is superior to mitomycin C in reducing tumour recurrence in high-risk superficial bladder cancer: a meta-analysis of randomized trials. *BJU Int.* 2004;93:485-490

38. Sylvester RJ, van der Meijden AP, Lamm DL. Intravesical bacillus Calmette-Guerin reduces the risk of progression in patients with superficial bladder cancer: a meta-analysis of the published results of randomized clinical trials. *J Urol.* 2002;168:1964-1970

39. Chang SS, Cookson MS. Radical cystectomy for bladder cancer: the case for early intervention. *Urol Clin North Am.* 2005;32:147-155

40. Hendricksen K, Witjes JA. Current strategies for first and second line intravesical therapy for nonmuscle invasive bladder cancer. *Curr Opin Urol.* 2007;17:352-357

41. Witjes JA, Kolli PS. Apaziquone for non-muscle invasive bladder cancer: a critical review. *Expert Opin Investig Drugs.* 2008;17:1085-1096

42. van Boven E, de Reijke TM, Vergunst H, et al. Phase II marker lesion study with intravesical instillation of Apaziquone for superficial bladder cancer: toxicity and marker response. *J Urol.* 2006;176:1349-1353

43. Colombo R, Salonia A, Da Pozzo LF, et al. Combination of intravesical chemotherapy and hyperthermia for the treatment of superficial bladder cancer: preliminary clinical experience. *Crit Rev Oncol Hematol.* 2003;47:127-139

44. Di Stasi SM, Giannantoni A, Giurioli A, et al. Sequential BCG and electromotive mitomycin versus BCG alone for high-risk superficial bladder cancer: a randomised controlled trial. *Lancet Oncol.* 2006;7:43-51

45. Prout GR, Marshall VF. The prognosis with untreated bladder tumors. *Cancer.* 1956;9:551-558

46. Stein JP, Skinner DG. Radical cystectomy for invasive bladder cancer: long-term results of a standard procedure. *World J Urol.* 2006;24:296-304

47. Koppie TM, Serio AM, Vickers AJ, et al. Age-adjusted Charlson comorbidity score is associated with treatment decisions and clinical outcomes for patients undergoing radical cystectomy for bladder cancer. *Cancer.* 2008;112:2384-2392

48. Stein JP, Skinner DG. The role of lymphadenectomy in high-grade invasive bladder cancer. *Urol Clin North Am.* 2005;32:187-197

49. Herr HW, Bochner BH, Dalbagni G, Donat SM, Reuter VE, Bajorin DF. Impact of the number of lymph nodes retrieved on outcome in patients with muscle invasive bladder cancer. *J Urol.* 2002;167:1295-1298

50. Haber GP, Crouzet S, Gill IS. Laparoscopic and robotic assisted radical cystectomy for bladder cancer: a critical analysis. *Eur Urol.* 2008;54:54-62

51. Turner WH, Studer UE. Cystectomy and urinary diversion. *Semin Surg Oncol.* 1997;13:350-358

52. Hautmann RE. Urinary diversion: ileal conduit to neobladder. *J Urol.* 2003;169:834-842

53. Soloway MS, van Poppel H, Thuroff J, et al. Muscle-invasive urothelial carcinoma of the bladder. *Urology.* 2007;69:3-16

54. Kuczyk M, Turkeri L, Hammerer P, Ravery V. Is there a role for bladder preserving strategies in the treatment of muscle-invasive bladder cancer? *Eur Urol.* 2003;44:57-64

55. Blank LECM, Koedooder K, van Os R, van de Kar M, van der Veen JH, Koning CCE. Results of bladder-conserving treatment, consisting of brachytherapy combined with limited surgery and external beam radiotherapy, for patients with solitary T1-T3 bladder tumors less than 5 cm in diameter. *Int J Radiat Oncol Biol Phys.* 2007;69:454-458

56. Holzbeierlein JM, Lopez-Corona E, Bochner BH, et al. Partial cystectomy: a contemporary review of the Memorial Sloan-Kettering Cancer Center experience and recommendations for patient selection. *J Urol.* 2004;172:878-881

57. Herr HW, Dotan Z, Donat SM, Bajorin DF. Defining optimal therapy for muscle invasive bladder cancer. *J Urol.* 2007;177:437-443

58. Advanced Bladder Cancer (ABC) Meta-analysis Collaboration. Neoadjuvant chemotherapy in invasive bladder cancer: update of a systematic review and meta-analysis of individual patient data. *Eur Urol.* 2005;48:202-205

59. Advanced Bladder Cancer (ABC) Meta-analysis Collaboration. Neoadjuvant chemotherapy in invasive bladder cancer: a systematic review and meta-analysis. *Lancet.* 2003;361:1927-1934

60. Winquist E, Kirchner TS, Segal R, Chin J, Lukka H. Neoadjuvant chemotherapy for transitional cell carcinoma of the bladder: a systematic review and meta-analysis. *J Urol.* 2004;171:561-569

61. Sternberg CN, Collette L. What has been learned from meta-analyses of neoadjuvant and adjuvant chemotherapy in bladder cancer? *BJU Int.* 2006;98:487-489

62. Advanced Bladder Cancer (ABC) Meta-analysis Collaboration. Adjuvant chemotherapy in invasive bladder cancer: a systematic review and meta-analysis of individual patient data. *Eur Urol.* 2005;48:189-199

63. Widmark A, Flodgren P, Damber JE, Hellsten S, Cavallin-Stahl E. A systematic overview of radiation therapy effects in urinary bladder cancer. *Acta Oncol.* 2003;42:567-581

64. Bochner BH, Montie JE, Lee CT. Follow-up strategies and management of recurrence in urologic oncology bladder cancer: invasive bladder cancer. *Urol Clin North Am.* 2003;30:777-789

65. Oosterlinck W, Lobel B, Jakse G, Malmstrom PU, Stockle M, Sternberg C. Guidelines on bladder cancer. *Eur Urol.* 2002;41:105-112

38

Prostate Cancer

Charles D. Scales Jr. and Judd W. Moul

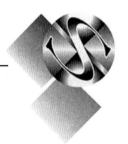

Introduction

Prostate cancer is the most common cancer among men in the United States. In 2010, an estimated 217,730 men will be diagnosed with the disease, and 32,050 will die from prostate cancer.[1] Despite a lack of consensus regarding optimal diagnosis and management strategies for prostate cancer, recent data suggest that prostate cancer mortality is decreasing, from 38.6 per 100,000 in 1990 to 25.5 per 100,000 in 2004.[1] The current chapter provides an overview of the epidemiology of prostate cancer, current strategies for screening and diagnosis, and treatments for both localized and advanced disease.

Epidemiology

Age

The risk of prostate cancer increases as men age, with 85% of men diagnosed after the age of 65, as compared to less than 0.1% of cases diagnosed among men under 50 years of age.[2] Autopsy series demonstrate an increasing incidence of microscopic foci of cancer without a peak or modal distribution. During the PSA testing era, an age migration at diagnosis has occurred, such that the age at diagnosis has significantly declined among men with prostate cancer. From birth to death, men in the United States have a one in six probability of developing prostate cancer.[1]

Race

Significant variation in prostate cancer incidence and mortality exists among various racial groups. The incidence of prostate cancer among African-American men is 1.6 times that of white American men, and the mortality from prostate cancer among African-American men is 2.4 times that of white American men.[1] Conversely, Asian-American men have a much lower incidence and mortality of prostate cancer as compared to white Americans, and Hispanic-American men have similar incidence and mortality to white Americans. The etiology for the differences among these groups, which are more cultural and social than biological, is likely multifactorial, including environment, access to care, and diet/lifestyle factors.

Geographic Variation

Significant variation exists in prostate cancer mortality and incidence between countries and ethnicities worldwide. North American and Scandinavian men experience the highest incidence and mortality from this disease, whereas the incidence and mortality are lowest in Asia.[3,4] The cause of this geographic variation is not entirely understood, but likely involves a number

C.R. Chapple and W.D. Steers (eds.), *Practical Urology: Essential Principles and Practice*,
DOI: 10.1007/978-1-84882-034-0_38, © Springer-Verlag London Limited 2011

of factors including environment, genetics, diet/lifestyle factors, and access to care.

Risk Factors and Prevention

Family History

Family history is a consistent risk factor for prostate cancer. Men with a single first-degree male relative (father or brother) have twice the risk of prostate cancer as men without this family history. The risk of prostate cancer increases with an increasing family history of disease.[5,6] Based on this familial association, several studies have investigated genes, particularly single nucleotide polymorphisms (SNPs) that may be associated with increased prostate cancer risk. These studies have noted associations with SNPs located in three regions of 8q24, and one region on 17q12 and 17q24.3, among others, and examined the potential for using these SNPs as screening markers for prostate cancer.[7]

Diet and Lifestyle

A number of dietary and lifestyle-associated risk factors for prostate cancer have been proposed, including dietary fat, smoking, alcohol consumption, and obesity. Unfortunately, epidemiologic studies examining the association between these factors and prostate cancer incidence have yielded mixed results. Therefore, definitive evidence linking these diet and lifestyle influences to the development of prostate cancer is lacking.

Prevention

Prostate cancer is an attractive target for chemoprevention efforts because of the dependence of prostate cancer development on androgens. Results from the Prostate Cancer Prevention Trial demonstrated a 24.8% relative reduction in the risk of prostate cancer among men randomized to daily finasteride as compared to placebo.[8] However, a reported increase in high-grade cancer detection in the finasteride group has hindered adoption of finasteride for this purpose. Recent PCPT follow-up studies suggest that the observation of high-grade cancers in the finasteride group may be a detection artifact.

The results of ongoing trials will hopefully clarify this unexpected finding.

Dietary factors have also been examined for prostate cancer prevention. Based on observational studies, both selenium and vitamin E were thought to potentially have a role in prostate cancer prevention. However, results of a recent randomized controlled trial demonstrated that neither selenium nor vitamin E, alone or in combination, decreased the incidence of prostate cancer as compared to placebo.[9]

Screening and Diagnosis

Current Screening Recommendations

Early detection of prostate cancer through annual PSA testing with digital rectal examination is a subject of active debate in the medical literature. The American Urological Association recommends that average-risk men 50 years of age or older with at least a 10 year life expectancy be offered PSA testing (with digital rectal exam) annually for the early detection of prostate cancer. For men at higher risk (i.e., African-American race or family history), PSA testing may be offered at a younger age. Similarly, the American Cancer Society suggests that men aged at least 50 years with a 10 year life expectancy be *offered* PSA testing with DRE to detect prostate cancer. Again, men with additional risk factors should be offered PSA testing at a younger age. With both groups, the emphasis is on a discussion of the potential risks and benefits between the patient and his physician, recognizing the limitations of sensitivity and specificity of PSA testing for prostate cancer,[10,11] overdetection of clinically insignificant disease,[12,13] and the uncertain benefit of early detection and treatment of prostate cancer.[14–16] The National Comprehensive Cancer Network has recently advocated a risk-stratification approach to PSA testing, wherein men with a PSA ≥ 0.6 ng/mL at 40 years of age are recommended to undergo PSA testing annually.[17] Early results of two randomized trials of prostate cancer screening demonstrate only a small mortality reduction, if any, to prostate cancer screening.[18,19] However, the results of the U.S. study are potentially limited by a high rate (up to 52%) of PSA testing in the "non-screening" arm.[18] Proponents of early detection for prostate cancer point out the significant stage migration and decreasing prostate cancer mortality since the widespread introduction of PSA testing as evidence supporting the continued use of PSA testing with DRE.

In contrast, in 2008 the United States Preventive Services Task Force (USPSTF) stated that the current evidence is insufficient to assess the balance of benefits and harms of prostate cancer screening among men aged less than 75 years. Among men over 75 years of age, the USPSTF recommends against screening, believing that the limited average life expectancy and known harms of screening outweigh the potential benefit of early detection of prostate cancer in these elderly men. PSA testing in elderly men is common and indiscriminate, so it is doubtful that these practice patterns will soon change.[20–22]

Additional tests may provide assistance when uncertainty exists as to whether a prostate biopsy is indicated. For men with a PSA level <10 ng/mL, a commonly employed test is the ratio of free/total PSA (percent free PSA). In men with no prior biopsy who have a PSA level of at least 4.0 ng/mL, a free PSA of less than 25% may indicate a 50–60% chance of prostate cancer. Among men with a prior negative biopsy, a free PSA <10% is an indication for repeat biopsy. PCA3 is a urine-based mRNA assay which may assist in determining whether men with a prior negative prostate biopsy should undergo repeat biopsy.[23,24]

Biopsy

When indicated, prostate biopsy is typically performed as an office procedure. Under ultrasound guidance, 8–12 tissue cores are obtained transrectally with an 18-gauge biopsy gun. Typically, this procedure is performed under local anesthesia (peri-prostatic nerve block with lidocaine). The primary side effects of prostate biopsy are hematochezia and hematuria lasting for 2–3 days. Hematospermia may last up to 4–6 weeks. Significant infection following prostate biopsy occurs in 0.5–1% of cases, with appropriate antibiotic prophylaxis.

If the prostate biopsy is negative, men should undergo continued monitoring of PSA and DRE annually, with rebiopsy as indicated by a rapid rise in PSA or a new abnormality on DRE. Men with high-grade prostatic intraepithelial neoplasia or atypical small acinar proliferation should undergo repeat biopsy in 3–6 months, as up to 30–50% may have prostate cancer on repeat biopsy.

Pathology

Almost all prostate carcinomas are adenocarcinoma. Other tumor types are rare, and include ductal carcinoma, mucinous adenocarcinoma, and transitional carcinoma of the prostate. Small-cell (neuroendocrine) tumors of the prostate are even less frequent. Both primary transitional carcinomas and small-cell carcinomas of the prostate are very aggressive and carry a poor prognosis. These tumors require aggressive surgical intervention for localized disease.

The histologic grade assigned to prostate adenocarcinoma is based on the system developed by Gleason. The Gleason grade is the sum of the most common cellular pattern (1–5) and the second most common cellular patterns (1–5) in the biopsy or surgical specimen. This histologic grade provides valuable prognostic information, in addition to the PSA at the time of biopsy and clinical stage.

Prognosis

Central to the management of the disease is an understanding of prostate cancer risk stratification, the patient's health status, and life expectancy. The TNM system is widely accepted for the clinical staging of prostate cancer (Table 38.1). Tumors confined to the prostate gland are T1 or T2, whereas once local extension occurs, tumors are classified as T3 or T4. Several systems have been developed for risk stratifying prostate cancer based on PSA, clinical stage, and Gleason score. The Partin Tables define the probability of organ-confined disease, extraprostatic extension, seminal vesicle invasion, and lymph node invasion.[26–28] Subsequently, D'Amico et al. developed risk groupings for newly diagnosed men with localized disease (Table 38.2). Three risk stratifications (low, intermediate, high) for relapse after initial local therapy are defined, again using clinical stage, Gleason grade, and PSA.[29,30] The D'Amico risk stratification system has come into widespread use for counseling and planning interventions. Finally, preoperative and postoperative nomograms predicting risk of

Table 38.1. TNM staging system of prostate cancer

Definition of TNM	
Primary tumor (T)	
Clinical	
TX	Primary tumor cannot be assessed
T0	No evidence of primary tumor
T1	Clinically inapparent tumor neither palpable nor visible by imaging
T1a	Tumor incidental histologic finding in 5% or less of tissue resected
T1b	Tumor incidental histologic finding in more than 5% of tissue resected
T1c	Tumor identified by needle biopsy (e.g., because of elevated PSA)
T2	Tumor confined within prostate[a]
T2a	Tumor involves one-half of one lobe or less
T2b	Tumor involves more than one-half of one lobe but not both lobes
T2c	Tumor involves both lobes
T3	Tumor extends through the prostate capsule[b]
T3a	Extracapsular extension (unilateral or bilateral)
T3b	Tumor invades seminal vesicle(s)
T4	Tumor is fixed or invades adjacent structures other than seminal vesicles: bladder neck, external sphincter, rectum, levator muscles, and/or pelvic wall

[a]*Note*: Tumor found in one or both lobes by needle biopsy, but not palpable or reliably visible by imaging, is classified as T1c

[b]*Note*: Invasion into the prostatic apex or into (but not beyond) the prostatic capsule is classified not as T3 but as T2

Pathologic (pT)	
pT2[a]	Organ confined
pT2a	Unilateral, involving one-half of one lobe or less
pT2b	Unilateral, involving more than one-half of one lobe but not both lobes
pT2c	Bilateral disease
pT3	Extraprostatic extension
pT3a	Extraprostatic extension[b]
pT3b	Seminal vesicle invasion
pT4	Invasion of bladder, rectum

[a]*Note*: There is no pathologic T1 classification

[b]*Note*: Positive surgical margin should be indicated by an R1 descriptor (residual microscopic disease)

Regional lymph nodes (N)	
Clinical	
NX	Regional lymph nodes were not assessed
N0	No regional lymph node metastasis
N1	Metastasis in regional lymph node(s)

Table 38.1. (continued)

Pathologic	
pNX	Regional nodes not sampled
pN0	No positive regional nodes
pN1	Metastases in regional node(s)
Distant metastasis (M)[a]	
MX	Distant metastasis cannot be assessed (not evaluated by any modality)
M0	No distant metastasis
M1	Distant metastasis
M1a	Nonregional lymph node(s)
M1b	Bone(s)
M1c	Other site(s) with or without bone disease

[a]*Note*: When more than one site of metastasis is present, the most advanced category is used. pM1c is most advanced

Source: Used with the permission of the American Joint Committee on Cancer (AJCC)[25]. Published by Springer Science and Business Media LLC www.springerlink.com.

Table 38.2. D'Amico risk stratification for clinically localized prostate cancer

Risk group	Criteria
Low	Diagnostic PSA <10.0 ng/mL and highest biopsy Gleason score ≤ 6 and clinical stage T1c or T2a
Intermediate	Diagnostic PSA >10 but <20 ng/mL or highest biopsy Gleason score = 7 or clinical stage T2b
High	Diagnostic PSA >20 ng/mL or highest biopsy Gleason score ≥8 or clinical stage T2c/T3

recurrence after radical prostatectomy have been developed by Kattan et al.[31] All of these tools provide the clinician with information to counsel patients regarding treatment decisions following a diagnosis of prostate cancer.

Understanding a patient's likelihood of prostate cancer mortality, that is, the natural history of the disease, is central to balancing life expectancy and overall health status with the need to treat (or expectantly manage) prostate cancer. For example, men with Gleason grade 2–4 disease may be expected to have a very indolent disease course, with only a 4–7% chance of dying from their disease within 15 years (Table 38.3). In contrast, men with high-grade disease may

have a risk of prostate cancer mortality as high as 87%, if left untreated.

Another indicator of prognosis following treatment for prostate cancer may be the velocity of PSA rise prior to treatment. In large, retrospective cohorts, men with a PSA velocity of >2 ng/mL/year face a greater risk of prostate cancer death following radical prostatectomy as well as radiation therapy.[33,34] Therefore, pretreatment PSA dynamics may be considered during patient counseling and treatment planning for multimodal therapy, in addition to the risk stratification schemes outlined above.

Treatment of Prostate Cancer

A variety of treatment options exist for prostate cancer, which should be appropriately employed considering the patient's disease state, preferences, and overall health status and life expectancy. Conceptually, prostate cancer treatments may be categorized into those for localized disease, locally advanced disease, recurrent disease, and metastatic disease. For localized disease, management options include surgical therapy, radiation therapy, and active surveillance. Locally advanced prostate cancer is best managed by a multidisciplinary, multimodality treatment approach. Management of recurrent prostate

Table 38.3 Risk of dying of clinically localized prostate cancer without definitive locoregional therapy

Gleason score	Age			
	55–59	60–64	65–69	70–74
2–4	4%	5%	6%	7%
5	6%	8%	10%	11%
6	18%	23%	27%	30%
7	70%	62%	53%	42%
8–10	87%	81%	72%	60%

Source: Adapted from Albertsen et al.[32]

cancer following treatment for localized disease is characterized by lack of consensus and active investigation. The mainstay of treatment for metastatic prostate cancer remains androgen deprivation, with chemotherapy reserved for androgen-independent prostate cancer.

Treatment for Localized Prostate Cancer (T1, T2)

Several management options exist for localized disease, including radical prostatectomy, external beam radiation therapy (EBRT), brachytherapy, or active surveillance, as described in a recent guideline from the American Urological Association.[35] No randomized controlled trials during the PSA era exist to compare treatment outcomes among these options. However, outcomes for surgical and radiation therapy, when stratified by risk, are similar across several retrospective cohorts. Again, patients may be classified into risk groups according to clinical stage, pretreatment PSA, and Gleason grade. Large series of low-risk groups exhibit approximately 85–90% freedom from biochemical recurrence, as compared with 75% and 35–50% for men with intermediate- and high-risk features, respectively. Recent data suggest that pretreatment PSA velocity (>2 ng/mL/year) and PSADT may also have prognostic significance, although further research is needed to clarify how this information should be incorporated into pretreatment risk models.[33,34]

Radical Prostatectomy

Radical prostatectomy is the mainstay of surgical therapy for prostate cancer, and is typically performed using a retropubic approach, although some practitioners will perform perineal prostatectomy in selected patients. The retropubic approach permits sampling or removal of the pelvic lymph nodes. In low-risk men, node sampling may not be necessary, but should be considered in intermediate risk patients, and is considered standard of care for men with high-risk disease. Perioperative morbidity and mortality for the procedure are low, with operative mortality <0.05% at centers of excellence. Data from Medicare claims suggest that outcomes are better at facilities which perform at least 40 radical prostatectomies annually.

The major adverse effects of radical prostatectomy are incontinence and impotence. Patients may expect urinary incontinence during the first few months of recovery, but by 1 year after surgery, published series from expert centers typically report continence rates of 90–98%. Erectile function can be significantly impaired following radical prostatectomy. For men with low-volume disease, nerve-sparing prostatectomy offers the best opportunity for recovery of erectile function following surgery, with equivalent oncologic outcomes in appropriately selected patients. Among patients with good erectile function prior to surgery, expert centers report that 50–90% will recover significant erectile function with a bilateral nerve-sparing procedure. However, patients frequently note that the quality (rigidity and durability) of erections may not be equal to preoperative erectile function. A recent systematic review by the AUA Prostate Cancer Guidelines panel noted high variability in reporting of erectile function in radical prostatectomy series, with rates of "intact erectile function" ranging from 9% to 86%.[36] Recently, experts have advocated use of phosphodiesterase inhibitors, intracavernous or intraurethral delivery systems for prostaglandin E, and/or vacuum erection devices for rehabilitation of erectile function following radical prostatectomy, although evidence for this practice remains sparse.

Laparoscopic Prostatectomy (Robot-Assisted)

Robot-assisted laparoscopic prostatectomy has rapidly grown as a surgical treatment for prostate cancer. For example, among Medicare beneficiaries, the laparoscopic approach was used in over 30% of cases in 2005, as compared with only 12% of cases in 2003.[37] Reports of short-term outcomes (<12 months) from expert centers suggest similar oncologic efficacy to the open approach, but longer-term data on biochemical recurrence and prostate cancer mortality are lacking. One claims-based analysis suggests that salvage radiation therapy is more common following minimally invasive radical prostatectomy, although at high-volume centers the risk for salvage therapy was similar between the open and laparoscopic approach.[37] Functional outcomes (continence and potency) have not been well documented using validated instruments comparing subjects to baseline status, and thus further investigation of this approach to radical prostatectomy is needed.

EBRT

Radiation therapy of all types uses high-energy particles (typically photons) to damage cellular DNA and induce apoptosis in cancer cells. One of the oldest techniques for the treatment of prostate cancer is external beam radiation therapy (EBRT). Most institutions today use 3D conformal EBRT or intensity modulated radiation therapy (see below). 3D conformal EBRT uses CT images to create a high-dose treatment volume which conforms to the target shape (e.g., the prostate). Use of 3D conformal techniques allows greater radiation dose to the prostate while minimizing toxicity. For example, a recent randomized trial demonstrated that the use of 79.2 Gy of conformal therapy instead of 70.2 Gy resulted in a 49% decrease in biochemical failure rates.[38] The use of 78 Gy in multi-institutional trials has been associated with only a 3% incidence of significant acute gastrointestinal/ genitourinary toxicity. Thus, most centers today use a minimum of 75 Gy for 3D conformal techniques, with an expectation of increased efficacy and minimal increase in toxicity.

IMRT

Intensity-modulated radiation therapy (IMRT) uses nonuniform beam densities and multileaf collimation techniques to provide an even higher dose to the target while minimizing toxicity to surrounding structures. In recent series, doses between 81 and 86.4 Gy have been administered with late gastrointestinal or genitourinary toxicity in less than 1% of patients, while achieving good biochemical recurrence-free rates. IMRT is more labor-intensive than 3D conformal EBRT, but is rapidly becoming the standard of care at many institutions.

Brachytherapy

Implantation of interstitial radioactive elements offers the potential for targeted high-dose radiation to the prostate while minimizing exposure of surrounding tissues to radiation. The current approach to brachytherapy utilizes transrectal ultrasound-guided placement of radioactive elements in a template to maximize radiation exposure to the prostate. Because of rapid fall-off in radiation dose beyond the prostate, brachytherapy is most suitable for low-risk or highly selected intermediate-risk patients. In addition, large prostate glands (>60 g) may be difficult to optimally treat. Patients with intermediate- or high-risk disease may also be treated with a combination of brachytherapy with EBRT. To date, little data exists regarding the advantage of brachytherapy with EBRT as compared with conformal EBRT alone in the treatment of intermediate- and high-risk disease.

Treatment for Locally Advanced Prostate Cancer (T3, T4)

Treatment for locally advanced prostate cancer necessitates a multimodal, multidisciplinary approach, frequently involving urologists, radiation oncologists, and medical oncologists. The most commonly applied approaches include external beam radiation therapy combined with androgen-deprivation therapy, and radical prostatectomy.

EBRT with ADT

The physiologic rationale for combining androgen-deprivation therapy with radiation therapy is a potentially synergistic effect on prostate cancer cells. Androgen deprivation likely increases apoptosis in the irradiated field, and may also delay or prevent the development of metastatic disease. Clinical support for these hypotheses is provided by the results of two randomized controlled trials (RTOG 85–10 and EORTC), which suggests that immediate ADT with EBRT results in better outcomes than EBRT alone, among men with locally advanced or high-risk prostate cancer. Furthermore, secondary analyses of additional trials (i.e., RTOG 85–31) suggest that early indefinite ADT improves outcomes as compared with EBRT alone.

Radical Prostatectomy

Radical prostatectomy, with or without ADT, is a reasonable option for locally advanced (T3) prostate cancer. Well-differentiated T3 prostate cancers have a disease-specific survival following radical prostatectomy of approximately 76%. Androgen-deprivation therapy may improve outcomes following radical prostatectomy in this group, although further research is required to clearly define the role of androgen deprivation for locally advanced disease following radical prostatectomy.

Treatment for Recurrence Following Definitive Local Therapy

PSA Recurrence Following Radical Prostatectomy

Undetectable PSA levels are expected following radical prostatectomy, thus PSA is potentially a very sensitive marker for disease recurrence. However, some patients may develop very low levels of PSA following prostatectomy if benign prostate tissue remains. The AUA Prostate Cancer Guidelines panel systematic review noted significant variability in definitions of biochemical recurrence following radical prostatectomy, but endorsed the standard of PSA >0.2 ng/mL as representing biochemical failure, although not necessarily a threshold to initiate androgen-deprivation therapy.[39] Many clinicians regard a PSA level >0.4 ng/mL following radical prostatectomy as an indication for intervention (ADT), following appropriate staging evaluations. Tumor grade, time to PSA recurrence after surgery, and PSA doubling time are associated with the risk of prostate cancer mortality, and may be used to risk stratify those patients who may potentially benefit from early intervention following a biochemical recurrence.[40] A large, retrospective cohort study demonstrated reduced incidence of metastatic disease among high-risk (Gleason sum >7 or PSADT <12 months) men initiated on ADT for PSA recurrence following radical prostatectomy.[41,42] However, definitive data regarding the benefit of early versus delayed androgen deprivation in this setting is lacking. Men with short PSA doubling times (<15 months) appear to be at higher risk for disease-specific mortality.[43] Randomized trials are needed in this area to further define the role of ADT for PSA recurrence among men at higher risk for prostate cancer death.

PSA Recurrence Following Radiation Therapy

The 1996 consensus definition for PSA recurrence following radiation therapy is three consecutive increases in PSA, with the time of failure defined as halfway between the first rise in PSA and the prior measurement. As with PSA recurrence following radical prostatectomy, rapidly rising PSA is a harbinger of more aggressive disease and shorter time to distant metastasis. Androgen-deprivation therapy is most commonly used to treat PSA recurrence following radiation therapy. Salvage surgery has a very high complication rate, and a significant risk of incontinence, and is therefore rarely performed. Cryotherapy of the prostate is a relatively new option to treat postradiation PSA recurrence, so long-term data on outcomes is lacking.

Treatment for Advanced Prostate Cancer

Androgen-Deprivation Therapy

Deprivation of androgen stimulation is central to the first-line management of advanced (e.g., metastatic) prostate cancer. Several methods exist for androgen deprivation, including bilateral orchiectomy, LHRH agonists, and androgen receptor blockade (antiandrogens). With the rise of potent LHRH agonists and antiandrogens, surgical castration has rapidly been replaced by medical castration as the intervention of choice in this setting. LHRH agonists, such as goserelin and leuprolide cause a decline in testosterone levels by interfering with the normal pulsatile secretion of LHRH. However, a transient rise in testosterone occurs with initiation of these agents, so nonsteroidal antiandrogens (i.e., flutamide or bicalutamide) are frequently administered prior to initiation of LRHR agonists. Conflicting data exist over whether combined androgen blockade (LHRH agonist plus a nonsteroidal antiandrogen) improves outcomes. The most recent American Society of Clinical Oncology (ASCO) guidelines note that consideration of combined androgen blockade may be considered instead of monotherapy with an LHRH agonist.[44] For metastatic disease, initiation of immediate ADT, rather than symptom-onset ADT, offers no overall survival advantage due to an offset of increased prostate cancer-specific survival by a decrease in overall mortality.[44] Thus, ASCO does not specifically endorse early initiation of ADT, although this may be considered for men at high risk based on PSA kinetics or other parameters.[44]

Chemotherapy for Androgen-Independent Prostate Cancer

Some men with metastatic prostate cancer develop progressive disease on androgen-deprivation therapy, which has been termed androgen-independent prostate cancer. While many treatment options exist in this area (i.e., second-line hormonal therapy), the most definitive evidence supports the use of docetaxel-based chemotherapy. Randomized controlled trials suggest a 2–3 month survival advantage with the use of a 3 week course of docetaxel.[45] Data regarding the use of bisphosphonates in androgen-independent prostate cancer are conflicting, although a phase III trial of zoledronic acid demonstrated a reduction in skeletal-related events, but no improvement in quality of life. There is not a well-defined role for zoledronic acid in men with androgen-dependent prostate cancer, although these men are at higher risk for osteoporosis. Oral bisphosphonates may be a consideration in these patients, although level I evidence is lacking in this clinical setting.

Summary

Treatment of prostate cancer is an enterprise which mandates careful understanding of disease characteristics (aggressive versus indolent) as well as underlying patient health status. Quality-of-life considerations should also play an important role in counseling patients regarding treatment options. Many treatment options are available for the patient at all disease stages, and clinicians should be familiar with these options to enhance patient care.

References

1. Jemal A, Siegel R, Xu J, and Ward E. Cancer statistics, 2010. *CA Cancer J Clin.* 2010;60:277
2. Ries L, Melbert D, Krapcho M, et al. *SEER Cancer Statistics Review, 1975–2004.* Bethesda, MD: National Cancer Institute; 2007
3. Quinn M, Babb P. Patterns and trends in prostate cancer incidence, survival, prevalence and mortality Part II: individual countries. *BJU Int.* 2002;90:174
4. Quinn M, Babb P. Patterns and trends in prostate cancer incidence, survival, prevalence and mortality Part I: international comparisons. *BJU Int.* 2002;90:162
5. Bratt O. Hereditary prostate cancer: clinical aspects. *J Urol.* 2002;168:906
6. Bratt O, Damber JE, Emanuelsson M, et al. Hereditary prostate cancer: clinical characteristics and survival. *J Urol.* 2002;167:2423
7. Zheng SL, Sun J, Wiklund F, et al. Cumulative association of five genetic variants with prostate cancer. *N Engl J Med.* 2008;358:910
8. Thompson IM, Goodman PJ, Tangen CM, et al. The influence of finasteride on the development of prostate cancer. *N Engl J Med.* 2003;349:215
9. Lippman SM, Klein EA, Goodman PJ. Effect of selenium and vitamin E on risk of prostate cancer and other cancers: the selenium and vitamin E cancer prevention trial (SELECT). *JAMA.* 2009;30(1):39-51

10. Thompson IM, Ankerst DP, Chi C, et al. Operating characteristics of prostate-specific antigen in men with an initial PSA level of 3.0 ng/ml or lower. *JAMA*. 2005;294:66

11. Thompson IM, Pauler DK, Goodman PJ, et al. Prevalence of prostate cancer among men with a prostate-specific antigen level < or =4.0 ng per milliliter. *N Engl J Med*. 2004;350:2239

12. Etzioni R, Penson DF, Legler JM, et al. Overdiagnosis due to prostate-specific antigen screening: lessons from U.S. prostate cancer incidence trends. *J Natl Cancer Inst*. 2002;94:981

13. Draisma G, Boer R, Otto SJ, et al. Lead times and overdetection due to prostate-specific antigen screening: estimates from the European randomized study of screening for prostate cancer. *J Natl Cancer Inst*. 2003;95:868

14. de Koning HJ, Auvinen A, Berenguer Sanchez A, et al. Large-scale randomized prostate cancer screening trials: program performances in the European randomized screening for prostate cancer trial and the prostate, lung, colorectal and ovary cancer trial. *Int J Cancer*. 2002; 97:237

15. de Koning HJ, Liem MK, Baan CA, et al. Prostate cancer mortality reduction by screening: power and time frame with complete enrollment in the European Randomised Screening for Prostate Cancer (ERSPC) trial. *Int J Cancer*. 2002;98:268

16. Gohagan JK, Prorok PC, Hayes RB, et al. The prostate, lung, colorectal and ovarian (PLCO) cancer screening trial of the National Cancer Institute: history, organization, and status. *Control Clin Trials*. 2000;21:251S

17. Prostate cancer early detection. Practice guidelines in oncology. *NCC Network*. 2007. Published online by NCCN. http://www.nccn.org/professionals/physician_gls/PDF/prostate_detection.pdf

18. Andriole GL, Grubb RL III, Buys SS, et al. Mortality results from a randomized prostate-cancer screening trial. *N Engl J Med*. 2009;360:1310

19. Schroder FH, Hugosson J, Roobol MJ, et al. Screening and prostate-cancer mortality in a randomized European study. *N Engl J Med*. 2009;360:1320

20. Lu-Yao G, Stukel TA, Yao SL. Prostate-specific antigen screening in elderly men. *J Natl Cancer Inst*. 2003;95:1792

21. Scales CD Jr, Curtis LH, Norris RD, et al. Prostate specific antigen testing in men older than 75 years in the United States. *J Urol*. 2006;176:511

22. Walter LC, Bertenthal D, Lindquist K, et al. PSA screening among elderly men with limited life expectancies. *JAMA*. 2006;296:2336

23. Deras IL, Aubin SM, Blase A, et al. PCA3: a molecular urine assay for predicting prostate biopsy outcome. *J Urol*. 2008;179:1587

24. Sokoll LJ, Ellis W, Lange P, et al. A multicenter evaluation of the PCA3 molecular urine test: pre-analytical effects, analytical performance, and diagnostic accuracy. *Clin Chim Acta*. 2008;389:1

25. American Joint Committee on Cancer (AJCC). *AJCC Cancer Staging Manual*. 6th ed. Chicago, IL: American Joint Committee on Cancer; 2002

26. Partin AW, Yoo J, Carter HB, et al. The use of prostate specific antigen, clinical stage and Gleason score to pre-dict pathological stage in men with localized prostate cancer. *J Urol*. 1993;150:110

27. Partin AW, Kattan MW, Subong EN, et al. Combination of prostate-specific antigen, clinical stage, and gleason score to predict pathological stage of localized prostate cancer. A multi-institutional update. *JAMA*. 1997;277:1445

28. Partin AW, Mangold LA, Lamm DM, et al. Contemporary update of prostate cancer staging nomograms (Partin tables) for the new millennium. *Urology*. 2001;58:843

29. D'Amico AV, Moul J, Carroll PR, et al. Cancer-specific mortality after surgery or radiation for patients with clinically localized prostate cancer managed during the prostate-specific antigen era. *J Clin Oncol*. 2003;21:2163

30. D'Amico AV, Whittington R, Malkowicz SB, et al. Biochemical outcome after radical prostatectomy, external beam radiation therapy, or interstitial radiation therapy for clinically localized prostate cancer. *JAMA*. 1998;280:969

31. Kattan MW, Wheeler TM, Scardino PT. Postoperative nomogram for disease recurrence after radical prostatectomy for prostate cancer. *J Clin Oncol*. 1999;17:1499

32. Albertsen PA, Hanley JA, Fine J. 20-year outcomes following conservative management of clinically localized prostate cancer. *JAMA*. 2005;293:2095-2101

33. D'Amico AV, Chen MH, Roehl KA, et al. Preoperative PSA velocity and the risk of death from prostate cancer after radical prostatectomy. *N Engl J Med*. 2004;351:125

34. D'Amico AV, Renshaw AA, Sussman B, et al. Pretreatment PSA velocity and risk of death from prostate cancer following external beam radiation therapy. *JAMA*. 2005;294:440

35. Thompson I, Thrasher JB, Aus G, et al. Guideline for the management of clinically localized prostate cancer: 2007 update. *J Urol*. 2007;177:2106

36. Burnett AL, Aus G, Canby-Hagino ED, et al. Erectile function outcome reporting after clinically localized prostate cancer treatment. *J Urol*. 2007;178:597

37. Hu JC, Wang Q, Pashos CL, et al. Utilization and outcomes of minimally invasive radical prostatectomy. *J Clin Oncol*. 2008;26:2278

38. Zietman AL, DeSilvio ML, Slater JD, et al. Comparison of conventional-dose vs high-dose conformal radiation therapy in clinically localized adenocarcinoma of the prostate: a randomized controlled trial. *JAMA*. 2005;294:1233

39. Cookson MS, Aus G, Burnett AL, et al. Variation in the definition of biochemical recurrence in patients treated for localized prostate cancer: the American urological association prostate guidelines for localized prostate cancer update panel report and recommendations for a standard in the reporting of surgical outcomes. *J Urol*. 2007;177:540

40. Freedland SJ, Humphreys EB, Mangold LA, et al. Risk of prostate cancer-specific mortality following biochemical recurrence after radical prostatectomy. *JAMA*. 2005;294:433

41. Moul JW, Wu H, Sun L, et al. Early versus delayed hormonal therapy for prostate specific antigen only recurrence of prostate cancer after radical prostatectomy. *J Urol*. 2008;179:S53

42. Moul JW, Wu H, Sun L, et al. Early versus delayed hormonal therapy for prostate specific antigen only recurrence of prostate cancer after radical prostatectomy. *J Urol.* 2004;171:1141

43. Freedland SJ, Humphreys EB, Mangold LA, et al. Death in patients with recurrent prostate cancer after radical prostatectomy: prostate-specific antigen doubling time subgroups and their associated contributions to all-cause mortality. *J Clin Oncol.* 2007;25:1765

44. Loblaw DA, Virgo KS, Nam R, et al. Initial hormonal management of androgen-sensitive metastatic, recurrent, or progressive prostate cancer: 2006 update of an American Society of Clinical Oncology practice guideline. *J Clin Oncol.* 2007;25:1596

45. Tannock IF, de Wit R, Berry WR, et al. Docetaxel plus prednisone or mitoxantrone plus prednisone for advanced prostate cancer. N Engl J Med. 2004;351: 1502-1512

39

The Management of Testis Cancer

Noel W. Clarke

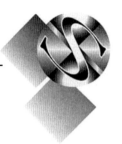

Presentation and Diagnosis

Testis cancer presents most commonly as a painless testicular mass but there are a number of other clinical scenarios. Approximately 20% manifest with scrotal pain and 10% will initially experience an acute orchitis.[1] The primary imaging modality in the first instance is ultrasound.[2] This has a sensitivity approaching 100% in experienced hands but there are circumstances where it is difficult to differentiate orchitis from tumor and in addition, small intratesticular lesions may produce considerable diagnostic uncertainty. Where precise clinical diagnosis is impossible and a lesion is suspicious, open biopsy or orchidectomy may be needed for definitive verification. If biopsy is to be undertaken, it is usually done using the Chevassu technique, bivalving the testis along its long axis on the opposite side to the epididymis. In these circumstances, surgical exploration should always be through the groin and testis conservation should be attempted where possible. It is inevitable that following surgery some lesions will ultimately prove to be benign: this should be explained to the patient preoperatively.

Serum Tumor Markers

Blood must be taken for marker evaluation before surgical removal of the testis. The main markers for non-seminoma are α fetoprotein (AFP), β HCG, and LDH. AFP is elevated in 50–70% of NSGCT, has a half-life of approximately 5 days, and is produced by yolk sac elements. It is not elevated in pure seminoma. βHCG is increased in 40–60% of NSGCTs and in up to 30% of pure seminomas. It is produced by trophoblastic elements in the tumor and has a half-life of 1 day. LDH is less specific but is more common in seminoma. Overall, 90% of NSGCTs elaborate at least one tumor marker, while in seminoma, markers are elevated in <40%.[1]

Primary Surgery

It is vital to undertake imaging of the scrotum with ultra sound prior to exploring *any* scrotal mass, thereby avoiding an inappropriate surgical approach through the scrotum (scrotal violation). If scrotal violation occurs, additional subsequent treatment may be required, often involving local radiotherapy to the scrotal area. This carries the potential for immediate compromise of fertility and a long-standing risk to the endocrine function of the contralateral testicle.

The standard primary treatment for a testicular tumor is radical orchidectomy. This involves a groin approach, opening the inguinal canal surgically and detaching the spermatic cord at the level of the internal inguinal ring before delivering the testis from the scrotum and removing the testis and cord en bloc (Fig. 39.1). If the patient wishes, a testicular prosthesis can be inserted safely at the same

C.R. Chapple and W.D. Steers (eds.), *Practical Urology: Essential Principles and Practice*,
DOI: 10.1007/978-1-84882-034-0_39, © Springer-Verlag London Limited 2011

Figure 39.1. Radical orchidectomy. Suspicious masses should be approached through the groin (**a**). The inguinal canal is opened and the cord mobilized (**b**) before transection at the level of the internal ring (**c**). The testis is then delivered from the scrotum, dividing the gubernacular attachments (**d**).

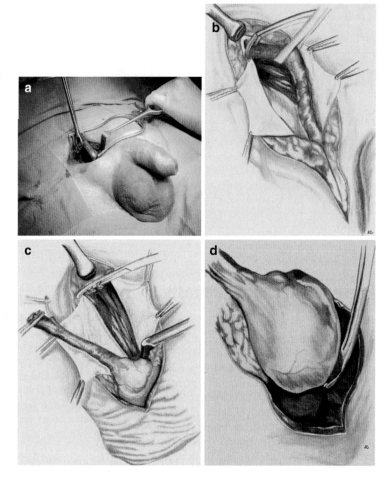

operation, although this should be avoided if the tumor is invading the scrotal wall or if there is preexisting infection.

Testis Preserving Surgery

This may be undertaken in specific circumstances, namely, the presence of synchronous bilateral tumors, development of a metachronous contralateral tumor, or in patients with a single testis. Conservative surgery is usually restricted to tumors of 2 cm or less although it may be possible to undertake local excision of larger tumors provided they are in the polar areas. It should be noted that testicular intraepithelial neoplasia (TIN) is present in up to 80% of patients undergoing testis preservation.[3,4] Sperm storage issues should be discussed prior

to surgery and the patient should be counselled about the long-term risks of tumor recurrence, long-term endocrine failure, and the requirement for subsequent radiotherapy or completion orchidectomy if TIN is detected.

Contralateral Testicular Biopsy and TIN

TIN is present in the contralateral testis of up to 5% of men presenting with testicular cancer. When present, it is associated with a high chance of progression to invasive disease. Treatment is usually by low dose irradiation of the affected testis after preliminary storage of semen.

In the case of primary orchidectomy, controversy surrounds the issue of whether synchronous contralateral testicular biopsies should be performed routinely. Because of this, the policy of contralateral biopsy at the time of primary surgery varies. High-risk cases can be identified, limiting contralateral sampling to those whose risk is greatest. The combined presence of maldescent, testicular atrophy and age <31 increase the chance of positivity for contralateral TIN significantly[5] and such cases should be considered for contralateral biopsy. When undertaking biopsies of this type, trans-scrotal "pinch" sampling technique should be used, taking a 2–3 mm sample of seminiferous tissue through a 2–3 mm incision in the scrotum. Diagnostic accuracy is improved if biopsies are taken from two separate places in the testis.[6]

If TIN is identified it should be treated with low dose scrotal radiotherapy. However, this treatment can be delayed in order to consider fertility issues. Prior to treatment, the patient needs to be informed that radiotherapy will lead to irreversible infertility. It is also important to be aware that following radiotherapy to the testis, even with the standard reduced dose of 18–20 Gy, about 30% of patients will develop Leydig cell insufficiency requiring testosterone substitution in the future.

Post-Orchidectomy Management

Histological classification and clinical staging is undertaken after primary surgery and subsequent management is predicated on its outcome. The disease stage is classified into two basic groups: clinical stage 1 (low and high risk) and stage 2 and above, subcategorized into three subgroups by the European Germ Cell Collaborative Consensus Group (EGCCCG) types.[7] These subclassifications are based on the findings of cross-sectional imaging and post-orchidectomy tumor marker levels. In these more advanced cases (clinical stage T2+), defined treatment schedules are followed according to specific protocols predicated on tumor type, marker levels at presentation, and the distribution of the disease (Table 39.1).

All patients undergoing orchidectomy must be staged clinically using cross-sectional imaging and tumor marker measurement. The imaging usually comprises CT scanning of the chest, abdomen, and pelvis as a minimum. The first-

Table 39.1. EGCCCG classification for advanced germ cell tumors

Subgroup	5 year OS	Definition
Good prognosis	90%	Testis or primary extragonadal retroperitoneal tumor and low markers AFP <1.000 ng/ml, ß-HCG <1.000 ng/ml (<5.000 IU/l) and LDH <1.5 × normal level and no non-pulmonary visceral metastases
Intermediate prognosis	75%	Testis or primary extragonadal retroperitoneal tumor and intermediate markers AFP 1.000–10.000 ng/ml ß-HCG 1.000–10.000 ng/ml, LDH 1,5–10 × normal level and no presence of non-pulmonary visceral metastases
Poor prognosis	50%	Primary mediastinal germ cell tumor or presence of non-pulmonary visceral metastases and/or "high markers" AFP >10.000 ng/ml, ß-HCG >10.000 ng/ml LDH >10 × UNL

order lymph nodes in the retroperitoneum are usually the initial site of metastatic spread although primary distal hematogenous dissemination can occur in up to 15% of men. CT scanning has its limitations: up to 30% of patients with negative CT scans will have positive lymph nodes detected subsequently at surgical staging. By contrast, up to 25% of patients may be radiologically overstaged, having abnormal nodes on CT staging, which are subsequently shown to be negative following surgical exploration. MR imaging has been used in this scenario although it is not proven to be more effective or reliable than CT scanning. PET scanning has significant problems with false negativity and is of limited utility in this setting. It does have some value in the post-chemotherapy assessment of the residual mass in seminoma (see below).

Once staging is completed, treatment plans can be formulated, preferably in a multidisciplinary forum in a center undertaking management of testis cancer cases in significant volume.

The strategies are discussed in greater detail below but in brief, these are subdivided into patients who are clinically stage 1 and those who have cT2 or greater staging. Those with clinical stage 1 seminoma or NSGCT have traditionally been managed by very different strategies, with options for radiation, low dose chemotherapy or surveillance and salvage therapy emerging for seminoma, and observation, low dose chemotherapy, or, in specific circumstances, primary RPLND for non-seminoma, depending on risk characteristics. If the disease is stage 2 or more, the standard treatment for most tumors is by combination platinum-based chemotherapy using bleomycin, etoposide, and cisplatinum (BEP) with subsequent surgical removal of postchemotherapy residual masses. This is undertaken for most NSGCT, while chemotherapy is used alone for most seminomas, with postchemotherapy surgery being indicated only for highly selected cases.[8]

Management of Clinical Stage 1 Disease

Non-Seminomatous Germ Cell Tumor (NSGCT)

Risk Stratification

Data from large multicenter studies correlating tumor-related factors with disease outcome has enabled stratification of clinical stage 1 NSGCT for risk.[9] The rationale for this is to identify men who truly have stage 1 disease and to separate these from those who are clinically stage 1 but have risk characteristics associated with the presence of occult microscopic metastases (pathological stage 2+). In this way, aggressive and potentially toxic treatments can be reserved only for those men who truly need them. Defined pathological findings in the primary are known to be associated with a high risk of occult metastatic spread in clinical stage 1 disease.[9,10] They are:

- Vascular and/or lymphatic invasion
- Absence of the yoke sac elements
- Presence of embryonal carcinoma

Patients with these primary characteristics are usually treated with a more aggressive therapeutic regimen or more intensive surveillance following initial orchidectomy, while those with lower-risk characteristics are entered into standard surveillance schedules. In this way, the toxicities of treatment are avoided in low-risk patients, while the potential for undertreatment of high-risk cases is minimized. Active treatment schedules involve the use of low dose adjuvant chemotherapy. Retroperitoneal lymph node dissection (RPLND) is still used in some centers (particularly in the USA), but its use is decreasing for the reasons set out below. The schemes of management are set out in the flow diagrams in Figs. 39.2 and 39.3.

Surveillance Versus Primary RPLND

Treatment strategies for clinical stage 1 disease have varied in different countries: for example, primary surgery has prevailed in the USA, while surveillance has been most commonly used in Europe. The rationale for primary RPLND is that up to 30% of patients will have microscopic evidence of disease in the retroperitoneal nodes. However, using risk stratification profiles based on histology, it is possible to predict with accuracy of approximately 80% that low-risk cases will not relapse[9] and furthermore, if they do, they can then undergo systemic treatment with chemotherapy with excellent results. Patients relapsing on surveillance are successfully treated with standard chemotherapy and have long-term cure rates of 98%, which is the same as that for primary surgery.[11] In addition, over 95% of patients who are going to relapse will do so within the first 2 years of diagnosis of their original cancer. Prolonged and intensive follow-up over many years is therefore not required although a degree of follow-up is needed because of the risk of late relapse. Surveillance is now the standard of care in most high volume centers.[7]

Primary RPLND

Existing noninvasive staging techniques fail to identify up to 30% of patients with positive nodes. This fact has provided a rationale for a surgical approach in clinical stage 1 testicular cancer. The procedure is usually carried out through a midline abdominal incision although an increasing number of reports have emerged relating to the use of laparoscopic techniques.

The traditional approach of standard bilateral lymphadenectomy is associated with loss of ejaculatory function in most patients. By contrast,

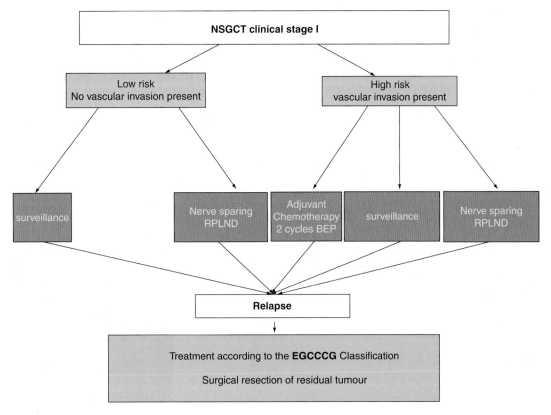

Figure 39.2. Strategies and outcomes for risk-adapted treatment of clinical stage 1 non-seminoma.

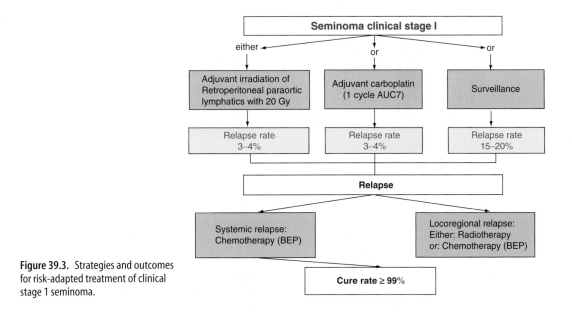

Figure 39.3. Strategies and outcomes for risk-adapted treatment of clinical stage 1 seminoma.

the use of "template"-based nerve sparing techniques (Fig. 39.4), utilizing knowledge relating to the course of ejaculatory nerves and the likely site of metastatic deposits has resulted in >75% of patients preserving ejaculatory function postoperatively.[12] The surgery required is major and there are significant complications even in expert centers (adhesion obstruction, wound infection, leg edema, etc.).[13] A further issue is the outcome relating to surgery; 70% will have no evidence of disease at lymphadenectomy and a significant number will have postsurgical relapse, 25% of which will be in extra-abdominal sites (mainly pulmonary) and up to 10% in the previously operated retroperitoneal sites.[11] Thus, despite the use of RPLND patients still need to undergo surveillance. For these reasons, the use of primary surgery has diminished in recent years, although there has been a rekindling of interest with the use of laparoscopic techniques. In most countries and high volume centers, surveillance for low risk is now the standard of care, with adjuvant intervention using chemotherapy or intensive surveillance for cases with high-risk features.

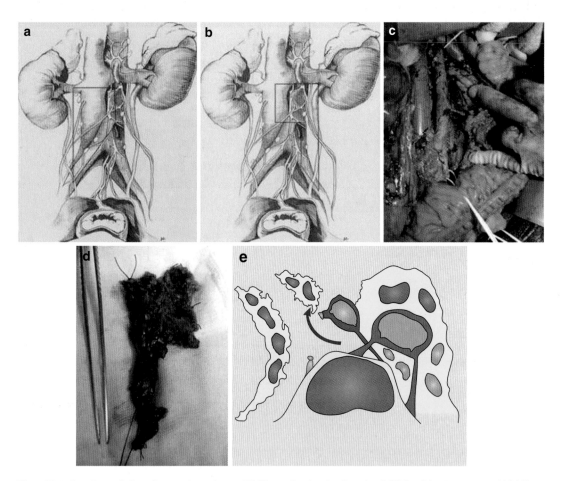

Figure 39.4. Template techniques for post-chemotherapy RPLND and the "split and roll" method. (a, b) Right and left templates for RPLND: Both templates remove tissue from the primary nodal landing sites including the interaorto-caval space. Right (a) and left (b) templates have "dogleg" extensions to the ipsilateral common iliac region, sparing the contralateral area, thereby preserving the ejaculatory nerve function. The final result is demonstrated showing the dissection field (c) and the tissue removed (d) following completion of a post-chemotherapy left template dissection. (e) The "split and roll" technique: lumbar branches of the aorta and vena cava are ligated and divided, enabling rolling and lifting of the great vessels off the anterior spinous ligament. This enables removal of the lymphatic tissue around and behind the aorta and IVC.

One specific indication for primary RPLND is where there are problems with patient compliance in attendance. This is known to present problems in certain circumstances, particularly when the distance patients have to travel to referral centers is great.

Adjuvant Treatment for High Risk

Many centers now use adjuvant reduced-intensity chemotherapy for high-risk cases, most commonly with bleomycin, etoposide, and cisplatin (BEP). Chemotherapy using a single cycle of BEP has been shown to be superior to primary RPLND (1% recurrence rate for chemotherapy vs 7.5% for nerve sparing surgery),[34] and 2 cycles of BEP have been proven to be superior than 1 (recurrence rate 0% for 2 cycles vs 3.5% for 1 cycle).[14] Another pragmatic approach adopted by many groups is to observe high-risk cases closely and treat relapsing patients with standard 3 cycle BEP on the understanding that while approximately 47% with vascular invasion will relapse,[9,14] over 50% will remain free of disease without the need for additional therapy. This strategy is viewed as safe on the basis that disease-free survival is equivalent whether the chemotherapy is given early or late, with long-term survival in the region of 98% in this group of patients.

Clinical Stage 1 Seminoma

Risk-Stratified Adjuvant Treatment

Because of the retroperitoneal relapse rate of 15–19%, the exquisite radio sensitivity of seminoma and the lack of serum tumor markers, adjuvant low dose abdominal radiotherapy has been used widely as an adjuvant treatment for this condition. However, more recent strategies involving the use of single agent chemotherapy with carboplatin have been adopted and these have been supplemented even more recently by the use of surveillance strategies.

Adjuvant Radiotherapy

Irradiation of the para-aortic and pelvic lymph nodes has been the most favored adjuvant treatment. The traditional standard approach involved irradiation of the para-aortic nodes with inclusion of the ipsilateral inguinal nodes ("dogleg" radiotherapy), but this has now been replaced with para-aortic treatment following studies showing no differences in survival/recurrence rates and reduced toxicity if the radiation field is limited to the para-aortic area.[15] Grade 1 complications such as nausea, vomiting, and GI ulceration are often seen with para-aortic XRT and a transient drop in sperm count can occur in a proportion. The decrease in sperm count will usually recover within 1 year. Using the low dose para-aortic regimen, acute toxicity is reduced and the effect on sperm count within the first 18 months is less profound. The dose of para-aortic radiation has also been reduced following publication of data comparing 20 Gy in 10 fractions versus 30 Gy in 15.[16] This study showed equivalence for both doses in relation to recurrence rates, with long-term radiation-induced toxicity occurring in less than 2%. Moderate chronic gastrointestinal (GI) side effects occurred in about 5% of patients, but with moderate acute GI toxicity in about 60%.

The main concern surrounding adjuvant radiotherapy is the increased incidence of radiation-induced secondary non-germ-cell malignancies. This represents a small but significant risk.[17]

Adjuvant Low Dose Chemotherapy

Studies using single agent chemotherapy with carboplatin as an alternative to radiotherapy have now shown that this therapeutic strategy is effective treatment for this type of disease. Pilot studies by Oliver et al. reported the relapse rate for patients treated with single dose carboplatin using a dose schedule known as "AUC7" was 4% (median follow-up of 51 months) and that 99% of patients remained disease free. These results were consolidated in the MRC TE19 study of carboplatin monotherapy versus adjuvant radiotherapy in clinical stage 1 seminoma. Results showed no statistical difference in recurrence rates. After a mean follow-up of >4 years, the relapse rate with a single cycle of carboplatin at 3 years was 5.2%.[18] There were, however, relapses occurring after more than 2 years and further long-term analysis of data is required to assess the true long-term outcome, particularly relating to toxicity and other late sequelae such as the induction of second malignancy, acquisition of drug resistance in recurrences, the effect on fertility, and the impact on quality of life.

Surveillance in Clinical Stage 1 Seminoma

Strategies have now emerged from Canada using a similar approach to those adopted for many years in clinical stage 1 NSGCT. Observation of clinical stage 1 seminoma patients has shown that about 16% of patients are at risk for recurrent disease: the median time to relapse is 12–15 months with 96% of these occurring in the retroperitoneum or inguinal region. In a multivariate analysis of several retrospective observation studies, a tumor size >4 cm and the presence of rete testis invasion remain adverse prognostic signs: these define a high-risk group for relapse. If both factors are present, patients have a risk of relapse during surveillance of 32%. If both factors are absent, a low-risk group can be defined with a relapse risk of only 12%.[19] Prospective studies using risk factors have now also been performed, for example, by the Spanish Testicular Cancer Group. One-third of the patients in this group's study had neither of the defined risk factors (rete testis invasion and a tumor size >4 cm):

they received surveillance only following orchiectomy. Only 6% of these patients relapsed after a median follow-up of 3 years. The remaining patients, with one or both risk factors, were treated with adjuvant carboplatin, and showed a relapse rate of 3.3%.[20] Studies of this type represent a significant way forward in targeting post-orchidectomy treatment for patients with clinical stage 1 seminoma who have a high risk of occult metastatic disease at the time of orchidectomy. Strategies to reduce immediate adjuvant treatment in as many patients as possible will confine treatment and treatment-related risk to those who need intervention most. This approach has been used to show that if the risk of relapse in patients managed with surveillance is under 10%, the number of follow-up investigations can be reduced.[7] It is, however, notable that in the Canadian surveillance series, patients needed up to 20 CT scans as part of their surveillance protocol and relapses occurred after more than 5 years of follow-up. Studies attempting to reduce the number of CT scans and also to replace CT with MR are currently ongoing (e.g., MRC TE20).

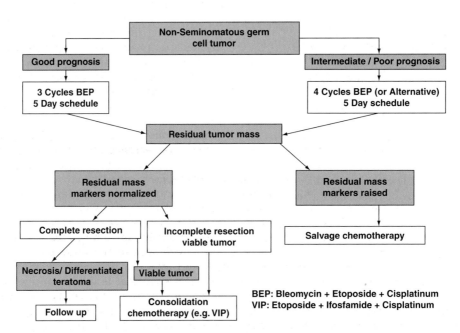

Figure 39.5. Management scheme for stage T2+ GCT. BEP: bleomycin + etoposide + cisplatinum; VIP: etoposide + ifosfamide + cisplatinum.

Management of Metastatic Testis Cancer

Primary Combination Chemotherapy

As with clinical stage 1 disease, the management of advanced disease is conducted according to risk-stratified protocols. These are based on the collective outcome of >5,000 patients with advanced disease, analyzed by the European Germ Cell Consensus Collaborators Group and published in 1997 (Fig. 39.5).[7] Good prognosis patients have the potential for good outcome, with a cure rate of >90% and even intermediate risk patients have a long-term survival >75%. However, patients with high-risk characteristics have a much worse prognosis, with <50% surviving at 5 years.

Standard treatment for seminoma and NSGCT is with combination chemotherapy. There is variation in the combinations used (e.g., addition of ifosfamide for bleomycin) but most groups adopt standard BEP regimens as exemplified by the Memorial Sloane Kettering group[21] as follows:

- Good Prognosis BEP × 3 Cycles or PE × 4 cycles
- Intermediate Prognosis BEP × 4 Cycles
- Poor Prognosis BEP × 4 Cycles or Trial-Based Drug Regimens

Treatment should, where possible, be given in high volume centers with multidisciplinary oncological teams incorporating surgery and nonsurgical oncology specializing in the management of testis cancer, as there is clear evidence that such centers have better outcomes than those dealing with low numbers of patients.[22] It is also important to emphasize that patients with high-risk disease should be referred to a specialist center immediately for evaluation and treatment. It is not always necessary to undertake an orchidectomy in such patients before initiating their primary chemotherapy.

There is variation in the chemotherapy dosage scheduling but most patients are treated as in-patients, with drugs given by centrally placed parenteral lines with added hydration, osmotic diuretics, antiemetics, and antibiotics (usually for the first cycle). Growth factor support is not usually necessary although it is used in some circumstances. Different combinations have been tried for good prognosis disease (e.g., the GETUG trial of 3 vs 4 cycles of BEP[23]), but to date, none of these has shown superiority in outcome without adding significantly to the toxicity profile. Studies of newer agents, such as taxanes are ongoing. In patients where there is concern about pulmonary function, bleomycin is used with caution or is omitted because of its known toxicity in inducing pulmonary fibrosis.

In intermediate and high-risk tumors attempts have been made to improve outcome in the primary setting by using different schedules and drug combinations and by increasing the dose of the drugs in "high dose" combinations. These have been disappointing overall in the studies done to date. An example of this is the US Intergroup trial of high dose versus standard in intermediate and high-risk disease. There was no difference in overall survival but there were differences in marker responses in specific patient types, suggesting that this approach may be appropriate for certain types of high-risk disease.[24]

Late Toxicity

Combination chemotherapy has resulted in dramatic improvements in cure rates for testis cancer but there are long-term toxicities related to treatment. While these are relatively low in frequency they can be significant. They include a doubling of the rate of long-term risks of treatment-related malignancy,[25,26] a doubling of the long-term cardiovascular risk,[27] and additional effects on long-term testicular endocrine and reproductive function. These must be borne in mind when counselling patients and when planning their long-term survivorship.

Post-Chemotherapy Resection of Residual Masses

The scheme followed by most groups for post-chemotherapy surgery is set out in Fig. 39.5. The rationale for post-chemotherapy retroperitoneal lymph node dissection (PC-RPLND) is to remove retroperitoneal lymph nodes that are persistently enlarged (>1 cm) following primary chemotherapy. This is undertaken because of the risk of persistent active disease, the presence of mature teratoma (problems associated with development of the "growing teratoma syndrome"), and the potential for de-differentiation or sarcomatous change over time in residual mature teratomatous masses: this can occur in up to 17% of residual masses left untreated.

PC-RPLND is not usually indicated in seminoma, where the incidence of fibrosis is very high and the technical challenges are greater because of fibrous fusion of the masses with the intima of the great vessels. Resection is only indicated in this setting if the residual mass is >3 cm in diameter and if the mass has positivity on FDG-PET scanning, although there is uncertainty even in this scenario, where it has been shown that there is a high false positivity with PET scanning. Its greatest value lies with a negative PET scan in the presence of a residual mass; this has a very high degree of accuracy in predicting fibrosis rather than active tumor.[28] In all other cases, the masses should be closely followed by imaging investigations and tumor marker assay.[29] Resection is indicated in NSGCT,[2] where the residual masses will contain mature teratoma in 30–40% and vital cancer in about 10–20%.[8] Resections in this setting are usually curative if all the residual disease is removed, and the overall outcome seems to be better if resection is undertaken early rather than when residual lesions show signs of progression.[30] Imaging is usually undertaken 6–8 weeks after the last chemotherapy cycle and surgery is not usually undertaken if the tumor markers have not normalized. In these circumstances, further chemotherapy is given before assessment of response and surgery if appropriate at that time. The surgery is technically challenging and should not be undertaken outside specialist centers. It involves full mobilization of the great vessels using the "split and roll" technique (Fig. 39.4e) and resection of concomitant structures (kidney/bowel/caval resection/aortic replacement) is required in some circumstances. There is debate as to whether bilateral or template-based PC-RPLND should be used. Bilateral procedures induce ejaculatory failure but there is a small risk of leaving vital disease using template methods in all cases. Data from the USA and Europe has now shown that template techniques are quite safe when used in selected cases.[8,31] Following resection, the long-term outcome is excellent if all disease can be resected, but if there is residual disease left after surgery, the long-term outcome is worse.

Salvage Strategies

Salvage treatment is used for early (<2 years) or late (>2 years) relapse. Early relapse is usually due to platinum resistance, which may be complete at the outset or apparent after an initial response to primary treatment. In establishing a diagnosis of "relapse," it is vital to be aware of the pitfalls that can mimic disease persistence or recurrence. These include the growing teratoma syndrome, whereby residual masses increase in size after chemotherapy because of cystic change and transformation from active to mature teratoma, false-positive marker relapse, new pulmonary nodules arising secondary to bleomycin, and elevations in tumor markers from a metachronous new primary testicular cancer. Approaches to treatment involve rechallenge with cisplatinum-based chemotherapy, acceleration of cisplatinum dose, use of newer drugs including combinations of ifosfamide, paclitaxel, gemcitabine, and oxaliplatin, high dose chemotherapy, and "desperation" surgery. There is evidence that high dose regimens may confer a benefit of around 14%[32] and that sequential high dose chemotherapy (HDC) may be advantageous.[33] However, these are toxic regimens and they carry a significant mortality of themselves. Salvage "desperation" surgery is indicated but only in the very limited circumstances where there is a feasible chance of resecting all residual tumor tissue. Patients generally do not benefit from this type of extensive surgery if all disease cannot be removed.

Conclusion

Testis cancer is an uncommon malignancy but it is the most common cancer in young men. With early diagnosis and appropriate treatment in expert centers, the long-term results are excellent in good prognosis cases. In intermediate prognosis disease, the considerable majority of patients are cured long term, but in poor prognosis testis cancer, mortality is still significant and new approaches are required. By comparison with the outcomes from recent history in this disease, the advances in the last 30 years of testis cancer treatment are a testimony to the benefits of collaborative translational science, clinical trial planning, and risk-adapted therapeutic approaches. As a consequence, this disease is now curable in the great majority.

References

1. Horwich A, ed. *Testicular Cancer—Investigation and Management*. 2nd ed. London: Chapman and Hall; 1996
2. EAU Guidelines on Management of Testis Cancer 2008; www.uroweb.org
3. Heidenreich A et al. Organ sparing surgery for malignant germ cell tumor of the testis. *J Urol*. 2001;166(6):2161-2165
4. Giannarini G et al. Organ-sparing surgery for adult testicular tumours: a systematic review of the literature. *Eur Urol*. 2010;57:780-790
5. Harland SJ et al. Intratubular germ cell neoplasia of the contralateral testis in testicular cancer: defining a high risk group. *J Urol*. 1998;160(4):1353-1357
6. Dieckmann KP et al. Diagnosis of contralateral testicular intraepithelial neoplasia (TIN) in patients with testicular germ cell cancer: systematic two-site biopsies are more sensitive than a single random biopsy. *Eur Urol*. 2007;51(1):175-183
7. Krege S et al. European consensus conference on diagnosis and treatment of germ cell cancer: a report of the second meeting of the European Germ Cell Cancer Consensus group (EGCCCG): part I+II. *Eur Urol*. 2008;53(3):478-513
8. Heidenreich A et al. Postchemotherapy retroperitoneal lymph node dissection in advanced testicular cancer: radical or modified template resection. *Eur Urol*. 2009;55:217-226
9. Read G et al. Medical Research Council prospective study of surveillance for stage I testicular teratoma. Medical Research Council Testicular Tumors Working Party. *J Clin Oncol*. 1992;10(11):1762-1768
10. Freedman L et al. Histopathology in the prediction of relapse of patients with stage I testicular teratoma treated by orchidectomy alone. *Lancet*. 1987;2(8554):294-298
11. Sternberg CN. The management of stage I testis cancer. *Urol Clin North Am*. 1998;25(3):435-449
12. Albers P. Management of stage I testis cancer. *Eur Urol*. 2007;51(1):34-43
13. Heidenreich A et al. *J Urol*. 2003;169:1710-1714
14. Tandstad T et al. Risk-adapted treatment in clinical stage I nonseminomatous germ cell testicular cancer: the SWENOTECA management program. *J Clin Oncol*. 2009;27(19):3263
15. Fossa SD et al. Optimal planning target volume for stage I testicular seminoma: a Medical Research Council randomized trial. Medical Research Council Testicular Tumor Working Group. *J Clin Oncol*. 1999;17(9):3004-3005
16. Jones W et al. Randomized trial of 30 versus 20 Gy in the adjuvant treatment of stage I Testicular Seminoma: a report on Medical Research Council Trial TE18, European Organisation for the Research and Treatment of Cancer Trial 30942 (ISRCTN18525328). *J Clin Oncol*. 2005;23(6):1200-1208
17. Travis SM. Risk of second malignant neoplasms among long-term survivors of testicular cancer. *J Natl Cancer Inst*. 1997;89(19):1429-1439
18. Oliver RTD et al. Radiotherapy versus single-dose carboplatin in adjuvant treatment of stage I seminoma: a randomised trial. *Lancet*. 2005;366(9482):293-300
19. Warde P et al. Prognostic factors for relapse in stage I seminoma managed by surveillance: a pooled analysis. *J Clin Oncol*. 2002;20:4448
20. Aparicio J et al. Risk-adapted management for patients with clinical stage I seminoma: the Second Spanish Germ Cell Cancer Cooperative Group study. *J Clin Oncol*. 2005;23:8717-8723
21. Carver B et al. Improved clinical outcome in recent years for men with metastatic nonseminomatous germ cell tumors. *J Clin Oncol*. 2007;25(35):5603-5608
22. Collette L et al. Impact of the treating institution on survival of patients with "poor-prognosis" metastatic nonseminoma. European Organization for Research and Treatment of Cancer Genito-Urinary Tract Cancer Collaborative Group and the Medical Research Council Testicular Cancer Working Party. *J Natl Cancer Inst*. 1999;91(10):839-846
23. Culine S et al. Refining the optimal chemotherapy regimen for good-risk metastatic nonseminomatous germ-cell tumors: a randomized trial of the Genito-Urinary Group of the French Federation of Cancer Centers (GETUG T93BP). *Ann Oncol*. 2007;18:917
24. Motzer RJ et al. Phase III randomized trial of conventional-dose chemotherapy with or without high-dose chemotherapy and autologous hematopoietic stem-cell rescue as first-line treatment for patients with poor-prognosis metastatic germ cell tumors. *J Clin Oncol*. 2007;25(3):247-256
25. Travis LB et al. Second cancers among 40,576 testicular cancer patients: focus on long-term survivors. *J Natl Cancer Inst*. 2005;97(18): 1354-1365
26. Belt-Dusebout AW et al. Treatment-specific risks of second malignancies and cardiovascular disease in 5-year survivors of testicular cancer. *J Clin Oncol*. 2007;25:4370
27. Huddart RA et al. *J Clin Oncol*. 2003;21(8):1513-1523
28. Hinz S et al. The role of positron emission tomography in the evaluation of residual masses after chemotherapy for advanced stage seminoma. *J Urol*. 2008;179(3):936-940
29. Schmoll HJ, EGCCCG, et al. European consensus on diagnosis and treatment of germ cell cancer: a report of the European Germ Cell Cancer Consensus Group (EGCCCG). *Ann Oncol*. 2004;15:1377-1399
30. Hendry WF et al. Metastatic nonseminomatous germ cell tumors of the testis: results of elective and salvage surgery for patients with residual retroperitoneal masses. *Cancer*. 2002;94:1668-1676
31. Beck SD et al. The role of postchemotherapy surgery in managing metastatic germ cell tumors. *Cancer*. 2007;110(12):2601-2603
32. Lorch A et al. *J Urol*. 2010;184(1):168-173
33. Lorch A et al. Single versus sequential high-dose chemotherapy in patients with relapsed or refractory germ cell tumors: a prospective randomized multicenter trial of the German Testicular Cancer Study Group. *J Clin Oncol*. 2007;25(19):2778-2784
34. Albers P et al. Randomized phase III trial comparing retroperitoneal lymph node dissection with one course of bleomycin and etoposide plus cisplatin chemotherapy in the adjuvant treatment of clinical stage I Nonseminomatous testicular germ cell tumors: AUO trial AH 01/94 by the German Testicular Cancer Study Group. *J Clin Oncol*. 2008;26(18):2966-2972

Index

A

Abdominal leak point pressures (ALPP), 281
Absorptive hypercalciuria, 152
Acid-base balance
　bicarbonate synthesis, 111
　CO_2/HCO_3 buffer system, 110
　filtered bicarbonate reabsorption, 111
　Henderson-Hasselbalch equation, 110
Acute bacterial prostatitis. *See* Prostatitis
　　syndromes
Adjuvant chemotherapy, 522
Adrenal glands, 41
Adult polycystic kidney disease (APCKD), 79
Agglutination, 188
Ambulatory urodynamics, 281
American Society of Clinical Oncology (ASCO)
　　guidelines, 537
American Urological Association (AUA)
　　guidelines, 512
Amiloride, 113–114
Anastomotic urethroplasty
　corpora cavernosa, 419–422
　dorsal onlay approach, 427
Androgen deprivation therapy (ADT), 537
　body composition, 230
　bone metabolism, 231
　cognitive decline, 230–231
　insulin resistance and metabolic
　　syndrome, 230
Androgen-independent prostate
　　cancer, 535
Angiomyolipoma, 73, 74
Anterior compartment repair
　arcus tendineus fascia pelvis, 475
　cystocele formation, 476
　techniques, 475

Anterior urethral pathology
　anatomy and function, 415
　management
　　optical urethrotomy/dilatation, 417
　　preoperative assessment, 418–419
　　urethral stents, 417–418
　pathophysiology, 415–416
　urethroplasty
　　anastomotic, 419–422
　　graft position, 427–433
　　grafts *vs.* flaps, 422–425
　　oral mucosal grafts, 425–426
　　substitution, 422
　　tissue engineering, 426–427
Antibiotics
　aminoglycosides, 99–100
　choice, 95
　collateral damages, 95
　cotrimoxazole, 100–101
　fluoroquinolones, 100
　fosfomycin, 96
　glycopeptides, 101
　groups and dosages
　　complicated UTI and uncomplicated
　　　pyelonephritis, 97
　　uncomplicated cystitis, 95–96
　α-lactam antibiotics, 96
　　carbapenems, 99
　　cephalosporins, 98–99
　　penicillins, 98
　linezolid, 101
　nitrofurantoin, 96
　pivmecillinam, 96
　trimethoprim, 100–101
Antibody-dependent cell-mediated cytotoxicity
　　(ADCC), 188

C.R. Chapple and W.D. Steers (eds.), *Practical Urology: Essential Principles and Practice*,
DOI: 10.1007/978-1-84882-034-0, © Springer-Verlag London Limited 2011

Antilymphocyte antibody, 191
Antimicrobials
    pharmacodynamics
        antimicrobial substances, 93–94
        minimal bactericidal concentration, 93
        minimal inhibitory concentration, 93
        and pharmacokinetics correlations, 94
    pharmacokinetic parameters, 94
    resistance patterns and bacterial spectrum, 94–95
    susceptibility and resistance
        clinical breakpoints, 92–93
        epidemiological breakpoints, 92, 93
        phenotypic expression, resistance
            mechanisms, 92
Apaziquone, 522
Apomorphine SL, 377–378
Aprepitant, 133
Arginine vasopressin (AVP), 108
Artificial urinary sphincter (AUS), 443, 444
Aspergillosis, 324
Autologous and allogeneic vaccines, 189

B
Bacillus Calmette-Guérin (BCG), 189, 518
Balanitis xerotica obliterans (BXO), 416
Ballistic lithotripsy, 407
Benign prostate enlargement (BPE), 212–213
Benign prostatic hyperplasia (BPH), 212–213,
        289, 353
    acute urinary retention, 362
    clinical manifestation, 361
    epidemiology, 361–362
    growth factors, 362
    incidence and prevalence, 361
    natural history, 361–362
    pathophysiology
        obstructive symptoms, 363
        prostatism, 362
        voiding symptoms, 362–363
    patient assessment
        bladder and prostate imaging, 364–365
        clinical history, 363
        endoscopy, 365
        frequency-volume charts, 363
        management algorithm, 364, 365
        physical examination, 363, 366
        post-void residual, 364–365
        prostate-specific antigen, 364
        symptom score, 363
        urinalysis, 363–364
        urodynamics, 365–366
    PSA concentration, 362
    treatment
        alpha1 adrenoceptor antagonists, 367
        antimuscarinics, 368
        5α-reductase inhibitors, 367–368
        holmium laser enucleation of the prostate,
            368–369
        microwave thermotherapy, 368

needle ablation, prostate, 368
        photo vaporization of the prostate, 368–369
        phytotherapy, 366–367
        prostate resection, 368
        watchful waiting program, 366
Bladder
    afferent signaling, 123–124
    CNS targets
        γ-amino butyric acid mechanisms, 132
        neurokinin and neurokinin receptors,
            132–133
        opioid receptors, 131
        serotonin mechanism, 131–132
    efferent signaling
        parasympathetic nerves, 124
        somatic nerves, 125
        sympathetic nerves, 124
    emptying phase
        vesico-bulbo-vesical micturition reflex,
            125–126
        vesico-spinal-vesical micturition reflex, 126
    functions, 123
    micturition, 123
    peripheral targets
        adrenergic receptors, 129–130
        afferent signaling mechanism, 126–127
        cholinergic receptors, 127–128
        phosphodiesterases, 130–131
        transient receptor potential receptors, 130
    storage phase, 125
Bladder cancer
    adjuvant chemotherapy, 522
    bladder-preservation treatments, 521–522
    CT-urography, 512
    cystoscopy, 512–513
    epidemiology, 511
    incidence, 175
    metastatic, 177–178
    muscle invasive, 176–177
    muscle-invasive bladder cancer, 523
    neoadjuvant chemotherapy, 522
    NMIBC
        cystectomy and CIS, 518
        device-assisted therapy, 520
        intravesical chemotherapy, 517–520
        intravesical immunotherapy, 518
        patient, follow-up, 522–523
        risk groups, 515–517
    non-muscle invasive (TaT1), 175–177
    pathology, 515
    preoperative radiotherapy, 522
    radical cystectomy, 520–521
    risk factors, 511
    screening, role of, 512
    sexual function-preserving techniques, 521
    signs and symptoms, 512
    transurethral resection
        bimanual examination, 514
        histopathological diagnosis, 514

PDD-assisted TUR, 514–515
  postoperative intravesical chemotherapy, 515
  recurrence, risk of, 514
  re-TUR, 515
urinary diversion, 521
urine tests, 513–514
UUT imaging, 512
Bladder injury
  adult and children, 503
  computed tomography, 503
  diagnosis and treatment algorithm, 503, 504
  DRE, 503
  formal repair, 505
  gross hematuria, 503
  initial management, 505–506
  retrograde urethrogram, 503
Bladder outlet obstruction index (BOOI), 212
Blastomycosis, 325
Boston Area Community Health (BACH) Survey, 437–438
Botulinum toxin (BTX), 442, 443
Brain lesions
  cerebellar ataxia, 459–460
  cerebral palsy, 459–460
  cerebrovascular accident, 457–458
  dementias, 459
  encephalitis/PML, 460
  epilepsy, 459–460
  Huntington's disease, 459
  multiple sclerosis, 459
  multisystem atrophy, 458–459
  normal pressure hydrocephalus, 459
  olivopontine cerebellar degeneration, 458–459
  Parkinson's disease, 458
  psychiatric disorders, 460
  ShyDrager, 458–459
  tumors, 460
Bulbospongiosus muscle, 419, 420

C
Calcium-based urolithiasis, 147–148
Calculi
  extracorporeal shock wave lithotripsy, 403–404
  flexible ureteroscopy, 407
  intracorporeal stone fragmentation devices
    ballistic lithotripsy, 407
    electrohydraulic lithotripsy, 407
    laser lithotripsy, 408
    ultrasound, 407
  percutaneous nephrolithotomy, 404–406
  renal stones
    calyceal diverticula stones, 410–411
    endoscopic management, 409
    flexible ureterorenoscopy, 410
    horseshoe kidneys and stones, 410
    lower pole stones, 410

  percutaneous surgery, 410
  staghorn calculi, 410
  stones and PUJ obstruction, 411
  semirigid ureteroscopy, 406
  ureteric stones
    endoscopic management, 408–409
    intervention, 412
    medical expulsive therapy, 411
    obesity, 412
    pregnancy, 412
    treatment outcomes, 411
Candidiasis, 323–324
Capsaicin, 442
Cerebrovascular accident (CVA), 457–458
Cervicitis, 344–345
Chancroid
  diagnosis, 342
  treatment, 342
Chemotherapy
  adjuvant, 175
  bladder cancer (see Bladder cancer)
  combination, 175
  penile cancer, 184
  prostate cancer (see Prostate cancer)
  renal cell carcinoma (see Renal cell carcinoma)
  side effects, 184
  testicular cancer (see Testicular cancer)
Chlamydia
  diagnosis, 345
  treatment, 345–346
Cholinergic receptors
  muscarinic receptors, 127–128
  nicotinic receptors, 128
Chronic bacterial prostatitis. See Prostatitis syndromes
Chronic diarrheal states, 155
Chronic pelvic pain syndrome (CPPS), 396. See also Prostatitis syndromes
Chronic prostatitis, 396
Coccidioidomycosis, 325–326
Codon, 165
Cognitive behavioral therapy (CBT), 389
Condylomata acuminata, 287
Congenital anomalies, 3–4
Congenital ureteral obstruction
  anomalies, 3–4
  megaureter-megacystis syndrome, 14
  pipestem megaureter, 13–14
  prune belly syndrome, 14
  vascular ureteral obstructions, 14–16
Cop's ring, 416
Corpora cavernosa, 419–422
Cryptococcosis, 324–325
Cyclosporine, 192
Cystine-based urolithiasis, 148
Cystinuria, 156
Cystourethroscopy
  flexible, 284
  rigid, 283–284

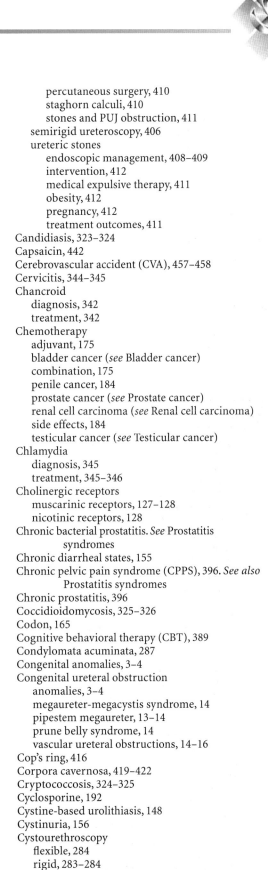

D

Dapoxetine
    clinical trials, 392–393
    patient reported outcomes, 393
    pharmacokinetics, 392
    regulatory approval, 394
    side effects, 393–394
Detrusor-bladder neck dyssynergia, 280
Detrusor sphincter dyssynergia (DSD), 215, 280
Dipstick hematuria, 352
Dipstick urinalysis, 354–355
Distal renal tubular acidosis, 155
Diuretics
    carbonic anhydrase inhibitors, 112
    loop diuretics, 112–113
    osmotic diuretics, 112
    potassium-sparing diuretics, 113–114
    thiazide diuretics, 113
DNA methylation, 165
Duloxetine, 132

E

Ectopic ureter
    embryology, 11
    location
        female, 11–12
        male, 11
    symptoms, 12
Ejaculation, 67
Ejaculatory function
    abnormal ejaculation, 143–144
    premature ejaculation, 143
Electrohydraulic lithotripsy, 407
Electromyography (EMG), 454
Embryology
    gonads
        anomalies, 21
        duct system, 23–25
        ovarian differentiation, 21
        testicular differentiation, 19–21
    kidney
        anomalies, 6–7
        development, 4–6
    prostate and urethral glands development, 23
    prostatic urethral valves, 24, 25
    ureteral development
        anomalies of number, 9
        anomalies of origin, 8–9
        complete ureteral duplication, 9–12
        congenital ureteral obstruction, 13–16
        incomplete ureteral duplication, 9
        ureteral orifices, 9
        ureteroceles, 12–13
        urogenital sinus, 7–8
    urinary bladder
        bladder duplication, 17
        cloacal duct anomalies, 17
        development, 16–17

        diverticula, 17–19
        extrophy, 19
        primitive cloaca, 16
        structure, 16
        urachal anomalies, 17
        urogenital sinus, 16
        urogenital sinus division, 16
Endocrinology
    clinical manifestation, 219
    kidneys
        endocrine functions, 231–232
        primary hyperparathyroidism and
            nephrolithiasis, 232
    paraneoplastic syndromes
        Cushing's syndrome, 234
        RCC, 233–234
    testis
        androgen deprivation therapy, adverse effects,
            230–231
        hypogonadism (*see* Hypogonadism)
        normal androgen metabolism, 219
        physiological actions and tissue targets, sexual
            hormones, 223–224
        testosterone replacement therapy, 229–230
Endoscopy
    cystourethroscopy
        flexible, 284
        rigid, 283–284
    nephroscopy, 285–286
    ureteroscopy and ureteropyeloscopy, 284–285
    virtual reality simulators, 286
Enteric hyperoxaluria, 155
Enterocele repair, 477
    goals, 477
    mechanisms, 476–477
    principles, 477
Epididymal appendages
    acute scrotum
        age, 314
        appendiceal torsions, 316
        bell clapper deformity, 315
        cryptorchid testis, 315
        Doppler vascular imaging, 316
        extravaginal torsion, 315
        history and physical examination, 314
        leukocytosis, 314
        testicular pain, 314–315
    spermatic cord torsion, 316–317
Epididymitis, 344
    clinical signs and symptoms, 311–312
    definition and etiology, 310–311
    diagnostic evaluation of, 312–313
    surgical treatment, chronic epididymitis,
        313–314
    treatment of
        acute, 313
        chronic, 313
        purulent and atypical, 314

Epirubicin, 515
Erectile dysfunction (ED)
    co-morbid PE, 395
    diagnosis
        cardiovascular system and sexual activity,
            374–376
        clinical evaluation, 373–375
        optional tests, 375–376
    modalities, 376–377
    pathophysiology, 374
    phosphodiesterase type 5 inhibitors,
        377, 379
    posttraumatic arteriogenic ED, 377
    risk factors, 373
    treatment
        apomorphine SL, 377–378
        inhibitors
        intracavernosal therapy, 378–379
        intraurethral therapy, 379
        lifestyle factors, 376
        pharmacokinetics, 379
        surgical therapy, 380
        treatment algorithm, 378
        vacuum constriction devices, 379–380
        yohimbine, 378
Erectile function, 142–143
Erection, 67
Everolimus, 172
External beam radiation therapy (EBRT), 535
External genital development
    anomalies, 26–27
    genital tubercle development
        female, 25, 27
        male, 25, 27
    hormonal influence, 25, 26
External urethral sphincter (EUS), 456–458
Extracorporeal shock wave lithotripsy (ESWL)
    complications, 404
    contraindications, 404
    electrohydraulic system, 403
    electromagnetic lithotripsy, 403–404
    implicit, 404
    piezoelectric lithotripter, 403
    principles, 403
Extracorporeal shock-wave therapy
        (ESWT), 381

F
Factitious hematuria, 352
Filariasis
    clinical manifestations, 334
    diagnosis of, 334–335
    treatment, 335
    Wuchereria bancrofti, 334
Fistula
    ureterovaginal fistula
        diagnosis and management, 489–491
        etiology and presentation, 489

urethrovaginal fistula
        diagnosis and management, 488–489
        etiology and presentation, 488
    uro-enteric fistula
        pyeloenteric fistula, 492
        urethrorectal fistula, 492–493
        vesicoenteric fistula, 491–492
    vesicouterine fistula, 491
    vesicovaginal fistula
        conservative management, 485
        cystoscopy, 484
        etiology and risk factors, 482–483
        evaluation and diagnosis, 483
        imaging, 484–485
        pelvic examination, 483–484
        surgical management, 485–488
        treatment, 485
Flap
    axial/random, 257–259
    island, 258–259
    peninsular, 258
Flap urethroplasty
    fistula, 424
    genital skin, 422
    glans torsion, 424
    hematoma, 424
    penile skin, 422–424
    sacculation, 424
    skin necrosis, 424
    subcutaneous tissue, 423
    types of, 422, 423
Flexible ureteroscopy, 407
Fournier's Gangrene
    anatomic barriers, 317, 318
    definition and etiology, 317
    infectious organisms associated
        clinical signs and symptoms, 318
        diagnostic evaluation, 318–319
        treatment, 319
    risk factors, 317
Frame shift mutation, 165

G
Gabapentin, 132
Galactorrhea, 234
Glial-derived neurotropic factor (Gdnf), 198
Glomerular filtration rate (GFR)
    autoregulation
        myogenic mechanism, 106–107
        tubuloglomerular feedback, 107
    creatinine clearance, 107
    filtration, 105–106
    hormones, 107
    protein intake, 107
    regression formula, 107
    renal blood flow, 106–107
    sympathetic control, 107
Glomerulotubular balance (G-T balance), 108

Gonads, 19
  anomalies, 21
  duct system
    anomalies, 24–25
    female, 23–24
    male, 23
    testosterone and MIF, 21–23
  ovarian differentiation, 21
  testicular differentiation
    caudal migration, gubenaculum, 21
    disorders, 23
    testis development, 19–21
Gonorrhea, 346
Gouty diathesis, 156
Grafts
  acellular collagen matrices, 257
  epidermal/epithelial layer, 255
  full-thickness, 255–256
  initial phase, 254
  inosculation, 254
  mesh, 256
  posterior auricular, 256
  rectal mucosal, 257
  split thickness, 255
  tunica vaginalis, 257
  urothelium and buccal mucosa, 257
  vein, 257

H
Hematuria
  aetiology, 352
    benign prostatic hyperplasia, 353
    drugs, 353
    infection and inflammation, 353
    malignancy, 352
    nephrological causes, 353–354
    trauma, 353
    urinary calculi, 352–353
  classification of
    dipstick, 352
    factitious, 352
    macroscopic, 351
    menstruation, 352
    microscopic, 351–352
    pseudohematuria, 352
  intractable, 357–358
  investigations
    abdominal examination, 355, 356
    blood tests, 355
    computed tomography, 357
    dipstick urinalysis, 354–355
    flexible cystoscopy, 355
    IVU, 356
    KUB abdominal X-ray, 356
    molecular tests, 355
    MRI, 357
    renal biopsy, 357
    renal USS, 356

    retrograde urogram study, 357
    urine cytology, 355
  loin pain hematuria syndrome, 358
  nonurological/intrinsic renal causes, 357
  patient history, 354
  patients follow-up, 358
  pelvic examination, 354
Herpes simplex virus
  diagnosis, 339, 341
  treatment, 341–342
Histoplasmosis, 326
Holmium laser enucleation of the prostate
      (HoLEP), 368–369
Hormone refractory prostate cancer (HRPC), 178
  abiraterone, 179
  adverse events, chemotherapy, 178
  carboplatin and cisplatin, 179
  cyclophosphamide, 179
  epitholone B analog ixabepilone, 179
  estramustine, mitoxantrone, and docetaxel,
      178–179
  mitoxantrone plus prednisone, 179
Human papilloma virus
  diagnosis, 347
  treatment, 347–348
Hypercalcemia, 233
Hypercalciuria
  absorptive, 152
  renal, 152, 154
Hypersensitive bladder sensation, 276
Hypertension, 203, 233
Hyperthyroidism, 395
Hyperuricosuric calcium oxalate nephrolithiasis,
      155
Hypocitraturic calcium oxalate nephrolithiasis,
      155–156
Hypogonadism
  age-related, 221
    erectile and libido function, 221
    Leydig cells decrease, 221
    PDE5 expression regulation, 221
    testosterone deficiency syndrome, 221
    testosterone levels, 221
    testosterone regulation, 222
  androgen deficiency sign, 220
  causes, 220
  epidemiology, 221–222
  gonadotropin replacement, 220
  male
    biochemical assessment, 225–226
    clinical assessment, 224–226
    injectable preparations, 227
    oral androgen preparations, 227
    parenteral preparations, 228
    side effects and treatment monitoring,
        228–229
    testosterone preparations and recommended
        doses, 228

transdermal testosterone therapy, 228
treatment indications and pre-treatment
evaluations, 227
primary, 219
secondary, 219–220
sex steroid replacement, 220
Hypomagnesiuric calcium nephrolithiasis, 156
Hyposensitive bladder sensation, 276

I

Idiopathic hypocitraturic calcium oxalate nephrolithiasis, 155–156
Immunology, tumor and transplant
antibodies, 188
cytotoxic and T-helper cells
autologous and allogeneic vaccines, 189
Bacillus Calmette-Guérin, 189
immune reaction, 189
lymphokines, 189
MHC-peptide complex, 188–189
immune system, cancer therapy, 187–188
immunosuppression, 190
induction therapy
administer centre, 191
antilymphocyte antibody, 191
goal of, 190
monoclonal antibody, 190, 191
polyclonal antibody, 190–192
side effects, 191
innate immunity and physiologic response, 187
interleukin-2, 187
maintenance therapy
allograft, 192
azathioprine, 193
calcineurin inhibitors, 192–193
corticosteroids, 193
mycophenolate mofetil and mycophenolic
acid, 193
organ rejection
accelerated rejection, 193–194
acute rejection, 194
chronic allograft rejection, 194
hyperacute rejection, 193
posttransplant lymphoproliferative disease, 194
rejection, 193–194
skin cancers and lymphomas, 187
Immunosuppression, 190
Infection lithiasis, 156
Infectious urolithiasis, 148
Infective and inflammatory disease
acute pyelonephritis, 81, 83
emphysematous pyelonephritis, 83, 84
IVU/CT urography, 81
pyonephrosis, 83, 84
renal abscess, 83
ultrasound, 81
urosepsis, 81
xanthogranulomatous pyelonephritis, 83–84

Intensity-modulated radiation therapy
(IMRT), 535
International Continence Society (ICS), 437,
440, 441
Intracavernosal therapy, 378–379
Intracorporeal stone fragmentation devices
ballistic lithotripsy, 407
electrohydraulic lithotripsy, 407
laser lithotripsy, 408
ultrasound, 407
Intractable hematuria, 357–358
Intralesional drug therapy, 381
Intraurethral therapy, 379
Intravaginal ejaculatory latency time (IELT)
distribution of, 386
estimation, 387
incidence, 385
Intravenous urography (IVU), 356
Iontophoresis, 381

K

Kidney injury
endovascular therapy, 500
expectant management, 499
flank tenderness/ecchymosis, 497–498
follow-up, 500–501
grading system, 498, 499
hematuria, 499
imaging guidelines, 498
indications, 499
nonoperative management, 498–499
operative intervention, 500
pediatric renal injuries, 501
renal exploration and repair, 500
reno-vascular injuries, 501
Kidneys
anomalies
renal agenesis, 6
renal aplasia, 6
renal ectopia, 7
renal fusion, 7
renal hypoplasia, 6–7
columns of Bertin, 30
development
mesonephros, 4
metanephros, 4, 6
pronephros, 4–5
ureteral bud and collecting system, 5
Wolffian body, 4
endocrine functions
calcitriol, 231–232
erythropoietin, 231
renin, 232
functions, 29
Gerota's fascia, 30, 33
inferior vena cava and abdominal aorta, 29, 31
nephrolithiasis, 232
paraneoplastic syndromes

clinical manifestation, 232–233
Cushing's syndrome, 234
RCC, 233–234
primary hyperparathyroidism, 232
renal collecting system, 37–38
renal parenchyma, 30–33
renal vasculature
inferior vena cava and abdominal aorta,
31, 35
intrarenal arterial anatomy, 36
rotation, 32, 34, 35
segmental renal arterial circulation, 35–36
venous drainage, 36–37
retroperitoneal lymphatics, 39
retroperitoneal nerves, 39–40
structure, 29
surgical anatomy
anterior and posterior Gerota's fascia,
31, 33
open/laparoscopic approach, 32, 35
rotational axes, 32, 34
transverse section, 32, 34

L

Laser lithotripsy, 408
Lasers
clinical application of
benign prostatic hyperplasia, 289
condylomata acuminata, 287
ureteral and urethral strictures, 290
urolithiasis, 287–288
Einstein's concept, 286–287
mode of emission, 287
physical properties of, 287
power output, 287
wavelength of, 287
Loin pain hematuria syndrome, 358
Lower urinary tract (LUT), 456
anterior abdominal wall
female pelvis, 44–45
male pelvis, 45–46
robotic-assisted radical prostatectomy
site, 45
structures, laparoscopic view, 44
tissue folds, 44
bladder neck, 53
deferent duct, 49
Denonviellers' fascia, 49
dorsolateral course, 49, 52
3D reconstructions nerve, 52
external urethral sphincter, 53–54
historiography, urology, 43
pelvic floor, 46–47
prostate
blood supply, 49
laparoscopic lymphadenectomy, 51
lymph node, 49, 50
nerve system, 49, 51–52

radical prostatectomy, 49, 51
zones, 48
puboprostatic ligaments, 49
pudendal arteries, 49
radiological image, sentinel lymph nodes, 50
retropubic radical prostatectomy, 49, 51
seminal vesicles, 49
situs laparoscopic lymphadenectomy, 49, 51
sphincter mechanism, 51–53
urethra (*see* Urethra)
urethral wall component, 53
urinary bladder, 47–48
Lower urinary tract dysfunction
abnormal function, 275–278
bladder outflow tract dysfunction
detrusor-urethral dyssynergia, 280
during micturition, 279–280
during storage, 279
complex urodynamic investigation
neurophysiological evaluation, 281–282
urethral pressure measurement, 280–281
detrusor motor function disorders, 278–279
diagnostic patient evaluation
cystometric findings, 269, 271–274
during storage phase, 274–275
urodynamic assessment, 269
videocystometrography, 270–271
during voiding phase, 275
lower urinary tract symptoms, 261, 262
micturition, 263
milkback, 263
sensation disorders, 276
storage phase
bladder compliance, 261
frequency, 262
incontinence, 262–263
nocturia, 262
urethra and sphincteric mechanisms, 262
urgency, 262
urodynamic techniques
pad testing, 264–265
post voiding residual, 267–269
typical test schedule, 265–266
uroflowmetry, 266–268
volume voided charts, 263–264
voiding phase, 263
Lower urinary tract obstruction
anatomical constriction/distortion, 216
BOO diagnosis
detrusor contractility, 209–210
flow rate and post-void residual, 211
post-micturition symptoms, 210, 211
storage phase symptoms, 210–211
voiding cystometry, 211–212
voiding symptoms, 210, 211
female
functional causes, 214
vs. male, 215–216

pelvic organ prolapse, 214
    stress incontinence surgery, 214
  male
    benign prostate enlargement, 212–213
    urethral strictures, 213
  mechanisms of obstruction, 207
  neurourology, 214–215
  normal lower urinary tract
    anatomy, 207
    neural control, 208–209
    storage function, 208
    voiding function, 208–210
  sphincter activity, 216
  symptoms, 207
Lymphogranuloma venereum
  diagnosis, 343
  treatment, 343–344
Lysis, 188

M
Macroscopic hematuria, 351
Male reproductive system
  accessory sex glands
    bulbourethral glands, 66
    prostate, 65
    seminal vesicles, 65–66
  blood supply of testicle, 62
  blood–testis barrier, 63
  epididymis and ductus deferens
    characteristics, 63
    clinic, 64
    ductuli efferentes, 63
    ductus epididymis, 64
    mucosa, 64
    spermatic cord, 64–65
  lymphatic drainage, 63
  nerves, 63
  penis
    anatomy, 66–67
    erection and ejaculation, 67–68
  spermatogenesis
    genetic regulation, 62
    hormonal regulation, 61–62
    meiosis and mitosis, 59
    seminiferous epithelial cycle, 60–61
    seminiferous epithelium, 59–60
    spermatogonium, 60
  testicular artery, 62
  testis and scrotum
    clinic, 57
    descensus, 57–58
    description, 57
    male genital organ development, 59–60
    male genital organs, 57–58
    origin, 58
    sexual differentiation, 58
    testis and layers comparison, 59
Megaureter-megacystis syndrome, 14

Menstruation, 352
Metastatic germ cell tumours
  advanced metastatic disease, 182–183
  low-volume metastatic disease (stage II A/B), 182
  salvage chemotherapy, relapsed or refractory disease, 183
Metastatic testis cancer
  late toxicity, 547
  post-chemotherapy resection, 547–548
  primary combination chemotherapy, 547
  salvage strategies, 548
Microscopic hematuria, 351–352
Missense mutation, 165
Mitomycin C (MMC), 515
Mixed urinary incontinence (MUI), 448
Modification of Diet in Renal Disease (MDRD) trial, 107
Monoclonal antibody, 170, 190, 191
Monocyte chemoattractant protein-1 (MCP-1), 199
Morphine, 131
Multiple sclerosis (MS), 459
Multisystem atrophy (MSA), 458–459
Muscle-invasive bladder cancer, 523

N
Narrow band imaging (NBI), 513
Neoadjuvant chemotherapy, 522
Nephrolithiasis, 149, 232
  hyperuricosuric calcium oxalate, 155
  hypocitraturic calcium oxalate, 155–156
  hypomagnesiuric calcium, 156
Nephroscopy, 285–286
Neurogenic bladder
  autonomic pathways, 456
  brain lesions
    cerebellar ataxia, 459–460
    cerebral palsy, 459–460
    cerebrovascular accident, 457–458
    dementias, 459
    encephalitis/PML, 460
    epilepsy, 459–460
    Huntington's disease, 459
    multiple sclerosis, 459
    multisystem atrophy, 458–459
    normal pressure hydrocephalus, 459
    olivopontine cerebellar degeneration, 458–459
    Parkinson's disease, 458
    psychiatric disorders, 460
    ShyDrager, 458–459
    tumors, 460
  classifications, 455–456
  examination and diagnostic tests
    electromagnetic stimulation, 454
    history and physical examination, 453
    imaging, 453–454
    urodynamics, 454, 455

peripheral neuropathies
    infections/autoimmune peripheral
        neuropathies, 461
    metabolic neuropathies, 461
    pelvic surgery, 461–462
  Pontine Micturition Center, 457, 458
  somatic pathways, 456–457
  spinal lesions and pathology
    intervertebral disk prolapse, 460
    spinal cord injury, 460–461
    transverse myelitis, 461
  treatment, 462–463
  urine storage and release, 457
Neutralization, 188
Nonbacterial infections
  filariasis, 334–335
  fungal
    aspergillosis, 324
    blastomycosis, 325
    candidiasis, 323–324
    coccidioidomycosis, 325–326
    cryptococcosis, 324–325
    histoplasmosis, 326
    radiographic findings, 326
    risk factors, 323, 324
    treatment of, 326–328
  onchocerciasis, 335
  schistosomiasis, 332–334
  tuberculosis (*see* Tuberculosis)
Non-seminomatous germ cell tumor
    (NSGCT)
  adjuvant treatment, 545
  risk stratification, 542
  surveillance *vs.* primary RPLND, 542–545
Nonsense mutation, 165
Normal pressure hydrocephalus (NPH), 459

O
OCT. *See* Optical Coherence Tomography
Olivopontine cerebellar degeneration (OPCD),
    458–459
Onchocerciasis, 335
Onlay substitution
  dorsal, 427, 428
  lateral, 427, 428
  ventral, 427, 428
Opsonization, 188
Optical Coherence Tomography (OCT), 513
Optical urethrotomy, 417
Oral mucosal grafts, 425–426
Orchitis
  clinical signs and symptoms, 309
  definition and etiology, 309
  diagnostic evaluation, 310
  treatment of
    infectious, 310
    noninfectious epididymorchitis, 310
Ovarian differentiation, 21

Overactive bladder (OAB)
  cause of, 439
  treatment of, 441
Oxytocin receptor antagonist, 396

P
Papaverine hydrochloride, 379
Paraneoplastic syndromes
  clinical manifestation, 232–233
  Cushing's syndrome, 234
  RCC
    chorionic gonadotropin, 234
    galactorrhea, 234
    hypercalcemia, 233
    hypertension, 233
    nonmetastatic hepatic dysfunction, 234
    polycythemia, 233
    signs and symptoms, 233
Parapelvic renal cysts, 80, 81
Parkinson's disease (PD), 458
Patient-reported outcomes (PRO), 440
Pelvic floor muscle training (PFMT), 445
Pelvic organ prolapse (POP), 214
  anatomy, 466–467
  biomaterials, 474
  clinical evaluation, 467–469
  clinical manifestation, 465
  conservative management, 473–474
  cystourethrogram, 470
    grading system, 471
    outcome, 472
    voiding, 471
  defecography/culpocystodefecography,
    470
  diagnosis, 467–469
  epidemiology, 465–466
  indications, 474
  MRI, 470, 472
  outcome measures, 469–470
  pathophysiology, 466–467
  recurrence, 465
  risk factors, 465
  surgical management
    anterior compartment repair, 475
    enterocele repair, 476–477
    uterine/apical prolapse, 475–476
  synthetic meshes, 474–475
  urodynamics, 472–473
Pelvis
  female
    pelvic fascia, 45
    peritoneal pelvic cavity, 44–45
    rectouterine folds, 45
  floor
    pelvic diaphragm, 46
    urogenital diaphragm, 46–47
  male, 45–46
Penile cancer, 184

Penis
  amputation, 506–507
  anatomy, 66–67
  erection and ejaculation, 67–68
  fracture, 506
Percutaneous nephrolithotomy (PCNL)
  access, 405
  complications, 406
  instrumentation, 405
  nephrostomy drain post, 405
  principles, 404
Peripheral transcutaneous nerve stimulation
      (PTNS), 443
Peristalsis
  autonomic nervous system, 116
  infection, 120
  mediators, 115–116
  modulation, 116–118
  pregnancy, 120
  prostaglandins, 117
  sensory nerves, 116–117
  smooth muscle-neurotransmission
        coordination, 115
  structural changes, 117–118
  ureteral obstruction, 118
  ureteral pacemaking, 116
Peyronie's disease (PD)
  clinical workup, 380
  diagnosis, 380
  extracorporeal shock-wave therapy, 381
  intralesional drug therapy, 381
  iontophoresis, 381
  oral drug therapy, 381
  prevalence, 380
  radiation therapy, 381
  surgical therapy, 381–382
  symptoms, 380
Phagocytosis, 188
Phosphodiesterase type 5 (PDE 5) inhibitors,
      377, 379
Phosphodiesterase type-5 isoenzyme (PDE-5)
      inhibitors
  PE, 394–395
Photodynamic diagnosis (PDD), 515
Photo vaporization of the prostate (PVP),
      368–369
Pipestem megaureter, 13–14
Plastic surgery
  flap
      axial/random, 257–259
      direct cuticular axial, 258
      fasciocutaneous, 258
      island, 258–259
      muscuocutaneous, 258
      peninsular, 258
  genitourinary reconstruction
      bladder, 252
      buccal mucosa, 252, 253

grafts
      acellular collagen matrices, 257
      epidermal/epithelial layer, 255
      full-thickness, 255–256
      initial phase, 254
      inosculation, 254
      mesh, 256
      posterior auricular, 256
      rectal mucosal, 257
      split thickness, 255
      tunica vaginalis, 257
      urothelium and buccal mucosa, 257
      vein, 257
  reconstructive ladder, 252
  tissue characteristics, 252–255
  tissue transfer principles, 252
Polyclonal antibody, 190–192
Polycythemia, 233
Pontine Micturition Center (PMC), 457, 458
Posterior urethra injury
  antegrade cystoscopy/cystogram, 505
  endoscopic realignment, 505–506
  immediate management, 505
  retrograde urethrogram, 503–504
  staging, 504
Postobstructive diuresis, 203
Posttransplant lymphoproliferative disease
      (PTLD), 194
Posttraumatic arteriogenic erectile
      dysfunction, 377
Potassium balance
  potassium distribution, 109–110
  potassium excretion, kidneys, 110
  significance, 109
Potassium para-aminobenzoate (PotabaT), 381
Precipitation, 188
Premature ejaculation (PE)
  a1-adrenoceptor antagonists, 391
  acquired PE, 386
  chronic prostatitis, 396
  clinical manifestation, 385
  co-morbid ED, 395
  dapoxetine, 392–394
  definition, 387
  distress, 388
  epidemiology, 385
  etiology, 388–389
  hyperthyroidism, 395
  intracavernous injection, vasoactive
        drugs, 394
  intravaginal ejaculatory latency time, 387
  lifelong PE, 385–386
  natural variable PE, 386
  oxytocin receptor antagonist, 396
  pharmacological treatment, 389
  phosphodiesterase inhibitors, 394–395
  premature-like ejaculatory dysfunction,
        386–387

562

INDEX

psychosexual counseling, 389
selective serotonin reuptake inhibitors
    daily treatment, 389–391
    on-demand treatment, 391–392
sexual satisfaction, 388
SSRIs and 5-HT1A receptor antagonist, 396
surgery, 397
topical local anesthetics, 394
tramadol, 394
voluntary control, 387–388
Prenatal hydronephrosis, 197
Primary hyperparathyroidism, 154–155, 232
Progressive multifocal leukoencephalopathy
    (PML), 460
Prostate
    afferent nerves, 240–241
    androgens, 240–241
    blood supply, 49
    catecholamines, 240
    dihydrotestosterone, 240, 241
    estrogens and adrenal steroids, 240
    free T enters cells, 240
    innervation
        afferent axons, 242
        CGRP-immunoreactive nerves, 243
        cholinergic fibers, 242
        micturition and sexual function, 242–243
        noradrenergic nerve fibers, 241–242
        sympathetic nerves, 241
    laparoscopic lymphadenectomy, 51
    LUTS treatment, BPH, 244–245
    lymph node, 49, 50
    nerve system, 49, 51–52
    neurophysiology and neuropharmacology, 243–244
    pharmacology, 240, 242
    physiology, 239, 241
    prostatic secretions, 240
    radical prostatectomy, 49, 51
    zones, 48
Prostate cancer
    androgen-deprivation therapy, 535
    androgen-independent prostate cancer, 535
    biopsy, 529
    brachytherapy, 533
    EBRT, 533
    epidemiology, 527–528
    hormone refractory (*see* Hormone refractory
        prostate cancer)
    IMRT, 533
    laparoscopic prostatectomy, 533
    pathology, 529
    prognosis, 529–531
    PSA recurrence, 536
    radical prostatectomy, 532–533
    risk factors and prevention, 528
    screening recommendation, 528–529
    treatment for, 531–532
    T3, T4 treatment, 533–534

Prostatic inflammation, 396
Prostatism, 362
Prostatitis syndromes
    bacterial prostatitis categories, 300–301
    classification system, 295, 296
    CP/CPPS
        alpha blockers, 302
        analgesics, muscle relaxants and
            neuromodulators, 303
        antibiotics, 302
        anti-inflammatory, 302
        conservative management, 301–302
        hormone therapy, 302
        phytotherapy, 302
        surgery, 303
        treatment goal, 301
    diagnosis
        evaluation, 298
        pain/discomfort, 298, 299
        quality of life, 298, 299
        symptoms, 298, 299
        urination, 298, 299
    etiology of, 296–297
    medical therapy for, 303–305
    prevalence and incidence, 296
    UPOINT system, 303, 305
Prune belly syndrome, 14
Pseudohematuria, 352
Pyeloenteric fistula, 492

R
Raman spectroscopy, 513
Renal cell carcinoma (RCC), 162–163
    angiogenesis inhibitor drugs, 180, 181
    chemotherapy, 179
    contrast injection, 72, 73
    immunotherapy, 180
    metastases, 72
    MRI, 73, 74
    mTOR pathway, 171–172
    prognosis, 179
    targeted therapy, 170
    T3 disease, 73, 74
    TNM staging, 72, 73
    tyrosine kinase inhibitors
        clinical utility, 170–171
        downstream signaling, 170
        sorafenib, 171
        sunitinib, 171
    ultrasound, 72
    VEGR and cell signaling
        angiogenesis, 168
        ligand-receptor interaction, 169
        Raf-Mek-Erk and PI3K-AKT-mTOR
            pathways, 169
        receptor and ligand, 168
        tyrosine kinases, 168–169
    VHL gene (*see* VHL gene)

Renal cysts
    benign renal cysts, 79, 81
    complex
        atypical features, 80
        Bosniak classification, 81–82
        CT images, 82
    hereditary
        adult polycystic kidney disease, 79
        parapelvic renal cysts, 80, 81
        von Hippel Lindau disease, 79
Renal hypercalciuria, 152, 154
Renal obstruction
    causes, 197, 198
    effects, prenatal development
        prenatal hydronephrosis, 197
        signaling pathways and tissue interactions,
            198
        spectrum, renal abnormalities, 197–198
    patient management
        antegrade urography, 202
        computed tomography, 202–203
        hypertension, 203
        intravenous urography, 202
        magnetic resonance urography, 203
        nuclear renography, 202
        postobstructive diuresis, 203
        ultrasound imaging, 202
        Whitaker test, 202
    renal functional changes
        current and future research, 200–201
        electrolyte transport/renal concentrating
            ability, 199
        glomerular development changes, 199–200
        inflammatory mediators, 199
        limitations, animal models, 200
        mechanical stretch, renal tubules, 200
        renal growth/counterbalance, 199
        unilateral vs. bilateral, 200, 201
        vascular changes, 199
Renal physiology
    acid-base balance regulation, 110–111
    body fluid compartments
        fluid composition, 107
        intracellular and extracellular
            compartments, 107
        osmolality, 108
        solute constituents, 107–108
        volume, 108
    body osmolality and body fluid volume control,
        108–109
    calcium balance regulation, 111
    daily renal turnover, 105, 106
    diuretics
        carbonic anhydrase inhibitors, 112
        loop diuretics, 112–113
        osmotic diuretics, 112
        potassium-sparing diuretics, 113–114
        thiazide diuretics, 113

    glomerular structure and function
        autoregulation, 106–107
        capillary layers, 106
        glomerular filtration rate (see Glomerular
            filtration rate)
        ultrafiltration, 105–106
    nephron, 105
    phosphate balance regulation, 111–112
    potassium balance regulation, 109–110
    sodium, chloride, and water reabsorption
        regulation, 108
    transport process, proximal tubule,
        105, 106
Renal stones. See also Stone disease
    calyceal diverticula stones, 410–411
    endoscopic management, 409
    flexible ureterorenoscopy, 410
    horseshoe kidneys and stones, 410
    incidence, 76
    lower pole stones, 410
    non-contrast CT
        flank pain, 79, 80
        multiplanar reformat, 79, 80
        renal enlargement, hydronephrosis, and soft
            tissue stranding, 78
        renal obstruction, 78, 79
        scout image, 78, 80
        sensitivity, 77
        ureteric edema, 78, 79
    percutaneous surgery, 410
    plain radiographs and IVU, 77, 78
    staghorn calculi, 410
    stones and PUJ obstruction, 411
    structural abnormalities, 76
    ultrasound, 77
Renin-angiotensin system (RAS), 199
Resistive index (RI), 202
Retroperitoneal lymph node dissection (RPLND),
    542–545
Retroperitoneum, 29–30
    lymphatics, 39
    nerves, 39–40

S
Sacral nerve stimulation (SNS), 443
Sacral parasympathetic nucleus (SPN),
    456, 460
Scabies
    diagnosis, 348
    treatment, 348
Schistosomiasis
    clinical manifestations, 332
    diagnosis, 333
    Schistosoma haematobium, 332
    treatment, 333–334
Seminal vesicles, 65–66
Semirigid ureteroscopy, 406
Serum chemistry, 150

564

INDEX

Sexual desire/arousal
    CNS drugs, 141
    dopamine, 141
    enzyme-inducing antiepileptic drugs, 141
    neurohormones, 140
    phases, 139
    serotonin, 141
    steroids
        estrogens, 140
        hypogonadism, 140
        testosterone, 139–140
Sexually transmitted infections
    cervicitis, 344–345
    chlamydia, 345–346
    epididymitis, 344
    genital ulcers, 339–341
        chancroid, 342
        herpes simplex virus, 339, 342
        lymphogranuloma venereum, 343–344
        syphilis, 342–343
    gonorrhea, 346
    human papilloma virus, 347–348
    scabies, 348
    trichomoniasis, 346–347
    urethritis, 344
Sirolimus, 192–193
Small intestinal submucosa (SIS), 427
Sorafenib, 171
Spermatogenesis
    genetic regulation of spermatogenesis, 62
    hormonal regulation of spermatogenesis,
        61–62
    meiosis, 59
    mitosis, 59
    seminiferous epithelium, 59–60
    spermatogonium, 60
    stages of seminiferous epithelial cycle, 60–61
Sphincter
    anatomy and function, 52–53
    muscular structures, 51–52
Spinal cord injury (SCI), 460–461
Spinal lesions
    intervertebral disk prolapse, 460
    spinal cord injury, 460–461
    transverse myelitis, 461
Spironolactone, 113–114
Stage I non-seminomatous germ cell tumours
        (NSGCT), 182
Stauffer syndrome, 234
Stone disease
    calcium-based urolithiasis, 147–148
    conservative management
        citrus juices, 151
        dietary restrictions, 151–152
        increased fluid intake, 151
        restricted oxalate diet, 152
    cystine-based urolithiasis, 148
    epidemiology, 147

infectious urolithiasis, 148
    metabolic evaluation
        calcium stone formers, 149
        chemical analysis, 150
        first time stone formers, 149
        goal of, 149
        medical history, 150
        nephrolithiasis and urolithiasis, 149
        physical examination, 150
        radiologic imaging, 151
        serum chemistry, 150
        stone analysis, 150
        urine evaluation, 150–151
    selective medical therapy
        absorptive hypercalciuria, 152
        cystinuria, 156
        enteric hyperoxaluria, 155
        gouty diathesis, 156
        hyperuricosuric calcium oxalate
            nephrolithiasis, 155
        hypocitraturic calcium oxalate nephrolithiasis,
            155–156
        hypomagnesiuric calcium nephrolithiasis, 156
        infection lithiasis, 156
        medication, 152–154
        primary hyperparathyroidism, 154–155
        renal hypercalciuria, 152, 154
    stone composition and clinical associations, 147, 148
    uric acid urolithiasis, 148
Stress urinary incontinence (SUI)
    female therapies
        duloxetine, 445–446
        estrogen receptors, 446
        PFMT, 445
        TOT, 446–447
        TVT, 446
    International Continence Society, 446
    male therapies
        AUS, 444
        detrusor hypocontractility, 444
        periurethral bulking agents, 443
Sunitinib, 171
Syphilis
    diagnosis, 342–343
    treatment, 343

T
Tacrolimus, 192
Temsirolimus, 172
Tension-free vaginal tape (TVT), 446, 447
Testicular cancer
    metastatic germ cell tumours, 182–183
    stage I non-seminomatous germ cell tumours, 182
    stage I seminoma, 182
Testicular differentiation
    caudal migration, gubenaculum, 21
    disorders, 23
    testis development, 19–21

Testicular torsion. *See* Epididymal appendages
Testis
    androgen deprivation therapy, adverse effects
        body composition, 230
        bone metabolism, 231
        cognitive decline, 230–231
        insulin resistance and metabolic syndrome, 230
    clinic, 57
    descensus, 57–58
    description, 57
    hypogonadism (*see* Hypogonadism)
    male genital organ development, 59–60
    male genital organs, 57–58
    normal androgen metabolism, 219
    origin, 58
    physiological actions and tissue targets,
        testosterone
        bones, 223–224
        brain, 223
        cardiovascular system, 224
        erythropoiesis, 224
        metabolic syndrome, 224
        muscle mass and adipose tissue, 223
        prostate, 223
    sexual differentiation, 58
    testis and layers comparison, 59
    testosterone replacement therapy
        BPH progression, 229
        prostate cancer, 229–230
Testis cancer
    clinical stage 1 seminoma
        adjuvant low dose chemotherapy, 545
        adjuvant radiotherapy, 545
        risk-stratified adjuvant treatment, 545
        surveillance, 546
    contralateral testicular biopsy and TIN, 540–541
    metastatic testis cancer
        late toxicity, 547
        post-chemotherapy resection, 547–548
        primary combination chemotherapy, 547
        salvage strategies, 548
    non-seminomatous germ cell tumor
        adjuvant treatment, 545
        risk stratification, 542
        surveillance *versus* primary RPLND,
            542–545
    post-orchidectomy management, 541–542
    presentation and diagnosis, 539
    primary surgery, 539–540
    serum tumor markers, 539
    testis preserving surgery, 540
Testosterone replacement therapy, 227
    BPH progression, 229
    prostate cancer, 229–230
Thiazide-induced hypocitraturia, 155
Thymoglobulin
    down-modulation, 192
    T-cell depletion, 190–191

Thyroxine, 395
Tissue transfer
    flap (*see* Flap)
    grafts (*see* Grafts)
    principles, 252
    tissue characteristics, 252–255
Tramadol, 131, 394
Transobturator tape (TOT), 446–447
Transurethral microwave thermotherapy (TUMT), 368
Transurethral needle ablation of the prostate
    (TUNA), 368
Transurethral resection (TUR), 516
    bimanual examination, 514
    histopathological diagnosis, 514
    PDD-assisted TUR, 514–515
    postoperative intravesical chemotherapy, 515
    recurrence, risk of, 514
    re-TUR, 515
Trans-urethral resection of the prostate (TURP), 368
Trauma
    adrenal injury, 501
    American Association for the surgery of trauma
        classification, 87
    angiography, 87–88
    anterior urethral trauma, 506
    AV fistula/pseudoaneurysm, 88, 89
    bladder injury
        adult and children, 503
        computed tomography, 504
        diagnosis and treatment algorithm, 503, 504
        DRE, 503
        formal repair, 505
        gross hematuria, 503
        initial management, 505–506
        retrograde urethrogram, 503
    contrast-enhanced CT, 88
    CT-IVP (CT with delayed images), 507
    cystogram, 507–508
    haematoma, 88
    hematuria, 87
    injury management, 497
    IVU, 88
    kidney injury
        endovascular therapy, 500
        expectant management, 499
        flank tenderness/ecchymosis, 497–498
        follow-up, 500–501
        grading system, 498, 499
        hematuria, 497
        imaging guidelines, 498
        indications, 499
        nonoperative management, 498–499
        operative intervention, 500
        pediatric renal injuries, 501
        renal exploration and repair, 500
        reno-vascular injuries, 501
    one-shot IVP, 508
    parenchymal laceration, 88

penis
    amputation, 506–507
    fracture, 506
posterior urethra injury
    antegrade cystoscopy/cystogram, 504
    endoscopic realignment, 505–506
    immediate management, 505
    retrograde urethrogram, 503–504
    staging, 504
post iv contrast studies, 88
renal infarction, 88
retrograde pyelogram, 508
retrograde urethrogram, 508
scrotal and testicular trauma, 507
ultrasound, 88
ureter injury
    delayed diagnosis, 502–503
    diagnosis, 501–502
    treatment, 502
Triamterene, 113–114
Trichomoniasis
    diagnosis, 346–347
    treatment, 347
Tuberculosis (TB)
    clinical manifestations
        bladder involvement, 328, 330–331
        chronic granulomatous prostatitis, 330
        genitourinary, 328–330
        organ of involvement, 328
        penile, 330
        renal, 328, 330
        scrotal transmission, 330
    diagnosis, 331
    incidence of, 328
    Mycobacterium tuberculosis, 328
    treatment, 331
Tube substitution, 422
Tyrosine kinase inhibitors (TKI)
    clinical utility, 170–171
    downstream signaling, 170
    sorafenib, 171
    sunitinib, 171

U
Ultrasound lithotripsy, 407
United States Preventive Services Task Force
    (USPSTF), 529
Upper urinary tract
    anatomy, 69
    angiomyolipoma, 73, 74
    benign renal cysts, 79, 81
    complex renal cysts
        atypical features, 80
        Bosniak classification, 81–82
        CT images, 81, 82
    contrast issues
        cautions, 72
        gadolinium-based contrast agents, 72
        iodinated contrast, 71–72

CT, 70–71
hereditary renal cystic disease, 79–81
infective and inflammatory disease
    acute pyelonephritis, 81, 83
    emphysematous pyelonephritis, 83, 84
    IVU/CT urography, 81
    pyonephrosis, 83, 84
    renal abscess, 83
    ultrasound, 81
    urosepsis, 81
    xanthogranulomatous pyelonephritis,
        83–84
intravenous urogram, 70
kidneys (*see* Kidneys)
MRI, 71
nuclear medicine, 71
oncocytoma, 73
radiation issues, 71
renal cell carcinoma, 72–73
renal mass biopsy, 76
renal stone disease
    CT, 77–80
    incidence, 76
    plain radiographs and IVU, 77, 78
    structural abnormalities, 76
    ultrasound, 77
renal trauma, 87–21
transitional cell carcinoma
    clinical manifestation, 73
    CT, 75, 76
    filling defects, 74
    IVU, 74
    nonmalignant causes, 74, 75
    pyeloureteritis cystica, 74, 75
    renal pelvis mass, 74–75
    retrograde studies, 75–76
    urinary cytology, 74
ultrasound, 69–70
upper urinary tract obstruction
    CT, 85, 86
    hydronephrosis, 84–85
    intrinsic and extrinsic causes, 84–85
    IVU, 85, 86
    management, 86–87
    MRI, 85–87
    parapelvic cysts, 85
    percutaneous nephrostomy tube, 86, 87
    ultrasound, 85
    ureteric calculi, 85–86
    ureteric stents, 86–87
utreters, 38
Upper urinary tract obstruction
    CT, 85, 86
    hydronephrosis, 84–85
    intrinsic and extrinsic causes, 84–85
    IVU, 85, 86
    management, 86–87
    MRI, 85–87
    parapelvic cysts, 85

ultrasound, 85
ureteric calculi, 85–86
Ureteral and urethral strictures, 290
Ureteral development
    anomalies of number, 9
    anomalies of origin, 8–9
    complete ureteral duplication
        anatomic position, 10
        clinical symptoms and signs, 10–11
        ectopic ureter, 11–12
        symptoms, 12
        ureteral duplication, 9–10
        Weigert-Meyer law, 9–10
    congenital ureteral obstruction
        megaureter-megacystis syndrome, 14
        pipestem megaureter, 13–14
        prune belly syndrome, 14
        vascular ureteral obstructions, 14–16
    incomplete ureteral duplication, 9
    ureteral orifices, 9
    ureteroceles, 12–13
    urogenital sinus, 7–8
Ureteric stones
    endoscopic management, 408–409
    intervention, 412
    medical expulsive therapy, 411
    obesity, 412
    pregnancy, 412
    treatment outcomes, 411
Ureter injury
    delayed diagnosis, 502–503
    diagnosis, 501–502
    treatment, 502
Ureteroceles, 12–13
Ureteropelvic junction obstruction (UPJO), 197
Ureteropyeloscopy, 284–285
Ureteroscopy, 284–285
Ureterovaginal fistula
    diagnosis and management, 489–490
    etiology and presentation, 489
Ureters
    anatomy, 115
    blood supply, 115
    peristalsis
        autonomic nervous system, 116
        infection, 120
        mediators, 115–116
        modulation, 116–118
        pregnancy, 120
        prostaglandins, 117
        sensory nerves, 116–117
        smooth muscle-neurotransmission
            coordination, 115
        structural changes, 117–118
        ureteral obstruction, 118
        ureteral pacemaking, 116
    pharmacology
        alpha antagonists, 119
        calcium channel blockers, 119

COX-2 inhibitors, 118–119
        experimental agents, 120
        neurokinin receptor antagonists, 120
        nitric oxide neurotransmitter, 120
        opioids, 118
        phosphodiesterase inhibitors, 119
Urethra
    bladder neck, 53
    external urethral sphincter, 53–54
    male and female, 51
    sphincter
        anatomy and function, 52–53
        muscular structures, 51–52
    urethral wall, 53
Urethral pressure measurement
    abdominal leak point pressures, 281
    ambulatory urodynamics, 281
    technique, 280–281
    urethral pressure profilometry, 281
Urethral pressure profilometry (UPP), 281
Urethral stents, 417–418
Urethral strictures, 213
Urethritis, 344
Urethroplasty
    anastomotic, 419–422
    flap urethroplasty (see Flap urethroplasty)
    graft position
        application of chloramphenicol jelly, 430, 431
        complications, 433
        dorsal inlay graft, 428, 429
        onlay substitution, 427, 428
        second-stage reconstruction, 430
        second-stage tubularization, 432
        two-stage procedure, 428, 429
        ventral onlay graft, 428, 429
    grafts vs. flaps
        fistula, 424
        genital skin, 422
        glans torsion, 424
        hematoma, 424
        penile skin, 422–424
        sacculation, 424
        skin necrosis, 424
        subcutaneous tissue, 423
        types of, 422, 423
    onlay substitution, 422
    oral mucosal grafts, 425–426
    tissue engineering, 426–427
    tube substitution, 422
Urethrorectal fistula, 492–493
Urethrovaginal fistula
    diagnosis and management, 489–491
    etiology and presentation, 489
Urge urinary incontinence (UUI)
    conservative treatments, 441
    invasive/surgical therapies, 442–443
    pharmacotherapy
        anticholinergic drugs, 441
        capsaicin, 442

M_1 and M_2 receptors, 442
OPERA Study, 442
transdermal delivery systems, 441–442
Uric acid urolithiasis, 148
Urinalysis, 150
Urinary bladder
blood supply, 47–48
embroyology
bladder duplication, 17
cloacal duct anomalies, 17
development, 16–17
diverticula, 17–19
extrophy, 19
primitive cloaca, 16
structure, 16
urachal anomalies, 17
urogenital sinus, 16
urogenital sinus division, 16
lymph nodes, 47
neural system
anatomic nerve fiber, 47–48
sympathetic fibers, 48
structure, 47
Urinary incontinence (UI)
clinical assessment
PRO, 440
VLPP, 441
complications and consequences,
438–439
epidemiology and risk factors
BACH Survey, 437–438
bladder function, 438
EPINCONT study, 437, 438
mixed urinary incontinence, 448
pathophysiology
bladder dysfunction, 440
GABA, 439
myogenic theory, 439
neurogenic theory, 439
OAB, 439
TURP, 440
stress urinary incontinence
female therapies, 444–448
male therapies, 443–444
urge incontinence
conservative treatments, 441
invasive/surgical therapies, 442–443
pharmacotherapy, 441–442
Urinary tract infections (UTIs)
antibiotics
choice, 95
complicated and nosocomially acquired
UTI, 96–101
uncomplicated, community acquired
UTI, 95–96
antimicrobials testing
pharmacodynamic parameters, 93–94
pharmacokinetic parameters, 94

pharmacokinetic/pharmacodynamic
correlations, 94
susceptibility and resistance, 92–93
bacterial spectrum and antimicrobial resistance
patterns, 94–95
complicated, 91
pathophysiology, 91–92
prevalence, 91
uncomplicated, 91
Urine evaluation
twenty-four hour urine collections, 150–151
urinalysis, 150
urine cultures, 150
Urodynamic nomograms, 211–212
Urodynamics (UDS)
neurologic diseases, 454, 455
pelvic prolapse, 472–473
videourodynamic tracing, 454
Urodynamic techniques
pad testing, 264–265
post voiding residual, 267–269
typical test schedule, 265–266
uroflowmetry, 266–268
volume voided charts, 263–264
Urolithiasis, 287–288
calcium-based, 147–148
cystine-based, 148
infectious, 148
metabolic evaluation, 149
stone composition, 147, 148
uric acid, 148
Urothelial cell carcinomas (UCC), 513
Uterine/apical prolapse
hysterectomy, 476
indications, 475
minimally invasive techniques, 476, 477

V
Vacuum-assisted closure (VAC), 252
Vacuum constriction devices (VCD), 379–380
Valsalva leak point pressure (VLPP), 441
Vascular ureteral obstructions, 14–16
Vault prolapse repair, 475
Vesico-bulbo-vesical micturition reflex, 125–126
Vesicoenteric fistula, 491–492
Vesico-spinal-vesical micturition reflex, 126
Vesicovaginal fistula
conservative management, 485
cystoscopy, 484
etiology and risk factors, 482–483
evaluation and diagnosis, 483
imaging, 484–485
pelvic examination, 483–484
surgical management, 485–488
treatment, 485
VHL gene
chromosome 3p, 164
epigenetic change, 165

genetic changes, 164–165
germ line mutation, 164
HIFα
    accumulation, 167
    gene regulation, 166
    gene transcription, 166, 168
    genomics and proteomics, 167
    hypoxia response elements, 165–166
    normal regulation, 165, 166
    polymerase chain reaction, 167
somatic cell mutation, 164
tumor suppressor gene concept, 163, 164
Voiding
    bladder outlet obstruction
        cystometry, 211–212
        neurourology, 214–215
        post-void residual, 211
        symptoms, 209–211
    detrusor contraction, 208
    evaluation, 208
    men, 208, 209
    synchronous outlet relaxation, 208
    women, 210
Voiding cysto-urethrogram (VCUG), 484
Von Hippel Lindau disease, 79. *See also* VHL gene

W
Weigert-Meyer law, 9–10
Whitaker test, 202
Wound healing
    inflammatory phase
        hemostasis and wound sealing, 249
        macrophages, 250
        neutrophils, 250
        platelet aggregation and vasoconstriction, 249
        vasodilation, 249–250
    plastic surgery (*see* Plastic surgery)
    primary, 249
    proliferation phase
        angiogenesis, 250–251
        collagen, 250
        epithelialization, 251
        fibroblasts, 250
        vacuum-assisted closure, 252
        wound contraction, 251
    remodeling phase, 252
    secondary, 249
    tertiary, 249

Y
Yohimbine, 378